Documentation and Reimbursement for Behavioral Healthcare Services

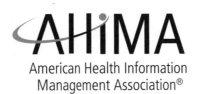

AHiMA

American Health Information
Management Association®

D1219344

ISBN 1-58426-130-7
AHIMA Product No. AB103505

AHIMA Staff:
Claire Blondeau, Project Editor
Melissa Ulbricht, Editorial/Production Coordinator
Michelle Dougherty, RHIA, Content Reviewer

*AHIMA strives to recognize the value
of people from every racial and ethnic background
as well as all genders, age groups, and sexual orientations
by building its membership and leadership resources
to reflect the rich diversity of the American population.
AHIMA encourages the celebration and promotion of human diversity
through education, mentoring, recognition, leadership, and other programs.*

American Health Information Management Association
233 North Michigan Avenue, Suite 2150
Chicago, Illinois 60601-5800

www.ahima.org

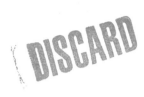

Contents

Preface

Clinical documentation and health records play a vital role in every aspect of healthcare delivery and decision making, no matter what the setting. Documentation also is a central focus in current efforts to improve healthcare quality and patient safety as well as the efficiency of the U.S. healthcare system. The development and implementation of electronic health record (EHR) systems promise to revolutionize the collection, use, and management of healthcare data over the next decade.

Ensuring the accessibility, accuracy, and integrity of health records has been the primary mission of health information managers since the profession emerged more than seventy-five years ago. Just as important, health information management (HIM) professionals continue to champion the protection of patient privacy and the confidentiality of health information. As experts in the documentation requirements of external government agencies and accreditation organizations, HIM professionals also play an invaluable role in managing their organizations' regulatory compliance and accreditation performance.

Documentation and Reimbursement for Behavioral Healthcare Services explains the importance of accurate and timely health record documentation in behavioral healthcare settings. However, many of the basic principles discussed also apply to other healthcare settings. Information on legal, regulatory, and accreditation requirements specific to this setting also is provided.

The paper-based forms in this book were designed specifically as examples of data capture and management tools and samples of appropriate health record documentation. In some cases, the sample forms have been simplified to fulfill educational purposes. They also have been sized and formatted to fit the printed book. Therefore, direct use for documentation of actual clinical services would not be appropriate. However, educators and students are free to copy and use the forms as part of their classroom activities. Any other usage would require the expressed permission of the American Health Information Management Association (AHIMA).

The goal of this publication is to help HIM practitioners and students understand the role of health records and clinical documentation in the delivery of direct client services and in the operations of behavioral healthcare organizations. Specifically, chapter 1, Documentation of Care, explains why healthcare information is documented and identifies its key users. It also describes various efforts to provide the healthcare industry with documentation guidelines and standards and discusses different documentation methodologies. Chapter 2, Content, Format, and Organization of the Health Record, explains what information is part of the health record and what is not. It also discusses the components of the acute care psychiatric health record. The electronic health record and its advantages and limitations are discussed in chapter 3, Understanding and Implementing the Electronic Health Record. The chapter also outlines steps for implementing the EHR and steps for selecting and contracting with vendors. Chapter 4, Record

Review and Analysis, examines the documentation challenges that are unique to behavioral healthcare. It explains how to conduct a clinical pertinence review and focuses on the importance of organizational health record policies and procedures and staff training. Chapter 5, Coding and Reimbursement, describes different clinical vocabularies and discusses different types of reimbursement systems, methodologies, and support processes. Chapter 6, Data and Information Management, defines the terms *data, information,* and *knowledge.* It also draws attention to the importance of ensuring data quality and describes various data and information management initiatives as well as information management systems. Healthcare regulation is the focus of chapter 7, Regulatory and Accreditation Requirements. The chapter discusses quality improvement organizations and the role of health information management professionals in the accreditation, certification, and licensure process. Chapter 8, Compliance, overviews the primary components of compliance using examples and citations drawn from the *Federal Register.* Chapter 9, Confidentiality, Privacy, and Security of Protected Health Information, discusses these issues as they are addressed in the behavioral healthcare setting. This chapter draws heavily from the Health Insurance Portability and Accountability Act (HIPAA) privacy and security rules. Finally, chapter 10, Outcomes Management and Performance Improvement, introduces different performance improvement models and the various measures that organizations can use to assess quality improvement program effectiveness.

This publication also includes ten appendixes. Appendix A offers several examples of inpatient forms used in the behavioral healthcare organization, and appendix B contains numerous outpatient forms. Appendix C overviews standards and requirements governing the form and content of the behavioral healthcare record. Appendix D contains principles of form and screen design to assist professionals in developing documents for their organizations. Two *Federal Register* documents are contained in Appendix E: OIG Compliance Program Guidance for Hospitals, created in 1998, and the draft supplemental guidance, developed in 2004. These documents are referenced numerous times throughout the text. Two AHIMA Practice Briefs are located in appendix F: "Seven Steps to Corporate Compliance: The HIM Role" and "Developing a Coding Compliance Policy Document." Appendix G contains sample audit tools, forms, and worksheets, and appendixes H and I contain sample compliance plans and sample policies and procedures. Finally, appendix J contains a glossary of key terms mentioned throughout the book.

The American Health Information Management Association hopes that the publication of this book on documentation for behavioral healthcare services will help new professionals, as well as those already in practice, to meet the current demands and future challenges of health information management in this setting.

Acknowledgments

The publications staff of the AHIMA gratefully acknowledges the contributions of the following subject matter experts and manuscript reviewers. Without the help of these dedicated professionals, this publication would not have been possible.

Nalini Ambrose, MS
Continuous Quality Improvement Coordinator
Behavioral Health Services
Lake County Health Department and Community Health Center
Waukegan, IL

Charlene Dunbar, RHIA
Madonna Rehabilitation Hospital
Lincoln, NE

Polly Isaacson, RHIA, CPHQ
Partner
Healthcare Consulting Associates, LLC
Salt Lake City, UT

Tonia Poteet, RHIA
Director of Health Information Management
Lakeside Behavioral Health
Memphis, TN

Jeany Sheehan
HIM Consultant
INTEGRIS
Oklahoma City, OK

Chris Simons, RHIA
Director of HIM Services and Privacy Officer
Spring Harbor Hospital
South Portland, ME

Elizabeth Tetreault, RHIT
Director, HIMS
Connecticut Children's Medical Center
Hartford, CT

Tamar Thompson, RMA, CCS-P
Reimbursement Specialist
GE Healthcare
North Las Vegas, NV

Nancy Tracy, MEd, RHIT
Brewer, ME

Ann Waters, RHIT, CCS
Consultant
Innovative Coding and Documentation
Mount Vernon, WA
How to Use This Book

About the Chapter Authors

Margret K. Amatayakul, MBA, RHIA, CHPS, FHIMSS, has more than thirty years of experience in national and international healthcare information management. She is a leading authority on electronic health record (EHR) strategies for healthcare organizations and has extensive experience in EHR selection and project management. After having served as director of medical record services at the Illinois Eye and Ear Infirmary, associate professor at the University of Illinois Medical Center, associate executive director of the American Health Information Management Association, and executive director of the Computer-based Patient Record Institute, Margret formed her own consulting firm, Margret\A Consulting, LLC, in 1999. She provides information systems consulting services, freelance writing, and educational programming to the healthcare industry. Margret earned her bachelor's degree from the University of Illinois Medical Center and her master's degree in business administration, with concentrations in marketing and finance, from the University of Illinois at Chicago. She is a much-sought-after speaker and has published extensively. Moreover, Margret has an impressive list of professional service awards to her credit. Finally, she continues to serve the health informatics community as adjunct faculty of the College of St. Scholastica and the University of Illinois at Chicago. She can be contacted at margretcpr@aol.com.

Jill Burt, MA, RHIA, earned her master's degree in health information management in 2000. She holds a registration in health information administration (RHIA). With more than seventeen years of healthcare experience in health information management, Jill has worked as a director in both behavioral health and acute care. Currently, she is a clinical business analyst for the Minnesota Department of Human Services' State Operated Services Division.

Linda Cannon, RHIA, has been chief of medical record services for mental health services for the County of San Diego since 1987. She has been employed in healthcare for thirty years beginning as a medical record clerk in an acute care facility, first earning her ART and then her RHIA in 1981. Linda has served as a past board member and chair of the Behavioral Health Section of AHIMA. She also assisted in the 1990 publication of the Professional Practice Standards for Mental Health. In 1996, Linda spoke at the AHIMA convention in Orlando, Florida. She is active on the Legislative Committee of the California Health Information Management Association.

Rhonda Edgecomb, RHIT, is currently manager of health information management services and chief privacy officer for Community Health and Counseling Services (CHCS) in Bangor, Maine. She has worked in the HIM profession for the past fourteen years, the past seven of which have been in the behavioral healthcare sector. Rhonda has served on the board of directors for the Maine Health Information Management Association (MeHIMA) since 2000 and is preparing to take office for her second term as president of the association.

Pamela T. Haines, RHIA, earned her baccalaureate degree in health information management and systems from the Ohio State University in 1997. For the past five and a half years, she has worked as medical records administrator for Operation PAR, Inc., a large behavioral healthcare organization on the west coast of Florida that treats clients with a primary diagnosis of substance abuse. Additionally, she is a privacy officer and has spoken several times at the AHIMA national convention on topics related to substance abuse records and confidentiality. Moreover, Pamela has written, contributed to, and been featured in many articles in the *Journal of the American Health Information Management Association* and other professional magazines and bulletins. She is consulted for her expertise in 42 CFR, Part 2, the federal regulations that govern the confidentiality of drug and alcohol records and the HIPAA privacy rule, is a facilitator for the AHIMA BH Community of Practice, and is a volunteer on the AHIMA My PHR Task Force.

Cheryl Kester-Hoffman, RHIA, is the health information technology (HIT) program director at South Piedmont Community College in Charlotte, NC. She has been a member of AHIMA since 1984 and has been active in the Behavioral Health Community of Practice.

Anna Lattu, MA, RHIA, is currently director of information management at the Minnesota Department of Human Services' State Operated Services, managing information technology services and health information management. She has been employed by the state of Minnesota for thirteen years, working as a health information management (HIM) director in behavioral healthcare settings, including facility-based programs, community-based programs, and forensics. Anna received her master and bachelor's degrees in health information management from the College of St. Scholastica, where she is an adjunct instructor. She has been active in local and state HIM associations.

Ruby Nicholson, RHIT, has been director of quality improvement/health information at The Kent Center for Human & Organizational Development for the past sixteen years. In addition to her role as director of the quality improvement and HIM departments, she is responsible for the organization's accreditation process, compliance program, and human rights office. Ruby has been involved in many state and national public policy forums. She has served as a member of AHIMA's Public Policy Task Force, past chair of AHIMA's Behavioral Health Section, and president of the Rhode Island Health Information Management Association. In 2004 and in 1995, Ruby had the privilege to participate as a member of an HIM delegation to the People's Republic of China. Her enthusiasm and dedication to the HIM profession have been recognized by her peers both nationally and within her state. She was the recipient of AHIMA's Champion Award in 2000 and RIHIMA's Distinguished Member Award in 2003.

Janice L. Walton, MA, RHIA, CHP, CPHQ, is the principal of Physician Office Specialists, Inc. (POS, Inc.), a health information consulting firm founded in 1989. POS, Inc., provides services to a wide variety organizations with health information needs, including physician offices, behavioral health organizations, acute care hospitals, managed care organizations, and long-term care facilities. The focus of Jan's consulting is on performance improvement, privacy compliance, corporate compliance, training and education on medical record/health information functions, and accreditation/licensure processes. She has more than twenty years of HIM experience, with ten years in the acute care setting and the remaining years with the consulting company she founded.

RoseAnn Webb, RHIA, LHRM, is currently director of health information management and privacy officer at Boca Raton Community Hospital in Boca Raton, Florida. She has been employed in healthcare for twenty-eight years, beginning with the Department of Veterans Affairs where she worked for sixteen years. In 1992, RoseAnn received her degree in health information management and left the VA to begin her career in private industry. She has held several positions, from manager to director in both behavioral health and acute care. Currently, she is a director for the Florida Health Information Management Association and an adjunct instructor at Florida International University.

Reshia Wheeler, RHIA, is currently the privacy officer at Adult and Child Center, Inc., in Indianapolis. In 1995, Reshia earned her degree in health information administration from the Indiana University School of Medicine. She has held positions as director, practice manager, and consultant in behavioral health, acute, and long-term care. Additionally, she has taught coding as an adjunct faculty member for Indiana University and the Community College of Indiana. Reshia continues to consult in various positions related to health information administration.

Tammy Young Lyles, MEd, RHIA, is director of quality improvement and records management for Gateway Family Services, the oldest social services agency located in Birmingham, Alabama. Certified as an ART (Accredited Records Technician) in 1983, she began her career working in utilization management and quality assurance settings. While working in acute care hospital settings and inpatient substance abuse facilities, she completed a BS degree in allied health administration in 1989. Leaving the direct-care setting, she worked as a clinical case manager for a behavioral health managed care organization while completing an MA degree in allied health and hospital administration (1990) at the University of Alabama in Birmingham (UAB). Having maintained good standing as an ART, while completing additional degrees and continuing to work in the field, she passed the RHIA exam in 1999 and was certified as a registered health information administrator. In her current position, she established and supervises a centralized records department that is utilized by six of the agency's programs and focuses primarily on agency policies and licensure/accreditation of multiple (15) service modalities. She is the agency privacy officer and serves on the Corporate Compliance Committee. Locally, Tammy serves as a volunteer for The Red Cross of Central Alabama, the Alabama Symphony, and the Greater Birmingham Humane Society. She provides consultation to other agencies on quality improvement issues and also serves as a peer reviewer for the Council on Accreditation for Children and Family Services (COA) of New York.

Introduction

Rhonda Edgecomb, RHIT

Documentation and Reimbursement for Behavioral Healthcare emphasizes the importance of high-quality health information in the behavioral healthcare setting. In short, high-quality documentation yields positive outcomes with client care, organization reimbursement, and compliance with the various regulatory and accrediting bodies discussed throughout this textbook. This book explores best practice and current trends in documentation, data management, quality improvement activities, reimbursement, and privacy practices in the behavioral healthcare setting. It is written as a resource for use by the health information management (HIM) professional working in behavioral health, behavioral healthcare administrators, educators, and students.

Early History and Background of Mental Health

The earliest accounts of mental illness date as far back as the days of the ancient Greeks. Often misunderstood, individuals suffering from mental illness were perceived to be possessed or demonic and were often subjected to cruel and inhumane treatment in an effort to rid them of evil spirits. Care for the mentally ill typically was the responsibility of the immediate family and was provided mostly in the home. It was not uncommon for the mentally ill to be caged, chained, and/or isolated for significant lengths of time, hidden from the view of the community (Shorter 1997, 1–4).

During the sixteenth and seventeenth centuries, long before psychiatry was established as a formal discipline, treatment for the mentally ill was provided by physicians in general care hospitals. In this setting, the mad or the insane were separated from the medically ill in distinct wards. Individuals with mental illness were generally grouped together in these wards regardless of their condition. Early accounts of such hospitalization detail torturous flogging, painful restraints, and dysenteric environments (Shorter 1997, 6).

In the late seventeenth century, formal asylums for the insane were established to relieve families of the significant burden of caring for individuals with serious mental illness. For many residents, the asylum simply offered a grim alternative to passing the remainder of their days in cages or man-made pits. However, their time was still spent in almost absolute solitude.

Physical restraints and heavy sedation by means of potent medications, which caused undesirable side effects, were common treatments in the asylum era. Very little was done to determine the actual cause of an affliction, so diagnosis-specific treatment was still an unknown. Because there were no established admission criteria for institutionalizing an individual, the system eventually became abused. By the nineteenth century, it was common practice for a husband to commit his wife involuntarily to an asylum for demonstrating excessive emotional behavior or for exhibiting signs of depression following the birth of a child (Shorter 1997, 4–8).

Biomedical, Technological, and Theoretical Advances in Care

For centuries, experts have debated the origin of mental illness. In the beginning, experts focused on the "spiritual" aspect of the human existence and attempted to modify behavior or, rather, ill behavior through the use of religion, witchcraft, and other forces affecting spirituality. Little or no effort was made to identify the cause of exhibited symptoms; thus, the origin went undiagnosed and untreated.

In more recent times, the debate has been a little more scientific. Starting in the very early 1900s, experts began to study the impact of genetics and simple brain chemistry to determine the severity and course of mental illness in individuals. Formalized universities studied the poorly maintained clinical records of insane asylums to establish trends and patterns of inherited mental illness. During this era, experts hypothesized that mental illness was not only hereditary, but also might actually worsen with each generation. This research marked the onset of a more scientific approach to treating mental illness (Shorter 1997, 93–99).

In the late nineteenth century and into the early twentieth century, research took a bit of a turn when experts, including the psychoanalysis pioneer Sigmund Freud, began to focus on past traumatic events in an individual's life as a cause for mental illness and ill emotional behavior. This was referred to as the psychoanalytic era in the history of mental health. This era bore images of individuals lying on a couch in a psychiatrist's office detailing accounts of personality-altering childhood experiences and events. Memories that had left psychological scarring and a permanent residual impact on the psyche were uncovered and explored during such sessions. Clinicians of the day discovered that medication management, hypnosis, and extensive one-on-one therapy sessions were effective tools in the treatment of such residual effects (Shorter 1997, 145–160).

To this day, experts continue to debate the origin of mental illness. Regardless of the cause, however, the treatment for mental illness has advanced significantly. Gone are the inhumane asylums of the early days. Today's approach to treatment focuses on the specific symptoms, diagnosis, and circumstances of the individual. This individualized approach to treatment provides the mentally ill with the best possible care.

Today's Behavioral Healthcare Environment

Today, it is estimated that one in five Americans, roughly 22 percent, will suffer from a diagnosable mental illness in any given year (NIMH 2001). These conditions, which encompass a wide variety of cognitive, emotional, and behavioral illnesses, along with mental retardation, developmental disabilities, and substance abuse, are classified in the *Diagnostic and Statistical Manual of Mental Disorders, fourth edition* (DSM-IV). DSM-IV is the classification system utilized in the United States to diagnose and classify mental illness.

The Recipient of Behavioral Healthcare Services

According to the surgeon general, it is estimated that more than 54 million Americans are currently diagnosed with a mental health disorder. Mental illness is prevalent in all races, ages, and social settings and affects almost every family in the United States (USPHS 1999).

Today's healthcare system offers a number of mental health or "behavioral" healthcare services to individuals living with these conditions. The terms *mental health* and *behavioral health* may be used interchangeably throughout this textbook as both are frequently used in treatment settings around the country.

The individuals who seek these services are commonly referred to as clients, although it is not uncommon for them also to be referred to as patients, consumers, or recipients. These terms are used interchangeably throughout this textbook as well.

Types of Conditions Classified as Mental Disorders

Invididuals seek professional healthcare assistance for any number of mental health or behavioral conditions. In many circumstances, such people are diagnosed with more than one condition in the following categories:

- Depressive disorders affect more than 18 million adults in America and are fairly well managed with medication. Conditions in this category include general depression, major depression, and the depressed phase of bipolar disorder. Of interesting note is that nearly twice as many women as men suffer from depressive disorders (NIMH 2001).

- Schizophrenia affects more than 2 million adults in America. One of the more serious forms of mental illness, it is possibly the most disabling of all diseases of the brain, often causing the individual to exhibit psychotic symptoms such as delusions or hallucinations. Long misunderstood by the general public, schizophrenia often subjects its victims to an undeserving stigma. Although acute bouts typically require hospitalization, schizophrenia is commonly treated on an outpatient basis with antipsychotic medications, therapy, and counseling (NIMH 2001).

- Anxiety disorders affect approximately 19 million individuals in America and include such conditions as obsessive–compulsive disorder, panic disorder, social phobias, generalized anxiety disorders, and post-traumatic stress disorder. Individuals commonly suffer from more than one form of anxiety disorder at a time and generally are subject to other forms of mental illness, such as eating disorders or depressive disorders (NIMH 2001).

- Eating disorders afflict more women than men. Consisting primarily of anorexia nervosa and bulimia nervosa, they are among the leading causes of deaths of females between the ages of fifteen and twenty-four in the United States (NIMH 2001).

- Attention deficit hyperactivity disorder (ADHD) is one of the most common mental disorders among children and adolescents under age eighteen. Children are commonly hyperactive, unable to focus, or generally disruptive in social environments. Although ADHD can persist until adulthood, medication management has been very successful in treating individuals affected by this disorder (NIMH 2001).

- Alzheimer's disease and dementia affect more than 4 million individuals in America over the age of sixty-five. Organic in nature, there is no cure at this time and healthcare providers are limited to treating only the symptoms of the conditions (NIMH 2001).

- Substance abuse and/or chemical dependency affect more than 22 million Americans aged twelve and older. This number reflects the total population of individuals in America abusing illicit drugs and alcohol (SAMHSA 2003). Substance abuse is linked to more deaths and disabilities annually than from all other causes, and it costs the United States approximately $276 billion dollars each year in medical resources used for care, treatment, and rehabilitation (direct expenses) and reduced or lost productivity (indirect expenses) (NCADD 2002).

- Mental retardation affects more than 7 million individuals, according to the most recent survey conducted in the 1990s (Batshaw 1997). Individuals diagnosed with mental retardation generally have an intellectual functioning level (IQ) below 70 and significant limitations in two or more adaptive skill areas (daily living skills necessary to live, work, and play in the community). The onset must occur during childhood (before age 18) for the condition to be classified as mental retardation (AAMR 1992).

- Developmental disabilities affect approximately 17 percent of children under the age of eighteen in the United States. These physical, cognitive, psychological, sensory, and speech impairments include conditions such as autism, cerebral palsy, and specific learning disorders (CDC 2003).

Types of Care

Today's behavioral healthcare environment allows for a more individualized approach to treatment. Treatment is specifically prescribed after a diagnosis has been established, and careful consideration is given to the individual's social, medical, and financial circumstances and service needs. It may be provided by a psychiatrist, a psychologist, or a variety of rehabilitative or social work specialists. In many settings, a combination of these individuals is used.

Care typically is prescribed through a well-devised treatment or service plan developed by the provider or provider team in response to the individual's needs. In today's environment, the client and his or her family, if available, are often encouraged to actively participate in development of the treatment or service plan.

Types of Facilities

There are three basics types of behavioral healthcare settings: inpatient, residential, and outpatient.

- Inpatient facilities are able to provide the individual with around-the-clock care. They may be a dedicated portion of a hospital or may stand alone. In some circumstances, clients are in need of partial-stay services or partial hospitalization. Such services are provided to individuals who fall between the need for inpatient and outpatient services and would benefit from a short stay at an inpatient mental health facility or hospital. Partial stay provides individuals with mental health treatment that is more intense than the services provided on an outpatient basis. Most payers (including Medicare) cover this service when determined medically appropriate by the physician (CMS 2003).

- Often referred to as group homes or foster homes, residential facilities provide an alternative to the inpatient setting. Clients of such facilities are often encouraged to achieve independence in daily functions with little assistance from the provider. The residence provides a somewhat stable environment that helps many individuals with mental illness to assimilate into the "real world."

- Outpatient care provides clients with access to a stable treatment provider on an outpatient basis. Such care may occur in a formal office setting or in the comfort of the individual's home or residence. In some circumstances, outpatient services are provided in homeless shelters in an effort to reach the estimated hundreds of thousands of homeless individuals in America who suffer from mental illness (CMHS 1992).

Employers also are acknowledging the need for mental health services for their employees by providing access to Employee Assistance Programs (EAPs). These outpatient programs are designed to provide employees immediate access to psychological counseling on a limited basis and may be provided on-site or through a local provider.

Schools and universities also commonly provide outpatient mental health assistance to their students through formal clinics, guidance therapy, or direct collaboration with area community-based providers. Moreover, schools often provide crisis therapy or counseling to students exposed to significant trauma due to violence in the school or community or following major devastating events such as the terrorist events that occurred on September 11, 2001. Such therapy or counseling services are commonly provided by local mental health providers and/or local law enforcement.

Organization and Operation

Behavioral healthcare facilities may be private, stand-alone entities or affiliated with an area hospital or larger healthcare organization. In addition, some behavioral organizations are part of a chain, with a main corporate office and facilities in a specific region or throughout the nation. Many organizations today are owned, operated, and funded by the individual states or counties.

In most states, healthcare plans such as Medicaid or those run by individual counties are responsible for providing funding for individuals with behavioral healthcare problems. If an individual is fortunate enough to have private insurance that covers behavioral healthcare services, the state or local government may likely be responsible for paying the difference. Additional funding sources such as grants and other charitable organizations and their impact on the quality of care are discussed in chapter 10 of this textbook.

Forces Affecting Behavioral Healthcare

Numerous forces in the healthcare environment have an impact on behavioral healthcare. The following subsections describe some of these forces and their influence.

Quality Improvement Organizations

Quality improvement organizations (QIOs), formerly known as peer review organizations (PROs), are entities operating under the funding of the Centers for Medicare and Medicaid Services (CMS). Their primary function is to assess and improve the quality of healthcare provided to consumers. Oftentimes functioning as advocates for healthcare consumers, QIOs perform retrospective record reviews, conduct national and local quality improvement studies, and investigate consumer complaints regarding the quality of care provided in a number of settings.

Although QIOs do not specifically review mental health facilities, care provided to individuals with mental illness is monitored in other settings in which behavioral healthcare is sought. QIOs also protect the integrity of the Medicare funds by ensuring that services are provided only when medically appropriate or necessary. QIOs are dedicated to protecting the rights of individuals receiving behavioral healthcare services (CMS 2003).

Managed Care

As with other industries in the healthcare delivery system, behavioral healthcare must take measures to control the cost of services. Managed care entities have added behavioral health benefits to their plans and routinely monitor compliance with contractual agreements. Each year, more and more employers opt to contract with large managed care organizations (MCOs) to provide healthcare services to their employees. In many circumstances, however, benefits provided for behavioral health services are less than those provided for traditional medical treatment. For this reason, many employers have opted to establish EAPs to provide employees with access to brief and limited counseling or therapy services during times of need. This service is often fully paid for by the employer.

Integrated Delivery Systems

In today's healthcare environment, it is not uncommon for a provider or organization to offer a variety of healthcare services. For example, one organization may provide acute care services, home healthcare services, and behavioral healthcare services under the same organizational name. As with any other healthcare provider, access to health information is critical to the successful delivery of care in such an integrated delivery system (IDS). Reliable and timely access to information is essential for the delivery of high-quality client care and yet is one of the most significant challenges in this type of healthcare system.

It is not uncommon for the individual component disciplines to establish and maintain separate and distinct records of care (commonly referred to as clinical records) in the IDS. Thus, it is essential that the provider has a well-maintained information management system or other reliable client indexing system that allows for the identification of shared clients. This permits optimal communication among healthcare providers in each component discipline within the network or IDS arrangement and ensures continuity of care for the client.

Healthcare Reengineering

As with other industries in the healthcare delivery system, behavioral healthcare has been subject to attempts at reengineering throughout the years. Healthcare reengineering is an approach to improve client care quality through the restructuring of services and/or redesignation of staff responsibilities to provide optimal services while maintaining control of costs. For some industries, this system has worked successfully with little effort. For recipients of behavioral health services, however, reengineering may cause a threat to the stable provider–client relationship, causing undue stress on the client. For this reason, many behavioral health providers have opted to ignore the financial benefit of reengineering and have chosen, instead, to maintain the personalized treatment sought by so many individuals within the mental health population.

Performance Improvement

Performance improvement (PI) activities are an important aspect of any industry in the healthcare delivery system. Behavioral healthcare facilities accredited by the Joint Commission on Accreditation of Healthcare Organizations (JCAHO) or by the Commission on Accreditation of Rehabilitation Facilities (CARF) demonstrate an excellence in high-quality service provision by maintaining compliance with hundreds of quality standards developed by the accreditation bodies. Accrediting bodies such as JCAHO and CARF closely monitor organizational policies and procedures related to PI activities. Various PI strategies are discussed later in this book.

Outcomes Assessment and Management

Outcomes assessment is an effective tool used to monitor the success of a plan from beginning to end. In behavioral health, it is a way to determine if care and services were prescribed appropriately and provided to assist the client in achieving the expected or desired outcome (Rudman 1997, 81–85).

Although behavioral healthcare experts report that individuals suffering from behavioral health conditions may never be "cured" in the traditional sense of the word, it is highly accepted that many of them can achieve a fairly independent lifestyle when diagnosed and treated properly. Various methodologies for outcomes assessment and management for behavioral health are discussed later in this book.

Growth of Outpatient and Partial Treatment Settings

With the rising cost of inpatient services, many individuals are seeking behavioral health services through outpatient or partial-treatment settings. These options provide the client with a stable healthcare provider at a significantly lower expense. Unfortunately, the decision to move to the outpatient setting is not always made by the individual or provider but, rather, by the payer.

Health Insurance Portability and Accountability Act

In April 2003, administrators, providers, and HIM professionals throughout the healthcare industry faced one of the most significant laws ever to impact healthcare delivery. This law, known as the Health Insurance Portability and Accountability Act (HIPAA), forever changed the manner in which organizations use and disclose the confidential information that is collected and maintained for healthcare purposes.

For many HIM professionals working in the field of behavioral health, HIPAA was a welcome relief to the constant battle fought with other industries (both inside the healthcare continuum and out) over protection of the highly sensitive information generated in behavioral health encounters. For the first time in the history of healthcare, all providers were required to protect health information with the same respect and care that behavioral healthcare providers had been accustomed to doing for decades.

Professional Associations, Government Agencies, and Organizations Related to Behavioral Healthcare

Over the years, professional associations, government agencies, and organizations related specifically to behavioral healthcare have flourished. The discussions below focus on those with the greatest impact.

Centers for Medicare and Medicaid Services

The Centers for Medicare and Medicaid Services (CMS) is a division of the U.S. Department of Health and Human Services (HHS). Referenced throughout this book, CMS plays an integral role in the quality of care provided to those individuals utilizing the behavioral healthcare system. It monitors expenses related to behavioral healthcare and provides mental health benefits through its Medicare program to eligible recipients (CMS 2003). Additionally, CMS oversees the QIOs, which monitor medical necessity, quality of care, and the appropriateness of reimbursed services in behavioral healthcare settings.

National Alliance for the Mentally Ill

The National Alliance for the Mentally Ill (NAMI) is a nonprofit organization dedicated to providing advocacy and support to individuals affected by severe mental illness (schizophrenia, bipolar disorder, major depressive disorders, and so on). NAMI not only assists individuals with the mental illness but also works with their families and friends. NAMI's primary mission is to eradicate mental illness and improve the quality of life for those affected by it (NAMI 2003).

National Mental Health Association

The National Mental Health Association (NMHA) is a nonprofit organization created to assist the more than 54 million Americans with mental disorders. Through its public advocacy, education, and research programs, NMHA hopes to elevate public knowledge of mental health issues, encourage reform, and promote the effective use of qualified prevention and recovery programs (NMHA 2004).

Joint Commission on Accreditation of Healthcare Organizations

The Joint Commission on Accreditation of Healthcare Organizations is a not-for-profit organization dedicated to continuously improving the quality of care provided to individuals throughout the healthcare industry. It offers voluntary accreditation to healthcare providers and organizations through its rigorous evaluation and accreditation process.

The JCAHO bases its accreditation outcome on the ability of the healthcare organization to demonstrate compliance with specific performance standards. The accreditation process includes an on-site survey by an interdisciplinary survey team that evaluates ongoing compliance with the performance standards specific to the healthcare setting (JCAHO 2003). Specific interaction between the JCAHO and the behavioral healthcare system are discussed throughout this textbook.

Commission on Accreditation of Rehabilitation Facilities

The Commission on Accreditation of Rehabilitation Facilities is similar to the JCAHO in that it is a not-for-profit organization devoted to ensuring continuous quality improvement in healthcare, but CARF specifically accredits organizations for quality excellence in rehabilitative and human services. Like JCAHO, CARF has developed performance standards that must be met in order for a healthcare organization to pass the survey process (CARF 2004).

Substance Abuse and Mental Health Services Administration

The Substance Abuse and Mental Health Services Administration (SAMHSA) is a federal agency of the HHS established to focus on assessing and improving the lives of individuals with or at risk for mental illness and/or substance abuse disorders. SAMHSA also offers public programs and funding to provide treatment, prevention efforts, and rehabilitation services for substance abuse and mental illness (SAMHSA 2003).

American Health Information Management Association

The American Health Information Management Association (AHIMA) is the dynamic professional association that represents more than 46,000 specially educated HIM professionals who work throughout the healthcare industry. HIM professionals serve the healthcare industry and the public by managing, analyzing, and utilizing data vital for patient care and by making that care accessible to healthcare providers when it is needed most.

The Health Information Management Professional's Role in Behavioral Healthcare

The HIM professional is a vital part of any behavioral healthcare organization. From the onset of care, he or she is able to provide best-practice guidance and expertise on documentation issues, compliance issues, and general record maintenance issues.

Successful HIM practices throughout the continuum of care provided in the behavioral healthcare setting assist in the safety and quality of care provided to clients, effective outcomes monitoring, and positive customer satisfaction. As the keepers and manipulators of information and data, HIM professionals play an integral, indispensable, and powerful role in meeting these challenges.

To provide accurate and timely assistance, it is critical that the HIM professional understand the complexity of the behavioral healthcare system, its rules and regulations, and its unique position in the healthcare delivery system.

This book provides HIM professionals with the fundamental tools and resources necessary to gain a greater understanding of the fascinating world of behavioral health.

References and Bibliography

American Association on Mental Retardation. 1992. *Mental Retardation: Definition, Classification, and Systems of Supports,* 9th ed. Washington, DC: AAMR.

American Psychiatric Association. 1994. *Diagnostic and statistical manual of mental disorders DSM-IV,* 4th ed. Washington, DC: APA.

Batshaw, M. 1997. *Children with disabilities.* Baltimore: Paul H. Brooks Publishing.

Centers for Disease Control, National Center on Birth Defects and Developmental Disabilities. 2003. Developmental disabilities. Accessed on-line at http://www.cdc.gov/ncbddd.

Centers for Medicare and Medicaid Services. 2003. Medicare and your mental health benefits. Accessed on-line at http://www.nimh.nih.gov.

Center for Mental Health Services. 1992. Mental health information and statistics. Accessed on-line at http://www.mhsource.com.

Commission on Accreditation of Rehabilitation Facilities. 2004. What does CARF accredit? Accessed on-line at http://www.carf.org.

Joint Commission on Accreditation of Healthcare Organizations. 2003. Facts about the Joint Commission on Accreditation of Healthcare Organizations. Accessed on-line at http://www.jcaho.org.

National Alliance for the Mentally Ill. 2003. About NAMI. Accessed on-line at http://www.nami.org.

National Council on Alcoholism and Drug Dependence. 2002. Alcoholism and drug dependence are America's number one health problem. Accessed on-line at http://www.ncadd.org/facts.

National Institute of Mental Health. 2001. The numbers count. Accessed on-line at http://www.nimh.nih.gov.

National Mental Health Association. 2004. About NMHA. Accessed on-line at http://www.nmha.org.

Rudman, William J. 1997. *Performance Improvement in Health Information Management Services.* Philadelphia: W.B. Saunders.

Shorter, Edward. 1997. *A History of Psychiatry.* New York: John Wiley & Sons.

Substance Abuse and Mental Health Services Administration. 2003. Overview of Findings from the 2002 National Survey on Drug Use and Health. Office of Applied Studies, NHSDA Series H-21, DHHS Publication No. SMA 03-3774. Rockville, MD: Substance Abuse and Mental Health Services Administration.

U.S. Public Health Service. 1999. Mental health: A report of the surgeon general. Accessed on-line at http://www.surgeongeneral.gov/library/mentalhealth.

Chapter 1

Documentation of Care

Jill Burt, RHIA

A **health record** is a private document, either paper based or electronic, created in the normal course of **client** care. Its compilation may begin prior to admission and proceeds through to the conclusion or transfer of treatment and, ultimately, disposition. This collection of documents, often organized to reflect the order of care events as they occur, should be sufficiently comprehensive to support a client's **diagnosis,** plan of treatment, course of treatment, outcomes, and billing activity. **Behavioral health** has unique documentation challenges. Clients may be at high risk for suicidal or homicidal behavior. Often they are committed to a behavioral healthcare facility involuntarily or are required to receive treatment against their wishes. Clients who voice suicidal thoughts or exhibit suicidal behaviors present organization staff with significant challenges in terms of care and safety. Consequently, staff must have an organized system for documenting and addressing such behavior (Teich 1998).

The health record is the documentation of a client's physical and behavioral health and the healthcare **services** provided in any area of the healthcare delivery system or continuum. It consists of individually identifiable data. The term **individually identifiable data** refers to information that identifies, or could be used to identify, an individual. This information:

- May be kept, stored, maintained, and transmitted in any medium

- Is collected and used when providing or documenting care and treatment

Data that are not individually identifiable are known as aggregate data. **Aggregate data** are data extracted from individual client records that have been deidentified and combined. Uses for individual and aggregate data are summarized in table 1.1.

This chapter defines the purposes of healthcare documentation and identifies its key users. It also describes various efforts, legislative and otherwise, to provide documentation guidelines and standards for use by the healthcare industry. Finally, the chapter discusses different documentation methodologies and focuses on the importance of developing organization **policies** and **procedures** and documentation review practices and of implementing employee education and training on the documentation **process.**

Purposes of Healthcare Documentation

Documentation in the client behavioral healthcare record has multiple purposes. It:

- Serves as a basis for planning client care and ensuring continuity in the evaluation of the client's condition and treatment

Table 1.1.   Uses for individual and aggregate data

Individually identifiable data	• Client care and treatment • Billing
Aggregate data	• Research studies • Statistical data on use of services • Statistical data on treatment • Provider patterns • Help the facility plan for the future

- Furnishes documentary evidence about the client's evaluation, treatment, and change in condition during the treatment encounter as well as during follow-up care and services

- Provides a mechanism for communication among all the healthcare professionals contributing to the client's care

- Substantiates treatment and services provided for insurance claims

- Documents client involvement and, when appropriate, family members' involvement in the client's treatment program

- Assists in protecting the legal interests of the client, the facility, and the responsible practitioners

- Provides data for research

- Provides data for use in internal training, continuing education, quality assessment, and utilization review

Users of Healthcare Documentation

Many individuals and groups use healthcare documentation for myriad reasons. Some of the key users of healthcare documentation are discussed in the following subsections.

Organization Staff

Myriad staff members provide care and treatment to behavioral healthcare clients, including physicians, psychologists, nurses, social workers, chemical dependency counselors, rehabilitation therapists, mental health workers, and **case managers.** Staff in administrative support areas such as quality improvement, utilization management, and risk management use both individual client and aggregate data for review activities. Finally, administrative staff members use aggregate data for **strategic planning.**

Other Healthcare Providers

Complete and accurate documentation is essential to ensure the continuity of care for behavioral healthcare clients across the continuum. Behavioral healthcare services are provided at many levels—from acute inpatient treatment to in-home community-based services.

Billing and Third-Party Payers

An appropriately documented behavioral healthcare record can reduce many of the difficulties associated with claims processing and can serve as a legal document to verify the care provided. **Third-party payers** review care documentation to ensure that the services provided are:

- Appropriate for the client's condition

- Medically necessary

- Coded correctly

- Provided in the correct setting

Because payers have a contractual obligation to enrollees, they want to know that their healthcare dollars are well spent and may require reasonable documentation to show that services are consistent with the insurance coverage provided (St. Anthony Publishing 2001). The diagnostic and procedure **codes** on the health insurance claim form should reflect the documentation in the healthcare record. Therefore, the more completely and accurately the client encounter is described, the easier it is to code the diagnoses and the procedures properly.

Documentation of each client **encounter** or **visit** should include the:

- Reason for the encounter and relevant history, physical examination findings, and prior diagnostic test results

- Assessment, clinical impression, or diagnosis

- Evaluation and treatment procedures performed

- Plan of care

- Rationale for ordering diagnostic and other ancillary service

- Client's progress, changes in treatment and response to those changes, and any revision of diagnosis

- Time taken to perform the encounter

- Date and authentication (signature and credentials) by the healthcare professional

Regulatory Bodies

Regulatory bodies include accrediting agencies, and state and federal licensure bodies. These agencies and licensing bodies review behavioral healthcare record documentation to help determine whether the organization or agency under review is in compliance with applicable rules, **regulations,** and standards.

(See table 1.2 for a list of regulatory bodies and table 1.3 for a list of Web sites to access statutes, laws, and administrative code.)

Documentation Standards

Health information management (HIM) **professionals** have to keep current with a wealth of rules, regulations, and standards for behavioral healthcare record documentation. They should review the *Federal Register* for proposed rules and the state regulatory bulletins for changes to rules. Accrediting agency publications and standards should be reviewed on a regular basis for updates and additions. Professional associations such as the American Health Information Management Association (AHIMA) can be an excellent source of information on documentation standards. The health record serves as a legal business record for a healthcare organization, and the regulations and standards vary depending on practice setting, state statutes and rules, and applicable case law.

Table 1.2. Regulatory bodies that govern behavioral health documentation

Health Insurance Portability and Accountability Act (HIPAA)	U.S. Department of Health and Human Services http://aspe.hhs.gov/admnsimp/
Behavioral health standards manual	Rehabilitation Accreditation Commission www.carf.org
Behavioral health standards	Council on Accreditation www.coanet.org
Patient Self-Determination Act (42 USC 1395-1396) (advance directives)	The Office of the Law Revision Counsel http://uscode.house.gov/uscode-cgi/fastweb.exe?getdoc+uscview+t41t42+1960+0++%28%29%20%20A
Medicare and Medicaid program manuals	Centers for Medicare and Medicaid Services www.cms.hhs.gov/manuals/default.asp
Conditions of Participation for Hospitals (42 CFR 482)	National Archives and Records Administration, Code of Federal Regulations www.access.gpo.gov/nara/cfr/waisidx_01/42cfr482_01.html
PPS for inpatient psychiatric hospitals, proposed rule	Code of Federal Regulations, proposed rules www.access.gpo.gov/su_docs/fedreg/a031128c.html
Interpretive guidelines for hospitals	Centers for Medicare and Medicaid Services www.csm.hhs.gov/cop/1.asp
Medicare Interpretive Guidelines for Psychiatric Hospitals	Centers for Medicare and Medicaid Services www.csm.hhs.gov/cop/1.asp
Comprehensive Accreditation Manual for Hospitals	Joint Commission on Accreditation of Healthcare Organizations www.jcaho.org
Comprehensive Accreditation Manual for Behavioral Health Care	Joint Commission on Accreditation of Healthcare Organizations www.jcaho.org
Code of Federal Regulations (42 CFR 2)	National Archives and Records Administration, Code of Federal Regulations www.access.gpo.gov/nara/cfr/waisidx_01/42cfr2_01.html
Standards for the accreditation of managed behavioral healthcare organizations	National Committee for Quality Assurance www.ncqa.org

Table 1.3. State-by-state listing of Web sites to access statutes, laws, and administrative code

State	Web Source
Alabama	www.alabamaadministrativecode.state.al.us/about-code.html
Alaska	www.legis.state.ak.us/default.htm
Arizona	www.azleg.state.az.us
Arkansas	www.accessarkansas.org/
California	www.leginfo.ca.gov/calaw.html
Colorado	www.courts.state.co.us/siteindex
Connecticut	www.cga.state.ct.us/lco/statute_web_site_lco.htm
Delaware	www.delcode.state.de.us
District of Columbia	www.grc.dc.gov/laws1/site/default.asp
Florida	www.flsenate.gov/statutes/index.cfm
Georgia	www.legis.state.ga.us
Hawaii	www.capitol.hawaii.gov/site1/docs/docs.asp
Idaho	www.state.id.us/legislat/idstat.html
Illinois	www.legis.state.il.us/legislation/ilcs/ilcs.asp
Indiana	www.in.gov/legislative/ic/code
Iowa	www.legis.state.ia.us
Kansas	www.kslegislature.org
Kentucky	www.law.state.ky.us/office/links.htm
Louisiana	www.legis.state.la.us/
Maine	www.state.me.us/legils/lawlib/homepage.htm
Maryland	mlis.state.md.us
Massachusetts	www.state.ma.us/legis
Michigan	www.michiganlegislature.org
Minnesota	www.leg.state.mn.us/leg/statutes.asp
Mississippi	www.mscode.com/free/statutes/toc.htm
Missouri	www.moga.state.mo.us/homestat.asp
Montana	www.state.mt.us/govt/mca_const.asp
Nebraska	www.unicam.state.ne.us/laws/index.htm
Nevada	www.leg.state.nv.us/law1.cfm
New Hampshire	www.state.nh.us/government/laws.html
New Jersey	www.njleg.state.nj.us
New Mexico	www.state.nm.us/category/governmentnm.html#laws
New York	www.findlaw.com/11stategov/ny/laws.html
North Carolina	www.ncleg.net/statutes/statutes.asp
North Dakota	www.state.nd.us/lr/information/statutes
Ohio	www.legislature.state.oh.us/laws.cfm
Oklahoma	www.lsb.state.ok.us
Oregon	www.leg.state.or.us/ors/home.html
Pennsylvania	www.legis.state.pa.us
Rhode Island	www.rilin.state.ri.us/statutes/statutes.html
South Carolina	www.scstatehouse.net/code/statmast.htm
South Dakota	legis.state.sd.us/statutes/index.cfm
Tennessee	www.tennesseeanytime.org/laws/laws.html
Texas	www.capitol.state.tx.us/statutes/statutes.html
Utah	www.le.utah.gov/documents/code_const.htm
Vermont	www.leg.state.vt.us/statutes/statutes2.htm
Virginia	legis.state.va.us/laws/AdminCode.htm
Washington	www.leg.wa.gov/
West Virginia	www.findlaw.com/11stategov/wv/laws.html
Wisconsin	www.legis.state.wi.us/rsb/stats.html
Wyoming	www.courts.state.wy.us/
Web sites that list state laws, regulations, rules	www.alllaw.com type in name of state, www.law.cornell.edu/topics/state_statutes.html

Centers for Medicare and Medicaid Services

Behavioral healthcare organizations that participate in the Medicare program must comply with federal standards issued by the **Centers for Medicare and Medicaid Services** (CMS) called the *Conditions of Participation.* Part 482.61 of these standards addresses special medical record requirements for inpatient psychiatric **hospitals** and states that "the medical records maintained by a psychiatric hospital must permit determination of the degree and intensity of the treatment provided to individuals who are furnished services in the institution." In other words, the documentation must support the amount and level of services provided.

The standards go on to give specific content requirements of the medical record. Part 482.24 provides guidelines for inpatient hospital medical records.

Joint Commission on Accreditation of Healthcare Organizations

The **Joint Commission on Accreditation of Healthcare Organizations** (JCAHO) is a not-for-profit organization established more than fifty years ago to evaluate the quality and safety of healthcare. Its behavioral health accreditation program was established in 1972. Services currently accredited include mental health, addiction services, and child welfare and developmentally disabled care in a variety of treatment settings. Depending on the type of state licensure and the funding source, some behavioral healthcare organizations continue to be surveyed under the hospital standards instead of the behavioral health standards.

JCAHO accreditation includes an intensive on-site survey process at least once every three years. The JCAHO uses documentation review during the survey process to evaluate the quality of care and **patient** safety. It recently revised its record review process but, as of this writing, has not come out with the revised record review recommendations.

Commission on Accreditation of Rehabilitation Facilities

The **Commission on Accreditation of Rehabilitation Facilities** (CARF) is an independent not-for-profit accrediting agency. Founded in 1966, CARF uses a continuous quality improvement process for its accreditation process. The commission has specific behavioral health standards and surveys a variety of behavioral health settings, including mental healthcare, substance abuse care, and other addiction programs. The mission of CARF is to promote the quality, value, and optimal outcomes of services through accreditation that centers on enhancing the lives of the persons receiving services. Part of the CARF survey process includes a quality medical record review.

National Committee for Quality Assurance

The **National Committee for Quality Assurance** (NCQA) is an independent, nonprofit organization whose mission is to improve the quality of healthcare. NCQA started surveying managed behavioral healthcare organizations in 1997. Its survey process is voluntary. NCQA developed its Behavioral Health Accreditation Standards with the input of all affected stakeholders—consumers, employers, policy makers, health plans, managed behavioral healthcare organizations, and **providers.**

NCQA uses documentation review, in part, to foster accountability within managed behavioral healthcare organizations for the quality of care and services its members receive. It also uses documentation review to help determine effectiveness in the provision of behavioral healthcare.

Council on Accreditation

The **Council on Accreditation for Children and Family Services** (COA) is an international, independent, nonprofit child and family services and behavioral healthcare accreditation organization. An organization that undergoes COA accreditation is evaluated against best-practice standards. The COA standards include organizational and management standards along with service standards. These standards are designed to facilitate organizational improvement. The COA uses medical record review during on-site visits to verify that standards are being met.

Health Insurance Portability and Accountability Act of 1996 Privacy Rule

The **Health Insurance Portability and Accountability Act of 1996** (HIPAA) took effect on April 14, 2003. Its privacy rule created a basic set of standards for the privacy of individually identifiable **health information** and set out numerous requirements for the use and disclosure of such information. HIPAA applies to healthcare plans, healthcare clearinghouses, and healthcare providers who transmit specific transactions electronically. These entities are referred to as covered entities under HIPAA. Some state laws or rules are more restrictive, but HIPAA provides a baseline with regard to the protection and disclosure of **protected health information** (PHI).

HIPAA impacts HIM practice by requiring employee education on privacy, the designation of a privacy officer, and the tracking of disclosures of PHI. The act also requires documentation of notification to a client of his or her privacy rights.

Client Right to Access Healthcare Records

The HIPAA privacy rule established, at the federal level, a client's right to inspect and obtain copies of his or her PHI in all but a limited number of situations. Prior to the privacy rule, some state laws gave a client the right to access. One of the exceptions is the right to access psychotherapy records.

HIPAA defines psychotherapy records as notes recorded (in any medium) by a mental health professional documenting or analyzing the contents of a conversation during a private counseling session or a group, joint, or family counseling session that are separate from the rest of the client's healthcare record. Few healthcare organizations maintain psychotherapy records under the HIPAA definition. The HIPAA definition most likely applies to private therapy notes or raw data from client psychological testing.

Psychotherapy notes exclude medication prescription and monitoring, results of clinical tests, and any summary of the following items:

- Diagnosis

- Functional status

- Treatment plan, symptoms, prognosis, and progress to date

A healthcare organization also may deny a client access to his or her PHI when:

- A licensed healthcare professional has determined that the access is likely to endanger the life or physical safety of the client or another person. For example, if documentation reveals that the client's sister supports inpatient hospitalization for the client and her position is contrary to the client's wishes, the client may retaliate against the sister.

- The PHI makes reference to another person who is not a healthcare provider, and a licensed healthcare professional determines that access to the documentation is likely to cause substantial harm to the person referenced. For example, access granted to a parent to the records of a minor that document abuse would likely put the child in jeopardy.

The HIM professional should note and advise providers that even in these rare instances information can be compelled by a judge to be released to the patient or his or her lawfully authorized representative.

Patient's Right to Amend

The HIPAA privacy rule requires all behavioral healthcare organizations to have policies and procedures in place that address how a client or his or her legal representative can enter an amendment into the healthcare record. For HIM practitioners in some states, giving a client the right to amend his or her healthcare information is nothing new and has been a requirement under state law or rule for many years.

With few exceptions, the privacy rule gives clients the right to request that a covered entity— a healthcare provider that conducts electronic transactions, health plans, and clearinghouses— amend its healthcare information. The rule requires specific procedures and time frames for processing an amendment. (See figure 1.1.) Although not required, it would be prudent to ask that the request be made in writing. Developing a form for the client and the covered entity to facilitate a request for amendment is highly recommended. (See figure 1.2.)

A separate entry in the record should be used for client amendment documentation. The amendment should document the information believed to be inaccurate or incomplete and the information the client or legal representative believes to be correct or needs to be added to. The HIM professional should flag the entry in question by writing "See correction/ amendment" and by indicating the amendment with his or her signature and the date. The amendment form should be attached to the incorrect or amended entry. The documentation in question should never be removed or deleted from the healthcare record and must be disclosed when the original document is disclosed.

The privacy rule gives specific conditions under which the request to amend can be denied, for example, when the health information that is the subject of the request is not part of the individual's health record, was not created by the organization, or is accurate and complete. For example, if a client requests to amend information in his or her chart that was received from another healthcare provider, the facility that received the information would not be required to amend it. Individual state laws or regulations may address how amendments should be processed, and healthcare organizations must comply with those requirements if they happen to be more stringent than those outlined under the HIPAA privacy rule.

Client's Right to Refuse Treatment

Behavioral healthcare poses unique challenges to patient rights. Even though clients may be at high risk for suicidal or homicidal behavior as a result of mental illness, they have the right to refuse psychiatric treatment. Clients are often committed involuntarily to a psychiatric institution, and the institution must define the fine line between safeguarding the client's rights and protecting the interest of society. Clients who complain of suicidal thoughts or display overtly suicidal behaviors yet persist in refusing care present healthcare providers with significant care and safety challenges. Complete and timely documentation of these situations is critical.

Advance Directives

An **advance directive,** or healthcare directive, is a written legal document that communicates a client's healthcare decisions in the event he or she is unable to make them or appoints a person to make them on the client's behalf. Advance directives provide written instructions about the kind of care the client does or does not want when the client is no longer able to direct his or her care. Situations in which an advance directive may be used include the following:

- Schizophrenic patients who refuse medication because they hear command voices to harm themselves

- Patients who decide what medications to take and when

Figure 1.1.   Sample policy and procedure client request to amend

CLIENT'S REQUEST FOR AMENDMENT/CORRECTION
OF THEIR MEDICAL RECORD

PURPOSE

To establish the client's right to request to amend and/or correct protected health information (PHI) as long as the Center maintains the client record.

POLICY

It is the policy of the Center to determine whether to accept or deny any request for amendment and/or correction to the client record when the client believes information is incorrect or incomplete. It is the Center's responsibility to ensure that action has been taken within sixty (60) days of the request.

PROCEDURE

1. The client may contact his or her primary staff worker, author of the document requested, Director of Health Information Services/Privacy Officer or Designee to complete the Amend/Correct Client Record Information Form.
   a. The client will complete the Amend/Correct Client Record Information Form with distribution as follows:
      i. Original to author of the document
      ii. Copy to Health Information Services
      iii. Copy to client
   b. The author will review the Amend/Correct Client Record Information Form to:
      i. Complete the denied/accepted section
      ii. Make comments
      iii. Sign and date the form
      iv. Forward to Health Information Services to be filed and a copy sent to the client

2. A denial to any request to amend a client record can be made in one of the following circumstances:
   a. The document was not created at Center but was received as a request for information from an outside source.
   b. The documents/documentation is not considered part of the client record (designated record set) and would not otherwise be available for inspection.
   c. The Center determines that the information is accurate or complete.

3. If the Center denies a request for amendment in whole or part, the Center:
   a. Must provide the client a written denial statement explaining the reason for the denial
   b. Must describe to the client the process for submitting a Statement of Disagreement
   c. Must provide instructions on how the client may make a complaint to the Center regarding the denial
   d. May prepare a rebuttal to the Statement of Disagreement and must provide the client with a copy
   e. Must identify the location of the disputed amendment/correction and cross-reference the information that is being disputed for the purpose of future release of information

   When the denial process has been completed, the Center has the responsibility to notify:
   a. The client
   b. Individuals and organizations the client identifies
   c. Facilities and business associates that have the information subject to the amendment/correction and may have relied—or might rely—on the information to the detriment of the client

4. If the Center accepts a request for amendment/correction in whole or in part, the Center must:
   a. Make the amendment/correction*
   b. Identify the challenged entry as amended or corrected
   c. Indicate the location of the amended/corrected information and cross-reference the information that is being amended or corrected for the purpose of future release of information

   When the amendment process has been completed, the Center has the responsibility to notify:
   a. The Client
   b. Individuals and organizations the client identifies
   c. Facilities and business associates that have the information subject to the amendment/correction and may have relied or might rely on the information to the detriment of the client

*See Policy and Procedure Staff Process for Corrections and Amendments to the Client Record

Date Established:

Date of Last Review:

Date of Last Revision:

Approved by and Date:

Figure 1.2.   Sample form request for amendment of the medical record form

---

REQUEST FOR AMENDMENT OF THE MEDICAL RECORD FORM

Patient Name: _____ D.O.B: _____

Medical Record Number: _____

Address: _____

Phone Number: (H)_____(W)_____

Date of entry to be amended: _____

Type of entry to be amended: _____

Please explain how the entry is incorrect or incomplete. What should the entry say to be more accurate or complete?

_____

_____

_____

Would you like this amendment sent to anyone to whom we may have disclosed the information in the past? If so, please specify the name and address of the organization or the individual.

_____   _____
Name   Address

_____   _____
Signature of Client or Legal Representative   Date

For healthcare organization use only:

Date received: _____   Amendment has been: ☐ Accepted   ☐ Denied

If denied, check reason for denial:

☐ PHI was not created at this organization.   ☐ PHI is accurate and complete.
☐ PHI is not available to the client for inspection   ☐ PHI is not part of client's designated record set.
  as required by federal law (for example, psychotherapy notes).

Physician/Author Comments:

_____ In response to your request, a correction/addendum will be made part of your permanent medical record.

_____ Your request has been made a part of your permanent medical record.

Comments of Healthcare Practitioner:

_____

_____

_____

_____

_____   _____
Physician/Author Signature   Date

The **Patient Self-Determination Act** (PSDA), passed as part of the Omnibus Budget Reconciliation Act of 1990, requires hospitals and other healthcare organizations that receive Medicaid funding to give clients written information concerning their rights under state law to make decisions about medical care, including the right to accept medical treatment. In addition, clients must be given information about their rights to formulate advance directives such as living wills and durable powers of attorney for healthcare.

At the time of this writing, seventeen states allow mental health advance directives. These directives may include permission for treatment with neuroleptic medication and electroshock therapy. HIM professionals should know the laws related to advance directives in the state in which they are working and should understand the elements necessary for the advance directives to be legal. (See figure 1.3 for a sample advance directive form.)

State Regulations

Many states have their own regulations, rules, laws, or statutes on behavioral healthcare record documentation. (See table 1.3.) State law trumps federal law when state law is more stringent. It is important to be aware of the laws and to keep up with any changes. Often state regulations are enacted in response to a specific public concern and are strong, detailed, and aimed at the state's unique experiences. State regulations may cover a broad range of organizations or be specific to certain types of organizations, such as government agencies or hospitals.

Characteristics of Good Documentation

Although originally developed for use with paper-based health record **systems,** many of the guiding principles discussed above now can be applied successfully to documentation practices in an electronic healthcare record (Dougherty 2002b). The characteristics of good documentation are outlined in table 1.4. Poorly kept medical records or documentation can lead to the following consequences:

- Mistakes or delays in treatment because of missing or inaccurate information

- Loss of malpractice litigation

- Loss of licensure or accreditation status

- Loss of eligibility for reimbursement by Medicare or some other third-party payer

- Lack of data for research projects, client care evaluations, or quality improvement activities

AHIMA's House of Delegates published a table of best practices in 1999 for documentation and completion of the health record. These are shown in table 1.5.

Individualized Documentation

Each page in the behavioral health record must identify the client by name and by unique identification number (if one is assigned) (Dougherty 2002b). The unique identification number is used to facilitate record accessibility and retrieval in either a paper- or computer-based record system. Although records for inpatient and outpatient encounters can be separated, this method is not recommended due to difficulty in ensuring that all healthcare records are available for continuity of care. The unique identification number may be assigned automatically by a computer system, or some organizations use the client's Social Security number.

Figure 1.3.   Sample advance directive form

SAMPLE ADVANCE DIRECTIVE FORM

I, _____, being of sound mind, willfully and voluntarily execute this **mental health advance directive** to assure that if I should be found incompetent to consent to my own mental health treatment, my choices regarding my treatment will be carried out despite my inability to make informed decisions for myself. If a guardian, guardian advocate, or other decision maker is appointed by a court to make healthcare or mental health decisions for me, I intend this document to take precedence over all other means of determining my intent while competent. This document represents my wishes, and it should be given the greatest possible legal weight and respect. If the surrogate(s) named in this directive are not available, my wishes shall be binding on whoever is appointed to make such decisions. If I become incompetent to make decisions about my own mental health treatment, I have authorized a mental healthcare surrogate to make certain treatment decisions for me. My surrogate is also authorized to apply for public benefits to defray the cost of my healthcare, to release information to appropriate persons, and to authorize my transfer from a healthcare facility.

My mental healthcare surrogate is:

Name: _____

Address: _____

Day Telephone: _____ Evening Telephone: _____

If the person named above is unable or unavailable to serve as my mental healthcare surrogate, I hereby appoint and request immediate notification of my alternate mental healthcare surrogate as follows:

Name of Alternate: _____

Address: _____

Day Telephone: _____ Evening Telephone: _____

Complete the following or initial in the blank marked yes or no:

A.   If I become incompetent to give consent to mental health treatment, I give my mental healthcare surrogate full power and authority to make mental healthcare decisions for me. This includes the right to consent, refuse consent, or withdraw consent to any mental healthcare, treatment, service, or procedure consistent with any instructions and/or limitations I have stated in this advance directive. If I have not expressed a choice in this advance directive, I authorize my surrogate to make the decision that he or she determines is the decision I would make if I were competent to do so.

_____ Yes   _____ No

B.   My choices of treatment facilities are as follows:

1.   In the event my psychiatric condition is serious enough to require 24-hour care, I would prefer to receive this care in this/these facilities:

Facility: _____

Facility: _____

2.   I **do not** wish to be placed in the following facilities for psychiatric care (optional):

Facility: _____

Facility: _____

C.   My choice of a treating physician is:

First choice of physician: _____ Second choice of physician: _____

I **do not** wish to be treated by the following physicians: (optional)

Name of physician: _____ Name of physician: _____

D.   If I am incompetent to give consent, I want staff to immediately notify the following persons that I have been admitted to a psychiatric facility.

Name: _____ Relationship: _____

Address: _____

Day Phone: _____ Evening Phone: _____

Name: _____ Relationship: _____

Address: _____

Day Phone: _____ Evening Phone: _____

Figure 1.3. (Continued)

E. If I am not competent to consent to my own treatment or to refuse medications relating to my mental health treatment, I have initialed one of the following, which represents my wishes:

    1. _____ I consent to the medications that Dr. _____ recommends.

    2. _____ I consent to the medications agreed to by my mental healthcare surrogate after consulting with my treating physician and any other individuals my surrogate deems appropriate, with the exceptions found in #3 below.

    3. _____ I specifically do not consent and I do not authorize my mental healthcare surrogate to consent to the administration of the following medications or their respective brand name, trade name, or generic equivalent (list name of drug and reason for refusal): _____

    4. _____ I am willing to take the medications excluded in #3 above if my only reason for excluding them is their side effects and the dosage can be adjusted to eliminate those side effects.

    5. I have the following other preferences about psychiatric medications: _____

F. My wishes regarding electroconvulsive therapy (ECT) are as follows:

    1. _____ My surrogate may not consent to ECT without express court approval.

    2. _____ I authorize my surrogate to consent to ECT, but only (initial one of the following):

        a. _____ with the number of treatments the attending psychiatrist thinks is appropriate; OR

        b. _____ with the number of treatments that Dr. _____ thinks is appropriate; OR

        c. _____ for no more than the following number of ECT treatments: _____

    3. Other instructions and wishes regarding ECT are as follows:_____

G. Other instructions I wish to make about my mental healthcare are (use additional pages if needed):

_____ Check here ( ) if other pages are used.

Signature By signing here, I indicate that I fully understand that this advance directive will permit my mental healthcare surrogate to make decisions and to provide, withhold, or withdraw consent for my mental health treatment.

Printed Name (Declarant): _____

Signature: _____ Date: _____

Witnesses This advance directive was signed by _____ in our presence. At his or her request, we have signed our names below as witnesses. We declare that, at the time this advance directive was signed, the Declarant, according to our best knowledge and belief, was of sound mind and under no constraint or undue influence. We further declare that we are both adults, are not designated in this advance directive as the mental healthcare surrogate, and at least one of us is neither the person's spouse nor blood relative.

Dated at_____ This _____ day of _____, _____
              (County & State)   (Day)   (Month)   (Year)

Witness 1:   **Witness 2:**

_____

Signature of witness 1   Signature of witness 2

_____

Printed name of witness 1   Printed name of witness 2

_____

Home address of witness 1   Home address of witness 2

_____

City, state, zip code of witness 1   City, state, zip code of witness 2

Acknowledgment of Healthcare Surrogate/Alternate

I, _____, mental healthcare surrogate designated by

_____, hereby accept the designation.

_____

_____   _____

Signature of mental healthcare surrogate   Date

I,_____, alternate mental healthcare surrogate

designated by _____, hereby accept the designation.

_____

_____   _____

Signature of alternate mental healthcare surrogate   Date

To link documentation to a client, the client's name and unique identification number should be on both sides of a single sheet of paper in the record (Dougherty 2002b). In an electronic health record (EHR), the same information must be on each page or screen, as well as on each page of any paper report or record that is generated. The organization's name also should appear on each page or screen to help identify where records originated if they are ever sent outside the organization.

Table 1.4. Characteristics of good documentation

Individualized	To link documentation to a client, the client's name and unique identification number should be on each page.
Permanent	Cannot be erased, fade over time, or be water soluble.
Complete	Document all facts—who, what, when, where, how, and why.
Appropriate	Documentation that pertains to the client's care and treatment. Do not document complaints or gripes.
Concise	Documentation should be factual and objective. Use only facility-approved abbreviations.
Authenticated	Shows authorship and assigns responsibility.
Legible	Documentation must be readable by other caregivers.
Timely	Make all entries as soon as possible after an event or encounter.
Continuous	Paper-based notes and entries should not contain blank lines or spaces.
Truthful	Never erase or obliterate documentation.
Integrity	Ensure that documentation has not been altered or destroyed in an unauthorized manner.

Source: Adapted from Dougherty 2002b.

Table 1.5. Table of best practices

Consistent and standard documentation requirements	• Streamline regulatory activities. • Develop consistent and standardized documentation requirements with accrediting and regulatory agencies.
Innovative, quality, and cost-efficient clinical documentation practices	• Develop policies and procedures to facilitate timely completion of medical records. • Utilize the latest technology for authentication. • Make forms used for documentation user-friendly.
Promote complete, current, and high-quality healthcare information by developing and using appropriate measures and monitors to assess documentation quality.	• Educate staff on the importance of clinical documentation practices. • Secure physician champion for documentation improvement. • Streamline medical record completion guidelines.
Plan strategically.	• Develop a computer-based health record. • Develop processes to effectively transition to an integrated health delivery system.

Source: Fletcher 1999.

Permanent Documentation

Whether in paper or electronic format, all entries must be permanent. Black ink is preferred for handwritten records to ensure legibility when they are photocopied. Black ink also seems to remain the most legible if a health record gets wet. A pencil should never be used for documentation purposes. Because of fading over time, thermal paper should be copied and the copy, marked as such, should be placed in the chart. When using a printed computer entry for documentation, the print must be permanent and should remain intact despite rubbing or normal handling. Ink jet printers should not be used because the ink is water soluble (Dougherty 2002b).

Complete Documentation

Complete documentation is vital for the continuity of optimum-quality client care. Caregivers need to be complete in their approach and record everything significant to the client's condition, including answers to who, what, when, where, how, and why. If all staff caring for the client were to suddenly disappear, a new team should be able to immediately continue the best possible care just by reading the record. Each change in a client's condition or significant client issues should be documented. The medical record confirms the care and treatment provided to the client. If it is not documented in the medical record, it did not happen. (See table 1.6 for specific requirements for progress note documentation.)

Table 1.6. Requirements for documentation of progress notes

Requirement	Example
Be specific and avoid generalization. Record the facts. Don't draw conclusions. Use objective terms. Rather than stating that "the client is upset," state exactly what behavior the client is exhibiting.	At 10:00 a.m., client was heard yelling in the east hallway. Client was shouting in a loud voice that she did not want to be here and that she was not mentally ill. She was waving her arms above her head and stamping her feet.
Be complete. Record everything significant to the client's condition, including who, what, when, where, how, and why.	Client refused her 8:00 a.m. dose of Buspar. She is also refusing to eat breakfast and has been isolated in her room the entire shift. Client denies any thought of self-abuse.
Be sure to document atypical treatment together with reasons for it (for example, restraints). Enter any unusual occurrences together with responsive and corrective steps taken and follow-up of the client's condition.	At 6:00 p.m., client was observed to have five superficial scratches on her left wrist. Client admits to scratching herself with a plastic knife. Client turned knife in to staff. On-call psychiatrist was notified and gave telephone order for 15-minute checks.
Use quotes when appropriate. One quote may be worth a thousand words in trying to describe a client's emotional state.	While in the dining room eating lunch at noon, client quickly stood up, knocking over her chair. Client then threw her meal tray on the floor, yelling, "The food is poison."
Use specific time frames rather than vague terms such as "usually," "frequently," or "often."	Client has been to the unit office at least six times during this shift, stating that she is not mentally ill and wants to be discharged right now.

Source: Dougherty 2002.

Appropriate Documentation

The behavioral health record should contain only documentation that pertains to the care of the client. It is not the place to voice complaints or gripes about coworkers, employers, physicians, or staffing issues and should not include statements that blame, accuse, or compromise other healthcare providers, the client, or his or her family (Dougherty 2002b). Likewise, hearsay (for example, from a client's roommate) should not be documented. If the behavioral health record were to end up in court, unprofessional and inappropriate documentation could bring the entire record under suspicion.

Sometimes it is necessary to refer to another client in the health record. When this happens, the client's full name should not be used; rather, his or her health record number, initials, or first name should be used.

Concise Documentation

Documentation should be specific. General characterizations should be avoided because they can be confusing. Examples of generalized statements seen frequently in the behavioral healthcare record include "the client is uncooperative" or "the client is doing well." Documentation should reflect only factual information.

Although they may provide a timesaving benefit, abbreviations used in behavioral health records present potential patient safety issues. Only abbreviations approved by the behavioral healthcare organization should be used in the medical record. The JCAHO National Patient Safety Goal #2b requires that a list be developed of dangerous abbreviations that should not be used in the medical record. At the present time, five abbreviations must be on the dangerous abbreviation list, all of which deal with the administration of medication.

The Institute for Safe Medication Practices (www.ismp.org) also maintains a list of error-prone abbreviations, symbols, and dose designations. Organizations should limit the abbreviations used in the record to help avoid misinterpretation. Two examples of dangerous abbreviations are Q.D. (every day) and Q.O.D. (every other day), which can be mistaken for each other. Abbreviations specific to behavioral health should be avoided because healthcare providers outside the behavioral health arena may be unfamiliar with them and unable to interpret their meaning correctly. For example, SIB (self-injurious behavior) or BP (borderline personality) might be common abbreviations within the behavioral healthcare organization, but unknown to someone outside behavioral health.

Authenticated Documentation

Authentication shows authorship and **responsibility** for an entry and is the responsibility of the person providing the treatment or evaluation. It is used in behavioral healthcare entries to verify that they are complete, accurate, and final. There are multiple acceptable methods for authenticating an entry in the health record, including use of the first initial, last name, and title/credential or discipline and electronic/digital signatures.

Much debate has centered on compliance with authentication requirements, including the intent of the requirement and the labor-intensive process involved in being compliant. Each behavioral healthcare organization must identify the proper and acceptable method of authentication for the type of entry based on applicable regulations, laws, and payer requirements. Although accrediting agencies such as the JCAHO may no longer require authentication of behavioral healthcare entries, other accrediting agencies or state laws and regulations do. In general, the federal regulations and accreditation standards do not stipulate a specific time frame for authentication. The organization should research the requirements carefully before developing policies and procedures on authentication and acceptable methods of authentication (Welch 2002). It should contact the state licensing authority (usually the state health department's division of healthcare licensure) for specific requirements.

Documentation audits or reviews should include the need to assess the accuracy of entries that are not authenticated.

At a minimum, paper-based records should include the first initial, last name, and credential, or professional title (Dougherty 2002b). The signature should immediately follow the last word of the entry. Cosignatures, which are most likely required for residents and students, are used to demonstrate supervision by qualified, experienced, and responsible professional staff and should be used as required by state law and regulatory agencies. If initials are used to authenticate an entry, a corresponding master signature sheet with full identification of the initials should be included. Initials are used frequently to authenticate entries on flow sheets. Unless specifically prohibited by state regulations or behavioral healthcare organization policy, facsimile (fax) signatures are acceptable as long as the fax is not thermofax, which fades over time. Electronic and digital signatures are acceptable when allowed by state law.

When electronic signatures are used, the technology should follow the standards as outlined in the HIPAA security rule for message **integrity** and authentication. The security rule requires facilities to address implementation policies and procedures to protect electronic-protected health information from improper alteration or destruction. It also requires organizations to address mechanisms and procedures for both person or entity authentication and PHI authentication. Person or entity authentication is verification that a person or entity seeking access to electronic PHI is the one claimed. Electronic PHI authentication ensures that electronic PHI has not been altered or destroyed in an unauthorized manner. Rubber stamp signatures are acceptable when allowed by state and reimbursement regulations. Use of rubber stamps requires that a letter be kept on file stating that the individual whose name appears on the stamp is the only one who will use it. Autoauthentication, which allows a physician or provider to state, prior to review of an entry, that it is complete and accurate, is inconsistent with CMS requirements.

CMS

To participate in the Medicare program, behavioral healthcare organizations must comply with the Medicare *Conditions of Participation.* These federal regulations currently require authentication of various health record entries. The 42 **Code of Federal Regulations** (CFR), Paragraph 482.24, *Conditions of Participation for Hospitals,* Medical Record Services (a)(1) and (c)(1)(i), state in part:

> Entries in the medical record may be made only by individuals as specified in hospital and **medical staff** policies. All entries in the medical record must be dated and authenticated, and a method established to identify the author. The parts of the medical record that are the responsibility of the physician must be authenticated by this individual. When non-physicians have been approved for such duties as taking medical histories or documenting aspects of physical examination, such information shall be appropriately authenticated by the responsible physician. Any entries in the medical record by house staff or non-physicians that require counter signing by supervisory or attending medical staff members shall be defined in the medical staff rules and regulations.

The entry goes on to list what system would meet the authentication requirements, including signatures, written initials, or computer entry.

Legible Documentation

All entries must be neat and legible. Illegible documentation puts the client at risk. An Institute of Medicine (IOM) report entitled "To Err Is Human: Building a Safer Health System," published in 2000, estimates that as many as 98,000 people die each year from medical errors that occur in hospitals.

Other caregivers must be able to read and understand all prior documentation. Misspelled words and incorrect grammar create a negative impression, as does illegible handwriting. Caregivers should remember to use appropriate and correct capitalization, punctuation, and spelling. Careless documentation could imply carelessness or haste in the delivery of care.

Timely Documentation

The behavioral health record is a legal record. For it to be admissible in legal proceedings, documentation must specify when the encounter or event occurred. Charting that is not timely or is done in advance can lead to serious errors in patient care such as patient medication administration errors. Ongoing chronological entries should be made in behavioral healthcare records. All entries should be entered as soon as possible after the observation or encounter and never before the encounter. Memory recall is most accurate immediately after an encounter.

Timeliness is an area of focus for many accrediting and licensing agencies. Charting in advance compromises the credibility of the entire chart and of the staff member who made the entry. For example, the RN documents in advance that the client's 8:00 p.m. dose of Risperdal was given. However, the client attempts suicide at 7:00 p.m. and is admitted to the intensive care unit at the acute care hospital at 7:30 p.m. Because nurse documented the dose of Risperdal in advance, the credibility of the entire healthcare record is in jeopardy.

The date (month, day, and year) and time must be noted for each entry. Narrative documentation should reflect the actual time the entry was made. It is important to document when information was charted for continuity of care as well as to support the timely care and treatment of patients. It is unethical and against the law to pre- or backdate an entry. A sample policy on timeliness of medical record documentation is provided in figure 1.4.

In a computer-based health record system or a digital dictation system, an electronic time and date stamp is automatically put on documentation when created or saved.

When a client encounter entry is missed or not written in a timely manner, a late entry should be used to document it. A late entry is documented using the following steps:

1. Identify the new entry as a late entry.

2. Note the date and time of the current documentation as well as the actual date and time of occurrence.

3. Document late entries as soon as possible after the omission is discovered.

4. Note the circumstances of omission, if relevant.

5. Verify the signature of the author.

As more time passes, the reliability and validity of a late entry become more questionable; caregivers should avoid late entries as much as possible by using personal processes such as notes or reminders (Dougherty 2002b). Late entries should be avoided after an incident or occurrence to avoid the appearance of defensive documentation.

Continuous Documentation

When using paper-based progress notes, entries should be made on the next available line or space with no blank lines between notes, just as there should be no blank spaces before or after authenticating signatures. Drawing a single line through the balance of a blank line limits the possibility of changes being made to the documentation after the fact. All lines should be completed on a page before a new page is started. Blank lines imply that someone forgot to document (Dougherty 2002b). All blank lines on forms should be completed, or a field that is not applicable should contain some entry to that effect (for example, "not applicable or "N/A") to show that the field was reviewed. Blank fields or lines could suggest tampering. A staff member could insert an entry that puts the sequence of events into question.

Figure 1.4. Policy on timeliness of medical record documentation

---

TIMELINESS OF MEDICAL RECORD DOCUMENTATION

Purpose

To ensure timely and complete medical record documentation as it occurs. To support ongoing quality client care and to meet the regulatory requirements of accrediting agencies. To meet the documentation requirements for reimbursement by third-party payers and reduce risk to the client and the facility.

Policy

All medical record entries shall be written or entered as soon as possible after the encounter or observation, and never before the encounter. Medical record for the following documentation will be written or entered within the time frames as stated in federal and state regulations, accreditation agencies, and third-party payer requirements:

- The history and physical must be completed within 24 hours of admission.
- The psychiatric assessment will be completed within 60 hours of admission.
- The nursing assessment will be completed within 24 hours of admission.
- The provisional diagnosis shall be recorded in the medical record within 3 days of admission.
- The treatment plan will be completed within 7 days of admission.
- Informed consents for neuroleptic medication and invasive procedures will be obtained and signed prior to the dispensing of the medication or performance of the procedure except in emergencies.
- Progress notes must be entered at least daily for the first 30 days and at least weekly after that. Progress notes must include the name and credentials of the individual making the entry, the department/service of the individual making the entry, and the individual's signature. Progress notes must include month, day, year, and time for each entry.
- The entire medical record, including signatures, must be completed within 30 days of discharge.

Date Established:

Date of Last Review:

Date of Last Revision:

Approved By and Date:

Truthful Documentation

An error in documentation should never be erased, obliterated, or covered with ink or correction fluid. Such practices cast doubt on the chart's accuracy and damage the credibility of the staff member who made the erasure. The author of the original documentation may make corrections by drawing a single line through the original entry. He or she then should date and sign the edit, and state the reason for the change in the margin or above the note. (See figure 1.5 for a sample policy on this issue.)

When correcting an error in a computerized record system, the original entry should remain viewable, the date and time the correction was made should be recorded, the person making the correction should be identified, and the reason for the error should be documented. The functionality of making an addendum depends on the EHR system used. Some systems allow for making an addendum that is linked to the original documentation; others do not.

An addendum or clarification note may be needed to address a specific entry or to avoid misinterpretation of information previously documented. Such an addendum or note should document the current date and time, prominently indicate "addendum" or "clarification," and state the reason for the additional entry, referring back to the original entry as necessary. Addenda or clarification notes should be completed as soon as they are deemed necessary. Otherwise, the passage of time brings into question the reliability of the additional entry.

Integrity of the Information

The HIPAA security rule defines integrity as the property that data or information has not been altered or destroyed in an unauthorized manner. The organization must secure the record to

Figure 1.5. Staff process for corrections to client record entries

<table>
<tr><td colspan="2">**STAFF PROCESS FOR CORRECTIONS TO CLIENT RECORD ENTRIES**</td></tr>
<tr><td colspan="2">**PURPOSE**
The client record is a legal document and, as such, guidelines are needed to ensure the record's originality and provide means for corrections to the paper-based record.</td></tr>
<tr><td colspan="2">**POLICY**
The Center has established procedures for making corrections to the client record. These procedures have been established for the legal protection of the Center and staff and are the **ONLY** acceptable way to make such changes. It must be clear that no part of the original record can be erased, obliterated, torn out, or otherwise deleted or altered.</td></tr>
<tr><td colspan="2">**PROCEDURE**
1. The same person who made the original entry must make all corrections.
2. The procedure for correcting an error is as follows: Draw a single line through the incorrect word or phrase. (Under no circumstances is correction fluid to be used, nor the error erased or obliterated.)
    a. Write "error" beside or above the mistake.
    b. Make the correction.
    c. State the reason for the change.
    d. Sign and date the correction.</td></tr>
<tr><td colspan="2">Date Established:</td></tr>
<tr><td colspan="2">Date of Last Review:</td></tr>
<tr><td colspan="2">Date of Last Revision:</td></tr>
<tr><td colspan="2">Approved by and Date:</td></tr>
</table>

prevent destruction, improper alteration, or unauthorized use. (See chapter 9 for more information on security.) Policies and procedures should be in place to address all aspects of data integrity, specifying implementation mechanisms such as unique user identification, automatic log-off, and data backup and storage.

Verbal Orders

For verbal orders, the Medicare *Conditions of Participation for Hospitals,* Nursing Services, Paragraph 482.23 (c)(2), require that all orders for drugs and biologicals be in writing and signed by the practitioner(s) responsible for the care of the patient as specified under 482.12(c). When telephone or verbal orders must be used, they must be accepted only by personnel authorized to do so by the medical staff policies and procedures, consistent with federal and state law, and signed or initialed by the prescribing practitioner as soon as possible and used infrequently.

Further, each verbal order must be dated and identified by the name of the individual who gave it and the individual who received it, and the record must document who implemented it.

If the state in which the organization is located requires authentication of verbal orders within a specific time frame, accrediting and licensing agencies will survey for compliance with that requirement. The state licensing authority (usually the state health department's division of healthcare licensure) should be contacted for specific requirements. Fourteen to thirty days is the generally accepted time frame and should be specified in the organization's policy and procedure.

A Documentation Methodology: SOAP

Traditional progress notes frequently contain a combination of facts and opinions without delineating which is which. As a result, opinions are apt to be interpreted as proven facts. Recording only factual observations solves the problem but leaves the reader without the valuable interpretation of those facts by an on-the-spot person.

The problem-oriented healthcare documentation method, also known as the Subjective–Objective–Analysis–Plan, or **SOAP,** allows the inclusion of both objective and subjective data and the documenter's assessment of those data. In addition, the system actually encourages the development of responses to observations and assessments.

The *S* refers to subjective information. This includes statements made by the client or family such as descriptions of the client's symptoms or history and opinions concerning how the client is doing. Using direct quotations can be helpful so that other staff members can have a clear idea of what the client is saying. Moreover, this is the place to record hearsay evidence or hunches reported by others. If there are no subjective data in the report, the *S* should be eliminated or "none" should be written after it.

The *O* refers to objective material or measurable data. This includes factual observations made by the writer about events or client behavior. It also may include the results of psychological or medical tests and physical examination findings. Again, if there are no objective data, either the *O* should be eliminated or "none" should be written after the *O*.

The *A* refers to the author's analysis of the subjective and objective data combined. It can consist of opinions or impressions. If the author is unable to offer an assessment, he or she might write "none at this time" or "need more information before assessing."

Finally, the *P* is the treatment plan. This may include therapeutic interventions or patient education. The plan should be in sufficient detail to allow another care provider to follow it to completion. No further specific format for documentation is recommended and depends on the provider and the setting.

There are several variations of SOAP, including SOAPER with *E* for expectations and *R* for results. The DAP methodology (data, assessment, plan) also is used in behavioral healthcare. For practical examples of all of these documentation methodologies, see figures 1.6, 1.7, and 1.8.

Figure 1.6. Example of SOAP documentation methodology

S: The client's roommate reports concern that the client's voice is slurred and she seems to be very sleepy.

O: This staff member talked to the client in her room and confirmed that the client's speech does seem to be slurred. Explained my concern with her slurred speech. Questioned whether she had been using any alcohol or chemicals or meds other than those prescribed. At first, she denies, but after being asked several times admits that during an outing to the mall on December 22, she had a fake prescription filled for Xanax. The client admits to taking three Xanax pills earlier in the day.

A: Slurred speech. Probable ingestion of contraband Xanax pills. Blood pressure, 146/90; pulse, 96; respirations, 16; temperature, 99.6. Pupils equal and reactive.

P: Order obtained from Dr. Smith to do a urine drug screen with vital signs to be taken every two hours. Order obtained for a room search.

Figure 1.7. Example of SOAPER documentation methodology

S: Client states he is doing well and is ready to be discharged.
O: Met with client. Attention improved. No pressured speech. Client complains of dry mouth. Denies self-injurious ideation.
A: Bipolar.
P: Continue current meds. Sugarless candy given to improve dry mouth.
E: Client to continue with current meds and treatment plan.
R: No significant side effects. Previous complaints of lip smacking and stuttering are resolved.

Figure 1.8. Example of DAP documentation methodology

D: Client had complained of memory loss and dry mouth. He feels he is on too much medication. Client does believe he is bipolar. Client has demonstrated social interactions without becoming suspicious. Olanzapine and depakote levels drawn.
A: Client has demonstrated progress on all goals.
P: Notify Dr. Smith when lab results received. Encourage group attendance and interaction.

Internal Policies and Procedures

Policies provide guidance for staff and procedures operationalize policies. Policies and procedures should be the starting point for an ongoing monitoring system to ensure compliance. Policies need to be measurable, concise, and practical and need to define responsibilities. If staff members who need to comply with the policy do not understand what it means or how to handle hypothetical situations based on it, the policy should be clarified. Procedures need to be comprehensive. When writing procedures, a list or flowchart might be useful in detailing the steps to be completed. All supporting documents, such as forms, should be included along with the policy. Additionally, the latest version of policies and procedures should be made readily available to staff.

Policies and procedures that address documentation in the client's behavioral healthcare record and are based on all federal and state statutes and regulations, accrediting body standards, professional practice standards, and third-party payer requirements are essential. Internal policies and procedures and the training to properly disseminate them should be considered the cornerstone of good documentation practice.

The following activities should be taken when researching regulations and standards for the development of documentation policies and procedures:

- Applicable federal regulations should be researched. If the organization is not governed by federal law, accreditation standards, state regulations, and professional practice standards should be used.

- If the organization is accredited by a third party such as the JCAHO, CARF, or COA, applicable standards pertaining to documentation should be researched. Even if the organization is not accredited, standards can provide a good foundation for establishing policies and procedures.

- All applicable state statutes should be searched to determine if any state regulations govern the practice setting. Some states have regulations by practice setting or organization licensure (Smith 2001).

Policies and procedures should be reviewed at least annually but updated more frequently, as needed, to reflect changes in regulations, standards, or other requirements. In addition, HIM professionals should use their networking opportunities to share policies and procedures.

Documentation Review

A concurrent review process should be established to identify and promote improved documentation. "Staff need to be aware of the importance of documentation and they also need to be involved in the regular review and evaluation of the patient's medical record" (Wilson 1998, 797). Having professional and other staff members who document in the record creates an awareness of real-life issues and can serve as an opportunity to increase awareness and education on proper documentation.

The behavioral health record also should be reviewed to see whether:

- Information is recorded in an objective factual manner.

- The record contains complaints or other undesirable comments regarding the patient, family, physician, or staff.

- The record is legible.

The health record review should evaluate the presence, timeliness, completeness, and accuracy of documentation on an ongoing basis. The following steps describe the overall approach in a good record review process:

1. Gather a multidisciplinary review team to perform the reviews.

2. Use a sample size of approximately five percent of the organization's average monthly discharges.

3. Include a sample of both inpatient and outpatient health records from all treatment settings within the organization.

4. Perform reviews on a monthly basis.

5. Report the results of the review to the necessary committees.

6. Display supporting data in a visual or graphic format, making them easy to comprehend.

7. After reviewing the findings, develop a corrective action plan that includes recommendations for corrective action for all documentation deficiencies.

8. Present the corrective action plan to individual departments or individuals, specifying what actions are expected (Pinder 2003).

Education and Training

Staff education is critical to a successful documentation process. Educational opportunities include new employee orientation, annual mandatory training, and continuing education opportunities. The HIM manager should develop education programs that stress the importance of documentation in client care and increase sensitivity to the risk of poor documentation. A comprehensive education program should be targeted toward direct-care staff, including physicians, and should cover issues from proper documentation to the development of policies and procedures. If the organization has identified a problem area, mandatory education may be necessary to train employees in specific areas of documentation.

In an effective education program, the presentations are useful, informative, and entertaining. Education programs uniquely designed for specific target audiences also should be considered. Because of budget constraints, it may not be possible to do in-person training in a classroom setting, in which case computer-based training may be an alternative. A **train-the-trainer** program provides trainers with the skills, knowledge, and materials to train staff who work in various areas of the organization or on different shifts. Sample topics to include in documentation training include (Burt 2000):

-   Examples of less-than-desirable documentation

-   The purpose of the medical record

-   Basic guidelines for good documentation

-   Specific requirements for progress note documentation

-   The DOs and DON'Ts of daily charting

-   **Case studies** in documentation

Educational objectives for a documentation training session may include the following (Burt 2000):

-   Participants should be able to describe their responsibility for documentation in the medical record.

- Participants should be able to discuss the importance of proper documentation.

- Participants should be able to state the general guidelines to follow when making entries into the medical record.

The results of the documentation review should be used to determine what, if any, areas of documentation education need to be focused on. The documentation review process also is a good way to review the success of the training program.

Conclusion

Documentation is a critical component of the HIM profession. The need for HIM professionals working in the behavioral healthcare setting to have a thorough knowledge and understanding of documentation law, rules, regulations, standards, and best practices is crucial to the operation of the behavioral healthcare organization.

Various groups and different attempts at legislation have promulgated documentation standards for the healthcare industry as a whole. In addition, the industry recognizes myriad characteristics associated with good documentation procedures. Every type of healthcare organization should implement a formal documentation review process and establish policies and procedures to follow as well as offer education and training on the importance of accurate documentation to their employees.

References and Bibliography

Amatayakul, Margret. 2003. Practical advice for effective policies, procedures. *Journal of the American Health Information Management Association* 74(4):16A–D.

Burt, Jill H. 2000. *Behavioral Health Risk Management Program.* Duluth, MN: College of St. Scholastica.

Central State Hospital, Georgia. Documentation and professionalism article. Accessed on-line at http://centralstatehospital.org/HIMD%20forms/gooddocu.pdf.

Code of Federal Regulations. 2001. Title 42, Volume 3, Chapter IV, 42CFR482.60. Centers for Medicare and Medicaid Services. *Conditions of Participation for Hospitals: Special provisions applying to psychiatric hospitals.* U.S. Government Printing Office, 42CFR 482.

Commission on Accreditation of Rehabilitation Facilities. 2002. www.carf.org.

Council on Accreditation. 2003. www.coa.org.

Dougherty, Michelle. 2002a. It's time to finalize your privacy policies. *Journal of the American Health Information Management Association* 73(10):61–64.

Dougherty, Michelle. 2002b. Practice Brief: Maintaining a legally sound health record. *Journal of the American Health Information Management Association* 73(8):64A–G.

Dougherty, Michelle. 2001. AHIMA Practice Brief: Verbal/telephone order authentication and time frames. *Journal of the American Health Information Management Association* 72(2):72A–T.

Fletcher, Donna M. 1999. Practice Brief: Best practices in medical record documentation and completion. Available on-line at http://library.ahima.org.

Glondys, Barbara. 2003. Practice Brief: Ensuring legibility of patient records. *Journal of the American Health Information Management Association* 74(5):64A–D.

Health Care Financing Administration, Department of Health and Human Services. 2003 (February 20). Health Insurance Reform: Security Standards; Final Rule. 45 CFR Parts 160, 162, and 164. *Federal Register* 67, no 157. Available on-line at http://www.hhs.gov/ocr/hipaa.

Health Care Financing Administration, Department of Health and Human Services. 2002 (August 14). Standards for Privacy of Individually Identifiable Health Information; Final Rule. 45 CFR Parts 160 and 164. *Federal Register* 68, no 34. Available on-line at http://www.hhs.gov/ocr/hipaa.

Hughes, Gwen. 2002. Practice Brief: Laws and regulations governing the disclosure of health information. Accessed on-line at http://library.ahima.org/xpedio/groups/public/documents/ahima/pub_bok1_016464.html.

Hughes, Gwen. 2001. Patient access and amendment to health records. *Journal of the American Health Information Management Association* 72(5):64S–V.

Institute of Medicine, Committee on Quality of Health Care in America. 2000. *To Err Is Human: Building a Safer Health System,* ed. L. Kohn, J. Corrigan, and M. Donaldson. Washington, DC: National Academies Press.

Joint Commission on Accreditation of Healthcare Organizations. 2003. *2004 Comprehensive Accreditation Manual for Behavioral Health Care Organizations.* Oakbrook Terrace, IL: JCAHO.

Joint Commission on Accreditation of Healthcare Organizations. 2003. *2004 Hospital Accreditation Standards.* Oakbrook Terrace, IL: JCAHO.

LaTour, Kathleen, and Shirley Eichenwald, eds. 2002. *Health Information Management.* Chicago: American Health Information Management Association.

National Committee for Quality Assurance. 2003. www.ncqa.org.

Nelson, Mary, and Shari Aman. 2002. The pursuit of excellence in medical record reviews. *Journal of the American Health Information Management Association* 73(6):45–50.

North Carolina Medical Board. 2003. Position Statement: Medical record documentation. Accessed on-line at http://www.ncmedboard.org/.

Nursing World Reading Room. 1991. Position Statement: Nursing and the patient self-determination act. Accessed on-line at http://nursingworld.org/readroom/position/ethics/etsdet.htm.

Pinder, Ray. 2003. Record reviews: Clinician education form best defense. *Journal of the American Health Information Management Association* 74(4):25.

Schott, Sharon. 2003. How poor documentation does damage in the courtroom. *Journal of the American Health Information Management Association* 74(4):20–24.

Smith, Cheryl M. 2001. Practice Brief: Documentation requirements for the acute care inpatient record. *Journal of the American Health Information Management Association* 72(3):56A–G.

St. Anthony Publishing. 2001. *Coding and Payment Guide for Behavioral Health Services.* Eden Prairie, MN: St. Anthony Publishing.

Teich, C. 1998. Risk management in the psychiatric setting. In *The Risk Manager's Desk Reference,* 2nd ed., ed. B. Youngberg, 328–39. Gaithersburg, MD: Aspen.

Thieleman, William. 2002. A patient-friendly approach to the record amendment process. *Journal of the American Health Information Management Association* 73(5):44–47.

Welch, Julie J. 2002. Practice Brief: Authentication of health record entries (updated): *Journal of the American Health Information Management Association.* Accessed on-line at http://library.ahima.org.

Wilson, J. 1998. Proactive risk management: Documentation of patient care. *British Journal of Nursing* 7(3):797–98.

Chapter 2

Content, Format, and Organization of the Health Record

Linda Cannon, RHIA

Unlike its counterpart in physical health documentation, behavioral health documentation does not have the benefit of a lab report, x-ray, or pathology report to substantiate the diagnosis and justify subsequent services rendered.

The substantiation of the diagnosis and justification of type, level, and duration of services for behavioral health rests in the clear documentation of the observations, interventions performed, and the patient's response.

Ultimately, all of the following areas must match up to assure that documentation and reimbursement are appropriate:

1. Acceptable/Valid Diagnosis

2. Level of Service Code—Provider license/training meets criteria to provide that service

3. Documentation supports diagnosis, time spent, and level of service provided, including necessity

4. Billing documents completed by care providers who accept responsibility for correctness of diagnosis/service provided

5. Claim matches billing documents

6. Remittance advice matches claim and chart documentation

The patient record generally contains two types of data: clinical and administrative. *Clinical data* document the client's condition, diagnosis, and treatment as well as services provided. *Administrative data* include demographic and financial information as well as various consent and authorization forms related to the provision of care and the handling of confidential client information.

Following are examples of the minimum documentation requirements unique to the behavioral health inpatient setting as established by the Joint Commission on Accreditation of Healthcare Organizations (JCAHO) and federal regulations:

- Identification data

- Source of referral

- Reason for referral
- Client's legal status
- Client's rights
- Client education
- Advanced directive information
- All appropriate consents for admission, treatment, evaluation, and aftercare
- Admitting psychiatric diagnoses
- Psychiatric history
- Record of the complete patient assessment, including the complaints of others regarding the patient, as well as the patient's comments
- Medical history (table 2.1), report of physical examination (table 2.2), and record of all medications prescribed
- Provisional diagnoses based on assessment that includes other current diseases as well as psychiatric diagnoses
- Written individualized treatment plan
- Documentation of the course of treatment and all evaluations and examinations
- Multidisciplinary progress notes related to the goals and objectives outlined in the treatment plan
- Appropriate documentation related to special treatment procedures
- Updates to the treatment plan as a result of the assessments detailed in the progress notes
- Multidisciplinary case conferences and consultation notes, which include date of conference or consultation, recommendations made, and actions taken
- Information on any unusual occurrences such as treatment complications, accidents or injuries to the patient, death of the patient, and procedures that place the patient at risk or cause unusual pain
- Correspondence related to the patient, including all letters and dated notations of telephone conversations relevant to the patient's treatment
- Discharge or termination summary
- Plan for follow-up care and documentation of its implementation
- Individualized aftercare or posttreatment plan

This chapter distinguishes between documentation that is part of the health record and documentation that is not. It then specifies the components of the acute care psychiatric health record and discusses elements that are considered specialized health record content.

What Is Not Part of the Health Record

This book primarily discusses what is included in the health or patient record, but it also is important to document what is not normally considered part of the patient record. Additionally, it is important to consider individual state regulations because some states stipulate that any patient-specific record that relates to healthcare is part of the clinical record. Moreover, the concepts of discoverability and admissibility must be considered evidence of the patient record and other medical and administrative records in judicial proceedings.

Table 2.1. Information included in a complete medical history

Components of the History	Complaints and Symptoms
Chief complaint	Nature and duration of the symptoms that caused the client to seek medical attention as stated in his or her own words
Present illness	Detailed chronological description of the development of the client's illness, from the appearance of the first symptom to the present situation
Past medical history	Summary of childhood and adult illnesses and conditions, such as infectious diseases, pregnancies, allergies and drug sensitivities, accidents, operations, hospitalizations, and current medications
Social and personal history	Marital status; dietary, sleep, and exercise patterns; use of coffee, tobacco, alcohol, and other drugs; occupation; home environment; daily routine; and so on
Family medical history	Diseases among relatives in which heredity or contact might play a role, such as allergies, cancer, and infectious, psychiatric, metabolic, endocrine, cardiovascular, and renal diseases; health status or cause and age at death of immediate relatives
Review of systems	Systemic inventory designed to uncover current or past subjective symptoms that includes the following types of data: • General: Usual weight, recent weight changes, fever, weakness, fatigue • Skin: Rashes, eruptions, dryness, cyanosis, jaundice; changes in skin, hair, or nails • Head: Headache (duration, severity, character, location) • Eyes: Glasses or contact lenses, last eye examination, glaucoma, cataracts, eyestrain, pain, diplopia, redness, lacrimation, inflammation, blurring • Ears: Hearing, discharge, tinnitus, dizziness, pain • Nose: Head colds, epistaxis, discharges, obstruction, postnasal drip, sinus pain • Mouth and throat: Condition of teeth and gums, last dental examination, soreness, redness, hoarseness, difficulty in swallowing • Respiratory system: Chest pain, wheezing, cough, dyspnea, sputum (color and quantity), hemoptysis, asthma, bronchitis, emphysema, pneumonia, tuberculosis, pleurisy, last chest X ray • Neurological system: Fainting, blackouts, seizures, paralysis, tingling, tremors, memory loss • Musculoskeletal system: Joint pain or stiffness, arthritis, gout, backache, muscle pain, cramps, swelling, redness, limitation in motor activity • Cardiovascular system: Chest pain, rheumatic fever, tachycardia, palpitation, high blood pressure, edema, vertigo, faintness, varicose veins, thrombophlebitis • Gastrointestinal system: Appetite, thirst, nausea, vomiting, hematemesis, rectal bleeding, change in bowel habits, diarrhea, constipation, indigestion, food intolerance, flatus, hemorrhoids, jaundice • Urinary system: Frequent or painful urination, nocturia, pyuria, hematuria, incontinence, urinary infections • Genitoreproductive system: Male—venereal disease, sores, discharge from penis, hernias, testicular pain, or masses; female—age at menarche, frequency and duration of menstruation, dysmenorrhea, menorrhagia, symptoms of menopause, contraception, pregnancies, deliveries, abortions, last Pap smear • Endocrine system: Thyroid disease; heat or cold intolerance; excessive sweating, thirst, hunger, or urination • Hematologic system: Anemia, easy bruising or bleeding, past transfusions • Psychiatric disorders: Insomnia, headache, nightmares, personality disorders, anxiety disorders, mood disorders

Table 2.2.   Information documented in the physical examination report

Report Components	Content
General condition	Apparent state of health, signs of distress, posture, weight, height, skin color, dress and personal hygiene, facial expression, manner, mood, state of awareness, speech
Vital signs	Pulse, respiration, blood pressure, temperature
Skin	Color, vascularity, lesions, edema, moisture, temperature, texture, thickness, mobility and turgor, nails
Head	Hair, scalp, skull, face
Eyes	Visual acuity and fields; position and alignment of the eyes, eyebrows, eyelids; lacrimal apparatus; conjunctivae; sclerae; corneas; irises; size, shape, equality, reaction to light, and accommodation of pupils; extraocular movements; ophthalmoscopic exam
Ears	Auricles, canals, tympanic membranes, hearing, discharge
Nose and sinuses	Airways, mucosa, septum, sinus tenderness, discharge, bleeding, smell
Mouth	Breath, lips, teeth, gums, tongue, salivary ducts
Throat	Tonsils, pharynx, palate, uvula, postnasal drip
Neck	Stiffness, thyroid, trachea, vessels, lymph nodes, salivary glands
Thorax, anterior and posterior	Shape, symmetry, respiration
Breasts	Masses, tenderness, discharge from nipples
Lungs	Fremitus, breath sounds, adventitious sounds, friction, spoken voice, whispered voice
Heart	Location and quality of apical impulse, trill, pulsation, rhythm, sounds, murmurs, friction rub, jugular venous pressure and pulse, carotid artery pulse
Abdomen	Contour, peristalsis, scars, rigidity, tenderness, spasm, masses, fluid, hernia, bowel sounds and bruits, palpable organs
Male genitourinary organs	Scars, lesions, discharge, penis, scrotum, epididymis, varicocele, hydrocele
Female reproductive organs uterus, adnexa	External genitalia, Skene's glands and Bartholin's glands, vagina, cervix,
Rectum	Fissure, fistula, hemorrhoids, sphincter tone, masses, prostate, seminal vesicles, feces
Musculoskeletal system	Spine and extremities, deformities, swelling, redness, tenderness, range of motion
Lymphatic	Palpable cervical, axillary, inguinal nodes; location; size; consistency; mobility; tenderness
Blood vessels	Pulses, color, temperature, vessel walls, veins
Neurological system	Cranial nerves, coordination, reflexes, biceps, triceps, patellar, Achilles, abdominal, cremasteric, Babinski, Romberg, gait, sensory, vibratory
Diagnosis(es):	

In many cases, some administrative and business records include information that is so closely related to patient health information that it is frequently considered for inclusion in the clinical record. Included among the items that are often discussed in this regard are incident reports, financial information, peer review records, photographs/videotapes, psychiatric testing, and other miscellaneous records.

When deciding what is and is not to be filed as part of the patient record, the following should be considered:

- Record content standards (internal and external)

- Laws regarding discoverability of medical records

- Laws regarding discoverability of business and administrative records

- Uses and users of the medical record

- Duplication of data

Records from other organizations on which care has been based should be kept in, but not considered part of, the designated record set.

Incident Reports

An **incident report** is a tool used to collect data and information about a potentially compensable event. An event is any occurrence that is inconsistent with the normal operation of the program or a situation that has risk management implications. Incident reports can be used to:

- Notify administration and medical staff that an incident and/or a "near miss" has occurred

- Notify the health departments in some states of significant incidents

- Notify the organization's risk manager, attorney, and insurer that a possible **claim** may be filed

- Help in the postincident retrospective review to attempt to identify the root cause of the occurrence to prevent a repeat of the same or similar incident

Thus, an incident report is an administrative tool, not a clinical record. An incident report:

- Describes the condition of the subject (usually a patient, but could be a visitor or material object) before, during, and after the incident

- Describes the incident itself with as much objective, relevant detail as possible

- Includes relevant statements or observations by witnesses to the incident

- Describes the corrective action(s) taken (Bryant 1992, 16)

Because an incident report contains information that could potentially compromise the treatment program should litigation occur, it is generally considered inappropriate to file one in the patient record or even state in the patient record that one has been completed.

Two schools of thought prevail with regard to protecting incident reports from discovery: the doctrine of attorney–client privilege and the attorney's work product rule. However, it is becoming more and more difficult to win this argument during litigation proceedings. To minimize the potential for discovery, treatment programs should:

- Never file the incident report in the patient record. The reasoning for this is that patients may view their own record and/or ask for copies of it. Also, to qualify under attorney–patient privilege, only a limited number of individuals within a treatment program should have access to the report.

- The form itself should clearly state that it is not part of the medical record.

- The medical record should not reflect that an incident report has been completed. Stating that an incident report has been completed is a red flag for the plaintiff's attorneys alerting them that a document exists with information that could compromise the program. The medical record should reflect the events and not that an incident report was completed.

- Incident report content should be limited to facts. An objective narrative that focuses on just the facts without making assumptions or placing blame on the program or one of its employees is critical. All clinically relevant information must be included (for example, "Noted at 10 p.m. that 100mg Haldol administered. 10 mg ordered").

- To ensure that incident reports are not included or referred to in the patient record, a routine record review should be done for this item.

Billing and Financial Information

To be reimbursed, services rendered must be reasonable and necessary for the diagnosis or treatment of an illness. **Clinicians** are required to record in the patient record pertinent facts, findings, observations about the patient's health history (including past and present illnesses), examinations, tests, treatments, and outcomes.

All information submitted for payment must be legible and document the following information for each date of service:

- The billed services have been rendered.

- The services were appropriate for the client's condition.

- The services meet reasonable standards for medical care.

- For some payment sources, each entry must be able to stand alone. The record must indicate that the client has a psychiatric illness or demonstrates emotional or behavioral symptoms sufficient enough to intervene with normal functioning. In addition, it must include the time spent in the psychotherapy encounter and show that cognitive skills such as behavioral modification, insight and supportive interactions, and discussion of reality were applied to produce therapeutic change. For interactive psychotherapy, the medical record also must indicate that the client does not have the ability to interact through normal verbal communication means (for instance, art therapy or family therapy).

Bills and client account records are administrative in nature and thus rarely are combined into the medical record because of their different purpose, uses, and users. However, they may be considered part of the "designated record set" as defined by the Health Insurance Portability and Accountability Act (HIPAA), albeit stored separately.

Financial information collected from the client (usually upon admission to the program) is appropriate for inclusion in the medical record. Traditionally, financial information includes:

- Expected payer(s)

- Insured's name

- Insured's gender

- Client's relationship to insured

- Employment data and insurance numbers

Peer Review Worksheets, Reports, and Records

In the event of a lawsuit, the admissibility and discoverability of peer review records is similar to that of incident reports. To encourage open participation in peer review activities, these activities must be protected from discovery by litigants or from being admitted into evidence. Unfortunately, although many states do prevent discovery of peer review materials, not all courts apply the discovery rules the same and the protection of this information is often challenged. Normally, peer review minutes are kept in medical staff or administrative offices never to be included in the medical record.

Utilization review (UR) worksheets are case specific, and the argument is sometimes made that they could be filed in the client's record. However, like peer review minutes, UR worksheets are generated through staff peer review functions and should not be kept in the medical record.

Photography, Videotaping, and Other Imaging

The **American Health Information Management Association** (AHIMA) recommends in its professional practice brief published in 1999 on patient photography, videotaping, and other imaging that, although patient imaging is fairly common today, liability issues need to be considered and federal regulations observed.

The first step in developing policies with regard to photography, videotaping, and other imaging is to inventory the types and locations in which client photography might be done. Each provider then must determine under what circumstances it will allow clients to be photographed and the requirements of the client consent.

Whether to retain images as part of the client record or for non-client-specific purposes is a treatment program-specific policy decision. In making the decision, the first step is to develop a comprehensive policy describing the purpose of the material. After the purpose has been defined, policies and procedures must address client consent, storage, retention and release issues, and the HIPAA-mandated notice of information practices. The consent for treatment should include a statement about patient photography if it is done routinely at the organization. Programs also should obtain a signed confidentiality commitment from anyone conducting the filming or videotaping. Programs that serve the chronically mentally ill sometimes must resort to the retention of photographs in the archival medical record to positively identify clients upon readmission who are unable or unwilling to identify themselves and carry no identification or who are elopement risks.

Non-Client-Identifiable Photographs and Videotapes

Sometimes clients are photographed or videotaped for purposes of educating healthcare workers or for research or publicity. Although these documents generally are not client identifiable, the consent of the client still should be obtained. The following issues must be considered:

- Authorization: A written authorization, signed and dated by the client or legal representative, should be obtained. The signatures should be witnessed, and the witnesses' signatures should be included on the authorization form. The authorization should detail the reason for the videotape or photograph and include a clause whereby the client waives his or her future right to access the document. The written authorization form should be filed in the medical record.

- Storage: Photographs and videotapes that are not kept as part of the client record are usually stored in the program's library, audiovisual department, or the department in which they were generated. If not retained in the client record, the photograph should be cross-referenced to the client record. All images should be identified with the client's name, identification number, and the date the image was made. All images should be stored in a manner that ensures timely retrieval when requested.

- Retention: Programs that create photographs or videotapes and make them part of the client record should consult their specific state regulations regarding retention laws. In the absence of a specific law in this regard, images should be retained in the same period of time specified for other health information. Policies and procedures must make clear whether they can be destroyed when no longer needed.

- Release: Due to confidentiality concerns, the use of videotapes and photographs should be closely monitored.

Client-Identifiable Photographs and Videotapes

Clients may be photographed for purposes of identification, healthcare worker education, or research. The following issues must be considered:

- Authorization: A written authorization signed by the client or his or her legal representative should be obtained. The authorization should explain in detail the reason for the photographing or videotaping.

- Disclosure: The photograph or videotape must be made available to the client and/or his or her representative upon request.

Laboratory Test Requisitions

It is unnecessary to retain requisitions for laboratory tests and temporary results. Retaining the complete physician orders and final results for diagnostic tests is sufficient. The retention of extraneous and duplicative reports that do not add to pertinent data only adds bulk to the record and serves no purpose after the final documentation is received.

Correspondence

Requests and authorizations for release of information are usually kept in an administrative section of the client record. Although not required, it is the most practical and convenient way to retain this information. In general, correspondence is not included when responding to requests for client information because it is not considered part of the legal health record (LHR).

Psychological Assessment and Measurement Materials: Test Data

Test data refer to raw and scaled scores, client/patient responses to test questions or stimuli, and psychologists' notes and recordings concerning client/patient statements and behavior during an examination.

Psychologists sometimes disclose test data pursuant to a client release or, in the absence of a client release, do not disclose test data unless legally mandated to do so. They have the discretion to withhold test data "to protect a client or others from substantial harm or misuse or misrepresentation of the data or the test." Psychologists are charged with using their professional judgment and discretion in determining whether to release the information. (See the American Psychological Association Ethics Code, section 9.04, for further details on the release of test data and section 9.11 on maintaining test security.)

What Is Part of the Patient Record

The client's health record should contain administrative data, demographic and financial information, and clinical data. These parts of the health record are discussed in the following subsections.

Administrative Data

The first page of any health record contains the client's demographic and financial information as well as the reasons he or she is seeking treatment. Typically, a clerk asks the client or his or her representative for the administrative information needed to complete the admissions form.

Today, most healthcare organizations collect admissions information via computer-based systems. When clients return to the same facility, the admissions process is expedited because they often only need to confirm that their information has not changed. For healthcare organizations dependent on a paper-based health record system, a printout of the admissions information is placed in the health record. In both paper- and computer-based health record systems, the admissions information becomes a permanent part of the client's record. Admissions information may be referred to as a face sheet, a registration sheet, or a registration form.

Demographic and Financial Information

Demographics is the study of the statistical characteristics of human populations. Healthcare **demographic information** includes the client's:

- Full name
- Identification number or **health record number** assigned by the healthcare facility
- Address
- Date of birth
- Place of birth
- Gender
- Race or ethnic origin
- Marital status
- Next of kin's name and address

In addition, the demographic information includes date and time the patient is admitted; type of admission (inpatient or outpatient); and healthcare organization's name, address, and telephone number.

The financial information maintained in the health record is limited to insurance information collected from the patient at the time of admission. Insurance information includes:

- Name of the expected payer
- Name of the policyholder (or insured)
- Gender of the policyholder
- Patient's relationship to the policyholder
- Policyholder's employer
- Individual and group insurance policy numbers
- Patient's Social Security number

A uniform minimum data set is a minimum set of informational items that have uniform definitions and predefined categories. Uniform minimum data sets are designed to meet the essential information needs of multiple users in the healthcare system. The framework adopted to guide development of the data set for most services is based on the U.S. Department of Health and Human Services concept of a uniform minimum data set. The uniform minimum data set will not necessarily meet the total needs of any one organization or limit additional data collection by an organization to meet its specific information needs. It addresses data documentation and collection at both the organizational and individual patient levels (Abraham 2001, 3).

Clinical Data

The patient's attending or primary physician/clinician usually gives the healthcare organization preliminary information about the patient before the patient is admitted for treatment. Such information includes an admitting or working diagnosis that identifies the condition or illness for which the patient needs care. The information is recorded on the face sheet, which, as mentioned above, also includes the patient's demographic and financial data.

The following types of clinical data are documented in the medical record during the patient's hospital stay:

- Patient's medical history
- Report of the patient's initial physical examination
- Attending physician's/clinician's diagnostic and therapeutic orders
- Care plan
- Clinical observations of the providers who care for the patient
- Reports and results of every diagnostic and therapeutic procedure performed
- Reports of consulting physicians
- Reports of other members of treatment team
- Patient's discharge summary
- Final instructions to the patient upon discharge
- After-care plan

Content and Structure of the Acute Psychiatric Care Health Record

The acute psychiatric care health record contains a number of assessments and reports pertaining to the patient's treatment. Table 2.3 provides a summary of the basic components of an acute psychiatric care health record, and figure 2.1 shows a sample table of contents for an acute psychiatric care health record.

Psychiatric Assessment

This assessment identifies the client's physical, cognitive, behavioral, emotional and social status. It also identifies facilitating factors and possible barriers that prevent the patient from reaching his or her goals beyond the presenting problems. (See figure 2.2 for items to be included in the psychiatric assessment.)

Table 2.3. Basic components of the acute psychiatric care health record

Component	Function
Registration record	Documents demographic information about the client
Medical history	Documents the client's current and past health status
Physical examination	Contains the provider's findings based on an examination of the client
Clinical observations	Provide a chronological summary of the client's illness and treatment as documented by physicians, nurses, and allied health professionals
Physician's orders	Document the physician's instructions to other parties involved in providing the client's care, including orders for medications and diagnostic and therapeutic procedures
Reports of diagnostic and therapeutic procedures	Describe the procedures performed and give the names of clinicians and other providers; include the findings of X rays, mammograms, ultrasounds, scans, laboratory tests, and other diagnostic procedures
Consultation reports	Document opinions about a client's condition furnished by providers other than the attending physician
Discharge summary	Concisely summarizes the client's stay in the hospital
Client instructions	Document the instructions for follow-up care that the provider gives to the client or the client's caregiver
Consents, authorizations, and acknowledgments	Document the client's agreement to undergo treatment or services, permission to release confidential information, or recognition that information has been received
Care plan	Documents the specific goals in the treatment of an individual patient, amending the goals as the patient's condition requires, and assessing the outcomes of care
Assessment	

Medical and Psychiatric History

A complete history documents the client's current complaints and symptoms and lists his or her past medical, personal, and family history.

Physical Examination Report

The physical examination report represents the attending physician's assessment of the patient's current health status. This report should document information on all of the patient's major organ systems.

Mental Status Exam

The mental status exam is as crucial to psychiatry as the physical exam is to other areas of medicine. Adolf Meyer developed the mental status exam in 1918. He felt that it was important to ask the same questions of every patient so that certain standards could be achieved. The exam describes various mental functions, including appearance, speech, thought process, behavior, affect, orientation, memory, mood, motor skills, intellect, judgment, and insight.

Figure 2.1.   Sample table of contents for an acute psychiatric care health record

Inpatient Care
MEDICAL RECORDS TABLE OF CONTENTS

ADMISSION DATA

Episode Face Sheet
Discharge/Aftercare Plan (pp. 1 and 2)
   * Emergency unit discharge/aftercare plan
   * Disposition of client's personal medication
   * Discharge summary

ASSESSMENT

Psychiatric Assessment
   * Progress notes
Psychiatric Assessment Addendum
   * Mini mental status exam (abbreviated)
Emergency Unit Nursing Screening Assessment
Nursing Admission Assessment (pp. 1–3)
   * Pain assessment
   * Fall risk assessment
   * Violence risk assessment
Tuberculosis Clinical Assessment
History and Physical Examinations
   * Social work assessment
   * Activity therapy assessment/addendum
   * Nutritional assessment
   * Abnormal involuntary movement scale

TREATMENT PLAN

Treatment Plan
Treatment Plan Problem Sheet
   * Treatment plan update (narrative)

PROGRESS NOTES

Progress Notes
   * Individual/group education note
   * Transition team services

PHYSICIAN'S ORDERS

Emergency Unit Admission Order
Inpatient Admission Order
Physician's Order Form
Informed Consent for the Use of Psychotropic Medications
   (information and/or consent for antipsychotic medication)

LAB/CONSULT

   * Tests: Lab, X ray, and consultation
      * Lab results
      * Diagnostic testing (laboratory, EKG, X ray, EEG)
      * Infection control alert form
      * Tuberculosis suspect case report
      * Tuberculosis discharge care plan
      * Consent of HIV blood test
      * Consent for ECT
      * Medical consultation

NURSES' NOTES

Daily RN Assessment/Flow Sheet
   (nutritional supplements/somatic treatments/continuation)
Clinical Record
   * Intake and output record
   * Close observation record
   * Restraint or seclusion assessment
   * Restraint or seclusion flow sheet
   * Code blue response record (a and b)

Figure 2.1. (Continued)

MEDICATION AND TREATMENT	* Diabetic record Record of Routine Medication Record of PRN Medication PRN/STAT Medication

PATIENT'S RIGHTS	Consent for Involvement of Interested Party
	Patient Rights and Responsibilities (a and b)
	Patient's Rights Denial Monthly Tally (removed at time of discharge)
	   * Patient valuables and personal property record
	   * Patient valuables inventory
	   * Patient valuables deposit and/or withdrawal voucher
	   * Request by a patient for release
	   * Withdrawal of writ application
	   * Refusal of treatment

ADMISSION/LEGAL	* Application for voluntary emergency room treatment
	Request for Voluntary Admission or Involuntary Admission
	   * Ex parte order for evaluation or detention
	   * Ex parte petition for evaluation
	   * Order for psychiatric examination
	   * Transport sheet
	   * Application for 72-hour detention for evaluation
	   * Involuntary patient advisement
	   * Notice of certification
	   * Certification review hearing findings and order intensive treatment
	Petition of Treating Physician's/Treating Physician's Declaration Regarding Capacity to Consent or Refuse Antipsychotic Medication
	   * Recommendation for conservatorship of the person
	   * Declaration of the professional person re: conservatorship (exhibits A and B)
	   * Citation for conservatorship
	   * Ex parte petition for appointment of a temporary conservator and for conservator of the person
	   * Conservatorship investigation report
	   * Consent to admission and treatment
	   * Limitation of liability attachment to patient admission agreement
	   * Review committee electroconvulsive treatment
	   * Authorization to use/disclose patient protected health information
	   * Authorization and consent for photograph and publication
	An important message from Medicare
	Client financial information
	Advance directive notification form
	Waiver of responsibility
	   * Tarasoff report
	   * Mental health facilities report of firearms prohibition
	Patient Notification of Firearms Prohibition and Right to Hearing
	   * Medical care request

MISCELLANEOUS RECORDS	Correspondence Third-Party Information

*The forms with an asterisk (*) are not always included as part of the patient health record.

Figure 2.2.   Components of the psychiatric assessment

Component
Physical factors, including disabilities
Cognitive disorders
Behavioral disorders
Emotional disorders
Mental disorders
Communicative disorders
Social and environmental factors, including social status
Substance abuse, dependence, and other addictive behaviors
Developmental disabilities
Vision and hearing impairments and disabilities
Symptoms that may be associated with a disease, condition, or treatment

Diagnostic and Therapeutic Orders

Physician's orders are the instructions the physician gives to the other healthcare professionals who actually perform diagnostic tests and treatments, administer medications, and provide specific services to a patient. These orders must be written legibly and include the date and the physician's signature.

Standing orders are orders the medical staff or an individual physician has established as routine care for a specific diagnosis or procedure. Standing orders are commonly used in hospitals, **ambulatory surgery** facilities, and long-term care facilities. Usually standing orders are preprinted on a single sheet of paper. Like other physician's orders, they must be signed, dated, and filed in the patient's medical record.

Physicians may communicate orders verbally or via the telephone when the healthcare organization's policies and procedures or medical staff rules allow. State law and medical staff rules specify which practitioners are allowed to accept and execute verbal and telephone orders. How the orders are to be authenticated and the time period allowed for authentication also may be specified.

Restraint and Seclusion Orders

Specific documentation guidelines and procedures to follow with regard to the use of restraint and seclusion procedures vary by state. However, the guidelines to follow in these matters are those outlined in the JCAHO manual (JCAHO 2002):

> Restraint or seclusion use is limited to emergencies in which there is high risk of the client (patient) physically harming him/herself, staff, or others, and nonphysical interventions would not be effective. The client's family should be notified promptly of the initiation of restraint or seclusion. A licensed independent practitioner sees and evaluates the client in person. Written or verbal orders for initial and continuing use of restraint or seclusion are time-limited. Clinical leadership is informed of instances in which clients experience extended or multiple episodes of restraint or seclusion. Clients in restraints or in seclusion are assessed, assisted, monitored, regularly reevaluated. Restraint and seclusion use is discontinued when the client meets the behavior criteria for their discontinuation. Following the discontinuance of the restraint or seclusion the client and staff participate in a debriefing about the restraint or seclusion episode. Each episode of restraint use is documented in the client's medical record.
>
> The organization collects data on the use of restraint and seclusion in order to monitor and improve its performance of processes that involve risks or may result in sentinel events.
>
> Organization policy(ies) and procedure(s) address the prevention of the use of restraint and seclusion and, when employed, guide appropriate and safe use. Any use of restraint is initiated pursuant to either an individual order or an approved protocol.

Consultation Reports

Consultation reports document clinical opinions requested from physicians outside the case by the patient's primary or attending physician. They are based on the consulting physicians' examination of the client and a review of his or her health record.

Diagnostic and Therapeutic Procedure Reports

The results of all diagnostic and therapeutic procedures are permanently filed in the patient's medical record. Diagnostic procedures include laboratory tests performed on blood, urine, and other samples from the patient.

Mandated Reporting

Many states mandate that certain types of reports be completed and forwarded to the appropriate authorities. Examples of mandated reports include, but are not limited to:

- Abuse reports (domestic, child, and elder abuse)

- Tuberculosis

- HIV

- Sexually transmitted diseases

- Legal/police reports, including recommendation to revoke a driver's license.

- Duty-to-warn reports: Mental health professionals have a duty to warn reasonably identifiable victims when there are known serious threats of violence against them. Most states title these reports differently (for example, in California, the Tarasoff Report) (*Tarasoff v. Regents of the University of California* 1976).

- Firearms prohibition: According to California statutory law (California Code of Regulations 2004), mental health organizations are required to submit these reports to the state to prevent clients from owning, possessing, receiving, or purchasing any firearm for a period of five years from the date of admission to the organization. This prohibition applies to all persons taken into custody as a danger to themselves or others; other states may have similar regulations.

Treatment/Care Plans

Treatment or care plans are developed based on the patient's needs as identified via the assessments. Plans must specify the patient's goals and objectives as well as the actions or interventions needed to meet them and time frames in which to accomplish them. Patients are to be involved in the formulation of their plans and asked for input. They also are asked to agree to the planned course of treatment, care, or services. In many jurisdictions, patients are asked to sign the care plan to indicate that they agree with it and are aware of its contents.

In addition, a plan for a rehabilitation program describes the strategy for providing specific skills and supports that will enable the patient to function in an environment that optimizes independence and choice. As patients improve over time, they are transitioned to increasingly less restrictive environments and are integrated into community settings. Ideally, rehabilitation programs not only offer access to community resources but also include continued goal achievement and independence after the client is discharged from the formal program. (See figure 2.3 for items to be included in treatment/care plans.)

Organization staff members facilitate planned actions or interventions outlined in the plans in accordance with the authorized scope of practice, appropriate policies and procedures, and standards of practice. Family members or other caregivers may perform some interventions after having received appropriate education.

Figure 2.3.   Information included in treatment/care plan

Clients care needs
Strategy to provide services to meet client needs
Treatment goals and objectives
Actions or interventions to meet goals and objectives
Criteria for discontinuing specified interventions
Indication that client agrees to plan

Each state defines the person in that state who may act as a case manager. Case managers prepare assessments and care plans, which then are included in the client's health record.

Care plans are updated when clinically appropriate and when required by organizational policy, state guidelines, and clinical path protocols.

Treatment/care plans may be documented via:

- Handwritten notes

- Electronic records

- Standards of practice

- Decision algorithms

- Care paths or maps

- Individualized preprinted plans of care

Outpatient Crisis Plan

Because of the nature of their mental illness, clients often develop a crisis plan with their therapist. A crisis plan might be viewed in the same way that an advanced directive is viewed for individuals in an acute care setting. It is the client's direction on what to do and whom to contact should he or she become mentally incapable of communicating his or her wishes. The crisis plan does not supercede an advanced directive but, rather, complements it.

Psychotherapy Notes

The special confidentiality protections afforded psychotherapy notes under HIPAA require programs to handle them in a special manner. For this reason, organizations must be clear in their understanding of HIPAA's definition of what constitutes psychotherapy notes.

Psychotherapy notes are what the "field" has historically called process notes. They capture the therapist's impressions of the client obtained from conversations during private counseling sessions or group, joint, or family counseling sessions. The notes contain details considered inappropriate for inclusion in the medical record and are used by the provider for future sessions. Psychotherapy notes exclude medication, prescription, and monitoring information; counseling session start and stop times; the modalities and frequencies of treatment furnished; results of clinical tests; and any summary of diagnosis, functional status, treatment plan, symptoms, prognosis, and progress to date.

Generally speaking, in order to qualify as psychotherapy notes, the notes must contain extended direct quotations from both client and therapist. In addition, they must include repeated and systematic references to interpretive insights to the client's intrapsychic dynamics as discussed in the therapy sessions. Finally, the documentation in the notes must weave together the client's unresolved past conflicts or issues with current difficulties. Notes that do not meet these criteria are much better identified as counseling progress notes, which are meant to be useful to the entire treatment team as well as the client.

This distinction is important because psychotherapy notes may not be released unless specifically identified on an authorization form and only with the author's permission.

However, not all therapy documentation requires special handling. Some therapy documentation may be released with a valid authorization. Such documentation includes:

- Records of the prescription and monitoring of medication

- Counseling session start and stop times

- Modalities and frequency of treatment

- Results of clinical tests

- Any summary of the client's diagnoses, functional status, treatment plan, symptoms, prognosis, and progress to date

Progress Notes

In psychiatric settings, clinical observations are typically documented in **progress notes.** The purpose of documenting the clinical observations of physicians, nurses and other caregivers is to create a chronological report of the patient's condition and response to treatment during his or her course of treatment.

The rules and regulations of the healthcare organization specify which **healthcare providers** are allowed to enter progress notes into the health record. Typically, these individuals include the patient's attending physician, any consulting physicians who have medical staff privileges, house medical staff, nurses, nutritionists, social workers, and clinical therapists. Depending on the record format used by the hospital, each discipline maintains a separate section of the health record or all provider observations are combined in the same chronological or integrated health record.

Progress notes serve to justify further treatment in the facility. In addition, they document the appropriateness and coordination of the services provided. For Medicare purposes, each note must be able to stand alone and justify medical necessity.

Nurses keep chronological records of the patient's vital signs (blood pressure, heart rate, respiration rate, and temperature) throughout his or her hospital stay. Moreover, it has increasingly become the practice to take vital signs routinely at outpatient care programs. Nurses often keep separate logs showing what medications were ordered and when they were administered.

Documentation of Medication Administration

Healthcare providers are required to obtain written consents and authorizations before providing treatment or disclosing confidential patient information. In addition, acknowledgments may be sought from the patient confirming that he or she has received specific information from the healthcare facility.

Consent to Treatment

Many healthcare facilities obtain a **consent to treatment** from patients or their legal representatives before providing care or services except in emergency situations. The consent to treatment documents the patient's permission to receive routine services, diagnostic procedures, and medical care (Abdelhak 2001, 91). The need to obtain the patient's consent before medical and surgical procedures is based on the legal concept of battery, which is the unlawful touching of a person without his or her implied or expressed consent.

Individual states may have laws or regulations that define the content of authorizations. When such laws or regulations exist, the treatment program should consult the HIPAA privacy rule to determine how to apply the state requirements.

Implied consent is assumed when a patient voluntarily submits to treatment. The rationale behind implied consent is that one can reasonably assume that the patient understands the nature of the treatment or would not submit to it. Expressed consent is a consent that is either spoken or written. Although courts recognize both verbal and written consent, verbal consent is more difficult to prove.

It is primarily the physician's responsibility to ensure that the patient understands the nature of the procedure, as well as alternative treatments, and its risks, complications, and benefits before it is performed. Medical staff rules or healthcare provider policies usually list the types of services and procedures that require written consent from the patient. Generally, procedures involving the use of anesthetics, the administration of experimental drugs, the surgical manipulation of organs and tissues, and significant risk of complications require written consent. In addition, some states have passed laws that require written consent forms for certain types of testing procedures (for example, HIV testing).

The original copies of consent forms should always be filed in the client's health record.

Acknowledgments of Client's Rights

Acknowledgment forms also are used to document the fact that information about the patient's rights while under care was provided to the patient. Hospitals and ambulatory facilities are not required to provide patient's rights information, but many do. However, federal law does require long-term care facilities to provide each resident with a patient's bill of rights.

When facilities do provide patient's rights information, there are two common ways to document them in the health record. First, the patient or his or her legal representative can sign indicating receipt of the bill of rights. Second, the facility can have the patient sign and date the actual bill of rights and file a copy in the health record.

Advance Directives

An **advance directive** is a written document that names the patient's choice of legal representative for healthcare purposes. The person designated by the patient then is empowered to make healthcare decisions on behalf of the patient in the event the patient is no longer capable of expressing his or her preferences. Living wills and durable powers of attorney for healthcare are two examples of advance directives.

The federal Patient Self-Determination Act (PSDA) went into effect in 1991. It requires healthcare facilities to provide written information on the patient's right to execute advance directives and to accept or refuse treatment. According to the PSDA, healthcare organizations that accept Medicare or Medicaid patients are required to:

- Develop policies that meet the requirements of state law regarding the patient's right to accept or refuse medical treatment and to develop advance directives

- Provide written information to the patient upon admission that describes the treatment decisions patients may make and the hospital's related policies

- Document the fact that the patient has an advance directive in his or her health record (although they are not required to make a copy of the directive a permanent part of the patient's health record)

Certifications for Holds, Restraints, or Seclusion

When a patient is found by his or her treating psychiatrist or psychologist to be a danger to others or himself or herself or to be gravely disabled as defined by state law, the patient may be held against his or her will for various periods of time, depending on state statute. In some states, the patient can request a judicial review. Patients also may petition the treating physician regarding capacity to consent or refuse antipsychotic medication.

Documentation of Conservatorship

When a person is unable to provide for personal needs such as food, shelter, or clothing as the result of a mental disorder, and thereby is gravely disabled and unwilling or incapable of accepting voluntary treatment, he or she may be recommended for conservatorship placement. Conservatorship documents become part of the medical record.

Documentation of Personal Property and Valuables

Healthcare organizations often document patients' personal property and valuables in the health record. Items such as eyeglasses, hearing aids, prostheses, and other special medical equipment should be documented. When the healthcare organization keeps items in a secure location, that fact should be documented on the property/valuable list. For residential or long-term care facilities, larger personal property such as furniture and electronics should be listed.

Discharge Summaries and Client Instructions

The **discharge summary** is a concise account of the patient's illness, course of treatment, response to treatment, and condition at the time of discharge from the service. The functions of the discharge summary include:

- Ensuring the continuity of future care by providing information to the patient's attending physician, referring physician, and any consulting physicians

- Providing information to support the activities of the medical staff review committee

- Providing concise information that can be used to answer information requests from authorized individuals or entities

The discharge summary must be signed by the attending physician. However, there are some exceptions to this rule. For example, some states allow nurses to sign discharge summaries in long-term care facilities and chemical dependency programs.

The discharge summary also includes instructions for the patient's follow-up care. It is vital that the client or his or her caregiver be given clear, concise instructions. Ideally, those instructions are communicated both verbally and in writing. The healthcare professional who provides them should sign the health record to indicate that verbal instructions have been issued. In addition, the person receiving the instructions should sign to verify that he or she understands them. A copy of the written instructions is then filed in the health record.

When someone other than the patient assumes responsibility for the patient's aftercare, the record should indicate that the instructions were given to the party responsible. Documentation of patient education may be accomplished through forms that prompt the person providing instruction to cover important information.

Despite the best efforts of hospital caregivers and physicians, some patients die while hospitalized. In such cases, the attending physician should add a summary statement to the patient's health record documenting the circumstances surrounding the patient's death. The statement can take the form of a final progress note or a separate report. It should indicate the reason for the client's admission, his or her diagnosis and course in the hospital, and a description of the events that led to his or her death.

Biopsychosocial Rehabilitation

Many providers in the United States have adopted a biopsychosocial approach to the care and treatment of serious mental illness. Professionals from all of the mental health disciplines, working collaboratively and harmoniously, can provide far more effective care and treatment than they can separately. Biopsychosocial rehabilitation helps people with mental disabilities to:

1. Learn to manage the symptoms of their disorder

2. Acquire and maintain the skills and resources needed to live successfully in the community

3. Pursue their own personal goals and recognize and celebrate their individual strengths

Psychosocial Rehabilitation and Recovery

The goal of psychosocial rehabilitation is to enable clients to compensate for or eliminate the functional deficits and interpersonal and environmental barriers created by mental disabilities and thus to restore their ability to live independently, socialize with others, and effectively manage their lives.

Psychosocial rehabilitation and recovery is a continuum of interventions that ranges from patient and support system education to individual treatment. It is designed to work with the whole person to improve individual functioning, increase the person's ability to manage his or her illness, and facilitate recovery. Everyone involved in service delivery must be able to work with the patient on an interpersonal level and with the patient's support systems to set goals and develop logical steps to meet them.

Specialized Health Record Content

There are differences as well as similarities among the health records maintained by different levels of care. The healthcare setting (acute care, outpatient, residential, group home, club house, day treatment, long-term care, and so on) is one factor. For example, the health records of residents in the long-term care setting often contain immunization records, but the health records of residents in the acute care setting do not.

A number of other factors can affect health record content in different healthcare settings, including variations in:

- Accreditation standards (for example, JCAHO health information standards for acute care hospitals versus Commission on Accreditation and Rehabilitation Facilities (CARF) standards for rehabilitation hospitals)

- State and local laws

- Federal funding (for example, federal regulations that apply only to organizations that treat Medicare enrollees)

- Type of medical services required (for example, schizophrenia versus depression)

- Duration of medical services (for example, long-term care versus emergency services care)

- Traits of individual patients (for example, age or functional status)

- Complexity of the client's condition

Information Pertaining to Emergency Care

The delivery of emergency care services occurs primarily in hospital-based emergency departments and freestanding psychiatric hospitals. However, it also occurs "in the field" with various outreach programs that include psychiatric emergency response teams working in conjunction with the police or emergency medical services. Emergency care documentation is limited to information about the patient's presenting problem and the diagnostic and therapeutic services provided during the episode of care. The services provided in emergency situations focus on diagnosing the problem and stabilizing the patient. Unlike physical illness in which minor injuries and illnesses may require no further medical treatment, psychiatric emergency patients must be referred to ambulatory care providers for follow-up care. Seriously ill patients are admitted to a hospital for ongoing acute psychiatric care treatment. At times, it is necessary to do this even against the patient's will. In this scenario, the client is determined to be incompetent to provide for his or her own care.

In emergency care records, it is extremely important to document the instructions given to the patient as well as the patient's presenting complaint, evaluation, and assessment. Thorough documentation is needed to justify reimbursement, to protect the organization or the patient in future legal proceedings, and to ensure continuity of care.

The following information must be entered into the patient's health record for each emergency care visit:

- Patient's identification (or the reason it could not be obtained)
- Time and means of the patient's arrival at the organization
- Pertinent history of the illness or injury and physical findings, including the patient's vital signs
- Emergency care given to the patient prior to arrival
- Diagnostic and therapeutic orders
- Clinical observations, including the results of treatment
- Reports of procedures, tests, and results
- Diagnostic impression
- Conclusion at the termination of evaluation/treatment, including final disposition, the patient's condition on discharge or transfer, and any instructions given to the patient, the patient's representative, or another healthcare facility for follow-up care
- Documentation of cases where patients left the hospital or emergency department against medical advice

Information Pertaining to Long-Term Care

Long-term care is provided in a variety of facilities, including:

- Skilled nursing facilities (SNFs)
- Nursing facilities (NFs) (also known as convalescent care centers)
- Intermediate-care facilities (ICFs)
- ICFs for the mentally retarded (ICF-MRs)
- **Assisted living** facilities
- State hospitals
- Institute of Mental Disease (IMD)
- Group home
- Residential care

The regulations governing long-term care settings have established strict documentation standards. Most providers are governed by both federal and state regulations. Assisted living facilities are usually governed only by state regulations. Most long-term care providers do not participate in voluntary accreditation programs.

The health records of long-term care patients are based on ongoing assessments and reassessments of the patient (or resident) needs. An interdisciplinary team develops a plan of care for each client upon admission, and the plan is updated regularly throughout the client's stay. The team includes the client's physician and representatives from nursing services, nutritional services, social services, and other specialty areas (such as physical therapy), as appropriate.

In SNFs, the care plan is based on a format required by federal regulations called the resident assessment instrument (RAI). The RAI is based on the Minimum Data Set (MDS) for Long-term Care. The overall RAI framework includes the MDS, triggers, utilization guidelines, and resident assessment protocols (RAPs). The client is reassessed on a quarterly and annual basis as well as whenever there is a significant change in his or her condition.

The RAI is a critical component of the health record. In addition to its role in the development of the care plan, the MDS form is used by Medicare to determine reimbursement. Many states also use it to determine Medicaid payments, and accreditation surveyors use it during the survey process.

The MDS is submitted electronically to each state health department and then on to the Centers for Medicare and Medicaid Services (CMS). At the CMS, demographic and quality indicator information is compiled and provided as feedback to each facility.

The physician's role in a long-term care facility is not as visible as in other care settings. He or she develops a plan of treatment, which includes the medications and treatments provided to the resident. He or she then visits the resident on a thirty- or sixty-day schedule unless the resident's condition requires more frequent visits. At each visit, the physician reviews the plan of care and physician orders and makes changes as necessary. Between visits, the physician is contacted when nursing identifies changes in the resident's condition.

Other specialized assessments and interdisciplinary progress notes are included in the long-term care health record. The following list identifies those that are most common:

- Identification and admission information

- History and physical and hospital records

- Advance directives and other legal records

- Clinical assessments

- RAI/MDS and care plan

- Physician orders

- Physician progress notes/consultations

- Nursing or interdisciplinary notes

- Laboratory, radiology, and special reports

- Rehabilitation therapy notes (physical therapy, occupational therapy, and speech therapy)

- Social services, nutritional services, and activities documentation

- Discharge documentation

Information Pertaining to Outpatient (Ambulatory) Care

The records of healthcare services provided in outpatient offices typically include the following:

- Registration forms

- Problem lists

- Medication lists
- History and physicals
- Progress notes
- Results of consultations
- Diagnostic test results
- Copies of records of previous hospitalizations
- Client history questionnaires
- Miscellaneous flow sheets (for example, pediatric growth charts and immunization records and specialty-specific flow sheets)
- Correspondence
- Authorizations to disclose information
- Advance directives

Many of the forms used in ambulatory care settings are similar to those used in acute care hospitals and have similar functions. For example, the registration form used in an outpatient setting includes the same demographic and financial information that a hospital admissions record does.

However, ambulatory care records do include several elements unique to the ambulatory setting. For example, they usually contain a problem list that facilitates ongoing patient care management. The problem list describes any significant current and past illnesses and conditions as well as the procedures the patient has undergone. Additionally, it may include information on the patient's allergies and drug sensitivities. Some ambulatory organizations place information about the patient's current prescription medications on the problem list; others maintain a separate medications list. These lists also should include any over-the-counter and herbal medications the patient takes.

Some ambulatory care settings use a structured form called a patient history questionnaire to collect past medical history information from the patient. When the patient completes the medical history information on the questionnaire, the treating clinician then must review and initial the form.

Outpatient Psychiatric Care

Outpatient psychiatric care falls into three categories: individual psychotherapy, group medical psychotherapy, and psychiatric pharmacotherapy.

Individual Psychotherapy

Psychiatric care consists of treatment methods directed toward identifying specific behavior patterns, factors that determine such behavior, and effective goal-oriented therapies.

Individual psychotherapy is a form of treatment that involves a therapist and a single client dependent principally on verbal interchange, including psychoanalysis, crisis intervention, insight-oriented behavior modification, and supportive therapy.

Group Medical Psychotherapy

In group psychotherapy, patients placed into a distinct group are guided by a psychotherapist for the purpose of enabling the group members to help each other effect personality change. By means of a variety of technical maneuvers and theoretical constructs such as intellectualization, ventilation, catharsis, instruction, and support, the leader uses the members' interaction to bring about change (National Heritage Insurance Company 2000).

Psychiatric Pharmacotherapy

Psychiatric pharmacotherapy is intended for medication-only patients and includes psycho-pharmacological management, which involves prescription use and routine review of medication. The psychotherapy provided is minimal and usually supportive only. Typically, the client is stable but requires pharmacologic regimen oversight. Services include an evaluation of the safety and effectiveness of the medication and/or a dosage adjustment to long-term medication. The prescription also may remain unchanged.

Most patients are managed with eighteen or fewer services in a twelve-month period, although there can be exceptions. In general, the administration and supply of oral medication is a non-covered service with few statutory exceptions (National Heritage Insurance Company 2000).

Information Pertaining to Day Treatment/Day Care/ Partial Hospitalization

Day treatment/day-care/partial hospitalization services include:

- Social and recreation activities for individuals who require general supervision during the day

- Psychosocial programs for social interaction

- Family counseling services directed toward a family member's problem in relation to the patient's condition

- Vocational training for employment opportunities, work skills, or work settings

Information Pertaining to Clubhouses/Peer Counseling

The Clubhouse approach to recovery and rehabilitation originated in the 1940s with a small group of psychiatric patients from Rockland State Hospital in New York State. This group founded the Fountain House, which has become the premier example of a Clubhouse model for mentally ill individuals. The Clubhouse model is a self-help group through which members provide aid and assistance to one another after leaving psychiatric hospitals. The principal purpose of the Clubhouse is to be a center for work, education, and entertainment activities organized and administered with the help of the members.

Information Pertaining to Rehabilitation Services

The documentation requirements for rehabilitation services vary because rehabilitation organizations provide care ranging from comprehensive inpatient care to outpatient services or special programs. Health record documentation reflects the level of care and services provided by the organization.

Many rehabilitation organizations are accredited through CARF. CARF requires the organization to maintain a single case record for any client it admits. Rehabilitation documentation standard for the health record includes the following requirements:

- Identification data

- Pertinent history

- Diagnosis of disability

- Problems, goals, and prognosis

- Reports of assessments and individual program planning

- Reports from referring sources and service referrals

- Reports from outside consultations and laboratory, radiology, orthotic, and prosthetic services

- Designation of a manager for the patient's program

- Evidence of the patient's or family's participation in decision making

- Evaluation reports from each service

- Reports of staff conferences

- Patient's total program plan

- Plans from each service

- Signed and dated service and progress reports

- Correspondence pertinent to the client

- Release forms

- Discharge report

- Follow-up reports

Conclusion

The patient health record generally contains both clinical and administrative information. However, there are exceptions and healthcare organizations must consider whether items such as incident reports, financial information, and other records should be kept as part of the health or medical record. Certainly clinical data, including health history, consultation reports, care plans, and psychotherapy notes are essential elements in medical record content. Medical records often also contain various patient consents to treatment, and authorizations concerning such matters as advance directives obtained by the healthcare organization are kept as part of the client's record. Moreover, the healthcare setting determines in large part the content of the health record because of the nature of the specific services each provides.

References and Bibliography

Abdelhak, Mervat, ed. 2001. *Health Information Management of a Strategic Resource.* 2nd ed. Philadelphia: W.B. Saunders.

Abraham, Prinny Rose. 2001. *Documentation and Reimbursement for Home Care and Hospice Programs.* Chicago: American Health Information Management Association.

American Psychological Association. 2002. *Ethical Principles of Psychologists and Code of Conduct.* Dated June 1, 2003. Accessed on-line at www.apa.org/ethics/code2002.html.

Bryant, L. Edward, Jr. 1992. Health law: Medical records and the law, the special incident report. *Journal of the American Health Information Management Association* 63(4): 16.

California Code of Regulations. 2004. Title 9: Rehabilitative and Developmental Services. Current as of Register 2004, No. 49. Dated December 3, 2004. Accessed on-line at www.calregs.com.

Centers for Medicare and Medicaid Services. 1995. *Conditions of Participation: Special Medical Record Requirements for Psychiatric Hospitals.* 482.60 Special provisions applying to psychiatric hospitals.

Code of Federal Regulations. 2001. Title 42, Volume 3, Chapter IV, 42CFR482.60. Centers for Medicare and Medicaid Services: Conditions of Participation for Hospitals; Special provisions applying to psychiatric hospitals. U.S. Government Printing Office, 42CFR 482.60.

Code of Federal Regulations. 2001. Title 42, Volume 3, 42CFR489.100. Public Health: General—Health Care, Department of Health and Human Services. U.S. Government Printing Office, 42CFR489.100.

Commission on Accreditation of Rehabilitation Facilities. 2000. *Behavioral Health Standards Manual.* Tucson, AZ: CARF.

Gitterman, Daniel, Richard Scheffler, Marcia Peck, Elizabeth Ciemans, and Darcy Gruttadero. 2000. *A Decade of Mental Health Parity: The Regulation of Mental Health Insurance Parity in the United States, 1990–2000.* NIMH Grant MH-18828-11. Berkeley: University of California.

Glondys, Barbara. 1996. *Documentation Requirements for the Acute Care Client Record.* Chicago: American Health Information Management Association.

Gorodezky, Michael J. 2003. Personal conversation discussing behavioral health information system consulting.

Hjort, Beth. 2001. Practice Brief: Patient photography, videotaping, and other imaging (updated). *Journal of the American Health Information Management Association* 72(6). Available at www.ahima.org.

Huffman, Edna K. 1990. *Medical Record Management.* Berwyn, IL: Physicians Record Company.

Joint Commission on Accreditation of Healthcare Organizations. 2002. *Comprehensive Accreditation Manual for Hospitals.* Oakbrook Terrace, IL: JCAHO.

Johns, Merida, ed. 2002. *Health Information Management Technology: An Applied Approach.* Chicago: American Health Information Management Association.

Jonas, Steven, and Anthony R. Kovner. 1999. *Health Care Delivery in the United States,* 6th ed. New York, Springer Publishing.

Meyer, Adolf. 1918. Mental health status exam. Accessed on-line at http://dcradar.org/doctors/picchio.

National Heritage Insurance Company. 2000. Billing guide for mental health services Medi-Cal Part B. Accessed on-line at www.medicarenhic.com.

National Institute of Mental Health. www.nimh.nih.gov/.

Roach, William H., ed. 1989. Legal Review: Hospitals Incident Reports. *Topics in Health Record Management,* September 1989.

Shale, Jack. April 2003. Personal conversation discussing psychotherapy notes.

Tarasoff v. Regents of the University of California. 1976. 131 Cal. Rptr. 14.

U.S. Department of Health and Human Services. 1999. *Mental Health: A Report of the Surgeon General.* Rockville, MD: U.S. Department of Health and Human Services, Substance Abuse and Mental Health Services Administration, Center for Mental Health Services, National Institutes of Health, National Institute of Mental Health. Accessed on-line at http://www.surgeongeneral.gov/library/mentalhealth/home.html.

Williams, Clemon W. 1985. Guide to hospital incident reports. *Health Care Management Review* 13.

Chapter 3

Understanding and Implementing the Electronic Health Record

Margret K. Amatayakul, MBA, RHIA, CHPS, FHIMSS

In his 2004 State of the Union Address, President Bush noted: "By computerizing health records, we can avoid dangerous medical mistakes, reduce costs, and improve care." This statement has been applauded by those people who recognize that electronic health records (EHRs) represent a huge opportunity to improve patient care and health system operations. However, efforts to achieve an EHR have represented a long journey from early visions to today's reality. The EHR is not a simple computer application; rather, it represents a carefully constructed set of systems that are highly integrated and require a significant investment of time, money, process change, and human factor reengineering.

This chapter focuses on the electronic health record, describing its components, origins, and vision. It also discusses different attempts at implementation and both the advantages and limitations of the electronic health record. Finally, the chapter outlines steps for implementing the electronic health record, including how to select and contract with vendors.

Electronic Health Record Definition

Defining the **electronic health record** (EHR) is not simple. Indeed, there is no standard definition. The EHR is not an **information system** (IS) that is purchased and installed as a word-processing package is, or even a billing system or laboratory system that may have to be connected to other information systems and devices and customized to a specific environment. The EHR is more of an information system framework that accomplishes a complete set of functions.

The Criteria for the Electronic Health Record

Possibly the simplest way to describe the EHR is to refer to the early work of the **Computer-based Patient Record Institute** (CPRI). The CPRI, now part of the **Healthcare Information and Management Systems Society** (HIMSS), identified three key criteria for an EHR. The electronic health record must:

- Integrate data from multiple sources

This chapter is derived from Amatayakul, Margret K. 2004. *Electronic Health Records: A Practical Guide for Professionals and Organizations,* 2nd ed. Chicago: American Health Information Management Association. For more in-depth information on electronic health records, please refer to this publication.

- Capture data at the point of care

- Support caregiver decision making

The intersection of these criteria may be considered the EHR, as illustrated in figure 3.1.

Components of the Electronic Health Record

Many organizations contemplating what an EHR is want to understand what information system (IS) components comprise an EHR. Figure 3.2 displays a conceptual model that depicts the technical system components that capture and integrate data and support caregiver decision making. However, because the EHR is as much a set of functions that provide value as it is technical system components, the conceptual model also shows the relationship of the technical components to the value of EHR. The value of integrating clinical, financial, and administrative data contributes significantly to improvements in quality, cost, and access to healthcare. Furthermore, the EHR is not limited to a single location but, rather, should include remote access for providers and consumers. Potentially, it should even be capable of integrating data across providers and from personal health records to form a longitudinal view of an individual's health status and healthcare.

Therefore, the technical system components of the EHR include:

- Source systems that *capture data* to support the EHR infrastructure. These source systems include all administrative, financial, and clinical department systems that relate in any way to the health record.

- Supporting infrastructure that *integrates data,* which may include a **data repository** that centralizes data from other components (or other means to integrate data); a **rules engine** that supplies programming logic for decision support, such as alerts and reminders, order sets, and clinical **protocols; knowledge sources** that make information available from various external sources; and **data warehouses** from which specific data can be mined (that is, aggregated and analyzed) to provide useful information.

- A **human–computer interface** that helps capture data *at the point of care* and, by virtue of access to data, rules, knowledge, and mined data, *supports caregiver decision making.* It may be any means by which users enter and retrieve data, such as a computer

Figure 3.1. EHR criteria

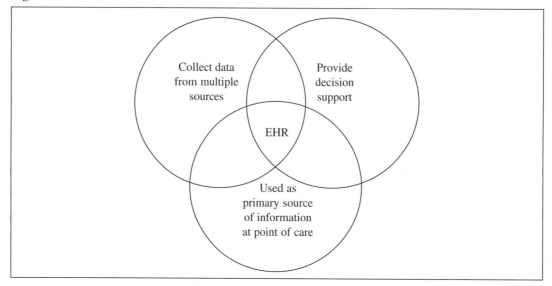

Figure 3.2.   Conceptual model of EHR

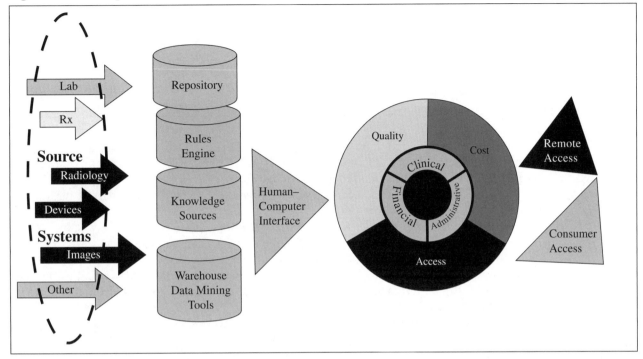

workstation, a personal computer (PC), a notebook computer, a personal digital assistant (PDA), a voice recognition system, a handwriting recognition system on a tablet PC, and so on.

The end result of implementing the technical components of the EHR is that quality, cost, and access to healthcare are enhanced through clinical, financial, and administrative data support. The American Health Information Management Association's (AHIMA's) Health Information Vision 2010 states that "health information will be used concurrently for multiple and diverse purposes, including healthcare delivery and treatment, outcomes measurement, finance, and support of health services and policy research, clinical trials, and disease prevention and surveillance at the individual, community, national, and international levels" (AHIMA 2003).

Origins of the Electronic Health Record

The concept of the EHR has existed since early use of computers in healthcare and has undergone a significant transformation over time. Figure 3.3 illustrates the major milestones in the history of EHR implementation.

Pioneers of the Electronic Health Record

The first major efforts to automate clinical information occurred in the late 1960s and early 1970s. Several forward-thinking universities and companies recognized the value of emerging **information technology** (IT) for healthcare.

Some of the early attempts at automating the health record were highly successful and are precursors of today's products. For example, efforts by Wiederhold at Stanford University and

Figure 3.3. History of EHR implementation

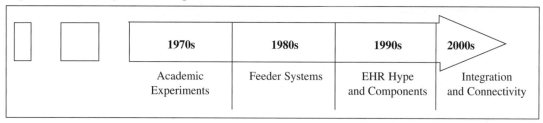

El Camino Hospital, conducted with scientists at the Lockheed Company, are often cited among the forerunners of the first commercial products. This early **clinical information system** (CIS) effort was subsequently taken over and further developed by the Technicon Corporation (subsequently TDS Healthcare Systems Corporation, which is now part of the suite of products available from Eclipsys, Inc.).

Another pioneering provider–vendor partnership took place at Latter Day Saints (LDS) Hospital, now Intermountain Healthcare, with the HELP system on which 3M has based products. Other organizations have contributed significantly to research in the design of CISs. Massachusetts General Hospital in Boston; Kaiser Permanente in Oakland, California; and Regenstrief Institute in Indianapolis have contributed significantly to the EHR body of knowledge (Shortliffe and Perreault 2001).

The National Library of Medicine (NLM) also has contributed greatly to early efforts and continues to play an extremely active role in data and vocabulary development. Its Integrated Advanced Information Management Systems (IAIMS) grants have helped—and continue to help—fund many EHR-related projects. (For a comprehensive history of medical informatics, see M. F. Collen's *A History of Medical Informatics in the U.S. 1950–1990.*)

Early Limiting Factors

For the most part, applicability of the early EHR projects was limited to the environments in which they were created. Products often could not be "commercialized" or made readily able to be implemented in other settings because they were so closely linked to processes at one organization.

Furthermore, in the early days of computer use, most healthcare organizations lacked the source systems—the laboratory, radiology, pharmacy, and other ancillary services—to supply an EHR with the data needed to provide users with much value. Thus, the automation that ensued in the 1980s focused on the relatively simpler, but critical, source systems and those that produced more immediate payback. Initially, these were administrative and financial systems such as registration–admission/discharge/transfer (R-ADT), master person index (MPI), and accounts receivable (A/R). Later, departmental systems for laboratory, radiology, pharmacy, dietary, materials management, and others were developed and implemented. In general, new interest in automating the health record itself waned as other systems were being implemented.

Landmark Effort

In the mid-1980s, frustrated by the inadequacies of the paper health record and slow progress toward automating clinical data, the Institute of Medicine (IOM) initiated a study on "improving the patient record in light of new technology." In 1991, the IOM released a report of its study entitled *The Computer-based Patient Record: An Essential Technology for Health Care.* The IOM coined the term "computer-based patient record" (CPR), more commonly referred to today as the electronic health record (EHR). At the time, the CPR represented a huge leap from the concept of documentation that primarily supported the provider to documentation that focused on the person receiving care. The IOM's landmark work laid the conceptual foundation for a vision of a system that would:

provide a longitudinal (that is, lifelong) record of events that may have influenced a person's health (IOM 1991, 137) and reside[s] in a system specifically designed to support users by providing accessibility to complete and accurate data, alerts, reminders, clinical decision support systems, links to medical knowledge, and other aids (IOM 1991, 11)

EHR Vision

EHRs may not yet be as widely implemented as the IOM would have desired, but the IOM vision remains firm. In 1997, a second edition of the original 1991 study report was undertaken. The result was retention of all original content as being valid and current for the time, with updates relative to implementations in the United States and Europe. The IOM vision for EHR remained committed to the use of IT for a number of purposes, including:

- To document all episodes of healthcare wherever they take place

- To provide immediate access to data

- To process data in a variety of ways to support better decision making for patient care and clinical and health services research

- To increase the efficiency of healthcare organizations and decrease the cost of services

- To ensure the confidentiality of data

- To improve the quality of care and promote the wellness of the population

The IOM's contribution was significant not only because it addressed a need, but also because it defined the scope of the transition to the EHR. This transition is characterized by the following key quotes from the IOM report:

- "Merely automating the form, content, and procedures of current patient records will perpetuate their deficiencies and will be insufficient to meet emerging user needs" (IOM 1991, 2)

- "The CPR encompasses a broader view of the patient record than is current today, moving from the notion of a location or device for keeping track of patient care events to a resource with much enhanced utility in patient care (including the ability to provide an accurate longitudinal account of care), in management of the health care system, and in extension of knowledge" (IOM 1991, 3)

- The CPR is "the core of health care information systems. Such systems must be able to transmit data to other types of clinical and administrative information systems within healthcare institutions; they must also be able to transmit data to and accept data from other healthcare institutions or secondary databases" (IOM 1991, 51)

EHR Terminology

A number of terms have come to be associated with the means to accomplish the IOM's goals. Some of these are generic; others are vendor specific.

As noted above, the IOM coined the term "computer-based patient record" (CPR), which it defined as "an electronic patient record that resides in a system specifically designed to support users by providing accessibility to complete and accurate data, alerts, reminders, clinical decision support systems, links to medical knowledge, and other aids."

Another popular term is **electronic medical record** (EMR). This term continues to be widely used, especially to describe systems based on document imaging or systems implemented in physician offices.

"Electronic health record" is the term used in this book and the term chosen in the IOM letter report, *Key Capabilities of an Electronic Health Record System,* which it submitted to the U.S. **Department of Health and Human Services** (HHS) in July 2003. Moreover, EHR is the term being incorporated into a standard description of an EHR being developed by Health Level Seven (HL7), a standards development organization, in collaboration with the IOM (Health Level Seven, 2004). EHR is believed to represent the most comprehensive vision of an information system that would support all types of caregivers, in all settings, including the individual who may be using it to record personal health status information.

EHR Migration Path

Although the variety of terms initially may have come about because of vendors attempting to differentiate their products, some in the industry have tried to use the different terms to describe either different visions or a **migration path** toward an ultimate vision.

The many functions that an EHR may address, from simple to sophisticated, include:

- Document-scanning/imaging systems

- Order communication/results retrieval (OC/RR) systems

- Clinical messaging systems

- Patient care charting

- Computerized physician/provider order entry (CPOE) systems

- Clinical decision support systems

- Provider–patient portals

- Personal health records

- Population health

These are the most common and significant functions. There are many other, more detailed functions—or at least subfunctions—that others might highlight.

Document-Scanning/Imaging Systems

Document-scanning/imaging systems represent a wide range of functionality. Some merely capture images of the forms in the paper record for storage in a computer system for later retrieval. Most systems today index the data on the forms to help retrieve specific data. Some document-imaging systems combine scanned forms with forms that have been computer generated. This is known as computer output to laser disk (COLD). Finally, document imaging can be integrated with work flow technology.

Work flow technology helps direct work on documents. For example, it can determine when a record is ready for coding and put it into the appropriate coder's work queue. Simultaneously, clinicians can view the documents when access is needed for subsequent patient care. The patient financial services department also may access the documents to generate a claims attachment. However sophisticated the ability to select blocks of text to view or how easily work may be distributed for processing, document imaging primarily affords access to what was originally paper record content from multiple locations.

Order Communication/Results Retrieval Systems

OC/RR systems provide the capability of transmitting orders to various ancillary departments and viewing results of laboratory and other diagnostic studies or the status of orders. OC/RR systems go a long way toward integrating the various source systems for operational purposes. However, they are essentially paper based because they rely on handwritten orders that are key-entered into a computer by clerical or nursing staff and diagnostic studies results that are typically generated in a paper format. These documents may be from ancillary information systems, such as laboratory systems, or from transcription systems where radiology and other reports are dictated and transcribed. Some organizations use COLD feed to compile these documents into a central automated archive; others merely file the documents into the paper **chart** folder.

OC/RR systems afford the functionality of automatically transmitting orders instead of telephoning, using a courier, or faxing, and of providing access to results from multiple locations.

Clinical Messaging Systems

Clinical messaging systems add to CR/RR systems the dimension of real-time interaction through Web-based technology. The Web-based technology may be applied within the organization's own internal **network**, or **intranet**, or may entail exchange of information through a secure Web portal from the Internet.

Clinical messaging systems enhance paper-based systems because they make available electronically the content of what would otherwise be on paper.

Patient Care Charting

Patient care charting is a system in which caregivers enter data (notes, vital signs, medications administered, and so on). Early patient care charting systems were focused primarily on nursing staff documentation but now have come to be used by any caregiver. Data entered into patient care charting systems may be structured or unstructured. Figure 3.4 illustrates both of these data-entry concepts, as further discussed below.

- **Structured data** refers to data that have been predefined in a table or checklist, such as shown in figure 3.4 for recording severity of symptoms. The user selects the data through the keyboard, touch screen, light pen, or any other human–computer interface via a checklist. In other cases, the user may be asked to enter a number or numeric score. For example, to record the severity of symptoms, a nurse may select a numeric score from 1 to 10 from a standard pain scale. It is important to note that the purpose of structured data entry is to help ensure standardization. It is interesting that in healthcare there are actually two pain scales. One consists of scores from 1 to 10 and is used by nurses; the other consists of scores from 1 to 4 and is used by physical therapists. When setting up structured data entry, it is important to ensure that the appropriate scale, scoring system, or code set is specified in some way. Structured data capture also may be accommodated through choices in a drop-down menu, such as the selection of a problem in the problem list in figure 3.4. Additionally, medical devices (such as cardiac monitors) or laboratory instruments generate structured data.

- **Unstructured data** essentially refers to narrative data, such as in the section for "presentation" in figure 3.4. Here, areas are reserved for caregivers to key in, dictate through voice recognition, handwrite through handwriting recognition, or even dictate and later have transcribed anything they wish to record. Such unstructured data are more difficult to use in searches and generally are not converted into tabular or graphical form.

Figure 3.4.   Structured and unstructured data entry in an EHR

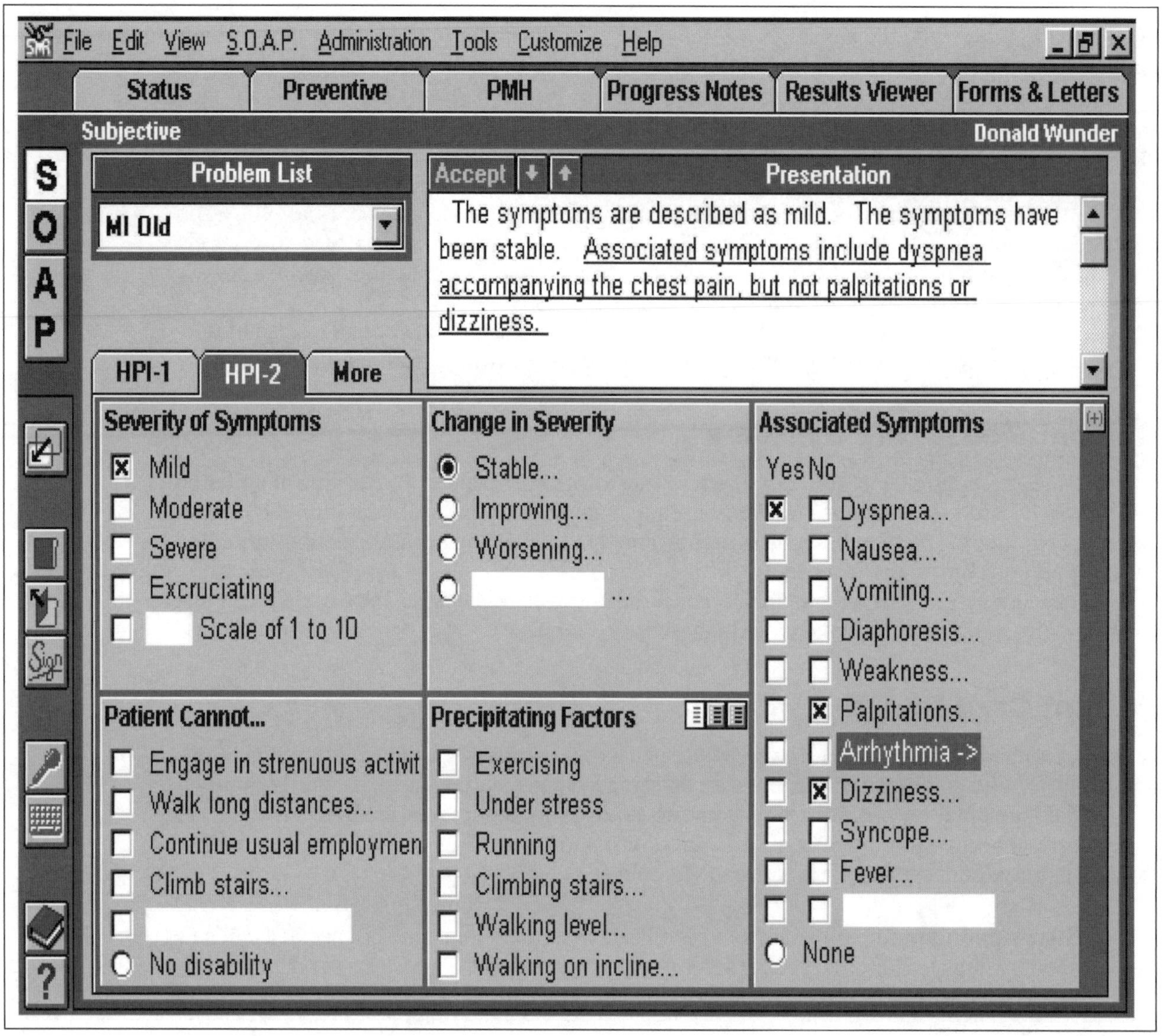

Early in their introduction, patient care systems required significant changes in **work flow.** They were often time-consuming and difficult to use. Attempts were made to use so-called bedside **terminals** because returning to a small number of terminals at a nursing station was inadequate. Today, patient care charting systems have become much more sophisticated. Data entry may be performed using handheld devices, many of which are wireless. Data also may be captured by using smart text (or what would be called macros in word processing), where only a few key letters have to be entered to represent an entire word or phrase. The most sophisticated systems would apply **natural language processing,** which permits narrative text to be converted to **discrete data** for processing by the computer. This last form of data entry is still very much in the developmental stage.

Computerized Physician/Provider Order Entry Systems

CPOE systems came about fairly recently as a result of the IOM's quality initiative, which began with the National Roundtable on Health Care Quality (1998) and subsequent studies on patient safety issues and medication errors in particular (*To Err is Human,* 1999; *Crossing the Quality Chasm,* 2001; and *Patient Safety: Achieving a New Standard for Care,* 2004). CPOE systems are intended for use by physicians and other providers to enter orders directly into the computer system and be given prompts, reminders, or alerts about the order entered. These systems enhance legibility to avoid errors, and their decision support capability enhances patient safety and healthcare efficiencies. Decision support might include calculating an appropriate dose and alerting the physician as the order is entered that, given the patient's weight, an alternative dose might be appropriate. Another example might be indicating that a prescribed medication is contraindicated under certain circumstances, such as when the patient is taking another medication or being prepped for a certain diagnostic study. The CPOE system might identify that a specific drug is not covered by the patient's insurance and might offer equivalents.

Some CPOE systems are more sophisticated than others. Some have minimal clinical decision support, such as merely checking an order against a **formulary**. In many of these less-robust implementations, physicians have complained that the order-entry process takes much longer than writing an order on paper and do not believe they are gaining any value.

Clinical Decision Support Systems

The term **clinical decision support system** (CDSS) is generally reserved to describe the help provided in association with data entry into an EHR system performed directly by the caregiver at the point of care. The help may come in the form of alerts or reminders that are generated by preprogrammed logic or rules. For example, if a patient has a diagnosis for which a certain medication has been found to be effective and no order has been given for that drug, the system could be programmed to suggest that the physician consider adding the medication to the patient's treatment regime. This is what supports the most sophisticated CPOE system. Another example might be support for coding in a physician office EHR system, where the complexity of the patient encounter must be reflected in the evaluation and management (E&M) CPT-4 code and ultimately contributes to the level of reimbursement for the visit.

The help provided through a CDSS also may be in the form of a **clinical practice guideline,** care path, or critical pathway. Moreover, the CDSS may tap external knowledge sources to provide more comprehensive information. For example, if a physician is unfamiliar with a new drug that is offered as an alternative suggestion, he or she may be able to click on a link to a reference that provides more complete information. A physician faced with an unusual set of symptoms and signs may look for reference material on the Web to develop a differential diagnosis. A pharmacist may need to make suggestions for alternative medications when a patient has an allergy, or research the efficacy of various drugs when there is an unusual diagnosis. The CDSS may produce tailored instructions to be given to the patient. Clinical decision support is considered concurrent (at the time data are entered) or even prospective (when presenting "best practices" in anticipation of care).

Clinical decision support should be contrasted with executive decision support, which is typically a stand-alone system that analyzes a large volume of aggregated data and provides trending information. Executive decision support is typically retrospective, providing quality improvement, productivity, staffing, and/or marketing information for executives.

Provider–Patient Portals

Provider–patient portals are the secure means to use the Internet for communicating protected health information (PHI) among providers, between provider and patient, or between provider and payer. In some cases, the provider–patient portal is used to support secure e-mail. In other cases, it may be used for remote connectivity to results retrieval systems (and **clinical messaging** systems). In still other cases, patient monitoring may be performed through such a connection. Some examples of areas where this is being used very effectively is for pacemaker monitoring in heart disease patients, blood sugar monitoring for diabetic patients, and breath sounds monitoring for babies at risk for sudden infant death syndrome.

Personal Health Records

Personal health records (PHRs) are systems designed to support patient-entered data. If they are associated with a provider, they may serve as a means for patients to access their own health records (or summaries of their records) or to provide information to their providers about their health status. In some cases, PHRs are integrated with the EHR and access is often provided through a Web portal. In other cases, typically when they are stand-alone systems not associated with a provider, they may be anything from a fax-back system to one that supports structured data entry by a patient on a Web site.

Population Health

Population health also is facilitated through accurate, complete, and timely capture and reporting of public health data, including data relating to homeland security. Population health data collection may be initiated in the provider setting and linked automatically to a state data collection system. Population health may be served by decision support that is provided to caregivers through alerts from public health departments, such as to notify them of a new strain of virus or to remind them to seek certain information from patients who present with certain symptoms. A precursor to population health may be disease management, wherein providers and health plans share data about patients/health plan members who would benefit from certain educational programs or special monitoring.

EHR Implementation Status

Electronic health record implementation has gone through a number of stages. Initial interest in its early history later led to disappointment, but eventually a better sense of reality.

Media Hype

The release of the IOM patient record study report in 1991 initially led to much media hype. Vendors flooded trade shows and publications with promotions for EHR products. Information systems leadership surveys conducted by HIMSS and other organizations made EHR projects the top priority for healthcare institutions.

It was assumed that an EHR product could be purchased and implemented in much the same way as other systems for keeping track of patient accounts, reporting laboratory results, and abstracting health records. Although many of these source systems now have become quite complex, they typically are more confined to a single department or a single set of functions.

Disappointment

As EHR project teams started evaluating institutional readiness for the EHR and assessing vendors' products, they found that the project was not as simple as buying software off the shelf or installing departmental systems. They came to understand that the EHR is a highly complex concept. Virtually every system in the organization would touch, and be touched by, the EHR. Many organizations simply had not integrated all the necessary source systems to support the EHR. Furthermore, for an EHR to provide benefit, all caregivers had to use it in place of the paper health record and use information in new and different ways. Caregivers had never before been touched by any system in the way they would be affected by an EHR.

Finally, vendor offerings were typically found to be less complete than anticipated. Early in the evolution of the EHR, many vendors developed only an EHR concept and were looking for organizations to be development partners. Some vendors had one component of the EHR but could not integrate it with other applications into an organization's total operations. Unfortunately, many vendors failed to recognize the complexity of the EHR system. Few vendors took the time to study the nature of clinical information or the flow of clinical data through the healthcare delivery system. Still fewer attempted to introduce a system that would truly improve clinical information management, not just duplicate the existing paper system. One vendor went so far as to advertise that its product would make significant improvements in productivity and the quality of care for physicians' offices—without changing a thing! The fundamental lesson learned from these early projects is that improvement requires change.

Reality

Since the IOM released its first study on patient records, hundreds of vendors have been selling what they have promoted as EHR products. Many of these vendors quickly went out of business or were sold to save their investment. Today the lure of the "better mousetrap" still attracts new vendors, but there is a more stable set of vendors with much more robust products.

The EHR market is beginning to settle down. Some of the early adopters have worked closely with vendors to develop mutually acceptable products. Although the market was segmented by acute care and ambulatory care in early systems, vendors now are acquiring companies and/or skills to develop systems that address the needs of integrated delivery networks (IDNs). EHR vendors are beginning to work on the key issues that have been stumbling blocks to success. Today's environment is much more realistic about what can be accomplished and what still needs to be done. When organizations undertake an EHR project today, they have a far greater understanding of what an EHR is and how it must be implemented. The jury may still be out on whether EHR systems pay for themselves directly, but many organizations are recognizing their strategic value and are planning to implement systems that address longer-term goals.

Because of the variability of terms used to describe EHR, the multiplicity of visions, and the migration path of functionality, it is difficult to determine the true status of EHR implementation. Indeed, some believe the success of achieving the IOM vision of an EHR may have been undermined by the multiplicity of visions associated with it and the wide variety of functionality available (Fox and Thierry 2003).

Currently, it is estimated that less than three percent of hospitals have a true EHR. A survey of 250 hospitals conducted by the Medical Records Institute in winter 2002 indicated that only four facilities had their "entire medical record computerized." Although this figure is probably about accurate, many would attempt to paint a rosier picture. The article describing this survey was accompanied by graphics describing the current status of computerized records in small, medium, and large hospitals. For example, it indicated that nearly half (45.2 percent) of the small hospitals surveyed have a computerized record but goes on to indicate that only a quarter of the computerization in these records was on-line. Clearly, many hospitals are starting down the path toward an EHR but are finding that automated components in themselves are not EHRs.

EHR Limitations

Designing, marketing, and implementing information systems that provide access to clinical data and process data into information that contributes to knowledge for improved quality of care has been challenging. A number of major stumbling blocks are being addressed in clinical and technological areas.

Clinical Data Limitations

Clinical data are textual and contextual, but computers have been designed primarily to manipulate discrete, factual data. Computers are very good at storing large volumes of data and performing mathematical formulas or clearly defined retrieval functions. However, they do not have the human capability of "thinking" or making associations or assumptions on their own. A lot of work is being done to program computers to perform more "reasoning" functions and to "learn" to offer decision-making support. But these functions are very sophisticated and still very much under development.

A good example of clinical data limitations may be to consider how a computer can process a simple statement such as "the skin is red." Interpretation of "red skin" depends on the context to define what is meant by "red." Does red describe a burned area, a rash, or an increase in temperature? What is the cause—fever, embarrassment, allergy, burn, high blood pressure, or something else? Unless we are satisfied with simply recording this information and making it available as documentary evidence of something caregivers observed, the field of computer science must learn how to structure data to associate them properly with other data for future processing.

One significant initiative that is helping the adoption of a standard, clinical vocabulary has been the licensure of the comprehensive Systemized Nomenclature of Human and Veterinary Medicine (SNOMED) vocabulary by the National Library of Medicine. Adoption of a standard vocabulary, such as SNOMED, and its use in structured data will open the door for much broader use of clinical decision support systems.

In addition to **data comparability** that could be achieved through adoption of a standard, comprehensive vocabulary, clinical practice requires more information today than it did in the past. First, there is much more to know—thousands of new drugs, new strains of viruses, and so forth. The field of medicine is continually changing and expanding. Physicians are having to track numerous diagnoses, procedures, diagnostic tests, clinical processes, devices, and drugs, and in many cases the payment rules associated with some of this. Just keeping up with the literature is daunting. For example, MEDLINE, an online bibliographic database of medical information compiled by the NLM, indexes nearly half a million new articles each year from biomedical literature alone. Connectivity to the Web and its resources has opened a huge opportunity to access information. Now the task is to convert that information into usable knowledge, which includes evaluating its reliability and validity.

Another factor that has presented limitations to clinical use of information systems includes the volume of patients and thus productivity concerns surrounding what typically has been a more time-consuming method to record information. It is not uncommon for a primary care physician to treat eighty patients per day during flu season. To quickly record data for this volume of patients, the way in which the caregiver enters or retrieves data from the computer (the human–computer interface) needs to be perfected. We are beginning to see many small, wireless input devices, including personal digital assistants (PDAs) and tablet computers.

Data reuse also is becoming popular. This refers to the ability to "cut and paste" data from templates, previous visit documentation, or even documentation developed for use in other patients' records. Obviously, this must be applied very carefully and cautiously to ensure that the same data directly apply to the current patient and episode of care. However, the function represents an opportunity that is important for adoption of EHRs (Amatayakul, Brandt, and Dougherty 2003).

A final clinical data limitation is that many caregivers find it foreign to rely on information systems for clinical decision support. But the IOM patient safety reports highlighting medication errors, and the subsequent efforts of employer groups and major corporations to sweeten contracts for those providers using IT to improve patient safety, has led to greater acceptance of clinical decision support systems.

Technological Limitations

Technological limitations have made clinical information systems difficult to use. Even as a new generation of caregivers emerges that is accustomed to using computers and engaging patients in their use, physical limitations still abound because healthcare is such a mobile profession. The care of patients requires direct interaction between patients and caregivers. Pen and paper that slip into a pocket are much easier to manage when a caregiver is making rounds and administering to patients. New, smaller, wireless devices, such as PDAs, notebook computers on carts, and even cellular phones with data capture capability and improvements in voice and handwriting recognition are beginning to address technological limitations. So, too, are efforts to redesign care processes that better incorporate the use of computers.

Another technological limitation is the extent to which disparate computer systems can be made to work together and exchange data. Standard protocols have been developed to help, but vendors must adopt the standards and conform to their requirements explicitly. In some cases, vendors have developed highly proprietary systems to encourage providers to buy all components from one vendor. When the vendor does not offer a specific component, the provider is faced with doing without until the vendor creates the component or buying the component from another vendor and hoping an interface (a special program to enable data exchange) can be written that will permit the data to flow across the two different vendor **platforms**. The lack of interoperability between systems has sometimes meant that providers have been unable to adopt EHR systems as rapidly as they would like.

Cost and Value Limitations

A major consideration for any provider adopting EHRs is cost. Today, all healthcare providers are seeing reduced revenue and increased costs. The Healthcare Financial Management Association (HFMA 2003) reports that providers are often strapped for cash and many have very limited access to capital. The EHR is considered an investment that must pay for itself. The systems undoubtedly cost a significant amount of money in addition to the time required to tailor them to the environment and to manage the degree of change they create. For example, it may be necessary to create interfaces enabling independent systems to communicate with one another and with the EHR. All of the application templates must be populated with the provider's specific requirements, clinical **practice guidelines,** any unique terminology, their own formulary and charge data, and many other requirements. In addition, although it generally does not take very much time to learn how to document in an EHR if it is properly designed, it does take time for the adoption process to occur and to manage work flow change.

Many have questioned whether the EHR can truly pay for itself. Part of the issue is that both cost and benefits are somewhat elusive. Because the EHR depends on the **integration** of all other clinical and administrative systems, sometimes some of this cost is attributed to the EHR when it should be attributed to processes that needed attention anyway. Although there are many direct, monetary benefits, many benefits either cannot be quantified or are very difficult to quantify—even when the effort is made to do so, which often is not the case.

Some initiatives have attempted to address the cost–benefit issue. For example, the Open Source EHR project spearheaded by the American Academy of Family Practice Physicians has attempted to significantly lower the cost of EHRs for physician offices by sharing the source code for development purposes. A number of industry awards that target the "most wired" or "exemplary implementations" have attempted to demonstrate the value of EHR systems (for example, "Most Wired" Hospitals and Health Networks, HIMSS).

Standardization Limitations

As alluded to in the preceding descriptions, the lack of standardization—to define the EHR, write interfaces, compare data, ensure data quality, and perform many other functions associated with EHRs—also has made it very difficult to achieve widespread adoption.

It is not that some standards do not exist. For example, there are standards for writing interfaces, but not every vendor is required to use them and they contain a high degree of optionality. Moreover, there are standard vocabularies, although their number, until recently converged into SNOMED, has equated to a Tower of Babel.

Even though every vendor should be able to apply its own "bells and whistles" to enhance and distinguish its products, standardization would at least achieve a baseline product expectation. The mark of a mature industry is when it can adopt standards that achieve baseline functionality, making the products it uses commodities. For example, the automotive industry has established a standard construct for what a car is. Yet everyone also knows the difference between a Chevy and a Cadillac. The EHR market needs to create a car to which vendors can apply more or less leather and chrome.

Change Limitations

Also alluded to in the above descriptions of limitations is the underlying issue of the degree of change imposed by EHR systems. Although somewhat dependent on the computer skills of healthcare professionals, the immensity of change begins with learning how to use a computer. Many healthcare professionals today still do not routinely use a computer at home or at work, and need basic computer skills. Work flows and processes in healthcare also represent enormous obstacles. Despite the fact that new procedures, tests, and drugs are constantly being developed, health professionals have a very ingrained sense of process. In fact, such habits enable them to react quickly to rapidly changing circumstances. It is extremely difficult to change these processes to accommodate what many healthcare professionals still view as "only" documentation rather than information that is a source of knowledge and value.

In fact, the extent to which the health profession rejects process change has resulted in many EHR product design efforts attempting to replicate the paper environment. This can be seen in screens that have "tabs," the volume of printouts generated in a paperless environment, and, essentially, the rejection of performing work that is typically viewed as clerical (such as order entry). When considered from a cost–benefit perspective, is it any wonder that executives question the value of a system that does nothing but automate today's environment?

The issue of change is something of a catch-22 in healthcare. The EHR should introduce sufficient change so as to improve quality, cost, and access to healthcare but still reasonably reflect processes essential to healthcare delivery.

Major Initiatives in Overcoming EHR Issues

The EHR projects the industry is now undertaking are based on the understanding that an EHR is not a turnkey product but, rather, is as much a **concept** as a set of interrelated systems. It is further recognized that technology alone is not the answer. It is possible to implement a well-designed EHR, but if the persons expected to use it are not engaged in selecting the system, do not aid in its design, are not properly trained, or are not supported by executive leadership, the system will likely either not be used or not be used effectively and thus fail to produce the anticipated value.

Creation of EHR systems depends on a thorough understanding of clinical data and how health professionals use information in clinical decision making. There must be support for adoption of data standards and data quality measures. The willingness to collaborate and share data, both among providers and between providers and patients, may be among the most difficult of the nontechnical issues to be addressed.

Private Efforts

Many provider organizations have made major strides in achieving the vision of the EHR. In some hospitals, 100 percent of the physicians use CPOE. Many hospitals have seen productivity increases from document imaging systems. Clinicians who have access to scanned documents or information through clinical messaging "will never return to paper." Home health agencies have benefited significantly from adoption of handheld devices to capture and submit data, either via telephone modem, docking to a PC, or wireless at a base station. Ambulance services are using not only telemetry, but also smart phones and other devices to quickly record their documentation. Each step along the migration path provides value. It should not be seen as necessary to wait to implement a comprehensive system in order to achieve benefits.

Federal Government Efforts

The federal government also has made EHR an initiative. The Department of Defense, the Veterans Administration, and the Indian Health Service are all focused on adopting some form of EHR. The National Committee on Vital and Health Statistics (NCVHS) has envisioned a National Health Information Infrastructure (NHII) in which health information would be available across the continuum of care for patient treatment as well as population health. The NCVHS also is responsible for overseeing implementation of the privacy, security, and transactions provisions of the Health Insurance Portability and Accountability Act of 1996 (HIPAA) and for developing recommendations for uniform data standards for the electronic exchange of patient medical record information (PMRI). NCVHS recommendations relative to data comparability were a significant driver in government licensure of SNOMED. Additionally, NCVHS has made recommendations relative to system **interoperability**, hoping to gain voluntary adoption of the latest versions of standards that would help interface disparate systems.

In 2003, the Secretary of the Department of Health and Human Services requested the IOM and HL7 to design a functional model and standard for the EHR. In response, senior executives and volunteer leaders from eight health-related professional and trade associations joined forces as the EHR Collaborative in July 2003 to further support the federal government's effort to advance toward the EHR. Members of the collaborative include the AHIMA, the **American Medical Association** (AMA), the American Medical Informatics Association (AMIA), the College of Healthcare Management Executives (CHIME), the eHealth Initiative (eHI), the Healthcare Information and Management Systems Society (HIMSS), and the National Alliance for Health Information Technology (NAHIT).

Private-Sector Organizational Efforts

In addition to the members of the EHR Collaborative, many other organizations have made EHR an initiative. As mentioned earlier, the CPRI was created based on the IOM patient record study; its work has since been transferred to HIMSS. The AHIMA was a contributor to the original IOM patient record study and has steadfastly taken many initiatives to support EHR and the use of health information management (HIM) professionals to support them. The Markle Foundation is another organization that contributed a project on Connecting for Health that carries some of the original CPRI work forward and promotes adoption of clinical data exchange standards, privacy and security, and personal health records. The Leapfrog Group is an organization of more than 150 primarily large companies that provide healthcare benefits to their employees. It promotes contractual incentives for hospitals that take specific steps to reduce harm to patients, most notably via CPOE. The eHealth Initiative is another group of healthcare stakeholders whose mission is to drive improvement in the quality, safety, and efficiency of healthcare through information and information technology.

Vendor Efforts

EHR vendors also have contributed significantly to research and development of EHR systems. Much of the existing standards development has come about through the dedication of vendor staff to the effort. Each product success and failure contains lessons learned. In addition, vendors have taken different approaches—some highly proprietary and others very open. This has provided the industry an opportunity to select applications that meet their specific needs.

EHR Implementation Stages

Much work remains to be done to achieve the fullest possible vision of the EHR. However, the vision expands as each new system is developed and implemented, and will continue to expand as new technology comes into being. Organizations desiring the quantitative and qualitative benefits of the EHR can choose from a variety of options. Historically, "build your own" was the mantra of many, but this mantra is rapidly being replaced with either buy or "borrow." Most providers today buy a commercial off-the-shelf (COTS) product, which is much more affordable and yet still highly customizable. Others acquire EHR functionality through a service, known as an **application service provider** (ASP), that maintains the system and leases usage. Whatever model is chosen to acquire an EHR, strategic planning and a carefully developed migration path need to be constructed. A summary of the implementation stages is provided in figure 3.5.

The stages are discussed briefly as follows:

1. Determine readiness for an EHR. Readiness for an EHR may need to be cultivated if there is resistance to computer use. Determine the readiness state and what needs to be done to ensure adoption by all. A key ingredient is user participation. Time and again, systems have failed to be adopted appropriately or yield their true results because the individuals required to use the system were not involved from the start.

2. Plan the migration path based on a shared vision of the ultimate goal, and then plot a migration strategy to achieve that goal. There may not be a quick fix or instantaneous solution. Although many might like a "big bang" that goes from minimal automation to the vision of the future, it is difficult to pull off in the best of environments. EHR achievement will more likely be an evolution rather than a revolution, although very recently some provider settings have been successful at achieving a revolutionary approach.

Figure 3.5. EHR implementation stages

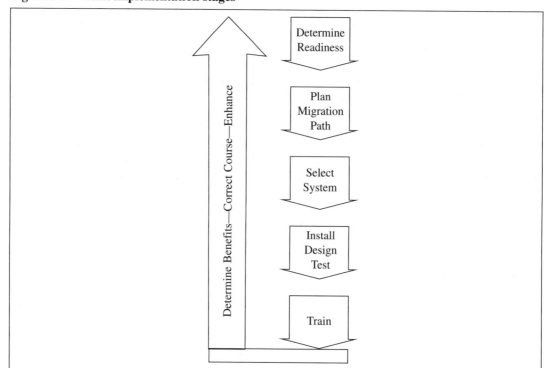

3. Select the EHR system that is right for the organization. Many providers are firmly entrenched with one major vendor, even though the vendor may not be the best for EHR. It may be necessary to compromise and extend the migration path until the vendor catches up, compromise the functionality (especially the customizability) to achieve the best integration with the incumbent vendor, or "bite the bullet" and switch vendors. The organization should conduct a thorough cost–benefit analysis to look at the overall picture.

4. Install, design, and test the system. Plan ahead to anticipate the impact on users, work flow, productivity, and patients. There are many issues, from whether and how implementation will be phased in to how past data will be integrated and old data retained

5. Train, train, and train. User involvement from the beginning is critical to success. So, too, is training. It is not unusual to have more trainers than staff on-site during the actual rollout of an EHR system. Plan for this, advise staff, and work with your vendor to ensure a smooth transition.

6. Determine benefits, correct the course if needed, and enhance the system. A benefits realization study is key to determining the payback. If this is not what was expected, it is a signal for course correction. When benefits are achieved, the results can justify further enhancements.

EHR Selection and Contract Negotiation

As momentum for the electronic health record (EHR) project grows, the selection process supplants planning as the project's critical component. It also is the riskiest component.

Since the IOM coined the term "computer-based patient record" in 1991, the number of vendors selling EHR systems has grown and been reshaped dramatically. In 1995, popular trade publications started listing EHR vendors. One list had eighty vendors, including most of the traditional hospital information systems and physician practice management vendors as well as numerous start-ups. By 2004, the same list had grown to more than 200 vendors, but, in any given year, only a very small percentage remained in business. It is estimated that over the eight years in which EHR vendor listings have been published, more than 500 companies have started selling EHRs and have either dropped out of the market, merged, or been sold (Hudson 2004). This instability in the marketplace, coupled with the complexity of the EHR, makes vendor selection challenging.

Executing EHR Planning

Although some would want to move into vendor selection quickly, the thoroughness of up-front **planning** without vendor influence pays tremendous dividends. EHR strategic planning ensures that the organization is clear about its vision for the EHR and that the EHR complements the organization's strategic initiatives and business plan. Executive management commitment and support are critical success factors in the EHR project. A sample tool for long-term EHR planning is provided in figure 3.6. Developing a migration path to achieve the vision of the EHR establishes a comprehensive plan and benefit expectations that can prevent premature adoption of system elements that might otherwise doom the project. Assessing the processes impacted by the EHR, identifying functional needs, and understanding the data and technology infrastructure help to clarify the functional requirements, establish design parameters, and commit users to change and to achieve specific, measurable return on investment (ROI).

Figure 3.6.   Sample tool for long-term EHR planning

MANAGEMENT INFORMATION SYSTEMS					
	Current	Available, Not Used	Wanted	Priority	Comments
Clinical Applications					
• Develop longitudinal integrated clinical record					
• Decision support					
• Diagnostic episode cluster analysis					
• Discharge plans					
• Disease management					
• Disease state criteria					
• Medication tracking					
• Client education features					
• Pharmacy system					
• Plan of treatment/care plans					
• Prescription assistance					
• Preventative medicine					
• Problem list with automatic updates					
• Protocol/critical pathways					
• Well-care coordination tracking—clinical					
Client Encounter					
• Shows history of present illness					
• Shows diagnostic tests					
• Shows medication profile					
• Client status updates					
• Shows conducted procedures					
• Shows therapies					
• Shows orders and treatment plans					
Laboratory					
• Allows for entry of lab test results that are done in-house					
• Provides an order-entry function for generating lab requests from outside laboratories. These requests can then be printed on forms, plain paper, and/or specimen labels.					
• Capable of interfacing with outside lab services for the electronic receipt of test results					
• Provides immediate, on-line display and long-term storage of lab test results					
• Can allow a staff person to flag lab results that need follow-up. The flags will interface with recall/system.					

Figure 3.6. (Continued)

MANAGEMENT INFORMATION SYSTEMS					
	Current	Available, Not Used	Wanted	Priority	Comments
Outcome					
• Define policy, protocols, and criteria for evaluating clinical outcomes and evaluation, working with the Family Service Team and affiliated agencies. Determine data elements to be collected.					
Communications					
• First generation: —Provide Web-enabled pilot for integrating information and providing linkages to other agencies —Link information/referral lines to enrollment application —Provide electronic communication between financial service center and providers (that is, e-mail, Web site, Internet applications)					
• Second generation: —Secure funding for integrated communication system —Develop integrated communication system —Maintain integrated communication system					
Practice Management Capabilities					
• Contract management	X				
• Data security	X				
• EDI functions for on-line eligibility and referral authorizations	X				
• Electronic claims submission	X				
• Electronic remittance capabilities	X				
• Fully integrated quality care guidelines with compliance tracking					
• HMO roster management					
• Hospital information system links					
• Incoming/outgoing referral tracking					
• Integrated claims adjunction					
• MSO reporting					
• Open item audit trail listing by line item					
• Client demographics					
• Client flow tracking					
• Supports MIP roll-up reporting					

(Continued on next page)

Figure 3.6. (Continued)

MANAGEMENT INFORMATION SYSTEMS					
	Current	**Available, Not Used**	**Wanted**	**Priority**	**Comments**
Functional Components					
▶ *Reports and Accreditation*					
• ORYX reporting—JCAHO					SDCPH using separate Vendor
• AAHP reports					
• Customer service					
• HEDIS reporting					
• Client satisfaction					
• OSHPD reporting					
Business Applications and Managed Care					
• Appropriateness and determination					
• Authorization					
• Benefits alert					
• Benefits management					
• Capitation					
• Carve-out population coordination					
• Case management					
• Catastrophic care coordination					
• Claim/case authorization					
• Claims management/review					
• Concurrent review					
• Contract/pricing management					
• Credentialing	X				
• Develop criteria, data requirements, and formats for management reports on claims, billing, collections, and overall program performance					
• Eligibility tracking	X				
• Episode management	X				
• Fee-for-service encounter	X				
• Membership enrollment	X				
• Precertification					
• Provide application data for processing claims from providers, including matching claims to authorizations and approving claims for payments					

Figure 3.6. (Continued)

MANAGEMENT INFORMATION SYSTEMS					
	Current	Available, Not Used	Wanted	Priority	Comments
Business Applications and Managed Care (Continued)					
• Provide application for compiling data and preparing management reports on claims, billings, and collections					
• Provide application for enrollment and data collection (IAR system)					
• Provide application for evaluating overall program performance outcomes					
• Provide application for paying provider					
• Provide application for submitting claims/bills to payers —Medi-Cal —Federal IV E —Private insurance, other payers					
• Provide applications for receiving payments from payers and reconciling to claims					
• Provide specifications for capability to interface with longitudinal integrated clinical record					
• Rate modeling					
• Referral tracking—to/from	X				
• Severity of illness					
• Third-party/client contract billing	X				
UM					
• Provide application for service authorization and approval					
▶ *Analysis*					
• Benchmarking	X				
• Case-mix analysis	X				
• Management reports	X				
• Medicaid	X				
• Medicare	X				
• Outcome analysis	X				
• Outcomes management					
• Provide capability to link to customer service databases					
• Profit/loss reporting					
• Results recording					
• Simulation					
• Ticklers/reminders					
• Time/effort tracking					

(Continued on next page)

Figure 3.6.   (Continued)

MANAGEMENT INFORMATION SYSTEMS					
	Current	**Available, Not Used**	**Wanted**	**Priority**	**Comments**
▶ *Administrative*					
• Call tracking					
• Inpatient					
• Letter/fax capability					
• Longitudinal management					
• Long-term care coordination					
• Outpatient					
• Risk management					
• Security					
• Scheduling					
Special Features					
• Clinical data repository					
• Clinical encounter documentation					
• Interfaces with electronic image processing					
• Interfaces to wireless, mobile, or handheld devices					
• Speech recognition interfaces					
• Supports provider interfaces					
• Enterprisewide capability					
• User-definable for different parameters					
• Locate client record capability					
• Referral analysis					
• Multiple-encounter support					
• Supports specific specialties					
• Stores provider demographic data					
• Stores client demographic data					
Other					
• ICD-9/CPT4 coding support					
• SNOMED coding system					
• Other coding support					
• Report generator					

Figure 3.6. (Continued)

MANAGEMENT INFORMATION SYSTEMS					
	Current	Available, Not Used	Wanted	Priority	Comments
Grant Billing					
• Can determine the grants for which a client is eligible based on the patient's registration data					
• Able to bill the eligible grant visits to grant sources that use a fixed-fee per visit reimbursement system. Because a client may be eligible for more than one source, the system must have a mechanism for prioritizing the allocation of visits to grant sources to optimize the use of grant funds without double billing for visits.					
• Can automatically compute contractual allowance on grant-billed visits, writing off the balances when the visits are billed					
Platform/Operating System					
• AIX, HP–UX, HP 9000, IBM RS/6000, Windows 3.1/3.11, 95, NT					
Programming Language/Database					
• C++, COBOL, Java, Visual Basic					
Technological Components					
• Client/server					
• Computer–telephony integration					
• Data warehousing/data mining					
• Document imaging/management					
• Electronic commerce					
• Groupware					
• Intranet/Internet	X				
• Mobile computing					
• Work flow					
Technology					
• Encryption technology					
• Object-oriented technology					
• Smart care technology					
• SQL-based technology					

Making the Build–Buy–Borrow–Blend Decision

It is critical that the planning be accomplished before any vendors are contacted. However, there is one other important decision to make prior to initiating a vendor selection process. This decision centers on *how* an EHR is going to be acquired, rather than on *what* the EHR is. Although some organizations are prepared to buy, others consider self-development or using an ASP or some form of outsourcing for their EHR. Often there also is a need to consider the extent of change from the organization's current vendor to a different vendor or mix of vendors.

Self-Development

The build or buy decision is a fairly historical decision. In the past, when there were few EHR vendors and products were not comprehensive, some organizations considered building their own EHR. Some of these systems were developed in academic medical centers or with a commercial partner who was interested in developing an EHR product. Indeed, many of these projects were forerunners to today's EHR systems. Today most organizations recognize that commercial products now can meet their needs and that most will far surpass the functionality that could be self-developed. Still, this decision is not totally dead. Some physicians are intrigued with developing their own, "perfect" system. Some hospitals have development teams they do not want to give up.

However, an organization's decision to build or buy should be based on a careful review of the marketplace because today it is generally more expensive to undertake self-development. Unless self-development is coupled with vendor partnership that leads to commercialization, a self-developed system also can be a drawback when attempting to integrate with commercial products when the organization grows, merges, or acquires affiliates.

ASP/Outsourcing Option

To buy or borrow is often an economic decision. Buying an EHR is a costly proposition. It requires considerable access to capital as well as considerable ongoing support for maintenance and upgrades. However, many organizations are considering outsourcing or ASP models as ways to borrow or lease EHR functionality. This acquisition strategy provides an EHR without the heavy capital outlays and IT staffing that buying an EHR entails.

Essentially, an ASP is an arrangement that involves a customer paying a fee to access a software application that resides on secure computers managed off-site by a vendor. This model of acquiring computing power is actually not new; many organizations shared computing services when computer mainframes were first being developed. Today new technologies have enhanced the basic service bureau business model of leasing access to sophisticated systems.

There is a variety of types of ASPs. One form hosts various applications developed by a number of software vendors from a remote data center and delivers them to its customers over a secure Internet connection or a private network. Another type of ASP manages and supports is own software applications while partnering with telecommunications and data center companies to deliver a complete solution to its customers. Another variation is the vertical service provider (VSP), which focuses on offering industry-specific application hosting services to customers in a particular vertical market, such as healthcare. VSPs may target specific applications such as diagnostics, medical record management, purchasing, claims processing, scheduling, or human resources.

Another option is outsourcing. **Outsourcing** is a contractual relationship with a specialized outside service provider for work traditionally done in-house. In some respects, it is broader than ASP because ASP generally refers to the utilization of computer services, whereas outsourcing can include both computer services and various management services. Outsourcing sometimes is equated with the use of offshore services. However, outsourcing does not have to be offshore or even off-premises. It can provide management of services directly at the provider's site.

There are advantages and disadvantages to the ASP/outsourcing model. These are summarized in table 3.1.

As with any set of advantages and disadvantages, careful management of the process can offset disadvantages and capitalize on advantages. Perhaps the most critical element of ASP/outsourcing is a strong service-level agreement (SLA) that establishes the terms of service the ASP/outsourcers will provide.

Best of Breed, Best of Fit, or Best of Suite?

Another consideration with respect to acquiring an EHR is whether to continue with an existing vendor's product line, mix vendor products, or scrap an existing set of vendor products for a new set. This decision occurs because many information systems (IS) products have been highly proprietary. This means that when a commitment is made to acquire, for example, a hospital information system (or a practice management system for a physician office) from one vendor, fitting products from other vendors becomes more difficult. "Best of fit," or single source, is a scenario in which the products in one vendor's suite of products fit well together and it is difficult to introduce other vendors' products. "Best of breed" is a situation where the best products are selected from various vendors. Unless best-of-breed products are open source—meaning the source code is readily available, is technology neutral, and does not restrict use of other software—they are more difficult to integrate (Open Source Initiative 2004; Briggs 2003).

Most healthcare organizations have tended toward best-of-fit scenarios, with only occasional use of another vendor for a very specific application, which usually is a stand-alone application. However, some vendors who offer very tightly integrated products (that is, highly proprietary) have not always kept up with the marketplace in the latest EHR technology. In this case, providers have had to think about compromising on functionality with their existing vendor or spending a lot of money on interfacing other products. Most providers are very reluctant to scrap an entire infrastructure, although doing so is not entirely unheard of, especially when the systems are very old or have not been regularly upgraded.

In deciding whether to wait out a best-of-fit vendor's EHR strategy, adopt a best-of-breed strategy, or literally switch to an entirely new vendor, "best of suite" is another option to consider. Best of suite is essentially a blend of one predominant vendor plus other niche vendors. Some vendors have recognized that they are unable to provide every solution for everyone and have been developing systems to accommodate a more blended approach.

Selecting a Vendor

Whatever decisions are made about building, buying, borrowing, or blending hardware, software, and peopleware to achieve the vision of the EHR, a purchase decision is generally involved. The organization must decide whether to select an ASP or outsourcing company, purchase additional components, and/or upgrade to entirely new system.

Table 3.1. ASP/outsourcing advantages and disadvantages

Advantages	Disadvantages
Lower up-front costs for hardware and installation	Loss of customizability
Software becomes an operating cost versus capital expenditure	Integration issues if ASP/outsourced functions must connect to in-house systems
Fewer data center headaches	Potential higher cost over long term
Access to new technologies	Loss of control/accountability issues

In going through a selection process, it is important to keep in mind that the vendors' marketing efforts are designed to show their products and services in the best light possible and to mask shortcomings (Reed 1998). The lack of objective information about EHR products makes it difficult for healthcare organizations to compare the capabilities of the various products currently available on the market.

Controlling the Selection Process

As the organization begins to undertake vendor selection, it should control interactions with vendors to ensure a fair, common representation of products and to keep marketing hype and accusations of competitive advantage to a minimum. Most organizations require all vendor interactions to go through one designated individual. The vendors that make the first cut should be treated evenly, with equal opportunity to demonstrate their products and interact with the selection team. In addition, the organization should select firm criteria.

The healthcare organization is buying a product or service, not salesmanship. This is as true for a poor salesperson as for a good one. Some have suggested that the more marketing techniques a salesperson must apply to the product, the less likely the product meets the requirements to sell itself. People can be highly swayed by friendliness, fancy dinners, and promises. Likewise, they can be turned off by surly salespersons who show little interest in the organization, even though their product may be outstanding.

Controlling the selection process is as much about *looking past* the salesperson as it is about *looking at* the product. The vendor's salesperson will *not* be responsible for installation, training, or ongoing support. A good salesperson represents the company as a whole and should be a member of a collaborative team that learns the buyer's needs, understands its business requirements, and offers proactive suggestions. However, the bottom line is that the salesperson's responsibility is sales. He or she will not be around when there are implementation problems.

In the EHR marketplace, it is important to recognize that the products are not commodities. Although many good EHR products are on the market, they differ from each other significantly. A good product for one organization will not necessarily be a good product for another. This fact emphasizes the need for thorough planning and a carefully controlled selection process.

Figure 3.7 provides a schematic of a process that most healthcare organizations find helpful in narrowing down the universe of potential EHR vendors. The process really is about using a set of filters to focus the candidate pool on the organization's specific requirements.

Most lists of EHR vendors include a wide variety of products and services, not just EHR products. In fact, some would suggest that an EHR product is as difficult to define as the EHR itself. Typically, however, an EHR product is considered to be one that provides data capture and retrieval at the point of care, integrates data from multiple sources, and supports evidence-based clinical decision making. This would mean that an EHR product needs a robust user interface, data integration and/or data repository functionality, and a rules engine and/or other analytical tools to support knowledge management.

Differentiating among Associated Products and Services

Associated products and services generally provide one, but not all, of the components inherent in an EHR product or provide supporting services. The vendors of associated products and services often include EHR consultants, systems integrators, component producers, and niche or specialty products.

EHR Consultants

EHR consultants provide everything from EHR strategic planning, process redesign, and vendor selection to system integration, implementation, and ASP services or outsourcing support. Any, all, or none of these types of consultants may be appropriate for your project.

Figure 3.7. Vendor selection process

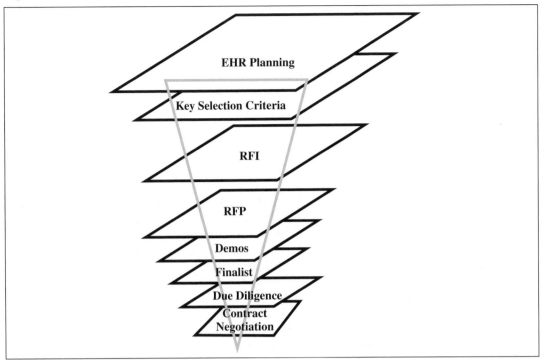

Many organizations find that a consultant is extremely helpful in facilitating definition of the EHR vision and overseeing process redesign efforts. A consultant for this aspect of the project should be open-minded, an excellent communicator, and someone who values details but is not mired in minutiae. The organization's users should take ownership of process redesign but will likely need direction and support.

Many organizations also prefer to have a consultant oversee the vendor selection process. In this case, the consultant should have a broad range of experience and be highly vendor neutral. Many organizations take as much care in selecting their EHR consultant as they do in selecting the EHR itself. However, many organizations also make the mistake of engaging a consultant who they perceive can carry them through all phases of the project—from visioning through implementation to ongoing support and benefits realization. This is often not the best strategy because a consultant who has sufficient experience in implementing a given product is likely to be highly biased toward that product and generally is not right for the planning stages.

Most organizations need to supplement their own staff with persons who can help implement the product. In many cases, the vendor itself supplies these persons. In other cases, the vendor outsources this function. In still other situations, the organization may decide to obtain its own consultants or use a mix of vendor and other resources. Too many different companies involved in the project can become a project management nightmare. However, where there are unusual interfaces to be developed, an accelerated time line, or special types of technology, it may be necessary to have multiple companies providing services.

Systems Integrators

Systems integrators are companies, or parts of companies, that specialize in getting disparate vendor products to work together. They may write interface programs or supply an interface engine, which is a software tool that manages connections among many disparate systems. Sometimes this is called middleware.

An interface engine supports multiple communications protocols, including (but not exclusively) HL7, by mapping data formats between two otherwise incompatible applications (for example, HL7 and XML). In addition to connectivity, an interface engine also supports enhanced security functionality. Within the clinical information **context,** CCOW is a vendor-independent standard developed by HL7 to support clinical application integration. CCOW stands for **Clinical Context Object Workgroup** and achieves simultaneous sign-on to multiple clinical applications by using mapping agents that map equivalent identifiers without sharing the same identification information for patients or users (often referred to as single sign-on) (CCOW 1999–2003).

Component Producers

Component producers sell products that support the EHR. Although the EHR relies on all source systems as well as point-of-care data capture for its data, there are a number of tools that manage the data in a variety of ways. Some of these may be data capture tools, such as document-imaging systems and voice recognition systems. Other tools serve to process the data. These might include an enterprisewide master person index or a data repository. The system integration tools mentioned earlier could be considered component products. Many of the CPOE, e-prescribing, and bar code medication administration (BCMA) tools are important components of an EHR.

Components may be sold separate and apart from EHR systems or be incorporated into EHR systems. When they are separate from an EHR system, they perform the one function they are designed to serve. When they are well integrated, they support much more robust functionality.

Niche or Specialty Products

Niche or specialty products provide EHR systems that are primarily designed for one type of clinical specialty. For example, the field of behavioral health services is quite different from that of general medical/surgical services. Certain vendors support EHRs exclusively for behavioral health services. Many specialty-based EHR products have been designed for physician office specialties. Still other products have been designed for cardiologists, nephrologists, family practitioners, and other specialties.

Narrowing the Universe of Vendors

No healthcare organization has the resources to evaluate hundreds of vendors to find one that will be the best fit. Most organizations narrow the universe of vendors by developing a short list of key criteria and then issuing a request for information (RFI) to some twenty to thirty vendors (at most) in an effort to focus on perhaps four or five to evaluate seriously. When the field is narrowed to a manageable number, the organization issues a **request for proposal** (RFP) to obtain more detailed information.

Key Selection Criteria

Organizations should draw from their planning activities to establish a set of initial vendor-screening criteria. Questions to ask include:

- Does the vendor share the organization's *vision* for the EHR?

- Does the vendor's product provide the key *functionality* needed to achieve the organization's vision?

- Does the vendor utilize the desired *technology?*

- Does the vendor qualify under the organization's *acquisition* policies?
- Can the vendor support the organization's desired *implementation* strategy?
- What is the vendor's track record for *operations and maintenance* support?
- What is the vendor's understanding of the *implications* of implementing an EHR system?

As discussed earlier, many healthcare organizations hire outside advisors to help them develop a short list of specific criteria and to evaluate the vendors against those criteria. Outside advisors often can help the EHR steering committee avoid becoming mired in detail at this stage. For instance, functionality is likely to be a key criterion and be substantiated by a long list of very specific functions the organization desires. At this stage, however, organizations should raise their level of evaluation to high-level functionality. For example, for a physician office EHR system, prescription refill, E/M coding support, and referral management might be the most important functions required in an EHR. For a hospital, the most important functions might be CPOE, bar code medication administration, and patient care charting. At this stage, it would be inappropriate to look at the format of the prescription refill request or the nature of the screen that provides patient care charting.

Request for Information

Many times, the external advisor sends out an RFI on the organization's behalf (without identifying the organization). In this way, the key criteria can be evaluated without the organization being inundated with vendors attempting to make sales calls. Generally, an RFI is limited to a two- or three-page set of questions on the following areas:

- *Company background:* To obtain information on the vendor's size and financial stability

- *Product information:* To obtain the product name, primary market, technical platform, and overview of product capabilities that will be matched with key functionality criteria

- *Market information:* To ask the vendor to identify its major competitors and explain how the vendor differs from them

- *Installed base and clients:* To identify the number of EHR products the vendor has sold, is currently implementing, and has fully installed

- *Special criteria:* To collect information on any unique features or functions the vendor has established as critical

Figure 3.8 is a vendor comparison map that can be used to plot the responses to the RFI. This tool helps narrow down a large list of vendors.

The vendor comparison map can accommodate any limited number of key criteria an organization desires. The figure illustrates the following hypothetical example:

A physician office has identified four major criteria to consider in making the initial cut. As an ambulatory care organization, its primary focus is outpatient work flow. Thus, it wants a vendor that can supply a full product suite in case the organization wants to replace its outdated practice management system. It also anticipates increased managed care contracting and thus wants to be able to move into that operation with the same vendor. Although wanting new technology, the organization is unwilling to risk accepting a new market entrant but, rather, prefers to buy from a stable vendor. Some sixteen vendors (labeled A through P for illustrative purposes) were considered likely candidates and plotted on a vendor comparison map. The vendors in the upper-right quadrant are the most suitable for the organization to evaluate further. In this case, five vendors will receive RFPs.

Figure 3.8.   Vendor comparison map

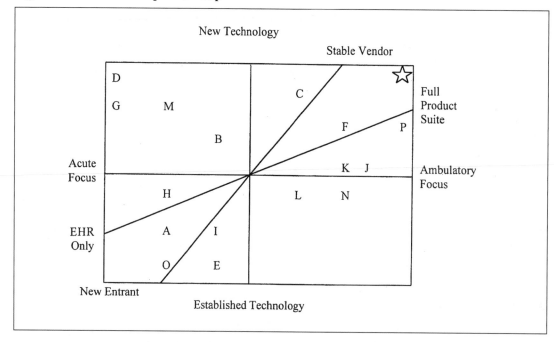

In making the initial selection of vendors to send RFPs to, external advisors can offer neutral and unbiased advice, generally based on their broader familiarity with the marketplace. In some cases, organizations may find that some of their staff members, especially those serving on the EHR steering committee and even some representatives of facilities within an integrated delivery system, may already have experience with one or more EHR products. Their experience may be as a direct user or the result of having seen product demonstrations at trade shows. However, sometimes these individuals can be blinded by the sales pitch or even have a vested interest in the selection of a particular vendor.

Request for Proposal (RFP)

An RFP is a formal document sent to vendors inviting them to submit bids for the organization's EHR project. Some industry observers suggest that RFPs no longer serve their intended purpose because they often lack substance. However, a well-constructed RFP serves two important purposes. First, it solidifies the planning information and organizational requirements into a single document. In a way, it is the culmination of the organization's strategic EHR planning. There is value in bringing this information together for the EHR steering committee and the organization as a whole. Second, when developed and managed correctly, the RFP provides valuable insights into the vendor's operations and products and tends to level the playing field in terms of asking all the vendors the same questions.

It requires skill to write an RFP that results in more than a set of checkmarks in a yes column on a form. The intent of the RFP should be to elicit a description of how the vendor believes its product solves the healthcare organization's specific problems and meets its requirements.

The RFP usually has some fairly standard components. Following are examples of RFP components:

- *Organizational profile:* The first section describes the healthcare organization, including its basic demographics, mission and goals, vision for the EHR, current information infrastructure, and specific constraints (such as its particular time line). This section also contains the organization's instructions for responding (for example, whom the bid should be sent to, how many copies, and how vendor questions will be handled).

- *Vendor information:* This section, which may be placed next or last in the proposal, asks the vendor for a description of its demographics. The description should include the vendor's size and longevity (years in business, revenues, profitability, number of employees), product research and development history and plans, types of installations (number, size, status), corporate composition (organizational makeup, employee qualifications and tenure, country in which the majority of work is performed), references, user group information (leader, size, frequency of meetings), and contract history (any defaults, pending lawsuits, IRS status).

- *Functional specifications:* In this section, the organization requests a description of functional capability, such as the process flows the product supports, and compares it against its redesigned processes. Alternatively, the organization may develop a script describing a scenario based on its redesigned processes and may ask the vendor how its product would perform them. This approach can be useful in avoiding yes and no responses but is difficult to write.

- *Operational requirements:* This section should elicit information on the EHR product's data **architecture**, analytical processes supported, necessary interfaces, reliability and security features, system capacity, expansion capabilities, response time, downtime, and other issues associated with system maintenance.

- *Technical requirements:* In this section, the vendor should propose the appropriate technical architecture to meet the organization's EHR functional specifications and operational requirements, delineating the specific hardware, networking, and software requirements.

- *Application support:* The vendor uses this section to propose an implementation schedule and to describe data conversion, acceptance-testing approach, training, and documentation, as well as the ongoing support, maintenance, and upgrades it will supply.

- *Licensing and contractual details:* In this section, the vendor is asked to supply one-time cost estimates and recurring costs based on the organization's requirements. This section also should include a request for the vendor's standard contract, financing arrangements, proposed relationships with hardware vendors, and warranty information. Some vendors enter into risk-sharing, risk/reward, outsourcing, or co-development contracts that relate payment directly to achieving goals (Schneider 1998). Moreover, this section should include clauses that protect the healthcare organization in the event the vendor goes out of business.

  Many organizations request that the pricing information be provided in a separate section of the response. Doing so removes the influence of cost from other critical factors. Pricing models vary considerably among vendors, and it is often easier for a financial specialist to attempt to normalize these for comparison purposes before the EHR steering or selection committee reviews them.

- *Evaluation criteria:* Some organizations add their evaluation criteria to the RFP so that the vendor knows up front the most important elements of the evaluation. This would indicate how the organization weighs various factors. For instance, evaluation criteria may identify that cost is weighed at 50 percent of the organization's decision-making criteria or that it is acceptable for the vendor to outsource interface development, but not maintenance.

Organizations and external advisors may have standard RFP formats or alternatives that they prefer to use.

Managing the Vendor Selection Process

Managing the RFP issuance, receipt, and evaluation is as important as preparing its content. RFPs should be sent to all vendors on the organization's short list at the same time, and all vendors should be given the same amount of time to respond. If a vendor requests an extension, it should be granted only for extenuating circumstances and only before any other vendor has submitted a response. All vendors then should be notified immediately that they have an equal extension period. (A request for an extension that is for anything other than perhaps a natural disaster or the death of the CEO should be viewed as a red flag for potential problems.)

Bergeron (1999) suggests that issuance of the RFP instantly establishes a "competitive feeding frenzy." The EHR steering committee should discuss the potential (inevitability) of this occurring and plan for it directly. Some organizations try to keep potential vendors' identities confidential; others include the potential vendors' names in the RFP. A middle ground is perhaps more common: The short list is not revealed, but respondents are not kept secret (which is virtually impossible anyway). Most organizations do not accept proposals from any vendor other than the ones to whom RFPs have been directed. If an exception is made, the EHR steering committee should vote on it and give the vendor no extra time, unless the committee deems the omission to be an oversight on the part of the organization. When sufficient planning and careful construction of the selection criteria have taken place, this should not occur.

Some organizations hold a bidders' conference to respond to questions about the RFP. In this situation, the RFPs include the specific date, time, and location for the conference. Any vendor may attend and ask questions. Thus, all vendors hear all questions and obtain the same answers, keeping the playing field even. Unfortunately, most vendors either do not attend or attend only to learn what other vendors are asking.

When no bidders' conference is scheduled, the organization should decide whether it will respond to questions, who will respond, and how. Notifying vendors that questions must be put in writing and that the questions and answers will be shared with all vendors receiving the RFP can serve the same purpose as a bidders' conference. How tightly the bidding process is controlled is up to the organization.

Evaluating the RFP

A first step in RFP evaluation may be to assess the vendor's overall response: Was it received early or on time? Did the vendor ask appropriate questions or simply questions to gain competitive advantage? Did the vendor follow the organization's instructions on how to respond? The answers to these and other such questions can be very revealing. The organization also may want to learn why certain vendors did not respond.

After obtaining some initial impressions, the organization should do an in-depth analysis of the responses and how they compare to the selection criteria. Because a comprehensive EHR is a big project, some organizations find it useful to allocate sections of it to different subject teams for in-depth evaluation. The teams then report back to the group as a whole. Many organizations use some form of scoring methodology to evaluate the proposal against the criteria and a formal group process technique to ensure everyone's input.

A Likert scale may be used to do a quantitative analysis on the results of the RFP. Figure 3.9 provides an example of a Likert scale, which compares six vendors (A through F) against ten weighted selection criteria.

The figure illustrates the following hypothetical example:

A hospital has prioritized ten criteria. It has assigned a simple numeric weight to each criterion, ranging from 1 (least important) to 10 (most important). (It is possible to use a different scale and assign different weights to each criterion. For example, a scale of 1 to 5 may be used. The first two criteria may be considered most important and both weighted as 5, the next three may be weighted as 3, and the remaining 5 weighted as 2.)

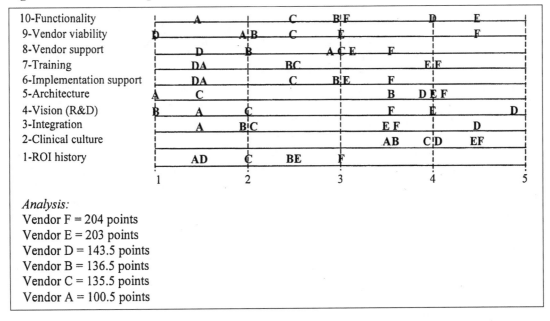

Figure 3.9. Vendor comparison on Likert scale

	1	2	3	4	5
10-Functionality	A	C	B F	D	E
9-Vendor viability	D	A B C	E		F
8-Vendor support	D	B	A C E	F	
7-Training	DA	BC		E F	
6-Implementation support	DA	C	B E	F	
5-Architecture	A C			B D E F	
4-Vision (R&D)	B A	C		F E	D
3-Integration	A	B C	E F	D	
2-Clinical culture				AB C D	EF
1-ROI history	AD	C	BE F		

Analysis:
Vendor F = 204 points
Vendor E = 203 points
Vendor D = 143.5 points
Vendor B = 136.5 points
Vendor C = 135.5 points
Vendor A = 100.5 points

To calculate each vendor's score, the sum of each criterion's weight is multiplied by the vendor's rating on that criterion. (In figure 3.9, vendor A earned 1.5 on the first criterion weighted 10, thus the 10 × 1.5 equals 15; it earned 2.0 on the second criterion weighted 9, the 9 × 2.0 equals 18; and so on. These are then totaled. In this case, vendor A earned a total of 100.5 points.)

In the final analysis, vendors F and E have the most potential for this organization because they are 60 points ahead of the next group of vendors consisting of D, B, and C.

At the conclusion of this evaluation, one vendor may rise to the top or several vendors may warrant further, in-depth review. At this stage, it is important to rule out any vendors who are below par.

One thing that few organizations discuss but that might be considered at this stage is the concept of good customership. Customers often chide vendors for their sales tactics and "vaporware," and yet vendors often expend considerable resources in responding to RFPs, conducting demonstrations, and performing other legitimate sales activities. Although these expenses are factored into the price of the product, frivolous demands should be avoided. When the organization is not serious about a particular vendor after reviewing the RFP, it should eliminate the vendor as politely as possible and extend appreciation for the vendor's response.

Determining the Vendor Finalist(s)

The next set of steps should culminate in identifying a single vendor with whom to begin contract negotiation. Some consultants suggest that the wisest approach is to narrow the field to two vendors and negotiate with the primary candidate first, leaving the second choice available in the event contract negotiations break down. Again, good customership is advised. If the process of contract negotiation is expected to be fairly rapid, a second vendor may be able to be managed. But there are many variables in contract negotiation and a second vendor kept waiting for a very long time may become frustrated and not provide the best second choice. If the negotiation fails with the first vendor, the organization may opt to begin the process again instead of returning to the second vendor (Cohen 2004).

Most organizations invite the vendors who have passed the initial RFP phase to conduct a demonstration of their EHR products on-site. Demonstrations are valuable for several reasons, even in cases where the organization has viewed demonstrations previously. First, the demonstration acquaints as many of the potential users as possible with the product to make everyone feel a part of the process and to obtain everyone's feedback. Potentially hundreds of persons may view a demonstration, and so a feedback mechanism should be devised to focus on the highlights. A second reason to conduct a demonstration is to evaluate products side by side. Finally, the demonstration illustrates the vendor's understanding of the organization's specific requirements. The requirements should be reflected in how the vendor conducts the post-RFP demonstration; earlier demonstrations probably would have been generic.

As with the RFP, one option for the organization is to prepare a script the vendor must follow during demonstrations to highlight the key processes the organization wants to observe. Although vendors will not be able to completely customize a product to match the script, through the use of PowerPoint® and Visual Basic® programming language, they should at least be able to simulate processes to meet the organization's requirements. This is an excellent test of whether the vendor fully understands the organization's situation. If the vendor cannot meet a specific requirement and indicates this fact during the demonstration, its honesty is certainly a point in its favor as long as the requirement was not a major factor.

However, it is important to be aware that just as vendors are easily able to create a simulation, they also can create an illusion. (After all, that is how they create vaporware. However, it is appropriate to remember that from the vendor's perspective, what organizations consider vaporware may be considered a prototype to evaluate response to product ideas.) The EHR product being demonstrated in response to the RFP should be based on the current, real release of the product, and any attempt to do otherwise should disqualify the vendor.

A demonstration is often conducted in several segments. One segment is for many users who will spend just five or ten minutes at the demonstration to get a sense of the look and feel of the product. A small, but important, use of the product should be scripted for such a purpose. Another segment might be a one- or two-hour demonstration of a more comprehensive scenario for members of the steering committee. In this segment, committee members should challenge the vendor and encourage the vendor to ask questions. The steering committee should include users of all types, including physicians, other clinicians, and administrative professionals. This ensures that all aspects of the EHR are thoroughly evaluated. A demonstration also may be planned for the organization's technical team to evaluate the interfaces, see the source code, understand modification procedures, and so on.

Vendors should be given adequate time to set up their equipment and test their software and network connections. Some organizations try to have all the vendors demonstrate at the same time but in separate locations. When this is not feasible, conducting the demonstrations as close together in time as possible is important for comparison purposes. As soon after the demonstrations as possible, evaluations should be collected and the selection committee debriefed.

Attending Site Visits

Organizations often visit vendor client sites that are similar to their own. The purpose of the visits is to assess the vendor's product in action. Site visits offer an opportunity to learn about the installation process and obtain feedback from direct users. Even though most vendors arrange site visits at their "best" sites, there are still valuable lessons to be learned. (The organization should pay for the trip and not accept the vendor's offer to do so.)

The site visit team should include a small (five to seven people), representative group composed of clinician users, information management representatives, and managers. Typically, this is a core group of the larger steering committee. It is preferable to have the same group go on all visits. Generally, one or two visits per vendor are made, and often visits are made to the clients of the two candidates that lead the field after the demonstrations.

It is advisable to establish an agenda for the site visit. The vendor may be present during introductions, but the rest of the site visit must be done without the vendor present. Team members should not hesitate to speak to people other than those scheduled (and potentially primed by the vendor). It is useful to observe as many people as possible who are not on the formal agenda. (Insofar as possible, these individuals should be typical users.) Even so, because the site needs its vendor to survive, people working at the site rarely give the vendor bad marks. In addition, questions will need to be crafted carefully so that the responses reveal important insights about the vendor's level of service and support without offending the vendor's representatives. Another reason to proceed cautiously is that vendors may have outsourced staff to the site; thus, it is possible that some of the IS staff, trainers, and others at the site may actually be employees of the vendor.

At the conclusion of each site visit, participants should be debriefed immediately before they forget their impressions or confuse their reactions with those they had at other site visits.

Checking References

At the same time that site visits are being conducted, reference calls should be made to as many of the vendor's other clients as possible. The organization has the right to ask for a complete list of the vendor's clients, and any vendor who does not provide a list at this point should be suspected of having something to hide.

As for site visits, an agenda should be established for conducting reference calls to ensure that no key questions are forgotten. A conference call or a series of calls to talk with equivalent users, technical staff, and administrators might be a useful tactic. Moreover, conversations with the leaders of the vendor's user group and reviews of agendas and meeting attendance lists can be helpful in supplementing reference checks.

Conducting Corporate Visits

If after site visits and reference checks it is still difficult to narrow the field to one vendor, a few other activities may be undertaken. One such activity is a corporate visit. Representatives from the healthcare organization, such as the CEO, the CFO, and medical director, meet with their counterparts at the vendor's company. The CIO may meet with the vendor's technical staff.

Corporate visits are particularly helpful when the organization is considering a codevelopment arrangement or some other special type of contract relationship.

Creating the Implementation Plan

Another activity that is useful in making the finalist selection is to request that the vendor's technical staff conduct a walk-through of the healthcare organization. This activity would help ensure that the vendors fully understand the technical infrastructure that exists and any customization that may be required. The walk-through should result in a detailed implementation plan and firm up any potential change in the initial cost estimates provided in the RFP.

Most organizations phase in EHR projects because EHR projects are so large and impose significant change. Some organizations may want to conduct a pilot program even before they consider phasing in a full implementation. Because the difference between conducting a pilot program and phasing in implementation can have a significant impact on contract negotiations, it is important to understand the purposes of both options.

A pilot program is a limited implementation of a proposed change for a selected group, after which the organization decides whether it will proceed with the rest of the project. A phased implementation is a confirmed project carried out in small segments over a period of time until all groups are implemented. Sometimes organizations can save money by having the vendor do the first few phases and then having the organization complete the rest. Phased implementation helps manage the impact of change on the organization whereas a pilot program is part of the decision-making process.

Healthcare organizations may decide to conduct pilot EHR programs for any number of reasons—for example, to determine the project's potential ROI, to compare the features of competing products, to determine the product's fit with the organization, to validate new hardware or software, to buy time to gain user acceptance, or to determine the organization's readiness for an EHR system. Often the underlying reason for conducting a pilot program, however, is other factors, including the fear of change, difficulty in managing change, insufficient funding, and uncertainty about whether any EHR will fulfill its potential. All of these factors are poor reasons to do a pilot; in such environments, pilots are likely to fail.

Another consideration is that for a pilot program to be successful, the vendor must install most of the product so that the organization can evaluate its interfaces and users can obtain the full value of data collection from source systems. Vendors recognize the issues presented by pilots and often steer clear of them. Unless a vendor is a new market entrant and needs a foot in the door, most vendors offer phasing and some have begun to offer risk-sharing contracts instead of pilots. A vendor that accepts a pilot contract will necessarily have to price the project higher than a phased project to overcome the risk. Sometimes the difference can be recouped by accepting the full product within a designated period of time (Amatayakul and Cohen 1999).

When an EHR project is phased in, consideration should be given to whether a direct cutover or parallel conversion will be used. The direct cutover has the advantage of not having to maintain two systems, but it requires considerable up-front preparation, including uploading data for active patients either before the cutover or as each patient is scheduled. Parallel conversion is more comfortable because the organization knows that everything is backed up, but it sometimes extends reliance on paper systems into perpetuity.

Often the nature of the organization (inpatient or outpatient, size, number of locations) and the extent of data already automated determine the form of conversion. Straight cutovers and parallel conversions are rarely done for an entire EHR implementation except in a small environment.

Making the Final Decision

Ultimately, the organization must narrow the field to a single vendor with which it will conduct final due diligence and contract negotiation. Usually the steering committee is responsible for recommending the finalist, although the decision is best made with input from all participants.

No product will meet all of the organization's requirements exactly. Customization is possible, but adapting the organization's requirements to adjust to a close match keeps costs down. Moreover, customization can have a long-term impact on the organization's ability to implement system upgrades successfully.

Even at this point in the project, the tendency may still exist to hold on to old, familiar ways. Vendors encourage the organization to recognize the need to redesign its processes. On its part, the organization has planned for a redesign and should be able to blend its generic redesign with the vendor's proposed solution in a way that satisfies most of the participants in the process.

Price should be the last factor considered in finalist selection. Many factors influence the pricing of EHR products. Hard-line negotiation seldom proves beneficial over the long term. At this point, prices should not be significantly different across the vendor finalists unless the products are significantly different. If the products are significantly different, the decision is often one of price versus functionality. When balancing functionality and price, the organization must consider its migration strategy carefully. It may be appropriate to phase in functionality, and good vendors should be able to show how this can be done. Alternatively, being penny-wise and pound-foolish can result in problems down the road, as the following hypothetical scenario illustrates:

A large group practice bought a comprehensive EHR system and expected to achieve significant cost savings through clinical decision support. Unable to fund workstations for every examining room, the practice decided to provide interim functionality through printouts and to have physicians use workstations centralized at the nurses' stations. Even though queues rarely formed at the workstations, physicians found the practice inconvenient and got their nurses to enter their data. Not only did this defeat the opportunity to benefit from clinical decision support at the point of care, but it also reduced the expected benefit to nursing personnel. The bottom line was that the physicians were essentially unhappy with the system. Although an investment in more workstations would have paid for itself, the physicians would not agree to the expenditure, seeing the entire system as being less than successful and beneficial only from an operational, not a clinical, view.

The following hypothetical example illustrates a successful implementation:

An integrated delivery system with many small- and medium-sized physician practice affiliates scattered across nearly an entire state needed a way to improve communications. Physician practices varied greatly, from not having an EHR to having fairly sophisticated systems. The IDS considered investing in the purchase of a single system for all affiliates. At the time, the cost was prohibitive, but supporting a Web-enabled system to exchange data and to begin feeding a repository was a significant advantage to all practices. Such a system also would accomplish a common look and feel among the hospitals and the practices. When practices wanted more functionality or upgrades for their current systems, they migrated to a common vendor.

Performing Due Diligence and Negotiating the Contract

The final steps before "signing on the dotted line" are final due diligence to investigate the vendor and contract negotiation.

Due Diligence

Demonstrations, site visits, and reference checks are all parts of due diligence. However, these activities focus primarily on the product. The healthcare organization also needs an in-depth understanding of the vendor company.

Credit checks on the company and its officers are essential. Depending on whether the company is public, some information may be easier to obtain than other information. Still, considering the size of the investment the healthcare organization is making, even a nonpublic company should disclose reasonable financial information at this point. The market status of other products in the vendor's product line is also a good indicator of its financial status and ability to meet its contractual obligations (Grams 1998).

Contract Negotiation

The following discussion is not a substitute for legal advice but provides some tried-and-true suggestions for effective contract negotiation.

Contract negotiation begins with folding in a copy of the original RFP and the vendor's response into the vendor's standard contract. The final implementation plan should be included in the contract because, by themselves, the vendor's response to the RFP and the organization's RFP are not legally binding documents.

Contracts should include a milestone-based payment schedule based on issues such as installation period, customer use, satisfaction, and projected savings. Compensation adjustments for product delivery delays and nonperformance should be specified. Maintenance contracts should include a clause that correlates problems with appropriate response times.

The Healthcare Financial Management Association (HFMA) has compiled a guide to IT contract negotiation that identifies ten critical components. These are included in table 3.2.

Table 3.2. Critical contract negotiation components

Component	Description
1. Product definition and contract structure	• Define the system components covered by the contract; include response to the RFP to ensure comprehensive functionality description • Determine whether software license agreement, maintenance provisions (including service-level agreement), and installation agreement are included in one contract or separate contracts
2. Scope of license	• Recommends a fully paid, perpetual, royalty-free, nonexclusive, nontransferable license for use by, or on behalf of, affiliates, as specified • Reviews a vendor's standard set of restrictions on licenses and negotiates incremental pricing, if necessary
3. Pricing structure	• One-time costs • Ongoing maintenance, including response to federal regulations • Operational changes
4. Implementation	• Includes specific work plan for implementation • Includes provisions for breach of agreement
5. Key personnel	• Qualifications • Replacement provisions • Third parties • Selection rights for key staff
6. Acceptance testing and payment terms	• Define testing stages (unit testing, integration testing, interface/network testing, stress testing, and live testing) • Define acceptance at each stage • Provide for correction of errors • Provide for resting and remedies
7. Performance warranties	• Response time • Uptime • Batch processing throughput assurance
8. Limitations on liability	• Ensure mutuality of liability • Insurances
9. Change in vendor control and product obsolescence	• Defines triggering events • Identifies remedies if a triggering event occurs • Identifies exclusions for limitation of liability
10. Dispute resolution and exit strategies	• Process • Mediation or binding arbitration • Exit clauses that outline right to deliverables and interim payment

Source: Adapted from HFMA 2004.

Conclusion

Planning and implementing an EHR system is a significant undertaking for any healthcare organization. Although the concept of the EHR is not new, the industry is now just beginning to fully appreciate the complexity of the integration required to achieve a comprehensive EHR. Indeed, many of the means to carry out the objectives of the EHR are still emerging. Major stumbling blocks in the form of content, value of information, and technological limitations are just beginning to be addressed. But there is no time like the present. Because of the rapid rate of change in information technology, putting off electronic health record implementation until "it becomes more affordable," "more proven," or "more acceptable" only puts off a new and different set of issues.

Although the EHR project is not just about vendor selection, vendor selection is its most obvious activity. Planning is critical to successful vendor selection. The organization that understands its environment, information needs, functional requirements, and ability to effect change will have a much easier time articulating its needs to potential vendors and helping users adapt to the system. Such planning reflects an organization that is well run and carries over into managing the selection process and the installation. Every element of planning has an impact on the selection and installation process.

Specific vendor selection is essentially the application of filters to the universe of vendors. The filters are formed through the organization's advanced planning and should be applied through unbiased facilitation.

The conclusion of the vendor selection process is successful contract negotiation, which also is the start of implementation and ongoing maintenance.

References and Resources

Altis, Inc. 1999–2004. Assessing an Interface Engine. Available on-line at www.altisinc.com/IE/assess.html.

Amatayakul, M., M. Brandt, and M. Dougherty. 2003. Cut, copy, paste: EHR guidelines. *Journal of the American Health Information Management Association* 74(9):72,74.

Amatayakul, M., and M. Cohen. 1999 (May 1). Conducting a successful EHR pilot. *TEPR 1999 Conference Proceedings*. Orlando, Fla.: Medical Records Institute.

American Health Information Management Association. 2003. A vision from the e-HIM future. *Journal of the American Health Information Management Association* 74(8):Suppl.

Aspden, P., J. M. Corrigan, J. Wolcott, and S. M. Erickson, eds. 2004. *Patient Safety: Achieving a New Standard for Care*. Washington, D.C.: National Academies Press.

Bates, G. W. 2001 (February). Transitioning to an electronic medical record: the essential elements to consider when choosing a system. *Group Practice Journal,* pp. 38–40.

Bergeron, B. 1999. A keystone in your change-agent strategy: the RFP. *ADVANCE for Health Information Executives* 3(3):65–70.

Briggs, B. 2003 (June). The main event: best-of-breed vs. single-source. *Health Data Management,* pp. 41–48.

CIO Executive Summaries. 2002. Service Level Agreement. Available on-line at www.cio.com/summaries/outsourcing/sla.

Clinical Context Object Workgroup. 1999–2003. Available on-line at www.hl7.org.

Cohen, M. 2004 (May 19). Negotiating successful CPR/EMR contracts. *TEPR 2004 Conference Proceedings*. Fort Lauderdale, Fla.: Medical Records Institute.

Collen, M. F. 1995. *A History of Medical Informatics in the U.S. 1950–1990.* Bethesda, MD: Hartman Publishing.

Computer-based Patient Record Institute. 1995–2004. *Annual Nicholas E. Davies Award Proceedings of the CPR Recognition Symposium.* Chicago: HIMSS.

Dickinson, G., L. Fischetti, and S. Heard, eds. 2003. HL7 EHR System Functional Model and Standard, Draft Standard for Trial Use, Release 1.0. and EHR Collaborative Report of Public Response to HL7 Ballot 1 EHR, August 29.

eHealth Initiative. 2004. *Who we are.* Available on-line at www.ehealthinitiative.org.

EHR Collaborative. 2004. *Who we are.* Available on-line at www.ehrcollaborative.org.

Fox, L. A., and P. Thierry. 2003. Multiple visions undermine success of EHRs. *ADVANCE for Health Information Management* 13(14):8–9.

Gillespie, G. 2003 (June). Doing your homework: Execs should analyze vendors' financial statement before they sign on the dotted line. *Health Data Management,* 11(6):56–64.

Grams, R. R. 1998. Shopping in the health care information systems market. *ADVANCE for Health Information Executives* 2(7):37–40.

Hagland, M. 2003 (June). Choosing a vendor. *Healthcare Informatics,* pp. 87–88.

Health Level Seven. 2004 (April). HL7 EHR Functional Descriptors, Draft Standard for Trial Use.

Healthcare Financial Management Association. 2004. Dotting the i's and crossing the t's: Ensuring the best IT contract. Promotional material. Westchester, IL: HFMA.

Healthcare Financial Management Association, in partnership with GE Healthcare Financial Services. 2003. *How are Hospitals Financing the Future? Access to Capital in Health Care Today.* Westchester, IL: HFMA.

Healthcare Information and Management Systems Society. 1995–2004. The Annual Nicholas E. Davies Award of Excellence. Available on-line at www.himss.org.

Healthcare Information and Management Systems Society. 1990–1999. *The Hewlett-Packard/HIMSS Leadership Survey.* Chicago: HIMSS.

Hjort, B. 2000. Surviving and thriving during contract negotiations. *Journal of the American Health Information Management Association* 71(7):73.

Hoppszallern, S. 2003 (July). Outsourcing information technology systems. *Hospitals and Health Networks,* Suppl.

Hospitals and Health Networks. *Most wired.* Available on-line at www.hospitalconnect.com.

Hudson, Vincent. 2004. POMIS, private conversation.

Hughes, G. 2003 (June). Practice Brief: Transfer of patient health information across the continuum (Updated). *Journal of the American Health Information Management Association.* Available on-line at www.ahima.org.

Institute of Medicine. 2003 (July 31). *Letter Report: Key capabilities of an electronic health record system.* Washington, DC: National Academies Press. Available on-line at http://www.nap.edu/books.

Institute of Medicine. 2000. *To Err Is Human: Building a Safer Health System,* eds. L. T. Kohn, J. M. Corrigan, and M. S. Donaldson. Washington, DC: National Academies Press.

Institute of Medicine. 1997. *The Computer-based Patient Record: An Essential Technology for Health Care,* eds. R. S. Dick, E. B. Steen, and D. E. Detmer. Washington, DC: National Academies Press.

Institute of Medicine. 1991. *The Computer-based Patient Record: An Essential Technology for Health Care,* eds. R. S. Dick and E. B. Steen. Washington, DC: National Academies Press.

Kibbe, D. 2003 (September 25). *Open source electronic health record for office-based medical practice.* American Academy of Family Physicians. Available on-line at www.aafp.org.

Medical Record Institute. 2002. Less than 3% of hospitals surveyed have completely computerized records. *Medical Records Briefing* (Winter).

Miranda, D. 1998. What works in point-of-care data collection systems. *ADVANCE for Health Information Executives* 2(4):37–40.

Mon, D. T. 2004. Setting the right expectations for the EHR standard. *Journal of the American Health Information Management Association* 75(3):52–53.

Monahan, T. 2001 (February). Nine hot trends. *Healthcare Informatics,* pp. 54–56.

Morse, D. 2003. White Paper: Looking outside: Using external capital sources to overcome budget constraints. HCT Project, GE Healthcare Financial Services. Available on-line at www.hctproject.com/white.asp.

National Committee on Vital and Health Statistics. 2001. *Information for Health: A Strategy for Building the National Health Information Infrastructure.* Washington, D.C.: National Committee on Vital and Health Statistics.

National Committee on Vital and Health Statistics. 2002 (February 27). Letter to Secretary Thompson, U.S. Department of Health and Human Services, on Recommendations on Uniform Data Standards for Patient Medical Record Information.

National Library of Medicine. 2003. *Fact Sheet: Integrated advanced information management systems* (IAIMS) grants. Available on-line at www.nlm.nih.gov/pubs/factsheet/iaims.html.

Open Source Initiative. 2004. Available on-line at www.opensource.org/docs/definition.

Reed, Tom. 1998. Lookout for lemons: How to buy an electronic medical record system—without getting sold. *Healthcare Informatics* June 1998(149).

Rhodes, H., and G. Hughes. 2003. Practice Brief: Redisclosure of patient health information (Updated). *Journal of the American Health Information Management Association* 74(4):56A–C.

Schneider, P. 1998. Partners in risk: Who pays when your systems don't? *Healthcare Informatics* 15(2):75–84.

Schooler, R., and T. Dotson. 2003. Rolling out the CIS. *ADVANCE for Health Information Executives* 7(10):51–58.

Sheridan, C. 2001. Do you need an ASP ASAP? *Journal of the American Health Information Management Association* 72(8):38–42.

Shortliffe, E. H., and L. E. Perreault, eds. 2001. *Medical Informatics: Computer Applications in Health Care and Biomedicine,* 2nd ed. New York: Springer-Verlag.

The Leapfrog Group for Patient Safety. 2004. *About us.* Available on-line at www.leapfroggroup.org.

Chapter 4

Record Review and Analysis

Reshia Wheeler, RHIA

Clear, concise, accurate documentation in the health record is vital for ongoing care, appropriate reimbursement, legal protection for providers and clients, and to meet regulatory and licensure requirements. Record reviews are vital to monitor documentation, develop improvement opportunities, and educate practitioners. Record review programs should include a representative sample of healthcare practitioners and services from each program.

This chapter discusses the challenges inherent in completing documentation in behavioral healthcare. It describes the objectives and components of conducting a clinical pertinence review, as well as the various methods used to track record completion performance over time. Finally, it discusses the importance of developing organizational policies and procedures regarding health record completion and training staff on the need to maintain accurate medical record documentation.

Documentation Challenges in Behavioral Healthcare

Healthcare providers are responsible for documenting the care they provide to clients. Clinical information must be captured during the normal course of business. Patient care, organizational decisions and planning, reimbursement, and regulatory compliance are all based on the quality and accuracy of documentation in the medical record.

Many governing bodies provide standards and guidelines for medical record documentation. These include the Joint Commission on Accreditation of Healthcare Organizations (JCAHO), the Commission on Accreditation of Rehabilitation Facilities (CARF), the Centers for Medicare and Medicaid Services (CMS), and state licensing agencies. The standards and guidelines promulgated by these agencies specify the minimum data elements that must be captured and the time frames for completion. All of these criteria must be considered and included in a record review program.

Provider and Setting Diversity

Behavioral healthcare is provided in many different settings, ranging from inpatient and partial hospitalization settings to outpatient **clinics**. Although documentation requirements vary from setting to setting, they share many similar attributes. The first step in developing a record review process is to assemble all the regulatory and licensure requirements and accreditation standards that apply to the specific healthcare setting. The medical staff rules and regulations and existing health information management (HIM) policies also should be reviewed. All applicable requirements and policies should be organized in a hard-copy format or into a file on the intranet for easy access.

Behavioral healthcare providers are equally diverse and include psychiatrists, psychologists, nurses, social workers, therapists, and case managers, among others. Moreover, a great range of training and competencies must be taken into consideration when reviewing record documentation. Documentation expectations must reflect the level of provider expertise.

Communication and Timeliness of Documentation

The health or medical record serves as a communication tool among healthcare providers for the current episode of care as well as for future treatment. Accurate and timely entries are vital for appropriate care. Organizations should follow the time frame requirements of their most stringent external agencies, whether federal or state regulations or standards of accrediting and licensing agencies. Table 4.1 outlines standard time frames for core documentation elements.

Record Review Guidelines

The *Comprehensive Accreditation Manual for Behavioral Health Care* requires that the clinical record be reviewed on an ongoing basis (JCAHO 2004). The tenth Element of Performance for IM.6.10 states: "Clinical/case records are reviewed on an ongoing basis at the point of care, treatment, and service and are based on organization defined indicators that address the presence, timeliness, readability (whether handwritten or printed), quality, consistency, clarity, accuracy, completeness, and authentication of data and information contained within the record, as well as appropriate scanning and indexing if document imaging is used." An M icon, which stands for measure of success, appears next to the tenth Element of Performance. A measure of success is defined as "a quantifiable measure, usually related to an audit, that can be used to determine whether an action has been effective and is being sustained."

Clinical Pertinence Review

Ongoing or concurrent record reviews are the best approach to ensure the presence, timeliness, completeness, and accuracy of documentation. Healthcare organizations must first decide on the purpose for their clinical pertinence review process in order to determine what criteria to audit against. A **clinical pertinence review** of medical records is done for a number of reasons, including:

- To provide supervision to staff in ensuring the quality of the clinical documentation

- To ensure that clinical documentation is completed in a timely manner

- To ensure that clinical documentation meets the requirements of all third-party payers

- To ensure that clinical documentation meets all regulatory standards, such as those determined by JCAHO and CARF

- To provide a mechanism for assessing clinician skills and an opportunity to provide education and training

When the organization has determined the purpose(s) for the clinical pertinence review, its requirements and policies should be reviewed to find criteria to audit against to fulfill each objective of the audit. For example, if the organization's objective is to meet regulatory and third-party payer requirements, those requirements must be included among the audit criteria.

Table 4.1. Standard time frames for core documentation elements

Documentation	Time Frame for Completion
Psychiatric assessment	24 hours after inpatient intake
Physical examination	24 hours after inpatient intake
Social assessment	72 hours after inpatient intake
Initial treatment plan	72 hours after outpatient intake
Treatment plan	Updated and signed by MD every 90 days for outpatient
Addictions treatment plan	Updated and signed by MD every 30 days for outpatient
Biopsychosocial assessment	Within 30 days of admission/intake
Client profile	Within 30 days of admission/intake
Nursing assessment	24 hours after inpatient intake
Progress notes	24 hours after visit
Discharge summary	Within 30 days of discharge/termination

Next, the organization should create a clinical pertinence review form that captures all of the elements to audit against. (See figure 4.1 for a sample form.) The medical record being audited should be identified at the top of the form with its number and the client's name. Other data that may be helpful to record include the date the record was reviewed; the reviewer's name and ID or staff number; the name of the primary clinician, case manager, or physician; the primary and secondary diagnoses; and DSM-IV codes. All the criteria should be set up in a yes–no–N/A format for ease of auditing and entering information into a database to run reports. The rest of the form should be divided into sections to easily identify specific data elements. The following subsections offer instructions on how to complete each section of the sample form in figure 4.1.

Client Identification Data

The registration paperwork or face sheet should be reviewed to see whether the data are complete.

Authentication and Legibility of Services/Documentation

All entries should be reviewed to ensure that they are signed and dated with the author's name and credentials. The entries also should be examined for legibility.

Consents

Consents to treatment should be signed and dated by the client or his or her current legal guardian. If the client is receiving medication, the medication consent should be signed and dated by both client and physician. If the client is receiving neuroleptic medications, a neuroleptic medication consent form should be present and signed by both client and physician every six months. The financial or fee agreement should be signed and dated by the client or his or her current legal guardian. Finally, any authorizations for the release of health information should be completed, signed, and dated.

Treatment Plan

The treatment plan should contain the client or current legal guardian's signature or a notation that the client or legal guardian refused to sign. It should be completed and signed by the clinician within 72 hours of admission or intake. Moreover, a physician should sign and update the treatment plan every 90 days (or within the time required by the most stringent third-party payer).

Figure 4.1. Clinical pertinence review form

Clinical Pertinence Review Form				
Client Name:		**Record #**	**Date of Review:**	
Clinician/CM:	**ID #:**	**Reviewer:**		**ID #:**
☐ Review of Non-QMHP	☐ Review of QMHP	☐ Reviewed in Peer Review Committee		
Primary diagnosis/DSM code:		**Secondary diagnosis/DSM code:**		

Client Identification Data			
Identification/registration data are complete.	☐ Yes ☐ No		

Authentication and Legibility of Services/Documentation			
All entries are signed (with credentials) and dated by clinical staff.	☐ Yes ☐ No		
All entries are legible.	☐ Yes ☐ No		

Consents			
Consent for services signed and dated by client or current guardian	☐ Yes	☐ No	
Medication consent signed and dated by client and physician	☐ Yes	☐ No	☐ N/A
Neuroleptic medication consent present	☐ Yes	☐ No	☐ N/A
Neuroleptic medication consent up-to-date (resigned by client/MD every 6 months)	☐ Yes	☐ No	☐ N/A
Fee agreement signed and dated by client or current guardian	☐ Yes	☐ No	
All necessary releases of information completed, signed, and dated	☐ Yes	☐ No	☐ N/A

Treatment Plan			
Client/current guardian signature on treatment plan or refusal to sign noted	☐ Yes	☐ No	
Initial treatment plan completed by clinician and authorized by physician within 72 hours	☐ Yes	☐ No	
Treatment plan updated and signed by MD every 90 days	☐ Yes	☐ No	☐ N/A
Addictions treatment goals identified if "Client Profile–History of Substance Abuse" form is present	☐ Yes	☐ No	☐ N/A
Treatment plan and staffing records signed by a QMHP	☐ Yes	☐ No	
Goals relate to problems/needs statement.	☐ Yes	☐ No	
Goals are stated in behavioral terms, focused on specific improvements that the client hopes to achieve through treatment.	☐ Yes	☐ No	
Objectives are measurable and written in behavioral terms.	☐ Yes	☐ No	
Objectives are achievable.	☐ Yes	☐ No	
Objectives are time limited with target dates.	☐ Yes	☐ No	
Treatment reviews adequately assess the success of treatment interventions in resolving identified treatment needs.	☐ Yes	☐ No	☐ N/A
Treatment reviews occur both at regularly scheduled intervals and in response to major changes in client status.	☐ Yes	☐ No	☐ N/A
Treatment reviews address changes in diagnosis.	☐ Yes	☐ No	☐ N/A
Treatment reviews reflect changes in the treatment plan.	☐ Yes	☐ No	☐ N/A

Figure 4.1. (Continued)

Client Profile			
Health screen completed and signed by MD	☐ Yes	☐ No	
Appropriate profile addendum(s) completed (child, addictions, adult general) and CAGE* for adults	☐ Yes	☐ No	☐ N/A
Profile is thorough and completed within 30 days.	☐ Yes	☐ No	
Profile summary and formulation adequately summarizes client needs.	☐ Yes	☐ No	
Profile summary and formulation adequately identifies the initial focus of treatment.	☐ Yes	☐ No	
Profile summary and formulation documents reasons for any deferred problems/needs	☐ Yes	☐ No	☐ N/A
Diagnosis is consistent with assessment findings.	☐ Yes	☐ No	
Client profile is updated annually or as diagnosis changes.	☐ Yes	☐ No	☐ N/A
Progress Notes/Services Delivered			
Treatment is appropriate to the diagnosis/identified functional needs and meets criteria for medical necessity.	☐ Yes	☐ No	
Frequency of contacts is appropriate to the identified functional needs.	☐ Yes	☐ No	
Progress notes correlate with problems and goals in the treatment plan.	☐ Yes	☐ No	
Progress notes are individualized and reflect the treatment issue for which services are being delivered.	☐ Yes	☐ No	
Progress notes reflect the response to treatment at the time of service.	☐ Yes	☐ No	
Progress notes at time of initial plan and plan reviews clearly indicate client involvement	☐ Yes	☐ No	
Initial note indicates that client rights were reviewed.	☐ Yes	☐ No	

Notes reviewed from _____ to _____

Comments:

CORRECTIONS/PAYBACK FOLLOW-UP

Corrections needed: ☐ YES   ☐ NO   **Payback needed: ☐ YES   ☐ NO**

QMHP audit form sent to clinician for corrections	Date _____
Corrections completed and returned to supervisor	Date: _____
Sent to Billing Department for payback	Date: _____
Processed by Billing Department for payback	Date: _____

*The four-question CAGE tool used to aid in the diagnosis of substance addictions.
1. Have you ever felt you should **C**ut down on your [substance]?
2. Have people **A**nnoyed you by criticising your [substance]?
3. Have you ever felt bad or **G**uilty about your [substance]?
4. Have you ever had an "**E**ye opener"—a [substance] first thing in the morning to steady your nerves?

The goals should relate to the problems/needs statement. They should be reviewed to ensure that they are stated in behavioral terms and focused on specific improvements the client hopes to achieve through treatment. The objectives should be measurable and written in behavioral terms. Moreover, they should be achievable and time limited with target dates.

Treatment plan updates should adequately assess the success of treatment interventions in resolving identified treatment needs. Treatment plan reviews should occur at regular scheduled intervals and in response to major changes in the client's status. Any changes in diagnoses should be addressed during the treatment reviews. The treatment reviews also should reflect any changes in treatment plan.

Client Profile

A physician should complete and sign the health screen. The appropriate client profile addendum (child, addictions, or adult) must be thorough and completed within 30 days. The profile summary and formulation should adequately summarize the client's needs and identify the initial focus of treatment. Moreover, the profile summary and formulation documents reasons for any deferred problems/needs. The diagnoses should be consistent with the **assessment** findings. The client profile is updated annually or when there is a change in diagnosis.

Progress Notes/Services Delivered

Progress notes should reflect that the treatment is appropriate to the diagnosis/identified functional needs and meets the criteria for medical necessity. The frequency of contacts is appropriate to the identified functional needs. The progress notes correlate with problems and goals in the treatment plan; they should be individualized and reflect the treatment issue for which services are being delivered.

Additionally, the response to treatment at the time of service should be indicated in the progress notes. Progress notes at the time of the initial treatment plan and treatment plan reviews clearly indicate client involvement. The initial note should indicate that the client's rights were reviewed during the first visit.

The Record Review Process

The next step is to establish a process for reviewing the medical records. All clinical staff should participate in the clinical pertinence review process in order to realize the full benefits of ongoing record review. Including ongoing record review in the staff's day-to-day functions will encourage them to view record reviews as part of their responsibility and heighten their awareness of the importance of maintaining high-quality documentation.

Role of the Qualified Mental Health Professional

Clinical pertinence reviews should be performed by qualified mental health professionals (QMHPs). QMHPs are clinicians who meet the organization's educational, work experience, and competency requirements and are granted appropriate credentials and privileges by the medical committee. (See figure 4.2 for a flowchart showing the QMHP process.) The supplemental provider manual issued by the CMS defines the QMPH as:

- A licensed psychiatrist

- A licensed physician

- A licensed psychologist

Figure 4.2. Flowchart of QMHP process

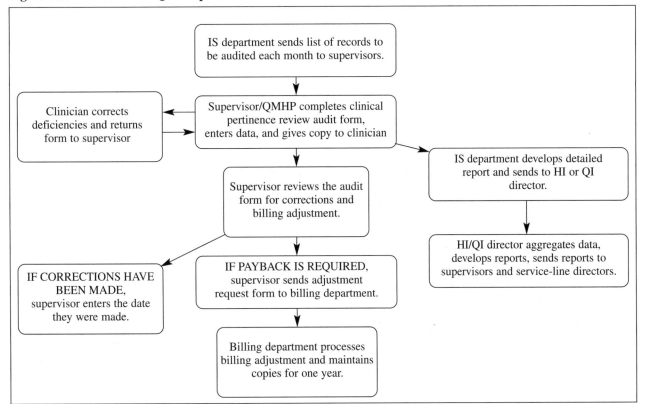

- An individual with at least two years of clinical experience working with persons with mental illness under the supervision of a mental health professional, such experience occurring after the completion of a master's degree or doctoral degree, or both, and who possesses one of the following sets of credentials:

  —A master's or doctoral degree, or both, in psychiatric nursing from an accredited university plus a license as a registered nurse

  —A master's or doctoral degree, or both, in social work from a university accredited by the Council on Social Work Education

  —A master's or doctoral degree, or both, in psychology from an accredited university and who meets the requirements for the practice of psychology

  —A master's or doctoral degree, or both, in counseling and guidance from an accredited university

  —A master's or doctoral degree, or both, in pastoral counseling from an accredited university; or a master's or doctoral degree, or both, in rehabilitation counseling from accredited university

  —A mental health professional with documented equivalence in education, training, and/or experience approved by the supervising physician

Only staff with QMHP status should conduct clinical pertinence reviews.

QMHPs at a supervisory level should be expected to complete a minimum number of reviews. Additional reviews may be performed at the supervisor's discretion to focus on problem areas. Performance of these reviews should be considered a job competency and included in the annual performance appraisal. The Peer Review Committee provides oversight of the process. Reviews should be completed at the following points of care:

- All of the clinical records prepared by staff other than QMHPs 30 days after case was opened should be reviewed by a QMHP.

- All of the clinical records prepared by staff other than QMHPs should be reviewed by a QMHP 180 days after the case was opened.

- For the records prepared by QMHPs, one clinical record per month should be reviewed by another QMHP.

Reports Resulting from Record Review

The clinical pertinence review form is completed for each audit, and the data from this form should be entered into an organizational database. This enables the information systems (IS) department or the health information management (HIM) department to generate detailed reports on a monthly basis. Any review resulting in the necessity of a billing adjustment due to an error or omission requires completion of an adjustment request form. (See figure 4.3 for an example of an adjustment request form.) The adjustment request then should be forwarded to the business office for processing.

Reporting the results of the reviews should be the responsibility of the IS department and the director of HIM or quality improvement. The director of HIM or quality improvement aggregates the data and issues a report that is used for performance improvement activities such as determining staff education and training needs. (See figure 4.4 for sample reports.) Training should be provided by individual supervisors or by the director of HIM or quality improvement after a staff member has been granted appropriate credentials and privileges as a QMHP.

Figure 4.3. Adjustment request form

Adjustment Request Form					
Due to results from a clinical pertinence review or a billing audit, a billing adjustment will be necessary for the following entries: Staff ID # _____					
Client name	**Record #**	**Date of Service**	**Service Activity Code**	**Time Spent**	**Reason for Adjustment**

Signature of Supervisor/Team Leader: _____ Date: _____

Signature of Service-Line Director:_____ Date: _____

FOR BILLING DEPARTMENT USE ONLY

_____ Adjustment required

_____ Refund required

_____ Not applicable   Staff name_____ Date: _____

Figure 4.4. Clinical pertinence review data

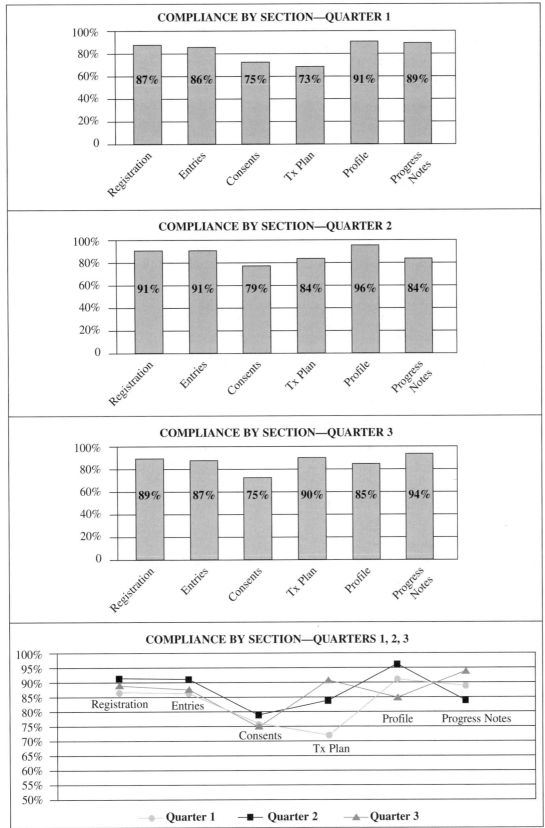

Peer Review Committee

The organization will need to set up a committee of multidisciplinary staff who will be responsible for monitoring clinical pertinence review activities. This committee might be called a Peer Review Committee, a Health Information Committee, or a Clinical Pertinence Review Committee. A sample committee description for a behavioral healthcare organization follows:

Name of Committee: Peer Review Committee

Purpose: To conduct **peer review** of medical records to monitor documentation compliance with regulatory bodies and third-party payers. The committee will discuss and make recommendations regarding issues pertaining to the medical records.

Responsibilities and Functions:

- To audit medical records on a monthly basis
- To provide peer review and feedback on clinical practice and documentation
- To assess compliance with admission, continuing stay, and discharge criteria for the various programs
- To provide oversight of the clinical pertinence review process

Reporting Relationships: This committee reports to the Clinical Leadership Committee.

Membership: Membership of the committee includes a psychiatrist, nurse, and a variety of clinical staff from the adult and children's service lines.

Facilitator: The committee is led by the director of Child/Adolescent Services.

Meeting Time/Frequency: The third Wednesday of each month from 12:00 p.m. to 1:30 p.m.

Performance Indicators Monitored: Compliance with established documentation guidelines and billing practices and clinical adherence to guidelines regarding admission, continuing stay, and discharge

Reporting Frequency and Schedule: The committee reports results on a monthly basis to the Clinical Leadership Committee.

Location of Minutes: The library

Closed-Record Review

The *Comprehensive Accreditation Manual for Behavioral Health Care* describes what must be included in a discharge summary and the time frame for completion of the record after discharge (JCAHO 2004). The seventh Element of Performance for I.M.6.10 states: "A concise discharge summary providing information to other caregivers and facilitating continuity of care, treatment, and services included the following:

- The reason for care, treatment, and services
- Significant findings
- Procedures and care, treatment, and services provided
- The client's condition at discharge
- Instructions to the client and family, as appropriate."

With regard to monitoring the timeliness of record completion, the ninth Element of Performance for I.M. 6.10 states: "The organization defines a complete record and the timeframe within which the record must be completed after discharge, not to exceed 30 days after discharge" (JCAHO 2004). A clear policy should be in place describing timely record completion and should be enforced without exception. Successful record completion programs motivate staff to complete their records in a timely and accurate manner and make the process as easy as possible.

Record Review Tools

A number of record review tools may be used to assist an employee at any level of the organization with process improvement efforts.

Richard Y. Chang's *Ten Tools for Quality* (1994) is a useful resource on how to collect and display data with graphs and charts.

Check Sheets

The **check sheet** is an important data collection tool. It is used to record how often or where an event or problem occurs over a designated period of time. The title and items to be measured are listed down the left side of the check sheet, and the day, time, or location of the monitoring function for each item should be listed at the top of the sheet. Tick marks might be placed under the appropriate column and row each time one of the items occurs. Occurrences should be recorded directly on the check sheet as they happen. Each row then should be totaled to compare the number of occurrences for each item.

Histograms

A **histogram** is a bar graph composed of horizontal and vertical axes that is used to show a range of various values. The horizontal axis contains ranges of values such as length of stay (LOS), and the vertical axis contains the number of observations, such as the number of clients. An LOS histogram would be created by collecting data on how many visits each client has during an episode of care and then dividing all of the clients during the recording period among the various ranges. For example, the LOS data collection for the month of July includes how many clients completed their treatment and how many visits were included during their LOS, as follows.

    1–2   visits   5 clients

    3–4   visits   10 clients

    5–6   visits   30 clients

    7–8   visits   15 clients

    9–10 visits   8 clients

    11–12 visits   3 clients

The data would be plotted on the histogram as shown in figure 4.5.

Run Charts

The **run chart** is used to track the performance of a process over a period of time. Run charts are helpful in tracking quality or productivity measures that will provide useful information in a decision-making process. Data for a particular **indicator** are tracked during a set period of time at certain time intervals (hourly, daily, weekly, or monthly).

Control Charts

A **control chart** is a run chart with lines on it called control limits. Control limits are lines that are drawn three standard deviations from the mean or average value in a series of numbers. The control chart provides information that can help predict the future outcome of a process with a high degree of accuracy.

Pareto Charts

A **pareto chart** is a bar graph listing the causes of a result along the horizontal axis from the most commonly occurring to the least commonly occurring. The left vertical axis shows the number of occurrences, and the right vertical axis shows the percentage of all occurrences that the number represents. A line is drawn on the chart from left to right showing the cumulative percentage of the reasons or causes. The purpose of the pareto chart is to create a graph that allows easy identification of the causes that are most responsible for a particular result. Table 4.2 shows an example of a data sheet. The pareto chart in figure 4.6 shows the reasons why someone is late to work.

Figure 4.5.   Length of stay histogram

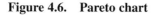

Table 4.2.   Data sheet

Reason for Being Late to Work	Number of Times Late	% of Times Late
Overslept	5	50%
Watch stopped	3	30%
Spilled coffee on self	1	10%
Car out of gas	1	10%

Figure 4.6.   Pareto chart

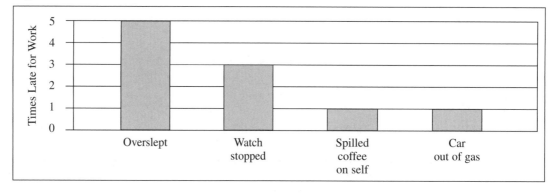

Deficiency Analysis

A **deficiency analysis** is an audit process designed to ensure that all services billed have been documented in the health record. There are two types of deficiency analyses: quantitative and qualitative.

Quantitative Deficiency Analysis

A **quantitative audit** (sometimes referred to as a billing audit) compares a report of services billed for a specific client and within a specific time frame against the health record documentation. Sometimes the report of services is referred to as an active caseload or billing report. (See table 4.3 for a sample report of services billed.)

The quantitative audit should be performed by a member of the HIM department. Job responsibilities include performing quantitative audits on all applicable staff members each month, writing and distributing audit reports to applicable administrative staff, and maintaining an audit schedule based on audit results. The HIM department may want to utilize a leveling system to determine how often individual staff are audited. Staff members who consistently meet the established documentation standards would be audited less frequently. Staff who are new to the organization or who have not yet achieved compliance with the standards would be audited more frequently. The leveling system would be used to determine the month in which an audit is due for a particular staff member. All staff would be categorized in one of the following audit levels based on their error rate in relation to documentation and billing standards:

Audit Level	Error Rate	Audit Frequency
Level A	Less than 4%	Semiannually
Level B	4%–9%	Quarterly
Level C	10% or greater	Monthly

A suggested audit sample would focus on thirty billed services per staff to establish a reliable and accurate compliance monitoring process. Staff members who do not regularly bill thirty events each month would be audited quarterly on the thirty billed services. All newly hired staff would be required to start at Level C and remain there for three months regardless of their calculated error rate. In addition, staff should not be able to advance to Level A until they have completed one full year of employment.

Staff may advance to a higher audit level after demonstrating an error rate below the required limits for three consecutive audits. For example, a staff member who is at Level C may advance to Level A after three consecutive audits showing an error rate of less than four percent. An error is defined as any deficiency in documentation noted during the audit. An

Table 4.3. Report of services billed

Case Number	Client Name	Event Date	Service	Service Description	Staff Code	Staff Name	Time	Fee
29847	Patient, Bob	3/5/03	112	Case management	854	Staffperson #1	12:15	27.00
29847	Patient, Bob	3/5/03	104	Partial day treatment	934	Staffperson #2	1:15	45.00
29847	Patient, Bob	3/5/03	108	Med Somatic	955	Staffperson #3	2:10	13.33
29847	Patient, Bob	3/5/03	112	Case management	854	Staffperson #1	2:00	216.00

error would be counted when any required element is missing (for example, the date, a signature, credentials, and so on). Only one error would be counted per required piece of documentation. For example, if a progress note was missing the date and signature, only one error would be counted. A staff member who has advanced to a higher audit level may be returned to a lower audit level if, during a subsequent audit, his or her error rate increases sufficiently. For example, a staff member at Level A whose error rate on a later audit is above 10 percent would return to Level C and be audited monthly until his or her error rate improves.

At a minimum, a quantitative audit should be conducted to ensure that:

- The intake and initial treatment plan is developed and/or reviewed.

- The intake and initial treatment plan is reviewed and signed by a physician within 72 hours of intake.

- Progress notes are present for all services billed by the staff member on his or her billing logs for the selected audit sample.

- Audited progress notes contain the following required elements:

    —Service code

    —Amount of time spent

    —Date of service

    —Time of day

    —Staff member's full name and credentials

- The treatment plan is updated by the clinician at least every 90 days

Regardless of the type of behavioral healthcare setting, all staff members are required to submit their billing information each day on some type of service activity log, sometimes referred to as a billing log or time sheet. (See figure 4.7 for a sample service activity log.) The service activity log contains data to enter into the billing system, such as date, staff identification number, staff name, service code, location, time spent, client name, record number, and signature.

One way to prevent missing documentation is to require staff to turn in their documentation with their service activity logs by 5:00 p.m. on the business day following the date of service. For example, the staff member would be required to turn in all documentation by 5:00 p.m. on Tuesday to support charges submitted on his or her billing logs for services provided on Monday. All supporting documentation should be attached to the service activity log and turned in with it. If some of the documentation was dictated, the staff member should write the word "dictated" next to the client's name. The service must be dictated before the service activity log is turned in for data entry.

The HIM staff member receiving the documentation reviews the service activity log to ensure that either documentation or the word "dictated" matches each service listed on the billing log. The documentation should be checked against the service activity log to confirm that the service codes, location, time spent, client name, and record number all match. If the documentation matches the service activity log, an "M" is written next to the client's name to confirm that the documentation was checked against the service activity log. The documentation then is detached for filing in the health record, and the service activity log is forwarded to the billing department for data entry.

If the service activity log is missing information, completed improperly, or submitted without the corresponding documentation, it should be returned with a missing/incorrect service activity log information form. (See figure 4.8 for a sample form.) The missing or incorrect information should be highlighted on the service activity log and a copy sent to the billing

Figure 4.7. Service activity log

Date		Staff ID	Staff Name		Signature	
	Location Code	**Service Activity Code**	**Time Spent**	**Client Name**		**Record #**
1						
2						
3						
4						
5						
6						
7						
8						
9						
10						
11						
12						
13						
14						
15						
16						
17						
18						
19						
20						

department for tracking purposes. The staff member must complete the missing/incorrect information immediately and return it to the person listed at the bottom of the form. The staff member then would have until the end of the following business day to complete the information. After that time, he or she is considered delinquent on that service activity log.

Qualitative Deficiency Analysis

Qualitative audits are a part of the clinical pertinence review process discussed earlier in this chapter.

Management of Incomplete Records

All healthcare organizations strive toward the common goal of maintaining complete health records. This challenge often falls on the shoulders of the HIM staff. A source of good ideas on how to manage incomplete records is *Mastering Records Completion: Successful Strategies from Medical Records Briefing* (Cofer 1998). The following sections contain a few suggestions to help HIM staff manage their incomplete records.

Figure 4.8. Missing/incorrect service activity log information

MISSING/INCORRECT SERVICE ACTIVITY LOG INFORMATION
The following information must be completed and returned with the original service activity log by the **end of the following business day.** If you are unable to provide the missing/incorrect information, the billing department or its representative must be notified immediately. Failure to provide the missing/incorrect information **by the end of the following business day** will result in a delinquent service activity log notification to your supervisor.
DATE RETURNED: _____
STAFF MEMBER: _____
SERVICE ACTIVITY LOG #: _____
SERVICE ACTIVITY LOG DATE: _____
The following missing/incorrect information must be completed and returned to the billing department representative immediately: • Missing progress note • Missing staff member signature • Missing/incorrect service activity code • Missing/incorrect time spent • Missing/incorrect client name and/or record number • Other_____
Health Information Staff

Storage, Retrieval, and Tracking of Incomplete Records

Large organizations may want to designate a section of their HIM department as an incomplete records area. This area would include all of the health records that are missing some type of information and waiting to be completed. Records in the incomplete record area should be filed in alphabetical or numerical order as they are in the permanent file area. Filing incomplete records by staff member name makes them difficult to locate. The incomplete record should be signed out from the permanent file area with a notation indicating that it now is located in the incomplete file area.

In one scenario for achieving ease of retrieval and completion, each staff member is assigned a color. When a deficiency is found in the record, a tab is attached to the edge of the deficiency that matches the color assigned to the staff member responsible the deficiency's completion. Thus, each staff member completes only the records tagged with his or her assigned color. This eliminates HIM staff from having to pull all the records each time a staff member is ready to complete his or her records. A list of the staff members' assigned colors should be posted in the incomplete records area to avoid confusion.

Small organizations may be able to hand-deliver incomplete health records to each staff member in the morning and retrieve them each evening. The records would include a tab where the staff member needs to complete a deficiency. This may be too cumbersome for larger organizations because of the time spent signing out and delivering records.

The easiest way for HIM staff to track incomplete records is via a computer-generated report. Such reports should be sent to staff members on a weekly basis to inform them of any deficient records located in the incomplete records area. Information on the report should include medical record number, client name, type of deficiency, staff member name, and number of days the record has been incomplete. This would help staff identify which records to complete first.

Policies and Procedures on Record Completion

The HIM director and the medical records director or the medical committee should develop a records policy that lists the responsibilities of the HIM staff and the medical and clinical staff. The medical director or medical committee should enforce the policy to alleviate tension between the two staffs. If the organization chooses to give rewards or punishments for record completion, the policy should include them as either incentives for high completion rates or suspension of privileges for excessive delinquencies.

Authentication of Medical Records

The purpose of authentication is to identify the source of an entry and to assign responsibility for it in the medical record. Every entry must be authenticated by the **author** and should not be signed by anyone other than the author. At a minimum, the signature should include the first initial, last name, and title/credential or discipline (Federal Regulations/Interpretive Guidelines for Hospitals 482.24[c][1]). An organization can choose a more stringent standard that requires the author's full name and credentials to assist in the proper identification of the author. Organizational policies should define the acceptable format for authentication of record entries (Welch 2000).

Authentication Requirements

The following subsections discuss authentication requirements issued by accreditation and licensing agencies.

Joint Commission on Accreditation of Healthcare Organizations

The *Comprehensive Accreditation Manual for Behavioral Health Care* (JCAHO 2004) requires the following for authentication of clinical record entries:

- Verbal orders: "Each verbal order must be dated and identified by the names of the individuals who gave it and received it, and the record must document who implemented it. When required by state or federal law and regulation, verbal orders are authenticated within the specified time frame. Medication orders must be authenticated."

- Clinical record entries: "Every clinical record entry must be dated, its author identified and, when necessary according to law or regulation and organization policy, is authenticated. The following entries must be authenticated either by written signature, electronic signature, or computer key or rubber stamp: history and physical examination, evaluations and assessments, progress notes, medication orders, and discharge summaries."

Centers for Medicare and Medicaid Services

The *Medicare Conditions of Participation for Comprehensive Outpatient Rehabilitation Facilities* (CMS 1993) published by the Centers for Medicare and Medicaid Services requires that "entries in the clinical record must be made as frequently as is necessary to insure effective treatment, and must be signed by personnel providing services. All entries made by assistant level personnel must be countersigned by the corresponding professional." Verbal orders are not mentioned in the Conditions of Participation.

State Laws and Regulations

The specific requirements for each state should be checked with the state licensing authority.

Recommendations on Creating Authentication Policies

All authentication requirements, such as state law, accrediting and licensing agency standards, and Medicare Conditions of Participation guidelines, should be reviewed for application to the healthcare organization. Organizational policy should reflect the most stringent requirement of all applicable authentication requirements. For example, if the state requires that verbal orders be authenticated within a specific time frame, accrediting and licensing agencies will check for compliance with that time frame during their survey. Staff must follow authentication policies by including this item in a quantitative deficiency audit or an ongoing record review.

Training for Record Review and Ongoing Performance Improvement

Time is a very important concern for behavioral healthcare professionals, and the documentation process is not an easy task. However, when healthcare professionals understand the value of documentation and, equally importantly, feel that the organization is sensitive to their time constraints, they are likelier to agree to undergo training in the documentation process. The most effective way to begin the process is to create a training plan.

The Training Plan

The training plan consists of the steps described in the following subsections.

Step 1. Choose an Appropriate Course Title

The first step of the training plan is to decide on a course title or topic to describe the main subject of the training.

Step 2. Determine the Target Audience

The next step is to determine the target audience of the training. For example, if the focus of the training will be on specific forms that only certain staff members will use, the target audience would be limited to those staff members. However, if discussion will center on documentation guidelines that apply to a large percentage of the clinical staff, the target audience will be much larger. Thus, the content of the training session (teaching new requirements, reminding staff about current policies, procedures, or forms, addressing poor record review scores, and so on) determines the target audience.

Learning Objectives

The training sessions should have learning objectives. It is important to motivate session attendees by showing them the benefits to be gained from the topic being discussed. For example, an in-service on the importance of documentation would stress that thorough documentation saves time in making client care decisions, improves reimbursement for services rendered, and eliminates negative survey or audit findings.

Method of Delivery

Several different methods of delivery or techniques can be used to turn a dry, formal lecture into a stimulating educational experience. Staff members who are not paying attention to the lecture certainly are not learning. It is important to give attendees something striking to look at or something to touch. They should be motivated to write and talk and become involved.

Interest can be stimulated through use of a training manual, handouts, table tents, or posters. The speaker might use a PC or Web-based presentation or show a videotape.

The facilitator should first introduce himself or herself, establishing his or her credibility by specifying his or her clinical record and documentation expertise. He or she then should explain the objectives of the training so that the attendees know what they are being taught and why.

A hands-on approach may be used by providing attendees with an exercise or group project. Contest-type exercises can be fun and create a great deal of enthusiasm. For example, the facilitator might give attendees a mock record with numerous documentation errors and offer a reward to the individual or group that finds the most problems.

Length of the Training Session

The last thing to decide is how much time will be needed to deliver the training session and achieve all the learning objectives without losing the attention of the session attendees.

Training of New Hires

All new hires should be required to attend a documentation training session as part of their orientation process. The session should review all the clinical forms and how to complete them. All policies and procedures regarding documentation also should be included in the orientation.

Retraining of Existing Staff

All existing staff should attend an annual documentation training to review any new requirements, forms, or policies and procedures. This training course acts as a refresher from the previous training they attended. A PC-based training session could be set up for staff to view at their convenience.

A posttest would need to be printed and filed in the employees' personnel file as proof of attendance for a PC-based training refresher course. Indeed, attendance logs should be maintained for all types of training sessions or in-services. This is the only way to prove that employees have attended required training sessions. Attendance logs and/or posttests should be retained for at least six years.

Awareness of Training

The organization can heighten the awareness of documentation requirements by hanging fliers or posters in all staff areas, sending reminder e-mails, giving handouts to staff, providing informational articles in the organization's newsletter, or providing short in-services with breakfast or lunch included.

Tracking of Productivity

Two methods for tracking clinical productivity are benchmarking and utilization review. These are discussed below.

Benchmarking

To track clinical productivity, the organization can establish productivity standards through a process called benchmarking. **Benchmarking** is a strategy of comparing internal performance against the performance of an external organization that has a similar background and offers similar services and programs. A program can be created to track each clinician's productivity level after the productivity standards are established. The data can be inserted into a graph that depicts productivity levels by staff, department, or team.

Supervisors and organizational leaders should review this information on a monthly basis. It should be a practice to conduct a quantitative (billing) audit on anyone whose productivity increases within a certain percentage from one month to another to ensure that no fraudulent billing is occurring.

Utilization Review

Criteria for admission, continued stay, and discharge for each level of care should be established to ensure the most effective and efficient use of treatment service resources. These criteria also will ensure that clients receive services of appropriate intensity and duration in the least restrictive and intrusive level of care possible. Utilization review can be monitored during the clinical pertinence review or a separate medical record review process. The organization should establish protocols and procedures for handling any clinical cases that fall outside the established criteria for a level of care.

These procedures should include a process through which clinicians can request exceptions to the established criteria for a level of care. Their requests should be evaluated and either granted or denied. (See figure 4.9 for a sample of level-of-care criteria for admission, continued stay, and discharge for serious mental illness, substance abuse, adult intermediate care, and child and adolescent intermediate care.)

Conclusion

The medical record is a prime communication medium for planning and ensuring excellent quality of care between and among providers. The medical record justifies admission, length of stay, and discharge for utilization management and for maximum reimbursement. Because of these reasons and many others that have been listed throughout the chapter, it is of utmost importance for practitioners to follow the standards and requirements set forth for documentation practices. It is up to the health information management administrators and staff at each organization to ensure that these requirements are met.

References and Bibliography

Centers for Medicare and Medicaid Services. 1993. *Medicare Conditions of Participation for Comprehensive Outpatient Rehabilitation Facilities.* 42 CFR Ch. IV, Paragraph 485.60(a).

Chang, Richard. 1994. *Ten Tools For Quality.* West Des Moines, IA: American Media.

Cofer, Jennifer I. 1998. *Mastering Records Completion: Successful Strategies from Medical Records Briefing.* Marblehead, MA: Opus Communications.

Dougherty, Michelle. 2002. Practice Brief: Maintaining a legally sound health record. *Journal of the American Health Information Management Association* 73(8):64A–G.

Haney, Pamela. November 4, 2003. Personal correspondence regarding record review and analysis.

Joint Commission on Accreditation of Healthcare Organizations. 2004. *Comprehensive Accreditation Manual for Behavioral Health Care.* Oak Brook Terrace, IL: JCAHO.

Schlosser, Jean. December 5, 2003. Personal correspondence regarding record review and analysis.

Scholtes, Peter. 1988. *The Team Handbook.* Madison, WI: Joiner Associates Inc.

Walsh, Tom. 2002. *Building Effective Training Programs to Make Cultural and Behavioral Changes.* Chicago: American Health Information Management Association.

Welch, Julie. 2000. Practice Brief: Authentication of health record entries. *Journal of the American Health Information Management Association* 71(3). Available at www.ahima.org.

Figure 4.9. Admission, continuing stay, and discharge criteria

Serious Mental Illness

Admission
- Adults age 18 years and older
- DSM-IV diagnosis, usually of a psychotic-level disorder, for example, schizophrenia, bipolar disorder, or recurrent major depression with psychotic features (295.xx – 296.xx) with or without associated diagnoses on Axis I or Axis II, and
- Duration of symptoms and/or impairment longer than 12 months, except if the client has sustained a severe situational trauma, and
- Demonstrated significant impairment in two or more areas of life functioning:
    Activities of daily living
    Interpersonal functioning
    Concentration, persistence, and pace
    Adaptation to change, and
- Assessed need for intensive community-based services to maintain stable housing, nutrition and/or safety, and
- GAF <65 and >25

Continuing Stay
- Primary DSM-IV Axis I diagnosis, with or without associated diagnoses, and
- Continued demonstration of impairment in areas of life functioning such that independent community adjustment is not possible, and/or
- Continued demonstration of symptoms and/or symptom control suggestive of a need for active monitoring
- Continued involvement in services, including residence within the service area and an assessed ability to be appropriate for available services
- GAF <65 and >25

Discharge
- Demonstrated ability to maintain independent community adjustment with only appointment-based supports for at least six months, and
- Willingness and ability to assume responsibility for self-monitoring of medications, finances, and activities of daily living, or
- Client moves out of service area, or
- Client voluntarily chooses to seek services elsewhere and is not under legal commitment for services
- GAF >55

Substance Abuse

Admission
- DSM-IV diagnosis of a substance use disorder (substance dependency or substance abuse) of a duration longer than 12 months, unless the person has experienced amnestic episodes, convulsions, or other serious medical consequences of withdrawal as a result of substance abuse, and
- Evidence of negative consequences in two or more areas of life function as a direct result of substance use:
    Activities of daily living
    Interpersonal functioning
    Concentration, persistence, and pace
    Adaptation to change, and
- Willingness and ability to be involved in active abstinence-based treatment, and
- Cognitive ability to understand and profit from structured, interactive therapies, and
- GAF >25

Continuing Stay
- DSM-IV diagnosis of a substance dependency of a duration longer than 12 months (may be in remission or partial remission), and
- Evidence of negative consequences in two or more areas of life function, and
- Continued need for active involvement in treatment to achieve and/or maintain abstinence and functional stability, and
- Evidence of involvement in treatment without deterioration of function to a point requiring a more restrictive level of care, and
- GAF >35

Discharge
- DSM-IV diagnosis of a substance use disorder in remission or partial remission, and
- Evidence of resumed function in key areas of life function, and
- Completion of required aspects of the treatment process with evidence of incorporation into daily functioning, as evidenced by no further negative consequences associated with substance abuse, or
- Persistent refusal to engage in and/or meet the expectations of treatment, or
- Client chooses to leave service area or seek another provider.
- GAF >60

(Continued on next page)

Figure 4.9.   (Continued)

Adult Intermediate Care

Admission
- Adults older than 18 years of age and younger than 65.
- Active DSM-IV Axis I and/or Axis II diagnosis (excluding a primary diagnosis of mental retardation), and
- Evidence of impairment in two or more areas of life function:
     Activities of daily living
     Interpersonal functioning
     Concentration, persistence, and pace
     Adaptation to change, and
- Prior treatment of the identified primary diagnosis, and
- Ambulatory status as defined by ability to access service locations on a regular basis, and
- Ability to maintain adequate independent housing, safety, and nutrition, and
- Freedom from active substance abuse or dependency that would represent the primary diagnosis, and
- Willingness to participate in services
- GAF >45

Continuing Stay
- Adults older than 18 years of age and younger than 65, and
- DSM-IV diagnosis with a duration longer than 12 months, and
- Continued demonstration of an ability to maintain independence in the community, and
- Freedom from active substance abuse or involvement in concurrent substance abuse treatment, and
- Continued willingness to participate in services
- GAF >45

Discharge
- No change in DSM-IV diagnosis in past 12 months, and
- Demonstrated community stability as evidenced by independent housing, control of finances, and maintenance of activities of daily life for at least 12 months, and
- Freedom from active substance abuse, and
- Stability of symptoms with adherence to prescribed medication regiment for at least 6 months, or
- Client moves from service area, or
- Client chooses to seek services from another provider
- GAF >65

Child/Adolescent Intermediate Care

Admission
- Children or adolescents older than three years and younger than 18 years of age
- DSM-IV Axis I diagnosis and/or code of 999.5x, and
- Persistence of symptoms for more than 12 months, unless directly tied to an identified trauma
- Clear indication of lack of success in one or more areas of developmentally appropriate functioning:
     Activities of daily living
     Interpersonal functioning
     Concentration, persistence, and pace
     Adaptation to change, and
- Family resources sufficient to support treatment process (i.e., stable housing, parent figure, and so on)
- GAF >25

Continuing Stay
- Active DSM-IV diagnosis as evidenced by child's reassessment as meeting diagnostic criteria, and
- Continued evidence of need for assistance to achieve success in one or more areas of developmentally appropriate life function, and
- Continued evidence of family/community support for services
- GAF > 35

Discharge
- Client older than 18 years of age (requires transfer to appropriate adult services), or
- No currently active DSM-IV diagnosis and/or child has demonstrated symptom stability for more than two months, and
- No significant impairments in developmentally appropriate community life function, and
- Child has established functional support systems capable of fostering strengths in all areas of life function, or
- Child's caretakers move from service area, or
- Child's caretakers and/or service coordinators seek services from another provider
- GAF >45

Chapter 5

Coding and Reimbursement

Cheryl Kester-Hoffman, RHIA

This chapter describes the evolution of clinical vocabularies and reviews the main components of each. It then presents encoders as an example of technology that has had considerable impact on the practice of coding. Finally, the chapter discusses different types of reimbursement systems, methodologies, and support processes.

Development of Clinical Vocabularies

The International Classification of Diseases (ICD) was first used by hospitals in the late 1940s. It was based on the Bertillon **classification system,** which had been used since 1891. The Bertillon system classified the causes of death. It was adopted by registrars in Canada, Mexico, and the United States and was revised every ten years. Revisions were actually completed in 1900, 1920, 1929, and 1938. In 1948, the sixth revision was published under the auspices of the World Health Organization (WHO) and for the first time included lists for the tabulation of morbidity as well as mortality.

In 1959, the *International Classification of Diseases, Adapted for Indexing Hospital Records by Diseases and Operations* (ICDA), was published and later revised in 1962.

The *International Classification of Diseases (ICDA-8), Eighth Revision, Adapted for Use in the United States,* was published in 1968 and served as the basis for coding diagnostic data for official morbidity and mortality statistics in the U.S. It also proved suitable for use by hospitals in indexing hospital records by diagnoses and operations. A variation of the ICDA-8 classification system was published in 1968 by the Commission on Professional and Hospital activities for use with its Professional Activities Study (PAS) data-recording system.

In 1979, the *International Classification of Diseases, Ninth Revision, Clinical Modification* (ICD-9-CM), became effective as the WHO statistical classification. The WHO revises the ICD every ten years for use throughout the world. However, this international version does not completely meet the needs in the United States because of its emphasis on more acute, infective processes seen in underdeveloped countries rather than chronic diseases. For that reason, it was modified for use in the United States in 1977 (Huffman 1990).

International Classification of Diseases, Ninth Revision, Clinical Modification

In February 1977, the National Center for Health Statistics (NCHS) convened a steering committee to provide advice and counsel in developing a clinical modification of ICD-9. Task forces on classification provided clinical guidance and technical input. These task forces were made up of participants from the Council on Clinical Classification's sponsoring organizations. The American Medical Record Association and the **American Hospital Association** (AHA) were participants in the task force.

As mentioned earlier, ICD-9-CM is a clinical modification of the WHO's ICD-9. ICD is a classification system for medical diagnoses and procedures. The term *clinical* is used to emphasize the modification's intent: to serve as a useful tool to classify morbidity data for indexing medical records, medical care review, and ambulatory and other medical care programs, as well as for basic health statistics. To describe the clinical picture of the patient, the codes must be more precise than those needed only for statistical groupings and trend analysis.

History

ICD-9-CM is the most common classification system used today. Through the NCHS, the federal government modified ICD-9 to create ICD-9-CM. The intent of this modification was to provide a classification system for morbidity data.

The NCHS is responsible for updating the diagnosis classification, and the Centers for Medicare and Medicaid Services (CMS) (formerly called the Health Care Financing Administration, or HCFA) is responsible for updating the procedure classification.

In 1985, the ICD-9-CM Coordination and Maintenance Committee was established. Cochaired by representatives of the NCHS and the CMS, the committee meets twice a year to provide a public forum for discussing possible revisions and updates to ICD-9-CM. These are advisory meetings only, with all final revisions determined by the director of the NCHS and the administrator of the CMS. Changes are reported in the *Federal Register.* (*The Federal Register* can be accessed on the Web at www.gpoaccess.gov/fr/index.html.) The changes are published in October of each year for implementation in January of the following year.

Purpose and Use

The central office of ICD-9-CM has designated the following uses of ICD-9-CM:

- Classifying morbidity and mortality information for statistical purposes

- Indexing hospital records by disease and operations

- Reporting diagnoses by physicians

- Storing and retrieving data

- Reporting national morbidity and mortality data

- Serving as the basis of diagnosis-related group (DRG) assignment for hospital reimbursement

- Reporting and compiling healthcare data to assist in the evaluation of medical care planning for healthcare delivery systems

- Determining patterns of care among healthcare providers

- Analyzing payments for health services

- Conducting epidemiological and clinical research

Structure

ICD-9-CM is published in three volumes. Volume 1 is the Tabular List. It contains the numerical listing of codes that represent diseases and injuries. Volume 2 is the Alphabetic Index. It consists of an alphabetic index for all of the codes listed in Volume 1. The Tabular List and

Alphabetic Index for Procedures are published as Volume 3. Volume 3 is not part of the international version of ICD-9 and is used only in the United States.

Volume 1

Volume 1 of ICD-9-CM is divided into three subdivisions: classification of diseases and injuries, supplementary classifications, and appendices. The classification of diseases and injuries is divided into seventeen chapters organized by types of conditions or by anatomical systems. For example, chapter 5, Mental Disorders, contains groups of diseases by type of condition.

The chapters are further divided into sections. Sections are groups of three-digit code numbers, for example, Organic Psychotic Conditions (290–294) in chapter 5.

Sections are subdivided into categories. Categories represent a group of closely related conditions or a single disease entity. Category 290, Senile and presenile organic psychotic conditions, is an example of a category in chapter 5.

Categories are further divided into subcategories. At this level, four-digit code numbers are used. The following is an example of a subcategory: 290.1 Presenile dementia.

The most specific codes in the ICD-9-CM system are found at the subclassification level. Five-digit code numbers represent this level. For example, code 290.10 represents a code at the subclassification level.

Two supplementary classifications are part of volume 1: the Supplementary Classification of Factors Influencing Health Status and Contact with Health Services (V Codes), and the Supplementary Classification of External Causes of Injury and Poisoning (E Codes).

V Codes

V Codes are used to classify occasions when circumstances other than disease or injury are recorded as the reason for the patient's encounter with healthcare providers. These encounters may occur as follows:

- A person who is not currently sick may encounter a healthcare provider for a specific reason, such as an organ donor, prophylactic vaccination, or discussion of a problem that is not a disease or injury.

- A person with a disease or injury, whether current or resolving, may encounter the healthcare provider for a specific treatment of the disease or injury (for example, chemotherapy or dialysis).

- A person may encounter a healthcare provider with a circumstance or problem that influences his or her health status (for example, personal history of mental disorder or lack of housing).

V codes are always alphanumeric codes. They begin with V and are followed by numerical digits, for example, V40.1, Problems with communication (including speech).

V codes are rarely acceptable as a principle diagnosis because third-party payers will only pay for designated ones. Carriers should be queried with regard to acceptable V Code use.

E Codes

E Codes provide a means to classify environmental events, circumstances, and conditions as the cause of injury, poisoning, and other adverse effects. These codes must be used in addition to codes from the main chapters of ICD-9-CM. E Codes provide additional information that is used by insurance companies, safety programs, and public health agencies to determine the causes of injuries, poisonings, or other adverse situations.

E codes begin with E and are followed by numerical characters. For example, E950.0 is the code for a suicide and self-inflicted poisoning—analgesics, antipyretics, and antirheumatics.

The E code is never a principle diagnosis. Organizational policy should clarify the use of E codes. Not all states require E codes. Some carriers may require them and you need to check with your carriers.

Volume 2

Volume 2 is titled Index to Diseases and Injuries. The main terms are arranged alphabetically by type of disease, injury, or illness. Subterms are indented under the main term.

Volume 3

Volume 3 of ICD-9-CM contains the tabular and alphabetic lists of procedures. Chapters in this volume are organized according to anatomical systems, except for the last chapter titled Miscellaneous Diagnostic and Therapeutic Procedures. The mental health information manager rarely, if ever, uses this volume.

Appendices

Volume 1 of ICD-9-CM has five appendices. Appendix B, Glossary of Mental Disorders, is the one that mental health professionals find most useful. (See figure 5.1 for an example of a glossary entry in appendix B of ICD-9-CM.)

Organizations should purchase or update their codebooks yearly because codes are constantly added, deleted, and revised. Failing to have the latest information may affect reimbursement and lead to denial of payment (Brown 2002).

ICD-10

ICD-10 will be modified and published as ICD-10-CM. CMS also is developing a new procedure coding system called ICD, 10th edition, Procedural Coding System (ICD-10-PCS). Both systems are alphanumeric to allow a greater number of codes than the primarily numeric system of ICD-9-CM could accommodate. These modifications of ICD-10 are slated for adoption early in the twenty-first century.

ICD-O-2

The second edition of the International Classification of Diseases for Oncology (ICD-O-2) is a system used for classifying incidences of malignant disease. Hospitals use ICD-O-2 to develop cancer registries.

History

The WHO published the first edition of the *International Classification of Diseases for Oncology* (ICD-O) in 1976. It was developed jointly by the United States Cancer Institute and WHO's International Agency for research on cancer.

Figure 5.1. Example of a glossary entry in appendix B of ICD-9-CM

Alcohol intoxication

acute: A psychic and physical state resulting from alcohol ingestion characterized by slurred speech, unsteady gait, poor coordination, flushed facies, nystagmus, sluggish reflexes, fetor alcoholica, loud speech, emotional instability (e.g., jollity followed by lugubriousness), excessive conviviality, loquacity, and poorly inhibited sexual and aggressive behavior.

idiosyncratic: Acute psychotic episodes induced by relatively small amounts of alcohol. These are regarded as individual idiosyncratic reactions to alcohol, not due to excessive consumption and without conspicuous neurological signs of intoxication.

pathological—see Alcohol intoxication, idiosyncratic

Purpose

ICD-0-2 was developed initially to provide a detailed classification system for coding the histology, topography, and behavior of neoplasms. The current version provides a detailed classification that is used by pathology departments, cancer registries, and healthcare providers that treat cancer patients. Mental healthcare organizations rarely use this classification system unless they are a unit of an acute care hospital.

Healthcare Common Procedure Coding System

The Healthcare Common Procedure Coding System (HCPCS) is a uniform method for healthcare providers and medical suppliers to report professional services, procedures, and supplies. The American Medical Association (AMA) first published CPT in 1966 in a volume containing primarily surgical procedures. The second edition, published in 1970, contained 5-digit CPT codes, replacing 4-digit codes, for diagnostic and therapeutic procedures in surgery, medicine, and the specialties. The third and fourth editions were released in the 1970s. In 1983, the then HCFA (now the CMS) included CPT as part of the HCPCS. In the mid-1980s, HCFA mandated CPT codes for reporting outpatient hospital surgical procedures and required state Medicaid agencies to use HCPCS.

Prior to its development, there was no uniform system for coding a procedure, service, or supply for reimbursement (Huffman 1990, 354–97). CMS has maintained the essence of HCPCS, which is to:

- Meet the operational needs of Medicare/Medicaid

- Coordinate government programs by uniform application of CMS policies

- Allow providers and suppliers to communicate their services in a consistent manner

- Ensure the validity of profiles and fee schedules through standardized coding

- Enhance medical education and research by providing a vehicle for local, regional, and national utilization comparisons.

HCPCS Levels of Codes

Each of the two HCPCS levels is a unique coding system. Levels I and II, also are known by the names shown here with the level numbers.

Level I: Current Procedural Terminology

Level I is the AMA's Current Procedural Terminology (CPT). The Level I codes include five-digit codes and two-digit modifiers, both with descriptive terms for reporting services performed by healthcare providers. Level I codes and modifiers are described in detail in the CPT book.

The AMA released its first edition of CPT in 1966 with the intention of simplifying the reporting of procedures or services rendered by physicians or healthcare providers under their supervision. Procedures are grouped within six major sections: **evaluation and management** (E/M), anesthesiology, surgery, radiology, pathology and laboratory, and medicine. The major sections are divided into subsections according to body part, service, or diagnosis (for example, mouth, amputation, or septal defect).

Level II: HCPCS National Codes

The CPT book does not contain all the codes needed to report medical services and supplies, so CMS developed the second level of codes. In contrast to the five-digit codes found in Level I, National Codes consist of one alphabetic character (a letter between A and V), followed by four digits. The codes are grouped by the type of service or supply they represent and are updated annually by CMS with input from private insurance companies. Level II codes are required for reporting most medical services and supplies provided to Medicare and Medicaid patients and by most private payers. All D codes have a copyright by the American Dental Association.

Level II of HCPCS also contains modifiers, which are either alphanumeric or two letters in the range from –AA to –VP. National modifiers can be used with all levels of HCPCS codes. The appendices include a complete listing of Level II modifiers.

In 2002, several Medicaid T codes were added. The T codes (T1001–T1015) are designed to report services furnished by nonphysician healthcare professionals and can be reported with the new modifiers.

CPT Codes for Psychiatric Services

CPT codes for psychiatric services include general and special diagnostic services as well as a variety of therapeutic services. By CPT manual definition, therapeutic services (for example, CPT codes 90842–90844) include psychotherapy and continuing medical diagnostic evaluation; therefore, CPT codes 90801 and 90802 are not billed with these services.

Interactive services (diagnostic or therapeutic) are distinct forms of services for patients who have "lost, or have not yet developed either the expressive language communication skills to explain his/her symptoms and response to treatment." Accordingly, noninteractive services would not be possible at the same session as interactive services and are not to be billed together with interactive services.

Drug management is included in some therapeutic services (for example, CPT codes 90842–90844, 90847, 90853), and thus CPT code 90862, Pharmacologic management, is not to be billed with these codes.

When medical services other than psychiatric services are provided in addition to psychiatric services, separate E/M codes cannot be billed. The psychiatric service includes the E/M services provided according to Medicare guidelines.

Psychiatry

Psychiatry is the study, treatment, and prevention of mental disorders. Psychiatric services include diagnostic and therapeutic services in the hospital, office, or other outpatient setting. The codes in this subsection of CPT are used to report general psychiatric, clinical psychiatric, and psychiatric therapeutic services and procedures. Key coding issues for therapeutic services are the type of psychotherapy, the place of service, the face-to-face time spent with the patient during psychotherapy, and whether E/M services are furnished on the same date of service as psychotherapy.

Following are some rules that apply when coding psychiatric services:

- Hospital care services reported by the **attending physician** in treating a psychiatric inpatient may use the full range of hospital E/M codes.

- If the physician is active in the leadership or direction of a treatment team, a code may be selected based on the services provided that day using **case management** codes from the E/M series 99361–99362.

- All procedures that are performed in addition to hospital care, such as electroconvulsive therapy or medical psychotherapy, should be listed in addition to hospital care.

- Psychiatric care may be reported without time dimensions, using codes 90845–90857.

- The modifiers –52, Reduced Service, or –22, Unusual Service, may be used to bill for services that were less or more lengthy than the time-specified codes define.

Psychiatric Consultations

Consultation for psychiatric evaluation of a patient includes examination of the patient, exchange of information with primary physician and others (for example, nurses or family members), and preparation of a report. Consultation services provided by psychiatrists are billed using CPT E/M consultation codes. Psychiatric consultation services are limited to initial psychiatric treatment.

SNOMED

The **Systematized Nomenclature of Human and Veterinary Medicine** (SNOMED) is a nomenclature of medical terms. The American College of Pathologists defines SNOMED as a systematized, multiaxial, and hierarchically organized nomenclature of medically useful terms.

The first edition of SNOMED was published in 1977 by the American College of Pathologists (ACP). It is based on the Systematized Nomenclature of Pathology (SNOP), which was published by the ACP in 1965 to organize information from surgical pathology reports. This nomenclature was widely used and accepted in the medical community and expanded for use in other specialties (Huffman 1990).

Clinicians may use different terms for the same medical condition. This makes it difficult to gather and retrieve information. Standardized **vocabulary** is needed to facilitate the indexing, storage, and retrieval of patient information.

Diagnostic and Statistical Manual of Mental Disorders, Fourth Revision

The **American Psychiatric Association** (APA) developed the *Diagnostic and Statistical Manual of Mental Disorders* (DSM-IV-TR) as a tool for providing a set of codes that could be used to aid in the collection of clinical data using stand-alone personal computers. This was used to track mental health diagnoses. Some states specifically use these data and provide monies to state facilities for patient care.

History

The APA published the first edition of *Diagnostic and Statistical Manual of Mental Disorders (DSM)* in 1952. The APA's Committee on Nomenclature and Statistics developed DSM from ICD. DSM-I contained a glossary of descriptions of mental disorders. DSM has been revised three times since 1952 and is now published as the fourth edition with text revision, or DSM-IV-TR.

To facilitate ease of use with ICD versions, the APA has worked closely with other organizations to make DSM-IV, ICD-9-CM, and ICD-10 fully compatible. All DSM-IV codes are ICD-9-CM codes.

Purpose and Use

The main purpose of DSM-IV-TR is to provide a way to record the data of patients treated for substance abuse and mental disorders. DSM-IV-TR provides the **nomenclature** for communicating diagnostic information, standardizing the diagnostic process for patients with psychiatric disorders and the recording of detailed psychiatric data.

DSM-IV-TR contains a listing of the criteria for diagnosing a mental disorder and the key clinical manifestations. Mental conditions are evaluated along five axes, of which the first three are the diagnostic evaluation. (See figure 5.2.)

Structure

The five axes used in DSM-IV-TR are used by clinicians to establish a systematic evaluation of patient symptoms and subsequent diagnoses. The diagnoses then are given a code or codes that are the same as ICD-9-CM codes. This ensures that information of value is gathered for use in planning treatment and predicting outcome.

Axis I includes all the mental health conditions except personality disorders and mental retardation. Axis II is used to report mental conditions that may be relevant to treatment of the mental health disorder. Mental health facilities use ICD-9-CM for coding Axis III general medical conditions. Axis IV is used to report psychosocial and environmental factors affecting the person. Examples of these factors include the following:

- Problems with primary support group (for example, divorce)
- Problems with social environment (for example, death of a friend)
- Educational problems
- Housing problems
- Economic problems
- Occupational difficulties
- Legal difficulties
- Transportation difficulties

These are some of the categories a clinician will examine to see how the client is doing in life situations. Axis V, Global Assessment of Functioning, is the clinician's best guess of the client's overall level of functioning.

This system is used in behavioral healthcare settings and includes definitions and diagnostic criteria for mental disorders in addition to code number for the diagnoses. All **diagnostic codes** in DSM-IV-TR are valid ICD-9-CM codes. The DSM is used by mental health professionals to determine a diagnosis and by HIM professionals to determine a code. It is used in **psychiatric hospitals,** community mental health centers, developmental disability (mental retardation) centers, and mental health units in hospitals. Because most insurance claims still require the ICD-9-CM code, DSM-IV-TR is not routinely used in all mental health settings. **Crosswalks** (lists of translating codes from one system to another) have been developed to

Figure 5.2. The five axes of DSM-IV-TR

Axis I	Clinical Disorders
Axis II	Personality Disorders and Mental Retardation
Axis III	General Medical Condition
Axis IV	Psychosocial and Environmental Factors
Axis V	Global Assessment of Functioning

allow coders to code with DSM-IV-TR and then use the crosswalk to determine the correct ICD-9-CM code for the bill.

Coding Technology: Encoders

Technology has changed many aspects of the health information management (HIM) profession. One of the primary areas that has been most affected by technology is coding. As early as the 1980s, information technology was applied to make the coding process more effective and efficient. The type of tool used to aid in the coding process is commonly referred to as an encoder. The development of other technologies, including natural language processing, will likely have an even greater impact on the coding process.

Use of Encoders

Encoders for ICD were developed in the early 1980s. Since then, greater sophistication has been built into these technology solutions. An **encoder** is computer software that assists in the assignment of codes. Initially, encoders were developed to assist coders in assigning ICD-9-CM codes; today, they provide assistance with other coding systems.

The information science and technology behind the encoding software varies from vendor to vendor. Some encoders are built using expert system techniques, such as rule-based systems. Other encoding software is more simplistic, merely automating a look-up function similar to the manual index in ICD or other coding classifications.

Encoders have many different types of interfaces, depending on the vendor. An **interface** may be defined as the total component of screens, navigation, and input mechanisms used to help the end user operate the encoding software. Some encoder systems have an interface that prompts the coder through a series of questions. As the coder answers the question, the encoder suggests code assignments for diagnoses and procedures.

Alternatively, other encoders allow coders to input classification codes directly into the system and then go through a series of edit checks to ensure that only allowable code numbers are entered. In more sophisticated software systems, the encoder also prompts the coder to review the sequencing of the codes that have been selected to optimize reimbursement.

Good encoding software should include edit checks to ensure data quality. For example, an inappropriate combination of codes or inconsistent data should be flagged for the coder's attention. Encoding software is frequently linked to other information systems such as billing and crosswalks (Johns 2002, 318).

Types of Encoders

There are two types of encoders. The first uses a branching logic system. Usually the coder enters the main term from the diagnosis or procedure to be coded and is guided through a series of questions resulting in a code assignment. The second type of encoder is more like an automated codebook with the screen looking like the actual alphabetic index and tabular list. More experienced coders often prefer the automated codebook encoder because they can code more efficiently using their current coding skills rather than working through all the questions in a branching logic system. In turn, most less-experienced coders prefer the branching logic system because it guides them through selection of a code. Encoders are available for both ICD-9-CM and HCPCS/CPT.

Most encoders integrate other software into the coding logic. Many now include on-line references from *Coding Clinic* and *CPT Assistant* to assist coders in utilizing the most up-to-date coding guidelines.

Reimbursement Systems

Reimbursement systems were developed in an effort to ensure that every American receives healthcare services. Systems in which people are able to pay for all or a portion of their healthcare treatment include commercial insurance plans and managed care plans. People unable, for one reason or another, to obtain private healthcare coverage are often eligible for healthcare services through government-sponsored programs.

Commercial Insurance

Most working Americans are covered under employer-provided health insurance plans. One type of plan is the standard indemnity policy, which gives people freedom to visit a healthcare provider of their choice. They pay for their treatment out of pocket and are reimbursed by the insurance plan for some portion of the cost. The other common plan is a managed care plan. Under this plan, medically necessary care is provided in the most cost-effective or least expensive way available. Plan members must visit healthcare providers chosen by the managed care plan. Generally, the patient pays a copayment, but sometimes all care received from providers within the plan is covered.

Blue Cross and Blue Shield Plans

Blue Cross and Blue Shield (BC/BS) is the nation's oldest and largest provider of prepaid health coverage. It is a federation of individual nonprofit community corporations. The term *prepaid* means the carrier pays for specified medical expenses if premiums are paid in advance. Local Blue Cross and Blue Shield corporations, which provide this coverage, are known as plans.

The BC/BS organization was developed from two kinds of healthcare programs: Blue Cross, which covered hospital services; and Blue Shield, which covered physician services. Today, Blue Cross coverage has expanded to include benefits for outpatient and home care services, as well as other kinds of institutional care. Blue Shield plans now offer dental, vision, and other outpatient benefits.

The first Blue Cross plan was founded in 1929 at Baylor University in Dallas, Texas. Teachers there agreed to pay six dollars per year in exchange for twenty-one days of care at the university hospital if the need arose.

Founded in 1939, the first Blue Shield plan was known as California Physicians' Service. Its membership was restricted to individuals who earned less than $3,000 per year. The first members paid a monthly premium of $1.70.

After these plans began, additional employee groups and healthcare providers joined and similar programs were started in other communities. Most BC/BS plans operate as joint corporations but remain separate organizations. They all belong to the Blue Cross and Blue Shield Association, the national coordinating agency of BC/BS plans. It administers Medicare and other federal and state health programs.

BC/BS plans differ from commercial insurance carriers in the following ways:

1. They operate as nonprofit corporations.

2. Healthcare providers sign unique contracts with BC/BS plans.

3. They often accept members that other carriers do not cover.

4. They cannot raise rates without state approval.

Managed Care Plans

What is now called managed care began in the 1940s with the creation of health maintenance organizations (HMOs). Families getting medical care at HMOs were urged to get yearly checkups and seek preventive care and early treatment in case of illness. This proved cost-effective, and as healthcare costs rose, employers began to sign contracts with companies offering to "manage" their employees' healthcare. Managed care companies organize doctors into cost-conscious groups. Since the 1980s, more and more employee benefit programs have contracted with managed care companies. Today, there are hundreds of them, but their rules differ and contracts change from year to year.

Type of Care Provided

Managed care organizations (MCOs) provide services in many states for low-income Medicare and Medicaid beneficiaries. Both types of private health coverage may offer some coverage for mental health treatment, but it often is not paid for at the same rate as other healthcare costs.

Managed care controls medical costs mostly by limiting hospitalization, applying "standards of care" for most conditions, and contracting with exclusive providers. MCOs seek to provide less expensive, less restrictive care. Managed care pays for healthcare that is "adequate" and "medically necessary," using the least costly alternative. In essence, managed care:

- Strives to control healthcare costs

- Discourages unnecessary hospitalization

- Discourages overuse of specialists

- Provides services dependent on the contract

The benefits and drawbacks of managed care are summarized in table 5.1.

Two types of managed care providers or networks are health maintenance organizations (HMOs) and preferred provider organizations (PPOs). An HMO is a prepaid health plan. For a fixed fee per year, it provides enrollees with a range of medical services, both inpatient and outpatient. Doctors, on salary or contract, may work in a central facility or in a number of different places. A PPO is a group of independent providers in private offices offering services at a discount to the MCO. The plan distributes a list of participating doctors. In both PPO and HMO plans with a point-of-service option, enrollees generally pay more if they use a doctor outside the plan.

Many plans ask enrollees to pay a fixed sum of money toward each bill. This fee, called a copayment or copay, may be five or ten dollars per visit or prescription. The copay may be higher for mental healthcare than for other services. Moreover, there may be deductibles,

Table 5.1. Benefits and drawbacks of managed care

Benefits	Drawbacks
Improved facilities: Consumers of public mental health services may have access to more attractive facilities and better trained medical providers, located closer to home.	If hospitalization is denied without offering alternatives for intensive care, a person's symptoms may get worse.
Expanded choices: There may be additional alternative service options in the community. These include treatment services (day treatment, residential services, intensive outpatient care, home therapy, telephone counseling) and support services (self-help centers, psychosocial programs).	People with long-term mental illness may need more than short-term acute care preferred by managed care.
	Continuity of care may be difficult when people get short-term treatments at different locations. Protecting confidentiality might be troublesome due to entities needing to know the nature of the treatment at different locations.
Money saved can be used to expand outpatient benefits, reduce member costs, or help make health insurance affordable to more people.	Companies managing the mental healthcare may change, potentially disrupting services.

where the enrollee pays a set amount for services before the plan begins to cover them. When benefits are used up, people go without care or pay the total cost out-of-pocket.

Mental Health Coverage under Managed Care

States now are looking to the **managed care** industry to provide public healthcare, including mental health and related services. In the past, state and local governments allowed service providers to bill Medicaid and Medicare directly, after the services were provided, on a fee-for-service basis. Under managed care, providers who contract with an MCO may find that it expects to authorize every piece of service it considers medically necessary.

Managing care is harder than managing dollars. For people with long-term mental illness, managed care is a new way of delivering services that has not been tried before.

With managed care, each benefit package is determined by a contract developed by an employer or the state. There is no standard. Thus, a beneficiary with a preexisting condition (such as mental illness) should make sure that treatment is covered. Mental healthcare or drug and alcohol treatment service benefits may be limited. A contract may allow up to 30 days of inpatient care and 20 outpatient sessions a year. A maximum sum of money may be available for care in a year or over the patient's lifetime.

Government-Sponsored Healthcare Programs

The federal government has created a number of programs to help people unable to purchase private insurance obtain healthcare services. The following subsections discuss these programs.

Public Assistance

People with severe mental illness may be eligible for several forms of public assistance, both to meet the basic costs of living and to pay for healthcare. Examples of such programs are Social Security, Medicare, and Medicaid.

Social Security

Social Security has two types of programs to help individuals with disabilities. Social Security disability insurance provides benefits for those individuals who have worked for a required length of time and have paid Social Security taxes. Supplemental security income provides benefits to individuals based on their economic needs (SSA 2004).

Medicare

Medicare is America's primary federal health insurance program for people who are 65 or older, some people with disabilities who are under 65, and dependent widows. It was first offered to retired Americans in July 1966. Retired and disabled Americans who are eligible for Social Security benefits automatically qualify for Medicare coverage, without regard to income. Medicare provides basic protection for the cost of healthcare and its regulations are uniform across all states.

Medicare offers two coverage programs:

- Part A is financed through payroll taxes. In the beginning, coverage was applied only to hospitalization and home health care. Eventually, extended care in nursing homes was included. Those needing kidney transplantation or dialysis for end-stage renal disease and those on Social Security disability payments of more than two years were added to coverage in 1973.

- Part B is optional. Beneficiaries pay premiums to supplement the federal funding. Part B is for physician's services, outpatient hospital care, medical services and supplies, and certain other medical costs not covered by Part A.

Moreover, two programs exist to help people with low incomes receive benefits:

- Qualified Medicare beneficiaries (QMBs) are those individuals whose resources are at or below twice the standard allowed under the supplementary security income program and incomes at or below 100 percent of the federal poverty level. For QMBs, Medicaid pays Part A and B premiums along with the Medicare coinsurance and deductibles, subject to limits that states may impose on payment rates.

- Specified low-income Medicare beneficiaries (SLMBs) include Medicare enrollees who have resources similar to the QMBs, but higher incomes (although still less than 120 percent of the federal poverty level). Medicaid pays only Part B premiums for SLMBs.

Yet another category of beneficiaries includes disabled and working people who previously qualified for Medicare because of their disability but lost their entitlement when they returned to work. They are allowed to purchase Medicare Parts A and B coverage. When their income falls below 200 percent of the federal poverty level (and they do not meet any other Medicaid assistance category), Medicaid also may pay their Medicare Part A premiums under the program for qualified disabled and working individuals (Johns 2002, 351).

Beneficiaries are responsible for 50 percent of approved charges for outpatient psychiatric services.

Medicaid

Medicaid pays for some healthcare costs for America's poorest and most vulnerable people. More information about Medicaid and eligibility requirements is available at local welfare and medical assistance offices. Although there are certain federal requirements, each state also has its own rules and regulations for Medicaid. In some states, a fiscal agent, an organization that processes claims for a government program, may administer Medicaid.

As part of the 1965 Social Security Act, federal law required the first Medicaid programs. Under the legislation, the federal government determines which kinds of medical services are covered and paid for by the federal portion of the program. States participate in their Medicaid programs two ways:

- They may authorize additional kinds of services or make additional groups eligible.

- They determine eligibility within federal guidelines.

Because of this participation by the state government, Medicaid programs vary widely from state to state.

Many mental health organizations participate because of their client population. Participating in the Medicaid program means agreeing to accept Medicaid reimbursement for covered services as payment in full. The organization must write off the difference between fees charged for services and amount reimbursed. The patient must not be billed for the difference. However, the client may be billed for services not covered by Medicaid.

According to federal guidelines, Medicaid pays for the following types of services:

- Physician services

- Laboratory and X-ray services

- Inpatient hospital care

- Outpatient hospital and rural health clinic services

- Home healthcare

- Care in a nursing facility

- Family planning

- Early and periodic screening, diagnosis, and treatment (EPSDT) for low-income children

The above services are termed mandated services and must be provided to the categorically needy.

Mental health services fall under the state portion of a Medicaid program and are included in a number of additional services under its federally funded Medicaid program. Mental health, developmental disabilities, and substance abuse services may be paid for through Medicaid funding.

TRICARE

TRICARE is the current name for CHAMPUS, which stands for the Civilian Health and Medical Program of the Uniformed Services (Army, Navy, Air Force, Marine Corps, Coast Guard, Public Health Service, and the National Oceanic and Atmospheric Administration). The program was phased in nationally by 1998. Expansion to overseas military is now complete. TRICARE offers three options: TRICARE Prime, TRICARE Extra, and TRICARE Standard.

The program covers medical expenses for families of active duty members of the uniformed services, retired military personnel, and their dependents. It also covers military retirees and their families, some former spouses, and dependents of military personnel who were killed while on active duty.

CHAMPVA

CHAMPVA stands for the Civilian Health and Medical Program of the Veterans Administration. The Veterans Administration has changed its name and is now called the Department of Veterans Affairs.

This program is for veterans with permanent service-connected disabilities and their dependents. CHAMPVA shares healthcare costs for families of veterans with 100 percent service-connected disability. It covers the surviving spouse and children of a veteran who dies from a service-connected disability. Some surviving spouses of a service member who died on active duty may be eligible for CHAMPVA. The Department of Veterans Affairs determines eligibility.

TRICARE and CHAMPVA will not duplicate benefits from another program or health plan. Moreover, there are regulations for cases involving third-party liability. If a beneficiary qualifies for Medicaid or is covered under a supplemental insurance policy, TRICARE or CHAMPVA is the primary payer. However, TRICARE and CHAMPVA are secondary payers when the patient is covered under another health plan or belongs to an HMO or PPO. Further, they will not pay for illnesses or injuries covered by workers' compensation unless compensation benefits have been exhausted.

Indian Healthcare Services

Another government-sponsored healthcare program that mental health information mangers might see is the Indian Health Service (IHS). IHS provides health services to American Indians and Alaska natives.

The patient population served by IHS is eligible to receive preventive healthcare services, primary medical services (hospital and ambulatory care), community health services, substance abuse treatment services, and rehabilitative services. Most services are delivered on Indian reservations in Indian and Alaska native communities. Other services may be provided on a contracted basis.

Workers' Compensation

People with job-related illness or injury are covered under workers' compensation insurance. Workers' compensation varies according to state law.

Reimbursement Methodologies

Reimbursement methodologies include claim forms, electronic data interchange, fee for service, and prospective payment systems.

Claim Forms

The type of service delivered to the client indicates whether the CMS-1500 or the UB-92 (HCFA-1450) claim form is used. The CMS-1500 is used for nonhospital services; the UB-82 is used for inpatient, outpatient, hospice, home health, and long-term care services.

CMS-1500

Many private insurance carriers have specialized insurance claim forms for their policyholders, most of which ask for the same basic information. Most carriers accept the universal health insurance claim form known as the CMS-1500. (See figure 5.3.) The CMS-1500 is approved by the AMA and used to obtain reimbursement for services provided by physicians and other allied health professionals. The general insurance carriers such as BC/BS, TRICARE, Medicare, and Medicaid accept the CMS-1500 form. Information about the various government programs appears on the back of the form.

Revisions to the CMS-1500 were made in 1990, and the form was printed in red ink to meet optical scanning guidelines. In May 1992, Medicare began requiring that all services except ambulance services be billed on the CMS-1500.

UB-92 (HCFA-1450)

The UB-92 (HCFA-1450) or Uniform Bill is submitted by psychiatric and drug/alcohol treatment facilities (inpatient and outpatient services) to third-party payers for reimbursement of client services. (See figure 5.4.) It is used by all medical and psychiatric entities and keeps billing uniform.

Electronic Data Interchange

The **electronic data interchange** (EDI) is the electronic transfer of information. The EDI allows healthcare entities to exchange medical and billing information to process transactions quickly and cost-effectively. Using the EDI reduces handling and processing time compared to paper and eliminates the risk of lost paper documents. It can eliminate the inefficiencies of handling paper documents, thus reducing the administrative burden, lowering operating costs, and improving overall data quality.

Fee for Service

Fee for service is the term assigned to the payment for services rendered by the healthcare provider, whether a physician, a healthcare organization, or another clinician. A comparison of fees in a geographic region would likely show that the fees for services are similar. By ignoring the very high and very low fees, it is be possible to determine the usual and customary fees charged in the region.

Figure 5.3. CMS-1500 claim form

PLEASE DO NOT STAPLE IN THIS AREA

CARRIER

PICA

HEALTH INSURANCE CLAIM FORM

PICA

1. MEDICARE   MEDICAID   CHAMPUS   CHAMPVA   GROUP HEALTH PLAN   FECA BLK LUNG   OTHER
   (Medicare #)   (Medicaid #)   (Sponsor's SSN)   (VA File #)   (SSN or ID)   (SSN)   (ID)

1a. INSURED'S I.D. NUMBER   (FOR PROGRAM IN ITEM 1)

2. PATIENT'S NAME (Last Name, First Name, Middle Initial)

3. PATIENT'S BIRTH DATE   MM   DD   YY   SEX   M   F

4. INSURED'S NAME (Last Name, First Name, Middle Initial)

5. PATIENT'S ADDRESS (No., Street)

6. PATIENT RELATIONSHIP TO INSURED   Self   Spouse   Child   Other

7. INSURED'S ADDRESS (No., Street)

CITY   STATE

8. PATIENT STATUS   Single   Married   Other   Employed   Full-Time Student   Part-Time Student

CITY   STATE

ZIP CODE   TELEPHONE (Include Area Code)   (   )

ZIP CODE   TELEPHONE (INCLUDE AREA CODE)   (   )

9. OTHER INSURED'S NAME (Last Name, First Name, Middle Initial)

10. IS PATIENT'S CONDITION RELATED TO:

11. INSURED'S POLICY GROUP OR FECA NUMBER

a. OTHER INSURED'S POLICY OR GROUP NUMBER

a. EMPLOYMENT? (CURRENT OR PREVIOUS)   YES   NO

a. INSURED'S DATE OF BIRTH   MM   DD   YY   SEX   M   F

b. OTHER INSURED'S DATE OF BIRTH   MM   DD   YY   SEX   M   F

b. AUTO ACCIDENT?   PLACE (State)   YES   NO

b. EMPLOYER'S NAME OR SCHOOL NAME

c. EMPLOYER'S NAME OR SCHOOL NAME

c. OTHER ACCIDENT?   YES   NO

c. INSURANCE PLAN NAME OR PROGRAM NAME

d. INSURANCE PLAN NAME OR PROGRAM NAME

10d. RESERVED FOR LOCAL USE

d. IS THERE ANOTHER HEALTH BENEFIT PLAN?   YES   NO   If yes, return to and complete item 9 a-d.

READ BACK OF FORM BEFORE COMPLETING & SIGNING THIS FORM.

12. PATIENT'S OR AUTHORIZED PERSON'S SIGNATURE I authorize the release of any medical or other information necessary to process this claim. I also request payment of government benefits either to myself or to the party who accepts assignment below.

SIGNED _____   DATE _____

13. INSURED'S OR AUTHORIZED PERSON'S SIGNATURE I authorize payment of medical benefits to the undersigned physician or supplier for services described below.

SIGNED _____

14. DATE OF CURRENT: MM   DD   YY   ILLNESS (First symptom) OR INJURY (Accident) OR PREGNANCY(LMP)

15. IF PATIENT HAS HAD SAME OR SIMILAR ILLNESS. GIVE FIRST DATE   MM   DD   YY

16. DATES PATIENT UNABLE TO WORK IN CURRENT OCCUPATION   MM   DD   YY   FROM   TO   MM   DD   YY

17. NAME OF REFERRING PHYSICIAN OR OTHER SOURCE

17a. I.D. NUMBER OF REFERRING PHYSICIAN

18. HOSPITALIZATION DATES RELATED TO CURRENT SERVICES   MM   DD   YY   FROM   TO   MM   DD   YY

19. RESERVED FOR LOCAL USE

20. OUTSIDE LAB?   YES   NO $ CHARGES

21. DIAGNOSIS OR NATURE OF ILLNESS OR INJURY. (RELATE ITEMS 1,2,3 OR 4 TO ITEM 24E BY LINE)

1. ____ . ____   3. ____ . ____

2. ____ . ____   4. ____ . ____

22. MEDICAID RESUBMISSION CODE   ORIGINAL REF. NO.

23. PRIOR AUTHORIZATION NUMBER

24. A DATE(S) OF SERVICE From MM DD YY To MM DD YY	B Place of Service	C Type of Service	D PROCEDURES, SERVICES, OR SUPPLIES (Explain Unusual Circumstances) CPT/HCPCS MODIFIER	E DIAGNOSIS CODE	F $ CHARGES	G DAYS OR UNITS	H EPSDT Family Plan	I EMG	J COB	K RESERVED FOR LOCAL USE
1										
2										
3										
4										
5										
6										

25. FEDERAL TAX I.D. NUMBER   SSN EIN

26. PATIENT'S ACCOUNT NO.

27. ACCEPT ASSIGNMENT? (For govt. claims, see back)   YES   NO

28. TOTAL CHARGE $

29. AMOUNT PAID $

30. BALANCE DUE $

31. SIGNATURE OF PHYSICIAN OR SUPPLIER INCLUDING DEGREES OR CREDENTIALS (I certify that the statements on the reverse apply to this bill and are made a part thereof.)

SIGNED _____   DATE _____

32. NAME AND ADDRESS OF FACILITY WHERE SERVICES WERE RENDERED (If other than home or office)

33. PHYSICIAN'S, SUPPLIER'S BILLING NAME, ADDRESS, ZIP CODE & PHONE #

PIN#   GRP#

PATIENT AND INSURED INFORMATION

PHYSICIAN OR SUPPLIER INFORMATION

(APPROVED BY AMA COUNCIL ON MEDICAL SERVICE 8/88)   **PLEASE PRINT OR TYPE**   APPROVED OMB-0938-0008 FORM CMS-1500 (12/90),   FORM RRB-1500, APPROVED OMB-1215-0055 FORM OWCP-1500,   APPROVED OMB-0720-0001 (CHAMPUS)

Figure 5.4.   UB-92 (HCFA-1450) claim form

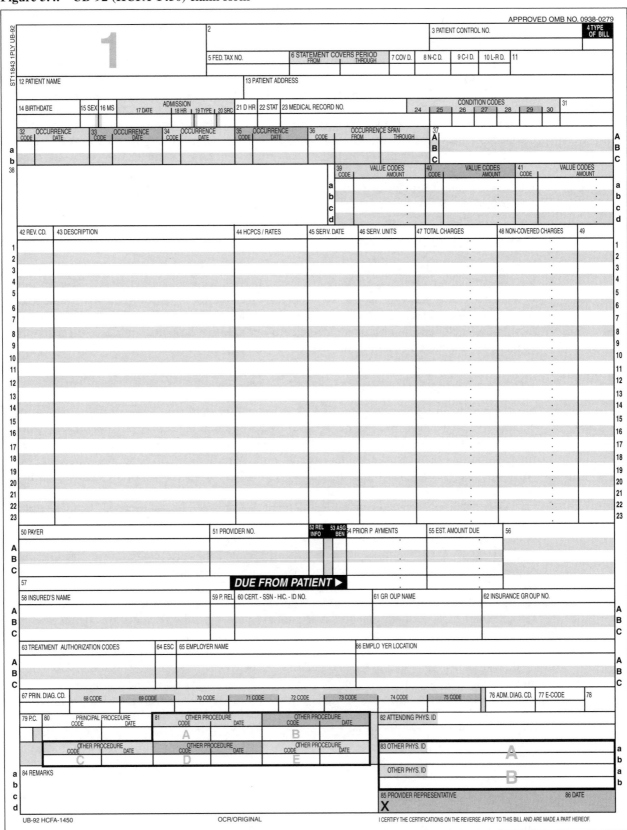

Before the widespread availability of health insurance coverage, individuals were assured access to healthcare only when they were able to pay for the services themselves. They paid cash for services on a retrospective fee-for-service basis. Under this system, the patient was expected to pay the healthcare provider after a service was rendered. Until the advent of managed care, capitation, and other prospective payment systems, private insurance plans and government-sponsored programs also reimbursed providers on a retrospective fee-for-service basis.

Today, fee-for-service reimbursement is rare for most types of medical services. Most Americans have some form of health insurance, and most health insurance plans compensate providers according to predetermined discounted rates. However, some types of care are not covered by most health insurance plans and still are paid for directly by patients on a fee-for-service basis. One example of such care is cosmetic surgery. Cosmetic surgery is not considered medically necessary and thus is not covered by most insurance plans. Many insurance plans also limit coverage for psychiatric services, substance abuse treatment, and the testing and correction of vision and hearing.

Prospective Payment Systems

Prospective payment is a method of determining reimbursement based on predetermined factors, not individual services. A number of insurance companies and the federal government use prospective payment systems (PPSs). Medicare uses the term *PPS* to describe its method of reimbursement to hospitals. Psychiatric hospitals and psychiatric units within a larger medical facility are excluded from Medicare acute care PPSs. Psychiatric hospitals are still paid on the basis of reasonable cost, subject to payment limits per discharge.

PPS Implementation for Psychiatric Hospitals

For the past twenty years, licensed inpatient psychiatry units and freestanding inpatient psychiatric hospitals have been exempt from DRG-based prospective payment for Medicare patients. However, in 2004, that began to change. In 2004, the CMS began to implement a PPS for psychiatric hospitals. Preliminary regulations were published in the *Federal Register* on November 28, 2003, and comments on the regulations were taken in an extended comment period through the end of February 2004.

As part of the Balanced Budget Refinement Act of 1999, hospital-based inpatient psychiatry units and freestanding psychiatric hospitals are required to move from cost-based reimbursement to PPS reimbursement for Medicare patients. The new PPS, which will affect approximately 2,000 facilities, is intended to promote long-term cost control and utilization management and will be implemented by CMS on a budget-neutral basis. Only licensed psychiatric hospitals and hospital-based psychiatry units will come under the new PPS, which will be phased in over a three-year period. General healthcare organizations that are not licensed for specialty care but occasionally treat patients with behavioral health or chemical dependency diagnoses will not come under the new PPS.

The psychiatric PPS system is different from the inpatient PPS for hospitals. PPSs implemented since 1983, including those based on DRGs, APCs, HHRGs, CMGs, and LTAC DRGs, all have been slightly different and yet use the same base DRG aggregate classification groups. The primary difference among systems centers on the formulas used to calculate reimbursement. The formulas are quite complex and will change over the three-year phase-in period in response to varying combinations of cost-based reimbursement and prospective payment calculation. Methods for treating outliers and transfers and for determining DRG assignment also will differ depending on the PPS.

Another way in which the proposed inpatient psychiatric regulations differ from other PPSs is in the limited number of diagnoses on which the inpatient psychiatric DRG is calculated. Over time, additional diagnoses, complications, procedures, and other factors of influence may be included in the PPS as it is put into practice.

Although the new PPS was originally projected for implementation on April 1, 2004, the extended comment period meant that the implementation date had to be pushed back. Upon the official implementation date in early summer 2004, inpatient psychiatry units and free-standing psychiatric hospitals will be reimbursed under the new PPS beginning on the first day of the organization's next fiscal year (for example, July 1, January 1) following publication of the final regulations.

Impact of the Psychiatric PPS System on Reimbursement

If the coding staff is experienced in ICD-9-CM coding and DRG grouping, little new education is needed. However, training may be required for psychiatric facilities that use DSM-IV clinical diagnostic assessment classifications for calculating reimbursement. DSM codes do not affect the DRG-based PPS system under the new regulations. In addition, good reference materials and resources and an encoding system are recommended to facilitate coding consistency, accuracy, and compliance. HIM departments also may want to consider additional tools to support grouping, reimbursement calculation, and data analysis and reporting so that the impact of the new PPS on facility revenues, for example, can be monitored over time.

The impact of the new PPS system on facility reimbursement may vary. When the inpatient DRG system was implemented twenty years ago, some hospitals experienced a decrease in reimbursement for Medicare patients and others experienced an increase. For a hospital to receive all the reimbursement it is entitled to under the psychiatric PPS, it must ensure that coding for its psychiatric patients is complete and accurate.

Many state Medicaid programs already reimburse for inpatient psychiatric care according to a DRG-based system. Previously, third-party payers had adopted other PPSs for reimbursement and so may consider using the inpatient psychiatric PPS when the efficacy of the system can be demonstrated.

The proposed inpatient psychiatric facility PPS rule and provider-related resources are available at www.access.gpo.gov/su_docs/fedreg/a031128c.html and www.cms.hhs.gov/providers/ipfpps.

Reimbursement Support Processes

Third-party payers routinely review and revise reimbursement support processes to control payments to providers. Healthcare organizations also conduct such support processes to ensure that they are receiving the appropriate level of reimbursement. Third-party payers revise fee schedules and healthcare facilities review chargemasters, evaluate the quality of documentation and coding, conduct internal audits, and implement compliance programs.

Revising Fee Schedules

A fee schedule lists the healthcare organization's services and procedures and the charges associated with each. Fee schedules are managed by the third-party payers and updated on an annual basis. Table of allowances is another name for fee schedule. The fee schedule is a representation of the approved payment levels for a given insurance plan.

Reviewing Chargemasters

The **chargemaster** contains the ICD-9-CM, CPT, and other HCPCS codes applicable to each charge. The HIM professional's knowledge of classification systems can be beneficial in ensuring that the chargemaster is current and accurate at all times. Organizations also may maintain an expanded list of activities and services that are performed but not billable. This expanded list helps to account for resources used. Because accuracy of the chargemaster helps to ensure appropriate billing, the chargemaster should be reviewed periodically.

Updating on a regular basis, especially when billing codes change, ensures that fees and associated costs are always current and accurate. Figure 5.5 lists fields that might appear in a chargemaster and explanations of what they mean.

The chargemaster (also known as the charge description master) includes a charge code (often linked to a HCPCS code), the associated charge, and any additional information necessary to process reimbursement. Services, supplies, and procedures included on the chargemaster generate reimbursement for almost 75 percent of UB-92 claims submitted for outpatient services alone.

Healthcare organizations use computer software to generate the chargemaster. Ongoing maintenance includes input and a review by billing, financial, and HIM personnel. Billing and financial personnel check on the accuracy of revenue codes and associated charges that appear on the chargemaster. As a bonus, they also monitor billing and reimbursement problems. HIM personnel are responsible for the accuracy of the ICD-9-CM and HCPCS codes that appear on the chargemaster. They verify that documentation supports the codes selected.

An inaccurate chargemaster adversely affects organizational reimbursement, compliance, and data quality. Third-party payers routinely review and revise reimbursement support processes to control payments to providers. Healthcare facilities also conduct reimbursement support processes to ensure that they are receiving the appropriate level of reimbursement.

In fee-for-service arrangements, healthcare organizations develop chargemasters that list the individual charges for every element involved in providing a service (room and board, nursing care, respiratory therapy, pharmaceuticals, medical equipment, and so on).

Certain negative impacts may result from an inaccurate chargemaster (Rhodes 1999). These include:

- Overpayment
- Underpayment
- Undercharging for services
- Claims rejections
- Fines
- Penalties

Because a chargemaster is an automated process that results in billing numerous services for high volumes of patients, often without human intervention, there is a high risk that a single coding or mapping error could spawn error after error before it is identified and corrected (Johns 2002).

Figure 5.5. Fields that might appear in a chargemaster

Field Name	Meaning
General ledger code	Internal code used by the facility's accounting department to track revenue and expenses
CPT/HCPCS code	Billing code for transmission to the insurer
Cost basis	Cost of the item to the facility
Charge	Amount facility charges for the item or service
Description	Definition or description of the item or service
Date	Date of the most recent update of the data for the item or service in the chargemaster

Evaluating Documentation and Coding Quality

Poor documentation leads to poor coding, which in turn leads to decreased reimbursement. Coding drives the reimbursement system in a facility. Physician, psychiatrist, psychologist, and clinician documentation needs to be as complete as possible in order for the coder to interpret it accurately for code assignment. The coder is an integral part of the staff in terms of knowledge of documentation requirements, which are rapidly changing in today's healthcare environment. The healthcare organization's reimbursement viability depends on providing the latest documentation information to staff in a timely manner.

Conducting Internal Audits

Coding activities require routine review. Insurers who identify a high percentage of coding errors may increase their audit activities, which places an administrative burden on the HIM department. Therefore, the HIM department should pay particular attention to the supervision, training, and development of its coders because of the critical role they play in reimbursement. Quality improvement studies and continuing education need to be ongoing in the department, and new coding directives must be shared with staff as soon as they are available. Money for this activity needs to be included in the department's budget.

Complying with Standards of Ethical Coding

Sometimes coders are faced with the dilemma of coding for accuracy versus coding for maximum reimbursement for the organization. The latter refers to manipulating codes when the codes assigned are not substantiated by the documentation provided in the medical record. This practice is unethical. Coders have a responsibility to assign codes that accurately reflect the documentation and provide the highest reimbursement supported by that information.

Each profession has a code of ethics and a set of standards that are imposed by the **credentialing** body and/or the licensing agency for that profession. HIM professionals must comply with AHIMA's Standards of Ethical Coding. (See figure 5.6.) In addition, AHIMA supports the profession through its issuance of a variety of publications designed to guide and promote excellence in professional practice. AHIMA regularly issues practice briefs, stating best practices in areas of interest to HIM professionals.

Ensuring Coding Quality

A coding supervisor can perform various reviews to ensure that coding is complete, accurate, and correctly abstracted and recorded. Sometimes, to ensure objectivity, outside auditors are contracted to perform coding reviews. There are two fundamentally different approaches to coding audits: general reviews of all records to identify potential problems and targeted reviews. Targeted reviews are important because they help identify coding mistakes by coder and thus highlight where training may be needed.

The following elements must be evaluated when assessing coding quality within the healthcare organization:

- Reliability: This is the degree to which the same results occur in repeated attempts. For example, different coders would assign the same codes to the same record or a single coder would assign the same diagnosis code to comparable records.

- Validity: Validity is the degree to which codes accurately reflect the patient's diagnoses and procedures.

- Completeness: Codes need to reflect all of the patient's diagnoses and procedures that apply to the encounter or admission.

- Timeliness: The record must be available for billing and retrieval after discharge.

Figure 5.6. AHIMA's Standards of Ethical Coding

In this era of payment based on diagnostic and procedural coding, the professional ethics of health information coding professionals continue to be challenged. A conscientious goal for coding and maintaining a quality database is accurate clinical and statistical data. The following **standards of ethical coding,** developed by AHIMA's Coding Policy and Strategy Committee and approved by AHIMA's Board of Directors, are offered to guide coding professionals in this process.

1. Coding professionals are expected to support the importance of accurate, complete, and consistent coding practices for the production of quality healthcare data.

2. Coding professionals in all healthcare settings should adhere to the ICD-9-CM (*International Classification of Diseases, 9th revision, Clinical Modification*) coding conventions, official coding guidelines approved by the Cooperating Parties,* the CPT (Current Procedural Terminology) rules established by the American Medical Association, and any other official coding rules and guidelines established for use with mandated standard code sets. Selection and sequencing of diagnoses and procedures must meet the definitions of required data sets for applicable healthcare settings.

3. Coding professionals should use their skills, their knowledge of currently mandated coding and classification systems, and official resources to select the appropriate diagnostic and procedural codes.

4. Coding professionals should only assign and report codes that are clearly and consistently supported by physician documentation in the health record.

5. Coding professionals should consult physicians for clarification and additional documentation prior to code assignment when there is conflicting or ambiguous data in the health record.

6. Coding professionals should not change codes or the narratives of codes on the billing abstract so that meanings are misrepresented. Diagnoses or procedures should not be inappropriately included or excluded because payment or insurance policy coverage requirements will be affected. When individual payer policies conflict with official coding rules and guidelines, these policies should be obtained in writing whenever possible. Reasonable efforts should be made to educate the payer on proper coding practices in order to influence a change in the payer's policy.

7. Coding professionals, as members of the healthcare team, should assist and educate physicians and other clinicians by advocating proper documentation practices, furthering specificity, and resequencing or including diagnoses or procedures when needed to more accurately reflect the acuity, severity, and the occurrence of events.

8. Coding professionals should participate in the development of institutional coding policies and should ensure that coding policies complement, not conflict with, official coding rules and guidelines.

9. Coding professionals should maintain and continually enhance their coding skills, as they have a professional responsibility to stay abreast of changes in codes, coding guidelines, and regulations.

10. Coding professionals should strive for optimal payment to which the facility is legally entitled, remembering that it is unethical and illegal to maximize payment by means that contradict regulatory guidelines.

Revised 12/99

*The Cooperating Parties are the American Health Information Management Association, American Hospital Association, Health Care Financing Administration, and National Center for Health Statistics. All rights reserved. Reprint and quote only with proper reference to AHIMA's authorship.

Source: American Health Information Management Association. 2000. Standards of ethical coding. *Journal of the American Health Information Management Association* 71(3).

Errors in coding may be caused by, but not limited to:

- Not reviewing the entire record

- Selecting an incorrect principal diagnosis

- Selecting an incorrect code

- Performing incomplete or inaccurate documentation

- Selecting codes the record does not validate

- Making data-entry errors to the database or bills

Implementing Compliance Programs

During the 1990s, the federal government increased pressure on healthcare organizations to demonstrate their commitment to data quality with billing accuracy being a thrust. The Department of Health and Human Services (HHS) Office of the Inspector General (OIG) has taken the lead in enforcing accurate billing through the process of audits and penalties. The Health Insurance Portability and Accountability ACT (HIPAA) of 1996 and the Balanced Budget Act of 1997 increased the penalties when an organization fails to comply with the regulations.

A corporate compliance program is facilitywide and comprises a system of policies, procedures, and guidelines that are used to ensure ethical business practices. A coding compliance program is part of a corporate compliance effort. It ensures accurate coding and billing through training, continuing education, quality assurance, and performance improvement activities (AHIMA 1999).

Coding routinely occurs three times during a patient's encounter with the healthcare organization, all of which relate to the physician's development of the diagnosis: upon admission, during the stay, and at discharge. When a patient is being admitted to a mental healthcare organization, he or she gives a reason for the admission. The psychiatrist also states the reason for admission in the form of a diagnosis known as the **admitting diagnosis.**

At admission, a code is assigned to the diagnosis to facilitate tracking during the patient's stay. If the admitting diagnosis is expressed only as a narrative, the computer will be unable to match and track the patient's diagnosis. This initial coding may rest with the patient registration/admitting department. If only narrative is used, the HIM department will have to assign the code after discharge. This negates the purpose of assigning an admitting diagnosis.

Conclusion

The coding process depends on the use of clinical vocabularies. Today's clinical vocabularies are based on the Bertillon classification system, first used in 1891. The most common classification system used today is the International Classification of Diseases, Ninth Revision, Clinical Modification (ICD-9-CM). Coding professionals use ICD-9-CM to classify morbidity data for indexing medical records, medical care review, and ambulatory and other medical care programs, in addition to basic health statistics.

Emerging technologies also have had a profound effect on the coding process. Beginning in the 1980s, information technology has been used to improve the coding process through the use of tools called encoders. Other technologies, such as natural language processing, will likely have an even greater impact on the coding process in the future.

The coding process is an extremely important part of ensuring that healthcare organizations are reimbursed appropriately for the services they provide. To that end, coding professionals must be familiar with the many reimbursement systems in place to provide Americans with healthcare services—systems that range from commercial insurance and managed care plans to government-sponsored programs. In addition to the accurate and timely reporting of coded data, this responsibility encompasses compliance with standards of ethical coding and adherence to the organization's corporate compliance program.

References and Bibliography

Abdelhak, M., S. Grostick, M. A. Hanken, and E. Jacobs. 2001. *Health Information: Management of a Strategic Resource,* 2nd ed. Philadelphia: W. B. Saunders Company.

American Health Information Management Association. 1999. Practice Brief: Seven steps to corporate compliance: The HIM role. *Journal of the American Health Information Management Association* 70(9).

American Medical Association. http://www.ama-assn.org/.

American Psychiatric Association. 2000. *Diagnostic and Statistical Manual of Mental Disorders* DSM-IV-TR (Text Revision). 4th ed. Arlington, VA: APPI.

Brown, Faye. 2002. *ICD-9-CM Coding Handbook, with Answers.* Chicago: AHA Press.

Centers for Medicare and Medicaid Services. http://www.cms.hhs.gov/.

Davis, Nadinia, and Melissa W. LaCour. 2002. *Introduction to Health Information Technology.* Philadelphia: W. B. Saunders Company.

Fordney, M. T. 1999. *Insurance Handbook for the Medical Office,* 6th ed. Philadelphia: W. B. Saunders Company.

Fox, L. A. 1992. An ethical dilemma: Coding medical records for reimbursement. *Journal of the American Health Information Management Association* 63(35).

Grzybowski, Darice. 2004 (May). PPS brings change to inpatient psychiatric facilities. *Journal of the American Health Information Management Association* 75(5): 64–66.

Huffman, Edna K. 1990. *Medical Record Management,* 10th ed. Berwyn, IL: Physicians' Record Company.

Johns, M. L., ed. 2002. *Health Information Management Technology: An Applied Approach.* Chicago: American Health Information Management Association.

Murphy, G. F., M. A. Hanken, and K. Waters. 1999. *Electronic Health Records: Changing the Vision.* Philadelphia: W. B. Saunders Company, 155–75.

National Center for Health Statistics. www.cdc.gov/nchs/.

Prophet, S. 1998. Coding compliance: Practical strategies for success. *Journal of the American Health Information Management Association* 69(1): 50–61.

Rhodes, Harry B. 1999. Practice Brief: The care and maintenance of charge masters. *Journal of the American Health Information Management Association* 70(7).

Scichilone, R. 1999. *CPT Coding Handbook, with Answers,* 1999 ed. Chicago: AHA Press.

Skurka, M. A. 1998. *Health Information Management: Principles and Organization for Health Record Services,* rev. ed. Chicago: American Hospital Publishing, 105–22.

Social Security Administration. 2004. Disability Programs. Available on-line at http://www.ssa.gov/disability/.

U.S. Government Printing Office. 1984. *Federal Register* 49(171): 34759.

World Health Organization. http://www.who.int/en/.

Chapter 6

Data and Information Management

Anna Lattu, MA, RHIA

Nearly all literature in the health information management field today emphasizes the importance of computerized patient information systems. The behavioral healthcare field, in general, has notably lacked in computerization. Information that is well organized, accessible, and accurate will effectively support behavioral healthcare entities by providing comprehensive, coordinated, intelligent, and cost-effective healthcare. Effective use of information can blend health knowledge, technology, and the human behavior.

This chapter clarifies the distinction among data, information, and knowledge and discusses the basic principles of information management. Further, it focuses on the importance of ensuring data quality and describes various data and information management initiatives and different information management systems.

Driving Forces

Data and information have become vital to the survival of healthcare organizations in the twenty-first century. Without high-quality data, and thus information, today's **behavioral healthcare organizations** would be unable to operate in an efficient and effective manner. The high demands of information today are driven by both external and internal forces. Some of these forces are described in the following subsections.

Institute of Medicine

The **Institute of Medicine** (IOM) released *To Err Is Human: Building a Safer Health System* in 2000, which revealed statistics on the number of people injured or killed as a result of medical errors. A follow-up report titled *Crossing the Quality Chasm* was issued by the IOM in 2001. This second report called for a redesign of the American healthcare system and offered key steps to strengthen clinical information systems. These two reports provide a push for the behavioral healthcare field to improve and expand its data and information management. Computerization is a key in providing high-quality, safe patient care.

Computer-based Patient Record Institute

The former Computer-based Patient Record Institute (CPRI) was an organization representing stakeholders in healthcare focused on clinical applications of **information technology** (IT) (HIMSS 2002). The CPRI was a strong leader in the push toward the electronic health record (EHR) and patient information systems. In 2002, it united with the Healthcare Information and Management Systems Society (HIMSS) to create the "definitive information resource" (HIMSS 2002).

The CPRI published numerous documents and toolkits focused on meeting patient information needs within a healthcare system. The fourth edition of the CPRI toolkit was published in 2003 with a focus on managing information security in healthcare.

Joint Commission on Accreditation of Healthcare Organizations

The **Joint Commission on Accreditation of Healthcare Organizations** (JCAHO) is another driving force in improving the management of data and information within the behavioral healthcare organization. The JCAHO places a major emphasis on patient safety and the role information systems can play in patient safety. The JCAHO's *Comprehensive Accreditation Manual for Behavioral Health Care* publishes standards addressing information management planning, clinical data and information, aggregate data and information, knowledge-based information, and comparative data and information. The JCAHO introduced the ORYX monitoring in 1997 and began using it in 2000 to assess the way healthcare organizations analyze and use performance management data.

Professional Organizations

Other external driving forces include professional organizations such as the American Health Information Management Association (AHIMA), the American Medical Association (AMA), and the North America Nursing Diagnosis Association (NANDA International). These organizations work independently—and together in some instances—to promote standards for the electronic patient record and **taxonomy** and to promote the use of electronic patient information. Such organizations place heavy emphasis on the importance of high-quality data and information and information systems.

Internal Sources within Behavioral Healthcare Organizations

Many behavioral healthcare organizations also have experienced strong driving forces in the management of data and information from internal sources. Many behavioral healthcare settings are publicly funded; thus, the demand for information has grown as more sources fight for the same dollar. As funds shrink, more efficient and effective means to provide data and information have grown. The manpower is not available to manually perform time-consuming data abstraction and analysis from paper records. In an electronic age, information must be available almost instantly.

Legislators and Administrators

Legislators and other public entities require information from behavioral healthcare entities to justify funding programs. Administrators and clinical leaders are forced to look at cutting programs that do not make money or are not serving clients effectively. Administrators in behavioral healthcare are actively exploring options to meet client needs in noninstitutional settings, often based on consumer and patient advocate demand. Administrators, state, county, and community officials require reliable data and information to make these difficult decisions.

Data, Information, and Knowledge

The distinction among data, information, and knowledge is shown in the hierarchical diagram in figure 6.1 (Johns 1997). This distinction provides the foundation for the design, development, and evaluation of information systems.

Figure 6.1.   Data, information, and knowledge hierarchy

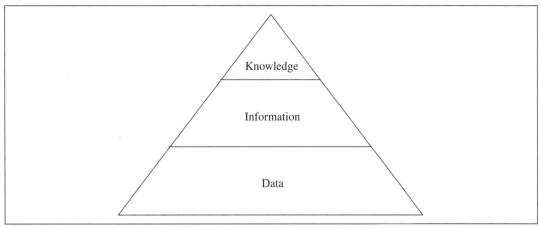

Source: Johns 1997.

Data are increasingly driving healthcare industry decision making. Information and the knowledge gained from data can be used for strategic, tactical, and operational purposes. Strategic decision making determines what goals are to be achieved by an organization. An example of a strategic decision would be that of developing an integrated information system (IS) to support clinical, financial, and management decisions (Johns 1997).

Tactical decisions determine how organizational goals are to be achieved, such as determining the need for a **computer-based patient record** (CPR) or a new pharmacy package or the need for a **decision support system** (DSS) to achieve the strategic decision (Johns 1997). Operational decisions based on data and information would include the day-to-day decisions that meet the organization's goals and keep the organization operating. Examples include scheduling employees, order entry, ordering supplies, caring for patients, and processing patient bills (Johns 1997).

What Are Data?

Data are discrete raw facts and figures, which, in isolation, have no meaning. They can consist of numbers, names, codes, words, narrative, images, or sounds. Data that are collected may or may not be useful depending on their intended purpose. They are noninterpreted and can have different meanings depending on the context in which they are displayed. Data may be found in numerous locations in a behavioral healthcare setting, including in assessments, care plans, progress notes, flow sheets, DSM-IV codes, billing systems, intake records, and orders. In essence, data are building blocks—the foundation for any IS.

Individual data are data that are patient specific or patient identifiable. Examples in behavioral health include basically the entire medical record, diagnosis, and any other data identifiable to an individual. In contrast, aggregate data are data on groups of people or clients without identifying information (Bowman 2002). Examples of aggregate data in a behavioral healthcare setting include **average length of stay** (ALOS), average age, most common diagnosis on Axis I and II, number of admissions and discharges, and average admission acuity level.

What Is Information?

Data become information when they are used for a specific purpose or task. **Information** consists of data or data sets that are placed in context for the intended audience. Meaning and context transform data into useful information. Data need to be formatted, filtered, and/or manipulated for the intended task or purpose in order to be converted to information (Johns 1997). Information is of central importance in problem solving and decision making. When correctly managed, information is one of the most important resources of a healthcare organization.

What Is Knowledge?

Knowledge is a "combination of rules, relationships, ideas, and experience" (Johns 1997). Information becomes knowledge when it changes or supports business decision-making processes. Knowledge provides the basis for reprogramming or redesigning business or even simple processes (Hackathorn 2001). Shams and Farishta (2002) describe knowledge as "the awareness and understanding gained through experience." Knowledge is information in context to produce an actionable understanding.

Knowledge Management

Knowledge management refers to the systematic processes by which knowledge needed for an organization to succeed is created, captured, shared, and leveraged (Rumizen 2002). Knowledge becomes meaningful in the larger context of our culture and our underlying beliefs and philosophy.

Knowledge-Based Assets

Knowledge-based assets fall into one of two categories: explicit or tacit. *Explicit knowledge* can be said, written down, and transmitted. It can be put into words, entered in a database, and archived. *Tacit knowledge* is what a person knows. It includes know-how, judgment, experience, insight, rules of thumb, and skills. Tacit knowledge exists within context. Santosus and Surmacz (2001) describe tacit knowledge as harder to grasp, with the challenge of figuring out how to recognize, generate, share, and manage it. Identifying tacit knowledge is a major hurdle for most organizations. Knowledge creation is a spiral of converting tacit knowledge to explicit knowledge and then back again (Rumizen 2002).

Basic Principles of Information Management

Information management is the function of collecting, managing, and utilizing information. JCAHO (2002, 2003, 2004) lists the key information management processes:

- Identifying information needs
- Designing the structure of the information management system
- Capturing, organizing, storing, retrieving, processing, and analyzing data and information
- Transmitting, reporting, displaying, integrating, and using data and information
- Safeguarding data information

For successful information management, Austin and Boxerman (1998) describe three key principles:

1. Treat information as an essential organizational resource. "Information resource management should receive the same care and attention that is given to human resources management, financial management, and materials management in an organization."

2. Obtain top executive support for IS planning and management. Top-level management should be knowledgeable and involved in IS planning and setting priorities.

3. Develop a strategic vision and plan. Like other healthcare organizations, behavioral healthcare organizations need an organizationwide vision of how information systems will support client care and **strategic management.** The IS **strategic plan** must be aligned with the organization's strategies. Strategic IS planning must be driven by business plans.

The healthcare organization must consider its data and information needs. Rather than just collecting any and all data, the organization should consider questions such as:

- Why are we collecting there data?
- Who will be using these data?
- Why will they be using these data?
- When are the data needed?
- How are the data needed?
- What is the best means to collect the data?
- Where are they collected elsewhere?

It is important to ask these questions to ensure that the right data are collected by the right people at the right time. It is more cost-effective to determine what data are needed early in the process of designing systems. On the other hand, it is costly and time-consuming to make program changes after systems are in place. Another risk an organization faces when the right questions are not asked ahead of time is that of collecting too much data. When the planning process has not been carefully thought out, data collection systems can grow to the point where more data are collected than can be handled to produce needed information. Table 6.1 lists the characteristics of information management (Austin and Boxerman, 1998).

Data Quality

HIM professionals are taught about, and are advocates for, the importance of complete, accurate, and timely documentation and the establishment of clear, standard data collection guidelines. (See table 6.2 for a list of data quality characteristics.) The principles applied to paper records also apply to computerized information systems. Teslow and Wilde (2001) indicate that the accuracy of data depends on the manual or computer IS design for collecting, recording, storing, processing, accessing, and displaying data as well as the ability and follow-through of the people involved at each phase of these activities. AHIMA (1998a) published the **data quality management** model, which encompasses four functions: application, analysis, collection, and warehousing. The four functions need to be used together when designing data and information systems.

Table 6.1. Characteristics of useful management of information

Information, not data	Data must be processed before they become useful information.
Relevant	Information must relate to the purpose for which it is to be used.
Sensitive	Information must provide discrimination and meaningful comparisons.
Unbiased	Information should not be collected or analyzed in a way so as to be prejudiced or impartial.
Comprehensive	All elements or components are visible.
Timely	Information must be presented to users in advance of the time when decisions or actions are required.
Action oriented	Information is designed to aid the decision maker directly in the decision process.
Uniform	Indicators can be compared over time both internally and externally.
Performance targeted	Information must be designed and collected in reference to predetermined goals and objectives.
Cost-effective	Anticipated benefits should be worth the cost of collecting and processing.

Source: Austin and Boxerman 1998.

Table 6.2. AHIMA's data quality characteristics

Accessibility	Data items should be easily obtainable and legal to collect.
Accuracy	Data are valid and have the correct values.
Comprehensiveness	All required data items should be included. The entire scope of the data should be collected and intentional limitations documented.
Consistency	The value of the data should be reliable and the same across applications.
Currency	The data should be up-to-date. A datum value is up-to-date if it is current for a specific point in time. It is outdated if it was current at some preceding time yet incorrect at a later time.
Definition	Clear definitions should be provided so that current and future data users will know what the data mean. Each data element should have clear meaning and acceptable values.
Granularity	The attributes and values of data should be defined at the correct level of detail.
Precision	Data values should be just large enough to support the application or process.
Relevancy	The data are meaningful to the performance of the process or application for which they are collected.
Timeliness	Timeliness is determined by how the data are being used and their context.
Validity	Validity is the extent to which data correspond to the actual state of affairs (Amatayakul 1999).
Reliability	Reliability is a measure of the consistency of data items based on their reproducibility and an estimation of their error of measurement (Amatayakul 1999).

Source: AHIMA 1998a.

Assessing data quality is an important part of the planning process when implementing an IS. Data quality is the stepping-stone to effective decision support and outcome assessment programs.

Establishing Data Quality Standards

Reliable information cannot be obtained from an IS if high-quality data are not entered into the system. When establishing data quality standards, an important consideration is the use of commonly used terms and their definitions. Examples of terms common to behavioral healthcare are **episode of care** and **length of stay** (LOS). During the planning phase of an IS, the definition of LOS must be established. Will the LOS calculation include short visits or overnights away from the facility? Does this term mean the same thing to financial management as it does to the HIM professionals?

Controlling Data Quality

Controlling data quality brings into focus AHIMA's data quality management model discussed above. In this model, AHIMA indicates that during the collection of data, "appropriate education and training and timely and appropriate communication of data definitions to those who collect data" are essential to ensuring **data accuracy.** An important part of data quality is the people skills necessary to manage data quality and the training and review that must go into an IS. When errors or trends of errors are found, appropriate action must be taken to correct them and turn them around.

In behavioral healthcare organizations that use real-time data collection, employees without the proper training often enter data into an IS. If the importance of the data is not emphasized, organizations will find errors and incomplete data in their information systems. Monitoring data quality is crucial to ensure high-quality information from a system.

Ensuring Data Integrity and Security

Federal and state regulations govern patient privacy and the security of patient information. The security and privacy standards promulgated by the Health Insurance Portability and Accountability Act (HIPAA) are receiving top priority in healthcare organizations today and must be met when designing patient information systems.

The HIPAA security standard, published in the *Federal Register* on February 20, 2003, is applicable to all healthcare information that is maintained electronically to protect its integrity, confidentiality, and availability (Nutten and Mansueti 2004). This standard applies to the information collected and used internally as well as information that is shared or maintained in conjunction with other entities. Each healthcare organization must assess the potential risks and vulnerabilities to the data it maintains in electronic form and develop appropriate security measures (Amatayakul 2000). Compliance with the security rules will rely heavily on the implementation of policies, procedures, plans, and other documentation (Walsh 2004).

Data integrity is ensuring that data are not altered or destroyed in an unauthorized manner or by an unauthorized user. Security measures must be in place to protect data integrity by preventing alteration or loss.

Data Security

Data security involves the employment of mechanisms to prevent unauthorized access to or use of health information. Information security often consists of both physical and technological mechanisms for preventing unauthorized data access (Knapp, Walter, and Renaudin 2000). Examples of data security efforts include the placement of computers in locations not accessible to unauthorized users; the use of passwords, key cards, or badges with access codes; and biometrics such as fingerprinting, voice or eye scan for user identification, automatic log-off, and **audit trails.** Data security mechanisms must be part of an IS system design.

Data Confidentiality

Data confidentiality is the right of an individual to control disclosure of his or her personal health information (PHI). Policies and procedures must be in place to govern the use of PHI, and employees must be trained on their application. Information systems must be created to ensure that client information is protected so that only authorized employees and those allowed by law have access to private data.

Data and Information Management Initiatives

The JCAHO, the Centers for Medicare and Medicaid Services (CMS), and professional organizations including AHIMA, HIMSS, and the AMA have placed emphasize on the importance of high-quality data and information and information systems. These organizations have focused on standardized assessments and data collection methods to improve the healthcare system and to compare indicators and outcomes across similar organizations.

Outcomes Monitoring

Outcomes monitoring evaluates the end results of treatment or intervention compared to preestablished criteria defining desired outcomes (Amatayakul 1999). Behavioral healthcare **outcomes** are designed to detect change as the result of an intervention. Behavioral healthcare organizations often utilize readmit data (30, 60, 90 days) and quality-of-life questionnaires to evaluate outcomes. (See the discussion below about the NRI and common outcome measures in behavioral healthcare.) Well-designed information systems assist clinicians in gathering and evaluating outcomes data. Using information systems, clinicians can compare how clients respond to specific treatments compared to other similar clients and also can monitor influences that may have an impact on treatment.

Evidence-Based Practices

Evidence-based practices refer to the use of decision support systems and **best practices** in medicine rather than relying on subjective information. Briggs (2004) explains evidence-based practice as "a means of evaluating the current best clinical practices and applying that information to the care of individual patients." With the help of information technology, large amounts of data can be sorted for easy access by the clinician. Data on best practices can be mined from internal and external sources so that they can be applied to an individual client (Briggs 2004). Utilizing decision support systems, clinicians are given objective data to treat clients.

Decision support systems in behavioral healthcare settings are not well established and often are met with caution based on the many individual differences and lifestyle influences in the behavioral healthcare client. Best practices in behavioral healthcare can be especially difficult to translate because outcomes tend to be difficult to measure. With a growing focus on quality and patient safety and outcomes, there is a growing interest in evidence-based practice.

JCAHO's ORYX Initiative

JCAHO introduced the **ORYX initiative** in 1997, a new set of performance and outcome measurement requirements, "to ensure a more thorough, continuous, and comprehensive accreditation process" (Zeglen 1997). This is accomplished by the ORYX program's objectives of establishing national comparative databases to support benchmarking, research, and internal performance improvement activities. Further objectives of the ORYX initiative are to foster the standardization of performance measures and to encourage the use of evidence-based treatment protocols (LaTour 2002). ("The initiative was named ORYX after an African animal that can be thought of as a different kind of zebra" [LaTour 2002]).

The ORYX initiative is intended to be a flexible and affordable approach for supporting quality improvement efforts to meet the needs of various types and sizes of healthcare organizations (JCAHO 2003). Further, the intent is to identify sound measures that support organizational process improvement. The JCAHO (2002) indicates that behavioral healthcare services are no longer required to report ORYX measurement data to the JCAHO as of Oct. 21, 2002. "This deferment acknowledges the slow pace of developing national standards in data collection and performance measures in non-hospital settings" (JCAHO 2002). The JCAHO continues to work with behavioral healthcare professionals and organizations to identify appropriate measures.

The National Association of State Mental Health Program Directors (NASMHPD) Research Institute (NRI) has committed to developing, maintaining, and improving an operational performance measurement system with the primary and most important purpose to assist states in meeting the JCAHO's ORYX initiative (NRI 2002). An NRI task force was charged with "developing a framework within which states and other providers of mental health services can identify and implement consistent measures of performance and outcomes" (NRI 2002). This framework provides the ability to benchmark critical measures of performance and outcomes and, ultimately, improve client outcomes.

Working with representatives from more than fifteen states, the NRI developed the NRI Behavioral Healthcare Performance Measurement System (BHPMS). Two sets of system measures were defined: initial reporting measures and assessment measures. These are summarized in figure 6.2.

Behavioral healthcare organizations participating in the NRI data collection submit electronic data monthly to the NRI. The NRI provides comparative statistics reports to authorized

Figure 6.2. NRI behavioral healthcare performance measurement system (BHPMS)

Initial Measures

- 30-day readmission rate
- Client injury rate
- Elopement rate
- Medication error rate
- New generation antipsychotic use
- Restraint use
- Seclusion use

Assessment Measures

- BPRS
- CBCL
- GAF
- CAFAS
- SF-12 or 36
- MCAS
- Client perception of outcome of care
- Client perception of dignity
- Client perception of rights
- Client perception of participation in treatment
- Client perception of facility environment
- Medication changes near discharge
- Mean new generation antipsychotic dose
- Concurrent antipsychotic treatment
- Mean number of scheduled treatment

Source: NRI 2002.

organizational personnel showing calculations for the prior twelve months together with national and state averages for the selected measures.

Information Management Systems

Before planning information management systems, organizations must review their strategic plans and determine how an IS fits into their overall **strategic planning.** Information management systems must be designed to complement and help meet the goals of the organization. For successful information management systems, organizations must have forward-thinking leaders in key information management positions. Organizations also must be willing to dedicate the necessary resources, in both dollars and personnel, to the information management system for success.

Systems Planning

All possible users and **stakeholders** of data must be considered when designing an information management system (IMS). Users and stakeholders include employees and clinicians within a behavioral healthcare setting, but also external people and entities. The users and stakeholders for behavioral healthcare entities include:

- Clinicians
- Billing specialists
- Payers
- Researchers
- Managers
- Governing board
- State healthcare agency
- State legislature and county boards

The needs of all of these users must be considered when designing forms, views, and reports (Teslow and Wilde 2001). Everyone involved in the design and use of these databases needs to understand how and why different end users search patient records and make those data easily available and accurate (Warren, Harris, and Warren 1999).

The process and techniques used in the design of an IS play a critical role in ensuring that work tasks, data, people, and technology are aligned appropriately to produce an effective and efficient IS (Murphy, Hanken, and Waters 1999). The focus of analysis is on work tasks and how they input, use, transform, or output data. Development of data flow diagrams (DFDs) is an integral part of analysis. DFDs document the flow, storage, creation, and transformation of data.

An example of a DFD would be the admission of a patient. (See figure 6.3.) In many behavioral healthcare settings, admission demographic and financial data are gathered prior to the actual admission from county workers or acute care general hospitals. If unavailable prior to admission, the data are gathered upon the arrival of the patient or others, depending on the patient's current psychiatric state. The demographic information is entered into the organization's information system. Clinicians perform assessments that are entered into the electronic health record. Diagnoses are established and recorded as part of the assessment process and entered into the IS.

Figure 6.3.   Data flow design

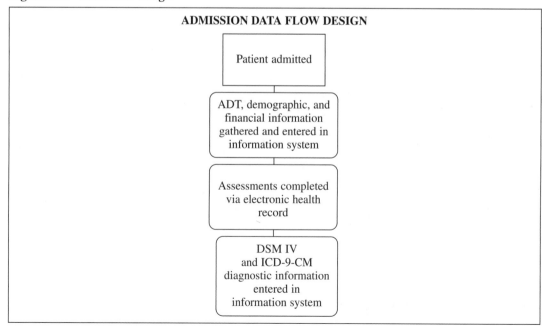

Initial and Ongoing Assessment of Data Needs

A **needs assessment,** a thorough evaluation of data and information needs, must be completed prior to IS development. Stakeholders and users from both within and outside the organization must be considered. The first step is to determine who the stakeholders are. When the stakeholders have been identified, the data and information needs of each must be determined. Accessibility and timeliness of the data and information must be addressed with the stakeholders. Data that are captured, but not accessible, or that are received too late do not meet stakeholder needs.

The needs assessment can be done using several methods. Connolly and Begg (1999) list the following ways to gather information required for **database** design:

- Interview individuals within the organization, particularly those who are regarded as experts within a specific area of interest.

- Observe the organization in operation.

- Examine documents, in particular those used to record or display information.

- Use questionnaires to gather information from a wide number of users.

- Use experience from the design of similar systems.

The more thoroughly users' information needs are determined before programming work begins, the better the results will be and the less time will be spent on reworking in the future. Adjustments and modifications to information systems can be very time-consuming and expensive.

As healthcare practices, medications, and regulations change, so will the needs of the stakeholders. Ongoing assessment and evaluation must be performed to ensure that the data and information needs of the stakeholders are being met. When identifying information needs, the JCAHO requires evidence of a planned approach that identifies the hospital's information needs and supports its goals and objectives (JCAHO 2004).

Data Capture and Collection

The use of data is driven by their availability (Warren, Harris, and Warren 1999). Computer-based systems expand research, decision support, outcome assessment, and program evaluation capability by giving users access to large quantities of information and making it less expensive and less time-consuming than with paper-based records. With its capability of querying large databases, retrieving data on **variables** being studied, and downloading data into statistical analysis programs, a computerized IS means that users will increase their demands for patient data and information. Collecting enough of the right type of data to satisfy this range of users clearly means defining the purpose (Teslow and Wilde 2001).

Manual and Automated Methods of Data Collection

Manual systems for **data collection** date back to the early days of the medical record profession. Data were—and in some cases, still are—collected on index cards and in logbooks. In the 1960s and 1970s, with the advent of computers, data were collected on paper or magnetic tape and punch cards. As personal computers became widely used in the late twentieth century, stand-alone computerized databases and spreadsheets became popular mechanisms to collect and store patient information. In today's healthcare organizations, data are collected and stored primarily on large servers where multiple users throughout the organization can access them.

Smaller organizations still rely heavily on stand-alone databases and spreadsheets to collect data. Users can quickly and easily design the databases and spreadsheets and use the data as needed. A major drawback to stand-alone systems is duplicate effort across organizations. Many employees collect the same information to meet their needs. Another drawback to stand-alone systems involves the inconsistencies found in the data. A **data element** may have different meanings depending on the person collecting it. For example, does marital status of single mean never married or not currently married (where the person could be widowed, divorced, or never married)? If definitions are not laid out across the organization, chances are that different definitions will be applied by those collecting the data.

Organizationwide information management systems, available to authorized users across the organization, decrease the amount of duplicate effort necessary to maintain data. When properly designed, and with the proper education and training, the data are more consistent in organizationwide IMSs than when maintained in stand-alone systems.

Analysis and Interpretation of Data

A major benefit of maintaining computerized data is the ability to analyze and interpret the data faster and in multiple ways. Analyzing and interpreting the data allow the user or the audience of the information to understand the data and place them in context. Table 6.3 describes the steps in analyzing data (Johns 1997).

Basic Tools for Data Analysis

Spreadsheet and statistical packages as well as report writer software are readily available off the shelf. Spreadsheet **software**, such as LOTUS 1-2-3 or Microsoft Excel, allows data to be entered and can perform basic statistical analysis as well as graph data for visual display. Statistical packages allow users to perform extensive statistical analysis on data and graphically display them. Report writer software allows users to perform **data analysis** and to design sophisticated reports from databases. These software packages can query or abstract the desired data from the database and/or information systems. Today's software comes with many preprogrammed statistical analysis and graphing and charting capabilities.

Table 6.3.   Steps to analyzing data

Step 1	Specify reason, theory, or hypothesis for which the data are being analyzed.	This step helps frame the request for data, giving parameters. **Example**: A physician asks for a list of all readmits. The list would not be meaningful without adding specifics for analysis. Is the physician looking for 30-, 60-, 90-day readmit patterns for a specific diagnosis or unit? Or any patient who has ever been to the facility before? Or other reason? By knowing the reason for pulling the data, parameters can be used to pull the data that better fits the requestor's need.
Step 2	Determine the variables that need to be gathered and analyzed.	Johns (1997) describes a variable as any "characteristic or property that can be classified into two or more groups." **Example:** The physician could select as variables, all readmits within 30 days where he is the attending physician with an Axis I diagnosis of 295.44.
Step 3	Select appropriate statistical procedures.	Once variables are selected, the analyst can determine which statistical procedure will answer the question being asked.

Source: Johns 1997.

Advanced Tools for Data Analysis

Advanced tools for data analysis include executive information systems, data-mining tools, and **on-line analytical processing** (OLAP) tools. These tools allow advanced data analysis to be performed. The user can pull data simultaneously from multiple sources and perform analysis in multiple views.

The **executive information system** (EIS) is an interactive interface with the databases or data warehouse that allows users easy access to information. The EIS is normally fed results from querying or reporting tools as mentioned above (such as Microsoft Access or Crystal Reports). The results are made available to users through the EIS. The EIS allows users to select from predetermined variables to meet specific reporting needs.

Data-mining tools search through large volumes of data, looking for trends and patterns. These tools do not tell users why trends are occurring but, rather, bring trends and patterns to the focus so that further analysis can be performed.

On-line analytical processing (OLAP) tools allow users to delve into the data to discover what is happening and why. OLAP tools allow users to look at data in different ways and at details under a summary that shows comparisons, trends, **variances**, and ranking. OLAP tools allow the data to be multidimensional, where dimensions represent various groups of data within the business. In behavioral healthcare, OLAP tools would allow users to access multiple databases and analyze clinical, physician, and financial data within one report.

Special Considerations about Data and Information for Mental Health and Substance Abuse

A challenge to the behavioral healthcare field in information management is continuity of care. Patients are often followed across many spectrums, depending on severity of illness, income level, and availability of services in the client's home area. So often, each behavioral healthcare provider maintains its own data and information without looking at client's continuum of care. As in other healthcare settings, the need for the longitudinal health record is great as more programs move from organization-based to community-based care with numerous providers caring for the behavioral healthcare client.

Conclusion

Numerous data and information concepts and processes must be considered by practitioners in the behavioral healthcare field. Having accurate and available data and information is vitally important to maintaining the care of patients being treated in behavioral healthcare organizations. Behavioral healthcare organizations must continue to place an emphasis on the data and information resources to survive and meet the challenges facing healthcare in the twenty-first century.

References and Bibliography

Amatayakul, M. 2000 (Winter). Security measures required for HIPPA privacy. *Journal of Healthcare Information Management* 14(4):5–8.

Amatayakul, M. 1999. *The Role of Health Information Managers in CPR Projects: A Practical Guide.* Chicago: American Health Information Management Association.

Amatayakul, M. 1997 (May). Making the case for electronic records. *Health Data Management* (5):56–58.

American Health Information Management Association. 1999 (March). Practice Brief: A checklist to assess data quality management efforts. *Journal of the American Health Information Management Association,* p. 3.

American Health Information Management Association. 1998c (November/December). Practice Brief: Data resource administration: The road ahead. *Journal of the American Health Information Management Association*, p. 11.

American Health Information Management Association. 1998a (June). Practice Brief: Data quality management model. *Journal of the American Health Information Management Association*, p. 6.

American Health Information Management Association. 1998b (May). Practice Brief: Designing a data collection process. *Journal of the American Health Information Management Association*, p. 5.

American Health Information Management Association. 1997 (July). Position Statement: Quality healthcare data and information. *Journal of the American Health Information Management Association*, p. 7.

Austin, C., and S. Boxerman. 1998. *Information Systems for Health Services Administration.* Chicago: Health Administration Press.

Bowman, E. 2002. Secondary records and healthcare databases. In *Health Information Management: Concepts, Principles, and Practice,* eds. K. LaTour and S. Eichenwald, 241–59. Chicago: American Health Information Management Association.

Briggs, B. 2004 (January). Working together: IT and evidence-based medicine. *Health Data Management,* pp. 24–26.

Bumby, K. M., and M. C. Maddox. 1999. Judges' knowledge about sexual offenders, difficulties presiding over sexual offense cases, and opinions on sentencing, treatment and legislation. *Sexual Abuse: A Journal of Research and Treatment* 11:305–15.

Computer-based Patient Record Institute. 1997. *Framework for Definition and Modeling of the Computer-based Patient Record Environment.* Bethesda, MD: Computer-based Patient Record Institute.

Connolly, T., and C. Begg. 1999. *Database Systems: A Practical Approach to Design, Implementation, and Management.* Edinburgh Gate, Eng.: Addison Wesley Longman Limited.

Grossman L. S., B. Martis, and C. G. Fichtner. 1999. Are sex offenders treatable? A research overview. *Psychiatric Services* 50:349–61.

Hackathorn, R. 2001 (January). The little BI versus big BI. *DM Review.* Available on-line at www.dmreview.com.

Haramati, N. 2000 (winter). HIPPA security: Compliance in radiology—an academic radiology department's plan contrasted with a small private practice. *Journal of Healthcare Information Management* 14(4):66–81.

Healthcare Information and Management Systems Society (HIMSS). 2002. Web site. www.himss.org.

Institute of Medicine. 2001. *Crossing the Quality Chasm.* Washington, DC: National Academies Press.

Institute of Medicine, Committee on Quality of Health Care in America. 2000. *To Err Is Human: Building a Safer Health System,* eds. L. Kohn, J. Corrigan, and M. Donaldson. Washington, DC: National Academies Press.

Johns, M. 1997. *Information Management for Health Professions.* Albany, NY: Delmar Publishers.

Joint Commission on Accreditation of Healthcare Organizations. (2004). *2001–2002 Comprehensive Accreditation Manual for Behavioral Health Care.* Oakbrook Terrace, IL: JCAHO

Joint Commission on Accreditation of Healthcare Organizations. 2003. *Facts about ORYX for Hospitals.* Oakbrook Terrace, IL.: JCAHO. Available on-line at www.jcaho.org.

Joint Commission on Accreditation of Healthcare Organizations. 2002. *Facts about ORYX for Behavioral Healthcare Organizations.* Oakbrook Terrace, IL: JCAHO. Available on-line at www.jcaho.org.

Knapp, T., J. Walter, and C. Renaudin. 2000 (Winter). Property rights and privacy principles. *Journal of Healthcare Information Management* 14(4):83–93.

Kohn, R. 1999 (July). Mainframes, client servers, Internet, intranet: Which one's for you? *Behavioral Health Management* 19(4):38–40.

LaTour, K. 2002. Healthcare information standards. In *Health Information Management: Concepts, Principles, and Practice,* eds. K. LaTour and S. Eichenwald, 127–28. Chicago: American Health Information Management Association.

Lattu, A. 2003. *Integrated Sex Offender Patient Information System.* Duluth, MN: College of St. Scholastica.

Loshin, D. 2002 (October). Knowledge integrity: What is knowledge integrity? *DM Review.* Available on-line at www.dmreview.com.

Martin, T., and S. Fuller. 1998. Components of the CPR: An overview. *Journal of American Health Information Management Association,* p. 9.

Murphy, G., M. Hanken, and K. Waters. 1999. *Electronic Health Records: Changing the Vision.* Philadelphia: W.B. Sanders Company.

NANDA International Web site. www.nanda.org.

National Association of State Mental Health Program Directors (NASMHPS) Research Institue (NRI). 2002. Web site. http://nri.rdmc.org/.

Nutten, S., and C. Mansueti. 2004 (February). An IT contingency plan to meet HIPAA security standards. *Journal of the American Health Information Management Association,* pp. 30–37.

Rhodes, H. 1998. The ORYX and other elusive quality animals. *Journal of the American Health Information Management Association* (6):64–65.

Rumizen, M. 2002. *The Complete Idiot's Guide to Knowledge Management.* Madison, WI: CWL Publishing.

Santosus, M., and J. Surmacz. 2001 (May). The ABCs of knowledge management. *CIO: Knowledge Management Research Center.* Available on-line at www.cio.com/research/knowledge.

Shams, K., and M. Farishta. 2002. Knowledge management. In *Health Information Management: Concepts, Principles, and Practice,* eds. K. LaTour and S. Eichenwald, 469–86. Chicago: American Health Information Management Association.

Shortliffe, E. H., and L. E. Perreault, eds. 1990. *Medical Informatics: Computer Applications in Health Care.* Reading, MA: Addison-Wesley.

Teslow, M., and D. Wilde. 2001. Data collection standards. In *Health Information: Management of a Strategic Resource,* eds. M. Adbdlhak, S. Grostick, M. A. Hanken, and E. Jacobs, 71–142. Philadelphia: W.B. Saunders Company.

Walsh, T. 2004 (February). The proof is in the policy. *Journal of the American Health Information Management Association,* pp. 24–28.

Warren, J., M. Harris, and E. Warren. 1999 (July–August). Mining the CPR (and striking research gold). *Journal of American Health Information Management* (7):50–54.

Yennie, H. 1997. MIS: Reviewing the basics. *Behavioral Health Management* (17):6–10.

Zeglen, M. 1997. Accreditation requirements for ORYX: The next evolution in accreditation. *Journal of American Health Information Management Association* (6):20–31.w

Chapter 7

Regulatory and Accreditation Requirements

Janice L. Walton, MA, RHIA, CHP, CPHQ

As the amount and complexity of healthcare documentation has grown over the years, so has the need to regulate healthcare organizations to ensure that the documentation is managed appropriately, not only with regard to accuracy and accessibility, but also with regard to confidentiality and security. Government at both the state and federal level and private accreditation agencies have developed standards to regulate the practice of healthcare throughout the industry.

This chapter describes the different types of healthcare regulation. It also discusses the purposes of quality improvement organizations and the role of health information management professionals in the accreditation, certification, and licensure process that healthcare organizations go through to prove compliance with the standards established by the five most widely accepted accrediting bodies in the United States.

Early Days of Health Information Documentation

Although the practice of health information documentation in the United States goes as far back as 1752, with Benjamin Franklin keeping logs of patient names, admission and discharge dates, and diagnoses, the need for regulation and standardization in this area was not formally recognized until 1913, when the **American College of Surgeons** (ACS) was founded by Dr. Franklin H. Martin. The lack of professional **standards** for surgeons as they related to patient outcomes was the impetus for the discussion and development of the ACS.

Dr. Martin's resolution for the ACS reflected that "some system of standardization of hospital equipment and hospital work should be developed to the end that those institutions having the highest ideals may have the proper recognition before the profession, and that those of inferior equipment and standards should be stimulated to raise the quality of their work. In this way patients will receive the best type of treatment, and the public will have some means of recognizing those institutions devoted to the highest levels of medicine" (Roberts, Coate, and Redman 1987).

As part of the evaluation process, candidates for ACS fellowship were required to submit records for the patients on whom they had performed procedures. The records could not supply enough information to describe the applicants' practices or support their competence. As a result, in 1917, the ACS developed "The Minimum Standards" for use in evaluating hospitals. These standards included "that accurate and complete records be written for all patients and filed in an accessible manner in the hospital—a complete case record being one which includes identification data; complaint; personal and family history; history of present illness; physical examination; special examinations, such as consultations, clinical laboratory, X-ray and other examinations; provisional or working diagnosis; medical or surgical treatment; gross and microscopical pathological findings; progress notes; final diagnosis; condition on discharge; follow-up and, in case of death, autopsy findings" (ACS 1930).

Despite the fact that the first surveys using these new documentation standards were performed in 1918 with only 89 of the 692 hospitals surveyed meeting the minimal standards, the standards became the benchmark of the accreditation process (AHIMA 2000).

Accreditation and regulation requirements for health information have changed to meet the needs of the medical profession since the early days and are playing an increasingly important role in all kinds of healthcare settings. However, it is interesting to note that today's standards, like those from 1918, still require records to be "accurate and complete."

Continuing to meet the needs of the medical profession and the general public has grown in importance for the specialty of behavioral health. This can be seen in the proliferation of standards, regulations, and laws to assess, evaluate, and protect the health information of patients receiving treatment for mental health and substance abuse. Because of the sensitive nature of the information contained in alcohol, substance abuse, and behavioral health records, as well as the past and oftentimes still current stigma associated with having been treated for these conditions and the inappropriate use of the health information, additional laws and regulations have been enacted.

Specifically, the Federal Confidentiality Regulations, **42 CFR Part 2,** provide a higher standard of confidentiality and protection for records of clients receiving treatment for alcohol or drug abuse–related conditions. Some states also provide for additional protection of behavioral health records. For example, the Michigan Mental Health Code prohibits acknowledging whether a client is being currently treated or has ever received treatment at a behavioral healthcare organization without his or her signed authorization.

Types of Healthcare Regulation

Healthcare regulation is—and continues to be—developed and refined by both government and private entities. These include the federal government and its agencies, individual state government agencies, accreditation organizations, and private for-profit and not-for-profit organizations such as insurance carriers and medical societies.

Standards and regulations also are referred to as performance standards, quality indicators, rules, practice guidelines, performance indicators, standards of care, performance measures, or other descriptive terms. Whatever name is used, standards criteria set an expected performance level that should be met in order for safe care to be provided. That the standards are met or to what extent they are exceeded tells us something about the quality of care at the organization. Standards relevant to accreditation and regulation include the following (Johns 2002):

- **Accreditation standards** are predefined criteria used to assess the performance of healthcare organizations participating in a voluntary accreditation process.

- **Certification standards** are detailed compulsory requirements for participation in Medicare and Medicaid programs.

- **Licensure requirements** set criteria that healthcare providers must meet to gain and retain state licenses to provide specific services.

Accreditation

Accreditation is a voluntary process, administered by private organizations, that healthcare organizations elect to undergo. Though voluntary, accreditation is required for reimbursement by Medicare and in some states by other insurers. The purpose of an accreditation survey is to evaluate systems and processes so that performance can improve. Surveys focus on answering the following questions:

- What is the organization doing right?

- How can it improve?

To answer these questions, the organization is compared against standards during a survey. Survey frequency varies by accrediting body. Traditionally, surveys have been announced. However, accreditors today frequently phase in unannounced surveys because some healthcare organizations "relax" after being accredited and do not strive to improve continuously throughout the accreditation cycle, focusing their attention, instead, on accreditation processes during the few months or weeks prior to an anticipated survey. Today's surveys are evolving to be a more consultative and educational experience with improvement as the value of the process and recommendations for improvement as the basis for the findings.

Upon successful completion of the survey, accreditation is awarded. For a number of states this is considered a **deemed status.** Generally, a healthcare organization that has been accredited by the Joint Commission on Accreditation of Healthcare Organizations (JCAHO) or the American Osteopathic Association (AOA) is considered to have deemed status and to meet the *Conditions of Participation* with the following exceptions (CMS 2003):

- The utilization review (UR) standards

- Any standard from the secretary of Health and Human Services (HHS) that is higher than an accreditation standard

- Any higher-than-national standard approved by the secretary of HHS for a particular state

- The special conditions for psychiatric hospitals (specifically, the medical record and special staff requirement standards)

Accrediting Bodies

Many different **accrediting bodies** exist for both healthcare and nonhealthcare organizations. The accreditation processes must be evaluated to determine which one will best serve an organization. Factors that influence this decision include the types of services the organization provides, its vision and mission, and the funding sources requirements or preferences. The goal of the accreditation process is to help organizations improve and facilitate quality changes. For behavioral healthcare organizations, there are five widely accepted accrediting bodies: the JCAHO, the AOA, the Commission on Accreditation of Rehabilitation Facilities (CARF), the National Committee for Quality Assurance (NCQA), and the Council on Accreditation (COA).

The history of accrediting bodies began as far back as the 1940s with the AOA and is as recent as the 1990s with NCQA. The rationale for the development of the accrediting bodies was to promote quality in care and practices within healthcare organizations. Accreditation is a voluntary process that many healthcare organizations choose to pursue for a variety of reasons, but it is not a requirement for operation.

Each of the accrediting bodies accredits a variety of different organizations or services, and each has its own approach to the accreditation process as well as specific references to behavioral health or mental health services either within the overall context of the survey or as a separate process. For example, one accrediting body may survey an entire hospital, including the behavioral health unit, and another may survey only specific components or programs within an organization.

Each accrediting body also defines its own eligibility requirements. Organizational values and mission as well as quality processes, provision of behavioral health services or other services for which the accrediting body has standards, length of time the organization has been in business, and whether the organization has fulfilled licensure requirements are some of the common elements that all accrediting bodies examine.

Table 7.1 provides a brief summary of the history of the different accrediting bodies, the types of organizations they accredit, their approach to the accreditation process, and their eligibility requirements.

Accreditation Standards

Each of the accrediting bodies uses a set of standards to measure a healthcare organization's compliance and quality. It is important that the health information management (HIM) professional become familiar with all aspects of the HIM-related standards as well as the other standards that apply to the organization. Having a well-rounded knowledge of all the standards by which the organization is evaluated makes the HIM professional a valuable asset.

Each accrediting body also has established specific standards for behavioral health services and programs. Some of the standards are embedded within the general provision of standards; others are very specific to behavioral health or distinct programs of behavioral health services. Moreover, each accrediting body has standards for health information management. Some accrediting bodies may have a specific chapter on health information; others may include the HIM standards in specific chapters or sections such as care and treatment or in other areas within the standards themselves.

Because standards are always being revised and updated, it is impossible to provide a summary of the current specific standards. Table 7.2 provides a general summary of the structure of the standards, the development of standards, current standards, and the frequency of updating for each of the identified accrediting bodies.

Survey Preparation

Common elements among the accrediting bodies for survey preparation include completion of an application and provision of supporting documents. Completion of a self-survey as part of the preparation is required by a portion of the accrediting bodies and is becoming more the rule than the exception.

A point person or contact for the accreditation process is assigned to assist with questions and preparation processes. In some instances, a consultation visit is required as part of the survey preparation process. Each accrediting body reinforces the importance of using the point person to facilitate the accreditation process. Not using the point person as a valuable resource can cause problems during the survey.

Most of the accrediting bodies provide a great deal of information in their manuals; on their Web sites; or through educational seminars, meetings, and publications. All recommend making the accreditation process an ongoing, continuous process that involves the full organization or program, as applicable. Maintaining focus on the process and having the skills to stay organized are identified by a majority of the accrediting bodies as key components.

Table 7.3 offers a summary of the application process, identifying time lines, the point person, and additional information to assist with survey preparation for each of the accrediting bodies.

Survey Process

All of the accrediting bodies use a survey team approach. Team membership varies depending on the services provided by a healthcare organization. Generally, at least administrative and clinical members represent the service aspects of an organization. Survey length also depends on the accrediting body and the organization being surveyed. On average, survey length ranges from one-and-a-half to four days but may be longer if the survey team finds it necessary.

Table 7.1. Behavioral healthcare accreditors

Accrediting Body	History	Types of Organizations Accredited	Accreditation Model or Approach	Survey Eligibility Requirements
JCAHO	Began accrediting hospitals in 1952. Began accrediting behavioral health organizations in 1971. Began surveys of managed behavioral health in 1997. Behavioral health accreditation includes mental health, developmental disabilities, child welfare, and addiction (JCAHO 2003b).	• Hospitals • Home care • Long-term care • Managed behavioral health • Ambulatory care • Behavioral healthcare • Preferred provider organizations (PPOs) • Assisted living • Critical access hospitals • Office-based surgery practices • Healthcare networks • Pathology and clinical laboratory services (JCAHO 2003b)	Medical Model, which includes a review of the entire organization as a whole entity inclusive of all services and programs provided by the organization (JCAHO 2003b)	Organization is within the United States or territories. If outside the U.S. or territories, it is operated by the U.S. government or under a charter of the U.S. congress or meets other applicable requirements for operating outside the U.S. or its territories. The organization has a process for assessing and improving service quality. Services provided are identified directly, contractually, or by other means. Services provided are those covered by JCAHO standards. Determining the standards applicable to an organization and how these will be used during the survey process also must be completed while determining eligibility (JCAHO 2003b).
AOA	AOA accredits organizations under the Healthcare Facilities Accreditation Program (HFAP). Developed in 1943 and implemented in 1945 for annual hospital surveys. HCFA (now CMS) gave AOA deemed authority to survey hospitals using the *Conditions of Participation* (COP) in 1965. Obtained deemed status for accrediting laboratories of AOA-accredited hospitals using the Clinical Laboratory Improvement Amendments of 1988 (CLIA) in 1995. Subsequently surveys were added for: • Mental health • Substance abuse • Physical rehabilitation medicine • Ambulatory care/surgery (AOA 2003)	• Osteopathic hospitals • Critical access hospitals • Mental health • Substance abuse • Physical rehabilitation medicine • Ambulatory care/surgery (AOA 2003)	A specific model was not identified. The approach is based on type of organization seeking accreditation (AOA 2003).	Meet state licensing requirements Bylaws that specify acceptance of the HFAP certification process Been in operation for at least three months prior to application Meet basic service requirements as well as requirements based on the type of organization seeking accreditation (AOA 2003)

(Continued on next page)

Table 7.1.   (Continued)

Accrediting Body	History	Types of Organizations Accredited	Accreditation Model or Approach	Survey Eligibility Requirements
CARF	Developed in the United States in the 1950s to promote quality services for rehabilitation services and patients with disabilities; it was formalized in 1966. Began accreditation services in Canada in 1969 with CARF Canada coming into existence in 2002. Began accreditation in Sweden in 1996 with accreditation moving to Western Europe. Merged with the Continuing Care Accreditation Commission (CCAC) in 2003 (CARF 2003).	• Behavioral health • Assisted living • Comprehensive blind rehabilitation services • Employment and community services • Medical rehabilitation • Network administration and access centers • Family services • Psychosocial rehabilitation • Alcohol and integrated behavioral health specific or core programs may be selected for accreditation also. Examples of these include: • Assertive community treatment (ACT) • Addictions pharmacotherapy • Assessment and referral • Case management/ services coordination • Children and adolescent • Community and housing • Community integration • Criminal justice • Crisis intervention • Crisis stabilization • Day treatment • Detoxification • Drug court treatment • Employee assistance • Inpatient treatment • Intensive family-based services • Juvenile justice • Out-of-home treatment • Outpatient treatment • Partial hospitalization • Prevention/diversion • Residential treatment • Therapeutic communities • Supported living • Employment and community services • Opioid treatment (CARF 2003)	Accredits human service and rehabilitation providing agencies using a rehabilitative model. Services or programs are accredited instead of organization as a whole (CARF 2003).	Eligibility requirements vary depending on the services or programs being selected for survey. Certain fundamental principles apply to all programs, including: • Demonstration of the organization's values and approaches to Leadership —Corporate compliance (U.S. only) —Information management —Fiscal management —Human resources —Communication —Accessibility —Health, safety, and transportation —Information analysis —Outcomes management —Quality record review —Rights —Program structure and staffing —Screening and access to services —Individual planning —Transition/recovery support —Pharmacotherapy —Seclusion/restraint —Records of persons served (CARF 2003)

Table 7.1. (Continued)

Accrediting Body	History	Types of Organizations Accredited	Accreditation Model or Approach	Survey Eligibility Requirements
NCQA	Established in 1990 with first managed care organization accreditation surveys in 1991. Developed Health Plan Data and Information Set (HEDIS) in 1992. Began accreditation program for Managed Behavioral Healthcare Organizations (MBHOs) in 1997. Began accreditation of PPOs in 1999 (NCQA 2003).	• Managed care organizations (MCOs) • Preferred provider organizations (PPOs) • Managed behavioral healthcare organizations (MBHOs) • Medical research facilities • Physician organizations • HEDIS auditors and software vendors • Utilization management or credentialing services organizations • Credentials verification organizations • Human research protection programs (NCQA 2003)	Based on specific organization type or services provided. For example, if providing medical care under an MCO and behavioral health services, standards for both the MCO and MBHO would be used in the survey (NCQA 2003).	Eligibility requirements are specific to the type of accreditation or certification being sought. For managed behavioral healthcare organizations, these include: • Implementing a quality improvement process for members • Having comprehensive services for members across the continuum of care • Being in operation at least 18 months • Having appropriate licensure and meeting state, local, and federal regulations, as applicable • Operating without discriminatory practices on the basis of gender, race, creed, or national origin. (NCQA 2003)
COA	Founded in 1977 by Child Welfare League of America and Family Services of America (COA 2003)	There are currently 76 programs or services that can be accredited under COA, including services for children, youth, and families and behavioral health. Those related to behavioral health include: • Mental health services • Psychosocial and psychiatric rehabilitation services • Case management services • Counseling services • Treatment/therapeutic foster care • Day treatment services (COA 2003)	COA accredits human service and behavioral healthcare organizations using a community-based social services model. The healthcare organization, in general, is accredited as well as specific individual programs (COA 2003).	Organizations seeking COA accreditation are both public and private and not-for-profit and for-profit and must provide at least one service COA has developed standards for. All required licensures or certifications must be obtained, and the organization must be able to demonstrate the ability to have independence for review as a legal entity (COA 2003).

Table 7.2. Structure, development, and frequency of accreditation standards

Accrediting Body	Structure	Standards Development	Current Standards and Frequency of Updating
JCAHO	JCAHO reviews organizations as a whole with the various sets of standards available. The 2004 behavioral health manual is divided into sections or chapters, including but not limited to: • Ethics, rights, and responsibilities • Provision of care, treatment, and services • Medication management • Surveillance, prevention, and control of infection • Improving organization performance • Leadership • Management of information management of the environment of care • Behavioral health promotion For 2004, JCAHO is implementing a new survey process that includes use of the tracer methodology and priority focus process (PFP). The plan also includes all surveys being announced by 2006 (JCAHO 2003b).	The Standards Interpretation Group assists organizations with standards and accepts suggestions for new and/or revised standards. Proposed standards have a field review via posting in the JCAHO Web site. The proposed standards then become draft standards and remain posted on the Web site until published in the *Perspectives* magazine and JCAHO manuals at which time they become official standards (JCAHO 2003b).	The current behavioral health manual is *Comprehensive Accreditation Manual for Behavioral Health.* Review for behavioral health services within an acute care hospital setting may be reviewed with the *Comprehensive Accreditation Manual for Healthcare Organizations* (JCAHO 2003b). JCAHO standards are updated annually.
AOA	AOA delineates standards by department or unit within each of the different types of organizations it accredits, including acute care hospitals and behavioral health facilities or services. Included with the standards is a crosswalk to the Medicare *Conditions of Participation* (COP) (CMS 1999b), which allows organizations to determine their compliance with both the AOA and COP standards. For acute care hospitals providing behavioral health services, survey standards include special provisions for psychiatric units, medical record documentation, and staffing requirements (AOA 2003).	Standards are updated when CMS updates its standards or when a significant change occurs necessitating a standards change. Updated standards are approved by the AOA Bureau of Accreditation and by CMS (AOA 2003). As CMS is a government agency, standards revision is a public process with CMS staff drafting new or revised standards. The proposed standards are published in the *Federal Register* with a comment period before being finalized and published in final format in the *Federal Register* (CMS 2003).	Revisions were made to the AOA standards manual subsequent to the September 11, 2002, event (AOA 2003). CMS standards have not had a comprehensive update in more than 10 years. The most recent change occurred in July of 1999 with implementation of the patient rights chapter (CMS 2003).

Table 7.2.   (Continued)

Accrediting Body	Structure	Standards Development	Current Standards and Frequency of Updating
CARF	CARF has standards for individual programs. These include Mental Health Family Services; Psychosocial Rehabilitation, Alcohol and Other Drugs/Other Addictions; and Integrated Behavioral Health. Each of these programs contains standards for specific services (CARF 2003). The current behavioral health standards include the following categories with subcategories further defining specific areas: • Business practices • Behavioral health leadership and management • General program standards • Behavioral healthcare program and specific population (for the programs or services, for example, case management, outpatient treatment) designation standards • Employment and community services Information management standards are listed as a separate subcategory under the business practice section as well as the behavioral health leadership and management section. The strategic plan for CARF includes a better understanding of the value of accreditation and outcome measurement management. The Research and Quality Improvement Division has been established since 1997 to facilitate the movement toward this goal (CARF 2003).	Development and revision of CARF standards is accomplished via leadership panels, advisory committees, focus groups, and field review. Organizations accredited by CARF, clients receiving services, and others are included in the development and revision (CARF 2003).	The current behavioral health standards are in the CARF 2003 *Behavioral Health Standards Manual.* The standards are published annually in January of each year with application beginning in July of that year. Publications are available in hard-copy format (CARF 2003).

(Continued on next page)

Table 7.2.   (Continued)

Accrediting Body	Structure	Standards Development	Current Standards and Frequency of Updating
NCQA	NCQA provides standards for the different types of healthcare organizations such as behavioral health, managed care, or preferred provider. If an organization has multiple services, the different sets of standards are used to include the various services. There are categories of standards for the following areas with multiple sub-categories for each: • Quality management and improvement, including behavioral health-care • Utilization management • Credentialing and recredentialing • Member's rights and responsibilities Health information management standards are included in the quality management and improvement category. In 1999, behavioral health standards were incorporated for coordination of care and appropriate service delivery (NCQA 2003).	The oversight and development of standards is done by NCAQ's Standards Committee. Membership includes representatives from purchases, consumers, and managed care organizations. A behavioral health stakeholders group was used in the development of the 1999 behavioral health standards (NCQA 2003).	NCQA standards and guidelines for the accreditation of MCOs, including behavioral health. Standards are updated annually (NQCA 2003).
COA	COA current standards in the 7th edition of COA's *Standards and Self-study Manual* (COA 2001) address the service standards and organization and management standards. The organization and management standards reflect eleven areas of standards that apply to all organizations. These include, but are not limited to: • Ethical practices, rights, and responsibilities • Continuous quality improvement • Intake, assessment, and service planning • Financial management • Service delivery • Quality of service environment The service standards contain standards for specific types of services. There are currently 38 sections with 60 different types of behavioral healthcare and social programs. Examples of these include: • Mental health services • Counseling services • Employee assistance programs • Day treatment services • Prevention and support services • Residential treatment services • Case management services • Crisis intervention (COA 2002)	Standards are developed and revised through standards advisory panels. Input is obtained from private and public organizations, advocacy groups, state departments, and national professional service agencies. The director of standards and evaluation at COA facilitates the process (COA 2003).	The current manual is the 7th edition, published in 1997 (COA 2003). The frequency of updates was not identified.

Table 7.3. Survey preparation

Accrediting Body	Application Process	Time Lines	Point Persons	Additional Resources/Information
JCAHO	For organizations seeking accreditation for the first time, early survey policy options are available or the organization can choose to have an initial survey. Early survey option 1 is a limited survey before the organization has opened. Early survey option 2 is a full survey after an organization has been open for at least one month. Each early option involves a second or follow-up survey to determine accreditation status. The initial survey consists of a full survey with applicable standards using a four-month time frame prior to the survey to determine compliance versus a twelve-month time frame for organizations seeking re-accreditation. Preparation for the survey includes completing an application. The application provides JCAHO with information about the organization and the services provided as well as evidence of required licensure. The application can be completed and mailed in, or an electronic version is available via the JCAHO Web site (JCAHO 2003b).	The survey for initial accreditation is conducted within six months of receipt of the application. For re-accreditation, the survey is scheduled either 45 days before or after the triennial due date. As a part of the survey process, an organization must notify the public about the upcoming survey. This includes notification within the facility for staff and people receiving services as well as notification to the community via newspaper, radio, Web site posting, or other notices. JCAHO recommends nine to twelve months' lead time for initial survey preparation. This allows time to review and understand the standards, perform a self-assessment, plan and implement improvements as identified from the survey, develop or revise any needed policies and procedures, and train staff (JCAHO 2003b).	An account representative is assigned to each organization seeking accreditation. The role of the representative is to assist with and facilitate preparation throughout the accreditation cycle (JCAHO 2003b). The JCAHO representative is a valuable resource for interpretating and understanding standards and helping organizations stay organized during preparation.	For organizations seeking re-accreditation, the best preparation technique is to work continuously throughout the three-year accreditation cycle to maintain and improve the organization's processes. This is not an easy task, and often the twelve months before the next survey become the focus of the organization's attention. Whether the organization and the HIM professional are able to keep focused on JCAHO throughout the three years or the last twelve months, staying organized, coordinated, keeping the tasks prioritized, and maintaining accountability are essential to having a meaningful and successful survey process. Additional tools or resources to use for either an initial survey or a re-accreditation survey include (JCAHO 2002): • Contact and network with colleagues. • Assess and reinforce staff understanding of the organization's processes. • Conduct a mock survey internally or hire an external agency to perform a mock survey. • Follow up on the findings of the mock survey.

(Continued on next page)

Table 7.3.   (Continued)

Accrediting Body	Application Process	Time Lines	Point Persons	Additional Resources/Information
AOA	The application packet must be completed and forwarded to AOA for review. Registration fees must accompany the application. Upon review and acceptance of the application and consultant's report, a survey is scheduled. Written notification is provided to the organization's administration of the survey date and schedule (AOA 2003).		For healthcare organizations seeking accreditation for the first time, a presurvey consultation is required. The consultant is an independent consultant who must be chosen from a list of consultants approved by the HFAP Bureau of Healthcare Facilities Accreditation (AOA 2003).	Obtaining the accreditation manuals that correlate with the organization and services being provided should be done when eligibility has been established. The AOA recommends healthcare organizations contact HFAP for advice on which requirements would apply (AOA 2003).
CARF	A multistep approach is recommended for preparing for a CARF accreditation survey. When the organization has made the commitment and decision to pursue the accreditation, it should request and submit the intent to survey. The resource specialist assigned to the organization must be contacted to obtain the form and will assist in completing it. The signed intent form must be submitted no less than three months before the two-month time frame the survey is requested in (CARF 20003).	The organization must complete a self-evaluation. Standards must be implemented for a minimum of six months prior to the survey and performance of the self-evaluation (CARF 2003).	The organization must contact CARF and have a resource specialist assigned. This person assists with determining exactly which standards will the used during the survey process and is available to interpret the standards and provide help during the initial phases of preparation and beyond (CARF 2003).	Prepare well in advance. Based on the self-assessment, the organization should determine which areas will take the most time to complete and begin with those. It should keep the plans for improving areas of non-compliance simple. Stay organized. The organization should index the standards into a matrix with their response to the standard and plan for complying with it and should maintain the index on an ongoing basis to assist with re-accreditation processes. Keep staff involved. Having staff at all levels of the organization involved in the preparation process is essential to a successful survey. Submit CARF survey fees. Fees are based on the number of days and surveyors needed to do the review (CARF 2003).

Table 7.3. (Continued)

Accrediting Body	Application Process	Time Lines	Point Persons	Additional Resources/Information
NCQA	Request an application from NCQA accreditation operations by either calling or from the Web site. Complete and submit the application to schedule the survey date. Complete and submit the preassessment information form. In addition, for behavioral health organizations, have the following information: • Organization chart • Narrative of the history and current structure of the organization • Narrative description of the quality improvement plan and committee • Sample pages of contracts • Specific standards for the organization • Satisfaction data • Complaint data • Copies of clinical practice guidelines • Descriptions of continuity and coordination-of-care processes • Treatment record documentation policies and procedures • Utilization management data • Credentialing and recredentialing data • Member rights and responsibility information • Preventive health information (NCQA 2003)	Submit financial arrangements and documents, as required, including a preassessment evaluation, and make arrangements for the survey team beginning twelve weeks before the survey (NCQA, 2003).	An accreditation survey coordinator is assigned approximately six months before the scheduled survey (NCQA 2003).	NCQA recommends the following steps in preparation for a survey: • Read and understand each of the standards that apply. • Include all departments/areas within the scope of the standard in the process. • Document how the organization has met each of the standards and substandards and include where the surveyors can find the documentation for verification purposes during the review. • Organize all the documentation into binders divided by specific category (quality improvement, utilization management, preventive health, and so on) and tabbed by standard. Have multiple copies available for survey team members (NCQA 2003)

(Continued on next page)

Table 7.3. (Continued)

Accrediting Body	Application Process	Time Lines	Point Persons	Additional Resources/Information
COA	Submit the COA application. Eight elements must be included with the application, including a description of each service or program the organization provides, the application fee, copies of all licenses, and the most current annual reports. Complete financial and accreditation agreements. The financial agreement formalizes the fees and payment between COA and the organization (COA 2003).	Complete the self-study. The self-study provides a framework to assist in identifying areas of compliance and areas for improvement. It is used by the survey team during the accreditation process. Completing the self-study takes four to eight months. The full accreditation process typically takes twelve to eighteen months. The accreditation agreement specifies the time frame in which the self-study must be completed. The self-study includes providing COA with notebooks for each of the programs or services with supporting documentation for each of the applicable standards (COA 2001).	Upon review and acceptance of the materials submitted, an accreditation coordinator is assigned to the organization. The accreditation coordinator determines, based on the program descriptions provided, which of the standards will be used for the survey. This information is incorporated into the accreditation agreement (COA 2003).	Keep organized. As the entire organization is the focus of the survey process, involvement with all areas or departments is necessary. Having a lead or point person to keep the preparation process on track with teams or groups of individuals assigned to specific tasks to facilitate the survey preparation process is one effective method of staying organized. Incorporating these activities into the day-to-day duties and functions is often the difficult part. However, the organization's commitment to quality should include the necessary resources for success (COA 2003).

The agenda of the survey comprises a variety of reviews, tours, interviews, and meetings, depending on the accrediting body. An opening conference or meeting is standard. The process for the rest of the survey can be predetermined and scheduled prior to the survey team's arrival or provided to the organization during the opening conference/meeting. An exit or closing conference also is a standard process.

Each of the accrediting bodies has established types of accreditation with lengths of time associated with each. A full or three-year accreditation and a denial of accreditation are recognized by all the accrediting bodies. Levels between these two, such as provisional or conditional, also are available and vary by accrediting body.

An appeals process for accreditation decisions is available with all the accrediting bodies. However, how an **appeal** is sought and the decision made depends on internal processes at each accrediting body.

HIM Involvement in the Survey Process

Involvement of HIM professionals in the survey process varies from one accrediting body to another and from organization to organization. Being prepared in terms of HIM policies and procedures, practice guidelines, and record processes is essential. Having knowledge of the care processes and how the resultant documentation completes the care process is of great value when working with survey team members. In the event there is a formal record review session, facilitating the session is a key HIM function. Accompanying surveyors during site visits is often beneficial because interviews or discussion often leads to a review of documentation.

JCAHO's Shared Vision Pathway

In 2003, the JCAHO made significant changes to its 2004 survey process with its Shared Vision Pathway. The new process includes the use of the tracer methodology and the priority focus process.

The **tracer methodology** selects patient or client records to use as a road map to review and evaluate compliance with standards and systems of care by retracing the specific care and services provided by each area or department the patient or client has contact with. Surveyors may identify performance issues that affect client care at a department-specific level or at an organizationwide systems level. When patterns are identified, the surveyors issue a requirement for improvement. The organization is required to submit evidence of standards compliance and identify measures of success in response to the requirement for improvement. Follow-up data submission also is required to show a track record of implementation and findings (JCAHO 2003a).

The **priority focus process** (PFP) gathers data, analyzes them through its automated rules, and uses the information to tailor the survey to the needs of the specific organization. The top clinical/service groups (CSGs) and **priority focus areas** (PFAs) are identified and used by surveyors in selecting the tracer clients used in the tracer methodology during the survey (JCAHO 2003a).

Table 7.4 provides a brief overview of the survey process, the different types or accreditation decisions, and the appeals process for all five accrediting bodies.

Licensure

Licensing reviews are mandatory for healthcare organizations and are completed by state government entities. Annual unannounced surveys are conducted with an emphasis on inspection. The focus of the survey is to determine what the organization is doing wrong by reviewing it against minimum expectations and looking for individual deficiencies. Survey processes compare an organization against the regulations with any adverse findings resulting in citations. Traditionally, the approach of the survey is to impose sanctions, penalties, and/or fines with the value of the process being enforcement. In some states, steps are being taken to move the licensure review toward a consultative and educational approach. Upon successful completion of the survey, **licensure** is awarded.

Licensing Bodies

The licensure of healthcare organizations includes hospitals with behavioral health inpatient units, partial hospitalization programs, crisis stabilization, and outpatient services. Outpatient facilities or clinics and individual behavioral health practitioners also are governed by individual state laws and standards. The requirements for specific types of services vary from state to state. In addition, some states provide specific requirements for behavioral health providers to meet within the Medicaid program. HIM professionals are encouraged to contact the agency responsible for licensure. Many states also have Web pages devoted to licensing requirements.

Licensing Requirements

Although each state has specific names for requirement manuals and guidelines, often they are referred to as the Public Health Code for healthcare facilities. A state Mental Health Code or a similarly named document under the auspices of the Department of Community Health or Mental Health also is used for licensure surveys of behavioral health entities. Additionally, a state's Medicaid requirements may contain parameters that must be met to serve this population of patients.

Table 7.4. Survey process

Accrediting Body	Agenda, Duration, and Survey Team Composition	Decision Types (including duration of accreditation)	Appeals Process
JCAHO	Composition of the survey team depends on the type and size of the organization being reviewed. For behavioral health organizations, team members are based on the specialty areas and service provision. This may lead to the inclusion of additional surveyors on the team. JCAHO announced a revision to the survey process that became effective January 2004. The survey process will focus on the organization's critical processes and systems versus standards compliance. Each organization will complete and submit a self-assessment for use during the survey. Education will become more of the focus during the survey process, as will increasing physician involvement in the process. The new agenda for the survey includes: • Opening conference and orientation • Survey planning session • Individual tracer activity and system tracer activity • Special issue resolution • Daily briefing • Competence assessment process • Medical staff credentialing and privileging • Environment of care session • Life safety code building tour • Leadership session • CEO exit briefing and organization exit conference (JCAHO 2003) The duration of the survey on average is two to four days (JCAHO 2003b).	The findings of the survey are forwarded to the JCAHO central office for review by the Accreditation Committee of the Board of Commissioners and accreditation decision. The decision can be for: • Full accreditation (three year) • Provisional accreditation • Conditional accreditation • Preliminary denial • Accreditation denial • Preliminary accreditation To continue assessing an organization, JCAHO may do unscheduled and unannounced surveys in response to reports of serious noncompliance. Generally a 24- to 48-hour notice is provided for these reviews. The review can be a full or a focused survey. Findings of the survey can affect accreditation status. Unannounced random surveys are also conducted on 5 percent of accredited organizations. There is no notice of an unannounced survey, and it is usually conducted nine to thirty months after the last survey. Fixed (preestablished) and variable (organization-specific) standards are used during the review (JCAHO 2003b).	With a denial of accreditation the appeals process consists of: • Evaluation by the Joint Commission staff • Review by the accreditation committee • Review of hearing panels • Second consideration by the Accreditation Committee • Review by the Board Appeal Review Committee • Final accreditation decision (JCAHO 2003b)

Table 7.4.   (Continued)

Accrediting Body	Agenda, Duration, and Survey Team Composition	Decision Types (including duration of accreditation)	Appeals Process
AOA	The survey team includes, at a minimum, an osteopathic physician, a nurse, and an administrator. Additional team members may be assigned depending on the type of services provided and the size of the organization. The length of the survey is generally three days. The schedule includes: • Introduction and document review • Meetings with medical staff and administration • Review of discharged/closed medical records • Touring and review of concurrent records within all units/departments • Preparation of initial report • Exit conference (AOA 2003)	Written results of the review are provided within sixty days. Identified areas of noncompliance are provided with the report, and a healthcare organization has sixty days to submit corrective action plans for each of the noted areas. The accreditation awarded is dependent on how the organization complied with the standards, the areas of deficiency, and the response submitted. Implementation of the corrective action plans is of great importance in determining the accreditation awarded. The Bureau of Healthcare Facilities Accreditation, a nine-member panel, makes the final accreditation determination. Four levels of accreditation are possible: • Three-year accreditation and re-survey • Two-year accreditation and re-survey • Conditional (provisional) accreditation with one year re-survey • Denial of accreditation Validation of the findings and accreditation surveys conducted by HFAP is completed by the Centers for Medicare and Medicaid Services (CMS) as part of an ongoing review of quality (AOA 2003).	An appeals process is available through the Bureau of Healthcare Facilities Accreditation. The full process includes: 1. Appeals committee hearing 2. Bureau decision 3. Appeal to AOA board with board committee hearing (AOA 2003)
CARF	The survey team selected by CARF to review an organization is based on the services and individual needs of the organization requesting the survey. Team members' area(s) of expertise are used in the selection process. The team reviews each service and program selected against the applicable standards by reviewing documents and records, observing services provided, and interviewing staff, people receiving services, and other organization stakeholders. Consultation will be provided by the team. The findings of the survey are provided at the exit conference. The duration of the survey depends on the services and programs selected for review, with one day as the least amount of time for a survey (CARF 2003).	The survey team submits the findings report to the CARF Board of Trustees where a final decision regarding accreditation is made. The options include: • Three-year accreditation • One-year accreditation • Provisional accreditation • Nonaccreditation The organization is notified approximately six to eight weeks after the survey and receives a written survey report. A quality improvement plan to provide action steps to address the recommendations made must be prepared and submitted within ninety days of receiving the report. For organizations that receive the three-year accreditation, an annual conformance to quality report must be completed and sent to CARF (CARF 2003).	A survey outcome can be appealed. The first step is through an appeals hearing process with the Accreditation Committee. If the organization disagrees with the outcome, it can bring the decision to the full Board of Trustees for review (CARF 2003).

(Continued on next page)

Table 7.4.   (Continued)

Accrediting Body	Agenda, Duration, and Survey Team Composition	Decision Types (including duration of accreditation)	Appeals Process
NCQA	The on-site survey assesses the organization's compliance with standards for each service. A 100-point rating system is used in evaluation. The scoring is used as a recommendation to the Review Oversight Committee. The survey team and the number of members depend on the intensity and service array of each organization. Minimally, the team consists of two reviewers, a physician, and an administrator. The length of a survey also varies but usually is from two to four days. The survey process includes a review of the systems in place for quality, credentialing, treatment records, rights, preventive programs, and utilization. This may include on-site observations; interviews with staff; a review of documents, including treatment records; credentials files; and administrative records. A review of the organization's operations for health and safety of its patients is incorporated throughout the survey process. Participation and data collection for the Health Plan Employer Data and Information Set (HEDIS) must also be evident and ongoing. HEDIS requirements include performance measures for several areas, including access to care, member satisfaction, and quality of care. A summation conference with a preselected administrative team is held at the end of the survey, providing a report of preliminary findings. A recommendation for accreditation is not made at this time (NCQA 2003).	The data and information obtained during the on-site review is taken back to NCQA, and a preliminary report is prepared and sent to the organization. The organization has fourteen days to respond to the report but may request an additional seven days, if needed. The amount of documentation that may be submitted is limited to 37 pages. The final accreditation determination is made by an independent review committee called the Review Oversight Committee. Four types of accreditation are awarded: • Full accreditation (three year) for organizations that meet NCQA's standards for continuous quality improvement. • One-year accreditation for organizations that meet most of the standards and have well-defined services and quality processes • Provisional accreditation for organizations that meet some of the standards and have adequate quality processes. One year is given to bring the organization into compliance. • Denial of accreditation for organizations that have not met the standards and systems for quality and have serious problems (NCQA 2003)	An appeals or reconsideration process is available for organizations with provisional or one-year accreditation status (NCQA 2003). The NCQA Reconsideration Committee, an independent review committee, is used for appeals and is the final decision-making entity (NCAQ 2003).

Table 7.4. (Continued)

Accrediting Body	Agenda, Duration, and Survey Team Composition	Decision Types (including duration of accreditation)	Appeals Process
COA	The site visit is conducted by a team of trained volunteer peer reviewers. A minimum of two reviewers makes up a review team. The spectrum of services provided by an organization is correlated with the reviewers' areas of expertise in the selection of the review team. The materials provided during the self-study are used extensively during the on-site review process. Though the schedule of activities during the review may vary, a general schedule would include: • Preentrance meeting with the management/leadership team • Tour of the organization • Visits to program/service locations • Interview of staff and governing body members. • Review of records, including medical records, personnel records, minutes, and so on • Observation of consumers in service • Interviews with consumers and community representatives • Exit conference Site visits last a minimum of one and one-half days. The total length of the visit depends on the size and number of programs and services offered by an organization. The visit may be lengthened by the review team, if necessary, to determine compliance with the COA standards (COA 2003).	The survey team provides a written preliminary accreditation report to the COA Accreditation Commission to evaluate when making the accreditation decision. For first-time accreditation reviews, there are two possible decisions: • Accreditation for either a three or four-year cycle. • Denial of accreditation For organizations seeking re-accreditation, a probationary accreditation status is possible in addition to the full accreditation and denial (COA 2003).	An appeal process is available for organizations to request additional review of the denial decision. Appeals processes are available for re-accreditation decisions as well (COA 2001).

Licensing Process

Each state establishes the process for the licensure survey. The organization of the state's departments dictates which regulations are used and how many surveys are conducted. For example, an acute care hospital with an inpatient adult psychiatric unit, a geriatric unit, adult and adolescent partial hospitalization programs, and outpatient behavioral health services may be reviewed by the state department responsible for monitoring implementation of the Mental Health Code. If a separate entity, the department responsible for the general hospital licensure may accept the results of the Mental Health Code survey and not re-review the behavioral health services or may choose to include the services in its annual hospital licensure survey.

The survey itself is dependent on the structures developed by each state. Generally, the surveyors review administrative, clinical, physical plant, and record-keeping policies and procedures. A tour of the service areas is conducted for environment, health, and safety. Should services be provided at alternate locations or through the use of contracted services, site visits can be expected. A review of medical records will be conducted. A representative sample of the services and programs is generally requested. However, the surveyors may choose to focus on a specific group, for example, child and adolescent, geriatric, or residential services. Areas of deficiency found in the previous year's survey are normally scrutinized closely. In all instances, if a **corrective action plan** (CAP) or similarly named document was submitted from the prior year, each of the elements will be revisited for compliance.

Each state has an approval or rating system. The system can be as simple as pass and fail or may be composed of a scale ranging from substantial compliance to noncompliance with one or more interim steps. A numerical rating scale may be used with an overall numerical rating for the organization.

The survey team's recommendations are sent to the state licensing board where the final decision regarding licensure is made, and a formal report is presented to the healthcare organization. Although the U.S. Postal Service has routinely been used, some states are beginning to provide electronic reports in place of hard copies. The time frame for receipt of the final report depends on individual state parameters.

When deficiencies are identified, a plan to remediate the findings and a CAP or a similarly named document is required. The development, approval, or need for revision of the plan and time frame for completion or correction of identified deficiencies is handled by each state's licensing department.

The HIM professional should obtain and become familiar with individual state licensure regulations and standards, as applicable. Having knowledge of the different agencies, specific requirements or standards, and the process is essential in facilitating a survey process and having a successful outcome. Not having the knowledge can result in a very difficult and frustrating survey process.

Certification

A survey conducted for **certification** has the same focus and methodology as that explained earlier for licensure.

Certification Bodies

The **Medicare *Conditions of Participation*** (COP) apply to healthcare organizations receiving funds from the federal government for providing services to Medicare and Medicaid patients. Because both federal and state monies fund the Medicaid program, the *Conditions of Participation* also apply to healthcare organizations serving Medicaid patients. The state portion of

Medicaid regulations differs from state to state and is not discussed in detail here. Information pertaining to specific state Medicaid guidelines and regulations can be obtained from individual state agencies (COP 2003).

Certification Requirements

Generally, a healthcare organization that has been accredited by JCAHO or the AOA is considered to have deemed status and meets the *Conditions of Participation* with the same exceptions as those indicated earlier in this chapter for accreditation (CMS 2003).

These additional regulations for behavioral healthcare organizations are contained in Subpart E of 42 CFR, specifically, Section 482.61, Conditions of Participation: Special medical record requirements for psychiatric hospitals; and 482.62, Conditions of Participation: Special staff requirements for psychiatric hospitals (CMS 1999b). In addition, Subpart C— Medicaid for Individuals Age 65 or Over in Institutions for Mental Disease, Section 441.106, Comprehensive mental health—and Subpart D—Inpatient Psychiatric Services for Individuals Under Age 21 in Psychiatric Facilities or Programs—provide additional regulations for healthcare organizations providing behavioral health services.

Appendix AA of the *Conditions of Participation* contains Psychiatric Hospitals Interpretive Guidelines and Survey Procedures. As with all regulations, these are updated on a continual basis. Additional information on and updates to these references can be obtained via the *Federal Register* or the Centers for Medicare and Medicaid Services (CMS) Web site.

Certification Process

Under the *Conditions of Participation,* healthcare organizations wishing to be certified must be in full operation to be considered for a survey. Enough patients will need to have been served for the survey team to determine whether the organization is in compliance with all of the regulations/standards. The process for certification varies by type of healthcare organization (hospital, long-term care, psychiatric, home health, and so on), but it generally includes (CMS 2003):

- Precertification assistance for prospective providers with the objective of helping applicants meet the requirements as quickly as possible

- Provision of documents substantiating a healthcare organization's eligibility under the *Conditions of Participation* (also known as designation requirements)

- Completion of the application packet

- Review of the application and, if needed, a request within thirty days of receipt of application for additional information

- Provision of additional information, if applicable

- Recommendation for approval

- On-site survey

- Final approval

Quality Improvement Organizations

Public Law 92-603 of 1972, under the direction of the Health Care Financing Administration (HCFA) (now the CMS), required the development of professional standards review organizations

(PSROs) for the review of Medicare and Medicaid inpatient services. The reviews focused on medical necessity, quality, and cost-effectiveness. In 1977, the Utilization Review Act was implemented and added fraud and abuse regulations (CMS 2003).

The peer review process was redesigned in 1982, with **peer review organizations** (PROs) replacing PSROs. With these changes, each state and territory implemented its own PRO. The focus of the reviews did not change; however, variations in decisions between and within PROs led to inconsistency and questions about the reliability of the data and the decisions being made (Huffman 1994).

In 1992, the PROs became **quality improvement organizations** (QIOs). Under contract with the federal government, they implemented the Health Care Quality Improvement Program (HCQIP). The focus of the program is to improve Medicare patients' health through evaluation patterns of care and changing the healthcare delivery system. Quality review studies under the Quality Improvement Program are to be conducted. The HCQIP regulations have defined these studies as "an assessment, conducted by or for a QIO, of a patient care problem for the purpose of improving patient care through peer analysis, intervention, resolution of the problem, and follow-up". Working with patients, providers, health plans, practitioners, and others who purchase services, the QIO attempts to:

- Develop scientifically based **quality indicators**

- Use carefully measured patterns of care to identify opportunities for improvement

- Communicate patterns of care to the appropriate professionals and providers

- Facilitate system changes to improve the quality of healthcare

- Perform follow-up reviews to evaluate success and identify areas for improvement

The current national review activities under the CMS focus on medical conditions as well as on reducing healthcare service differences for Medicare patients (CMS 2003). Psychiatric or behavioral health services are not currently within the scope of review. It is important that HIM professionals monitor QIO review activities for inclusion of aspects of behavioral healthcare.

Development of Policies and Procedures to Meet Multiple Standards

Maintaining a thorough knowledge of the different standards under which an organization is accredited, certified, and/or licensed is essential when developing good policies and procedures. Being aware of changes that occur and how they will affect an organization's operations (and subsequently policies and procedures) also is vital. Even though the requirements of the different regulatory agencies and accrediting bodies are similar, it is important to ensure that all the standards have been met, which can best be achieved by reflecting the most stringent standards in the healthcare organization's policies and procedures.

Role of the HIM Professional

The HIM professional has a very unique and important role to play with regard to regulatory and accreditation requirements. HIM systems and processes affect nearly all of an organization's departments. As a result, the HIM professional plays a vital role in ensuring that all of the regulations and standards are reflected in appropriate policies and procedures and, even more importantly, in monitoring practices within the organization.

Coordinating and monitoring the record review processes associated with each of the accrediting/licensing and regulatory bodies is a key role for the HIM professional. Through the use of a clinical record review, many of the key functions reviewed during a survey process are evaluated on an ongoing basis with continuous improvements made throughout the organization.

In an AHIMA practice brief, Dan Rode (2002) provides good insight into the role of AHIMA's policy and government relations. Although HIM professionals are not often seen in the actual creation of a specific law, interactions are seen in the comment period. HIM professionals, volunteers, and staff provide input and/or are contacted to provide input. Staying up-to-date and taking the lead within individual organizations with respect to new or changing regulations is equally as important.

Staying current with regulatory and accrediting requirements is difficult and time-consuming. However, staying current enables the HIM professional to be a valuable resource for the organization and helps to ensure the organization's success during the survey process. Excellent resources for staying up-to-date include the following:

- The Communities of Practice (COPs) within the AHIMA Web site are a good tool for obtaining published information specific to an area. The ability to post questions and obtain input from peers throughout the country dealing with the same or similar issues and problems is most helpful.

- State HIM organizations are excellent sources of information on regulatory requirements specific to a given region. On-line resources as well as seminars and meetings serve to assist HIM professionals in staying current.

- The accrediting body for an organization and certification and/or licensing agencies often have on-line resources as well as telephone and written resources available.

- In-house or contractual legal counsel and fellow staff members also are valuable sources of information.

- Related professional organizations such as the American Psychiatric Association (APA), the American Hospital Association (AHA), the AMA, and others offer a great of information for the HIM professional.

Tables 7.5 and 7.6 are provided to help organizations obtain current information and stay up-to-date. Table 7.5 lists accrediting and regulatory organizations, and table 7.6 lists accreditation and regulatory resources.

Conclusion

Regulatory and accreditation requirements have an impact on all healthcare organizations, but especially so in the specialty area of behavior health. The amount and intensity of accreditation and regulatory effect on a healthcare organization is not likely to decline in the years to come. Indeed, an increase in standards and rules is anticipated as the awareness of and need for quality continue to grow. The need for HIM professionals within the behavioral health setting to have a thorough knowledge and understanding of and expertise in the rules and regulations applicable to the setting is imperative for healthcare organizations and to the success of the HIM profession.

Table 7.5. Accrediting and regulatory organizations

Organization	Address/Telephone	Internet Address
Joint Commission on Accreditation of Healthcare Organizations (JCAHO) JCAHO's *Comprehensive Accreditation Manual for Behavioral Healthcare*	One Renaissance Boulevard Oakbrook Terrace, IL 60181 (630) 792-5000	www.jcaho.org
American Osteopathic Association (AOA)	142 East Ontario Street Chicago, IL 60611 (800) 621-1773	www.aoa-net.org
National Committee for Quality Assurance (NCQA) NCQA's standards for the accreditation of managed behavioral healthcare organizations	2000 L. Street NW, Suite 500 Washington, DC 20036 (202) 955-3500 or (888) 275-7585	www.ncqa.org
The Rehabilitation Accreditation Commission (CARF) CARF's behavioral health standards manual	4891 E. Grant Road Tucson, AZ 85712 (520) 325-1044	www.carf.org
The Council on Accreditation (COA)	120 Wall Street, 11th Floor New York, NY 10005 1-866-COA-8088	www.coanet.org
American Accreditation Healthcare Commission (URAC) Health utilization management standards	1275 K. Street NW Suite 1100 Washington, DC 20005 (292) 216-9010	www.urac.org
Centers for Medicare and Medicaid Services (CMS)	7500 Security Boulevard Baltimore, MD 21244-1850 (877) 267-2323 or 800-MEDICARE	www.csm.hhs.gov

References and Bibliography

Ambulatory Care Section of the American Health Information Management Association. 1997. *Ambulatory Care Documentation.* Chicago: AHIMA.

American Accreditation Healthcare Commission. 2003 (February). http://urac.org.

American College of Surgeons. 1930. *Manual of Hospital Standardization and Hospital Standardization Report.* Chicago: American College of Surgeons.

American Health Information Management Association. 2002a. *Practice Brief: Definition of the health record for legal purposes.* Available on-line at http://library.ahima.org.

American Health Information Management Association. 2002b. *Practice Brief: Maintaining a legally sound health record.* Available on-line at http://library.ahima.org.

American Health Information Management Association. 2001. HIM *Body of Knowledge: Winning "Joint Commission Jeopardy": Tips for success.* Available on-line at http://library.ahima.org.

American Health Information Management Association. 2000. HIM *Body of Knowledge: Accreditation: The journey continues.* Available on-line at http://library.ahima.org.

Table 7.6.   Accreditation and regulatory resources

Specific Reference	Source of Information
AHIMA	www.ahima.org Journal, Communities of Practice, FORE Library
State HIMA	Contact state and local health information management associations
State licensure law	State departments of licensure and/or regulation
Health Insurance Portability and Accountability Act (HIPAA)	www.cms.gov/hipaa www.hhs.gov/ocr/hipaa www.hipaadvisory.com
Recording and reporting of occupational injuries and illness	www.osha.gov/ 29 CFR Part 1904
Patient Self-Determination Act (PSDA)	Legal Information Institute www.law.cornell.edu/uscode/
Medicare and Medicaid program manuals, memorandums, and transmittals	www.cms.hhs.gov/manuals/cmstoc.asp www.cms.hhs.gov/manuals/memos/comm_date_dsc.asp
Psychology licensure, regulations, associations, and boards in 50 states	www.uky.edu/education/EDP/psyinfo2.html
American Psychological Association	www.psych.org
Healthcare providers credentialing standards	www.urac.org
Tracking legislative changes	http://thomas.loc.gov
American Hospital Association	www.aha.org
American Medical Association	www.ama-assn.org
National Council for Community Behavioral Health	www.nccbh.org
National Practitioner Data Bank and Healthcare Integrity and Protection Data Bank	www.npdb-hipdb.com
For the Record	Free publication for HIM professionals
Advance	Free publication for HIM professionals

American Osteopathic Association. 2003. www.aoa-net.org.

Centers for Medicare and Medicaid Services. 2003 (February). www.cms.org.

Centers for Medicare and Medicaid Services, 2001. *Medicare State Operations Manual. Section 2042, Psychiatric Hospitals, Section 2700, Conducting Initial Surveys and Scheduled Resurveys.* Washington, DC: U.S. Government Printing Office.

Centers for Medicare and Medicaid Services. 1999a. *Certification Surveys.* Washington, DC: U.S. Government Printing Office.

Centers for Medicare and Medicaid Services. 1999b. *Conditions of Participation, Subpart E.* Washington, DC: U.S. Government Printing Office.

Centers for Medicare and Medicaid Services. 1995. Appendix AA: Psychiatric Hospitals Interpretive Guidelines and Survey Procedures. *Medicare State Operations Manual Provider Certification.* Rev. 280. Washington, DC: Government Printing Office.

Commission on Accreditation of Rehabilitation Facilities. 2003. www.carf.org.

COP-Compliance. 2003 (December). Available on-line at http://www.cop-compliance.com.

Council on Accreditation. 2003 (January). http://www.coa.org.

Council on Accreditation. 2001. Standards and Self-Study Manual, 7th ed. New York: Council on Accreditation.

Huffman, Edna K. 1994. *Medical Record Management.* Berwyn, IL: Physicians' Record Company.

Johns, Merida L., ed. 2002. *Health Information Management Technology.* Chicago: American Health Information Management Association.

Joint Commission on Accreditation of Healthcare Organizations. 2003a (February). www.jcaho.org.

Joint Commission on Accreditation of Healthcare Organizations. 2003b. *Comprehensive Accreditation Manual for Behavioral Health.* Oakbrook Terrace, IL: JCAHO.

Joint Commission on Accreditation of Healthcare Organizations. October 2002. JCAHO's New Accreditation Process for 2004. *Perspectives:* 1–16.

National Committee for Quality Assurance. 2003 (January). www.ncqa.org.

Peer Review Organization Manual. 1999. Available on-line at www.cms.hhs.gov/manuals/19-pro/pr00.asp.

Roberts, James S., Jack G. Coate, and Robert Redman. 1987. A history of the Joint Commission on Accreditation of Hospitals. *Journal of the American Medical Association* 266(7):936–40.

Rode, Dan. 2002. HIM Body of Knowledge: Keeping current on legislation vital to HIM professionals. Available on-line at http://library.ahima.org.

The Rehabilitation Accreditation Commission. 2002 (December). www.carf.org.

Titzer, Anne, AOA accreditation program manager. Interview by author, March 25, 2003.

Tomes, Jonathan P. 1993. *Healthcare Records Manual.* Boston: Warren Gorham Lamont.

Chapter 8

Compliance

Ruby Nicholson, RHIT

Compliance is governed by a myriad of federal regulations that apply to all healthcare settings. Each healthcare provider has the opportunity to determine exactly how these components are translated into polices and procedures and implemented into the provider's organization. The challenge in behavioral healthcare organizations is the limited resources available to develop a compliance program and monitor its ongoing efforts.

This chapter provides an extensive overview of the primary components of compliance, closely referencing the federal regulations and first-hand examples of field implementation. Because compliance requires adherence to regulations, the basic design and explanation of the components of compliance are cited from the *Federal Register.* Additional information is available in the appendixes: See appendix E for the full text of the OIG Compliance Program Guidance for Hospitals (1998) and OIG Draft Supplemental Compliance Program Guidance for Hospitals (2004); appendix F for the AHIMA Practice Briefs: "Seven Steps to Corporate Compliance: The HIM Role" and "Developing a Coding Compliance Policy Document."

Goals of Compliance

Compliance is best described as "a formal program designed to prevent fraud and abuse and ensure the organization's commitment to uphold the laws and regulations governing the day to day operation of the provider"(Kent Center 2001).

The overall goals of an organization's compliance efforts are to:

1. Identify, investigate, and remediate any potential problems arising from auditing and monitoring

2. Ensure that the organization operates within the applicable rules and regulations

3. Clarify the organization's ethical standards and its commitment to honest/responsible conduct

4. Avoid or minimize any substantial fines or penalties that could occur as a result of an audit

5. Improve the work environment, including the financial performance of the organization

The purposes, components, implementation, and trends in compliance that support these overall goals are discussed later in this chapter.

Fraud and Abuse

If compliance is the prevention of fraud and abuse, then both must be defined in terms of their context to the healthcare industry. Medicare, Medicaid, and the industry have defined fraud as:

> Fraud is knowingly and willingly executing or attempting to execute a scheme or artifice to defraud any healthcare benefit program or to obtain, by means of false or fraudulent pretenses, representations, or any promises of the money or property owned by or under the custody or control of a healthcare benefit program (Kent Center 2001).

> Fraud is an intentional deception or misrepresentation made by a person with the knowledge that the deception could result in some unauthorized benefit to that person or entity or some other person or entity (CMS 2004).

> To purposely bill for services that were never given or to bill for a service that has a higher reimbursement than the service provided (Medicare 2004).

Simply put, fraud is an intentional act to defraud the healthcare system. Some examples of fraud are: a provider knowingly submits claims for procedures with a higher reimbursement code rather than the code appropriate for the procedures/services provided; a provider knowingly performs unnecessary services; a provider submits claims with false diagnoses. Improper billing practices, falsifying time sheets or encounter sheets, receiving kickbacks for referrals, charging for services paid for by Medicare or Medicaid, falsifying clinical documentation, unethical business practices, and similar activities can all be considered fraudulent activity.

Although fraud is an intentional deception, abuse is considered unintentional and more likely to be an error or omission. Note the difference in the following definitions of abuse:

> [Abuse is] payment for items or services when there is no legal entitlement to that payment and when the provider has not knowingly and/or intentionally misrepresented facts to obtain payment (Kent Center 2001).

> Abuse is provider practices that are inconsistent with sound fiscal, business or medical practice, and result in an unnecessary cost to the Government, or reimbursement for services that are not medically necessary or fail to meet professionally recognized standards for healthcare (Medicare 2004).

> Abuse is payment for items or services that are billed by mistake by providers but should not be paid for by Medicare (Medicare definition).

Abuse is considered to occur when a provider unknowingly receives payment for an error or omission. It can occur when a provider submits an incorrect code or diagnosis unknowingly, submits bills for the wrong client or service when documentation is insufficient to validate a service or medical necessity, submits incomplete documentation and/or incorrect coding assignment, and so on. Often most abuse issues are a result of either insufficient staff training and monitoring or human error. Compliance programs help providers assess these types of errors and provide opportunities for remediation and reduction of risk.

Common Types of Fraud and Abuse

The following list summarizes the most common types of fraud and abuse (U.S. Government Printing Office 1998):

- Misrepresentation of a diagnosis to justify services billed as well as services provided that are not medically necessary

- Billing for services not provided or covered

- Upcoding (billing for more complicated service than the one provided)

- Outpatient services rendered in conjunction with an inpatient stay (outpatient services of a provider could already be included in the inpatient billing, thus creating a duplicate bill)

- DRG creep (similar to upcoding billing for a DRG at a higher reimbursement rate)

- Unbundling (billing for an additional service that is already included in a "bundle" of comprehensive services)

- Billing for services without a valid treatment plan (Medicaid considers services not necessary if there is no prescribed course of treatment.)

- Not collecting deductibles and copays

- Incorrect coding of diagnosis and/or procedure (Behavioral health providers use DSM IV codes and activity codes specific to software or payer, which then have to be cross-walked to an ICD 9 CM and/or CPT code. Because an individual with no coding knowledge often does coding, errors can occur.)

- No documentation for services provided

- Inaccurate or incomplete documentation for services provided

- Conflicts of interests and kickbacks (pharmacies, labs, vendors, and so on)

- Charitable contributions vis-à-vis vendors (Contributions made by vendors could be in violation of antikickback **statutes.** Equally, solicitation to vendors for contributions could be in violation.)

- Marketing and fundraising practices (Providers need to be sure marketing and fund-raising activities do not violate antikickback statutes or create conflicts of interest.)

- Applying for eligibility programs not entitled to

Cooperating Government Components

There are several cooperating government agencies whose functions include monitoring healthcare compliance. The most important of these government agencies are discussed in the following subsections.

Centers for Medicare and Medicaid Services

The Centers for Medicare and Medicaid Services (CMS), formerly HCFA, is the agency within the Department of Health and Human Services (HHS) responsible for developing policies and ensuring that the Medicare, Medicaid, and State Children's Health Insurance Programs are run appropriately. CMS's mission is to "assure health care security for beneficiaries" (CMS 2004). Although CMS has several goals aimed at designing, promoting, and improving healthcare systems, a primary goal is to prevent fraud and abuse of the nation's healthcare system. As part of this effort, CMS provides guidance to states in developing systems that promote compliance with rules and regulations and encourages compliance program implementation within organizations.

Office of Inspector General

The mission of the Office of Inspector General (OIG) "as mandated by Public Law 95-452 is to protect the integrity of the Department of Health and Human Services (HHS) programs, as well as the health and welfare of the beneficiaries of those programs" (OIG 2004). Its primary focus is on Medicare, Medicaid, and Public Health Services.

The OIG investigates and conducts medical records and claims reviews to determine whether claims are correct and services were medically necessary, properly coded, and documented. As a division of HHS, the OIG reports to both the secretary of HHS and Congress on problems identified and makes recommendations for corrective action.

Federal Bureau of Investigation

Although several agencies are responsible for investigating healthcare fraud, the Federal Bureau of Investigation (FBI) is the only federal agency with authority to investigate offenses identified throughout the healthcare industry. Referrals may be made to the FBI by the OIG, the DCIS (Defense Criminal Investigative Service, which is responsible for the military health service system), CMS, private insurance companies, businesses, or individuals. Civil action suits for violations of the Federal False Claims Act made by private citizens or businesses also are referred to the FBI for investigation. Often this investigatory process is under way long before the healthcare provider is aware of any pending charges. Establishing a voluntary compliance program provides a way for a healthcare organizations to detect problems within its system and decrease the chance of a criminal investigation.

Department of Justice

The Department of Justice (DOJ) prosecutes charges of healthcare fraud and abuse and works in conjunction with the OIG and FBI in ensuring that convictions and penalties occur for individuals or organizations found guilty of healthcare fraud.

Medicaid Review Units

Medicaid fraud units, working out of each individual state's attorney general office, are responsible for investigating complaints of fraud or abuse of the state's Medicaid program. These investigations may occur as a result of an **audit** or **qui tam litigation.** Qui tam litigation allows whistleblowers, or individuals with knowledge of a provider's fraudulent or abusive practices, to file suit on behalf of the government as a civilian.

Quality Improvement Organizations

Various quality improvement organizations (QIOs), formerly called peer review organizations (PROs), conduct audits for private payers ensuring compliance with payer rules and regulations. These audits are usually random but often focus on a type of service identified by the payer as a high user of cost. Substance abuse treatment, services to children, day programs, and services provided by psychiatrists and psychologist are frequently a focus of review audits.

Audits

Auditing the organization's compliance with standards, policies, and payer rules is a compliance program's most costly and labor-intense activity. When establishing internal audit procedures, it is best to start with those areas of focus identified on the OIG's work plan. A copy of the OIG work plan is published annually and can be obtained from www.oig.hhs.gov/publications. (See figure 8.1 for the table of contents of the 2005 OIG work plan.)

When the specific areas for auditing have been determined, a schedule of audits should be established. Systems designed for auditing differ based on the organization's size and the type of services delivered (that is, inpatient rather than outpatient). Hospitals conduct a large number of audits prior to any bills being submitted whereas outpatient clinics may only conduct a limited number of retrospective reviews. Typically, this is because hospital-based programs have requirements, systems, and resources that support this process.

Figure 8.1. HHS/OIG Fiscal Year 2005 Work Plan—Centers for Medicare and Medicaid Services

Medicare Hospitals
Quality Improvement Organization Mediation of
  Beneficiary Complaints
Medical Education Payments for Dental and Podiatry
  Residents
Nursing and Allied Health Education Payments
Graduate Medical Education Voluntary Supervision in
  Nonhospital Settings
Postacute Care Transfers
Diagnosis-Related Group Coding
Inpatient Prospective Payment System Wage Indices
Inpatient Outlier and Other Charge-Related Issues
Inpatient Rehabilitation Facilities Payments
Inpatient Rehabilitation Payments—Late Assessments
Medical Necessity of Inpatient Psychiatric Stays
Consecutive Inpatient Stays
Long-Term Care Hospitals Payments
Level of Care in Long-Term Care Hospitals
Critical Access Hospitals
Organ Acquisition Costs
Rebates Paid to Hospitals
Coronary Artery Stents
Outpatient Cardiac Rehabilitation Services
Outpatient Outlier and Other Charge-Related Issues
Lifetime Reserve Days
Hospital Reporting of Restraint-Related Deaths
Medicare Home Health
Beneficiary Access to Home Health Agencies
Effect of Prospective Payment System on Quality of
  Home Health Care
Home Health Outlier Payments
Enhanced Payments for Home Health Therapy
Medicare Nursing Homes
Access to Skilled Nursing Facilities Under the
  Prospective Payment System
Use of Additional Funds Provided to Skilled Nursing
  Facilities
Nurse Aide Registries
Nursing Home Deficiency Trends
Nursing Home Compliance With Minimum Data Set
  Reporting Requirements
Nursing Home Resident Assessment and Care Planning
Enforcement Actions Against Noncompliant Nursing
  Homes
Nursing Home Informal Dispute Resolution
Nursing Home Residents' Rights
Skilled Nursing Facilities' Involvement in Consecutive
  Inpatient Stays
Imaging and Laboratory Services in Nursing Homes
Skilled Nursing Facility Rehabilitation and Infusion
  Therapy Services
State Compliance With Complaint Investigation
  Guidelines
Medicare Physicians and Other Health Professionals
Billing Service Companies
Medicare Payments to VA Physicians
Care Plan Oversight
Ordering Physicians Excluded From Medicare
Physician Services at Skilled Nursing Facilities
Physician Pathology Services
Cardiography and Echocardiography Services
Physical and Occupational Therapy Services
Part B Mental Health Services
Wound Care Services
Coding of Evaluation and Management Services
Use of Modifier –25
Use of Modifiers With National Correct Coding
  Initiative Edits

"Long Distance" Physician Claims
Provider-Based Entities
Medicare Medical Equipment and Supplies
Medical Necessity of Durable Medical Equipment
Medicare Pricing of Equipment and Supplies
Medicare Drug Reimbursement
Prescription Drug Cards
Employer Subsidies for Drug Coverage
Beneficiary Understanding of Drug Discount Card
  Program
Computation of Average Sales Price
Collecting and Maintaining Average Sales Price Data
Adequacy of Reimbursement Rate for Drugs Under
  ASP
Payments for Non-End-Stage Renal Disease Epoetin
  Alfa
Other Medicare Services
Laboratory Services Rendered During an Inpatient Stay
Laboratory Proficiency Testing
Independent Diagnostic Testing Facilities
Therapy Services Provided by Comprehensive
  Outpatient Rehabilitation Facilities
New Payment Provisions for Ambulance Services
Air Ambulance Services
Quality of Care in Dialysis Facilities
Monitoring of Market Prices for Part B Drugs
Follow-up on Medicare Part B Payments for Ambulance
  Services
Follow-up on Medicare Part B Payments for Radiology
  Services
Emergency Health Services for Undocumented Aliens
Medicare Managed Care
Benefit Stabilization Fund
Adjusted Community Rate Proposals
Follow-up on Adjusted Community Rate Proposals
Administrative Costs
Managed Care Encounter Data
Enhanced Managed Care Payments
Enhanced Payments Under the Risk Adjustment Model
Managed Care Excessive Medical Costs
Duplicate Medicare Payments to Cost-Based Plans
Prompt Payment
Marketing Practices of MCOs
Managed Care "Deeming" Organizations
Medicare Contractor Operations
Preaward Reviews of Contract Proposals
CMS Oversight of Contractor Performance
Program Safeguard Contractor Performance
Accuracy of the Provider Enrollment, Chain, and
  Ownership System
Handling of Beneficiary Inquiries
Carrier Medical Review: Progressive Corrective Action
Duplicate Medicare Part B Payments
Contractors' Administrative Costs
Pension Segmentation
Pension Costs Claimed
Unfunded Pension Costs
Pension Segment Closing
Postretirement Benefits and Supplemental Employee
  Retirement Plan Costs
Medicaid Hospitals
Medicaid Graduate Medical Education Payments
Hospital Outlier Payments
Medicaid Diagnosis-Related Group Payment Window
Disproportionate Share Hospital Payments
Hospital Eligibility for Disproportionate Share Hospital
  Payments

(Continued on next page)

Figure 8.1.   (Continued)

Medicaid Long-Term and Community Care
Payments to Public Nursing Facilities
Community Residence Claims
Assisted Living Facilities
Medicaid Home Health Care Services
Targeted Case Management
Personal Care Services
Home- and Community-Based Services Administrative
   Costs
Medicaid Eligibility and the Working Disabled

Medicaid Mental Health Services
Nursing Home Residents With Mental Illness and
   Mental Retardation
Claims for Residents of Institutions for Mental Diseases
Medicaid Services for Mentally Disabled Persons
Rehabilitation Services for Persons With Mental
   Illnesses
Community Mental Health Centers
Medicaid Reimbursement for Intermediate Care
   Facilities
Restraint and Seclusion in Children's Psychiatric
   Residential Treatment Facilities

Medicaid/State Children's Health Insurance Program
Duplicate Claims for Medicaid and State Children's
   Health Insurance Program
Enrollment of Medicaid Eligibles in SCHIP
State Evaluations of SCHIP Programs
Detecting and Investigating Fraud and Abuse in SCHIP

Medicaid Drug Reimbursement
Average Manufacturer Price and Average Wholesale
   Price
Medicaid Drug Rebates—Computation of AMP and
   Best Price
Oversight of Drug Manufacturer Recalculations for
   Medicaid Drug Rebates
Indexing the Generic Drug Rebate
Drug Rebate Impact From Drugs Incorrectly Classified
   as Generic
Dispute Resolution in the Medicaid Prescription Drug
   Rebate Program
Medicaid Drug Rebate Collections
Overprescribing of OxyContin and Other Psychotropic
   Drugs
Accuracy of Pricing Drugs in the Federal Upper Limit
   Program
Medicaid Drug Utilization Review Program

Other Medicaid Services
Family Planning Services
School-Based Health Services
Adult Rehabilitative Services
Controls Over the Vaccine for Children Program
Outpatient Alcoholism Services
Claims Paid for Clinical Diagnostic Laboratory Services
Payments for Services Provided After Beneficiaries'
   Deaths
Marketing and Enrollment Practices by Medicaid
   Managed Care Entities
Factors Affecting the Development, Referral, and
   Disposition of Medicaid Fraud Cases: State
   Agency and Medicaid Fraud Control Unit
   Experiences

Medicaid Administration
Contingency Fee Payment Arrangements
Upper Payment Limits
Calculation of Upper Payment Limits for Transition
   States
State Match for Medicaid Upper Payment Limit
   Reimbursement
Medicaid Provider Tax Issues
State-Employed Physicians and Other Practitioners
Skilled Professional Medical Personnel
Physician Assistant Reimbursement
Medicaid Claims for Excluded Providers
Administrative Costs of Other Public Agencies
Administrative Costs for Medicaid Managed Care
   Contracts
University-Contributed Indirect Costs
Federal Financial Participation for Medicaid Cost
   Allocation Plans
Medicaid Accounts Receivable
Section 1115 Demonstration Waiver
Medicaid Management Information System
   Expenditures
Appropriateness of Medicaid Payments
Medicaid FFS Payments for Beneficiaries Enrolled in
   Managed Care
CMS Oversight of Home- and Community-Based
   Waivers

Information Systems Controls
Security Planning for CMS Systems Under
   Development
Accuracy of the Fraud Investigation Database
Medicaid Statistical Information System
State Controls Over Medicaid Payments and Program
   Eligibility
Replacement State Medicaid System
Smart Card Technology
Compliance With the Health Insurance Portability and
   Accountability Act Privacy Final Rule—University
   Hospital
MCO's Compliance With HIPAA

General Administration
FY 2004 Medicare Error Rate Estimate
FY 2005 Medicare Error Rate Estimate
Group Purchasing Organizations
Contractual Arrangements With Suppliers
Corporate Integrity Agreements
State Medical Boards as a Source of Patient Safety Data
Payments for Services to Dually Eligible Beneficiaries
Nursing Home Quality of Care: Promising Approaches
Payments to Psychiatric Facilities Improperly Certified
   as Nursing Facilities

Investigations
Health Care Fraud
Provider Self-Disclosure

Legal Counsel
Compliance Program Guidance to the Health Care
   Industry
Resolution of False Claims Act Cases and Negotiation
   of Corporate Integrity Agreements
Providers' Compliance With Corporate Integrity
   Agreements
Advisory Opinions and Fraud Alerts
Anti-Kickback Safe Harbors
Patient Anti-Dumping Statute Enforcement
Program Exclusions
Civil Monetary Penalties

Source: HHS OIG 2005.

Outpatient programs not affiliated with a hospital organization have limited resources to conduct such audits prior to claims submission deadlines; therefore, **retrospective reviews** generally take place. Retrospective reviews do require strict attention to trends and remediation efforts in order to change problem areas and avoid consistent paybacks for recurring problems. When resources for compliance are limited, it may be necessary to schedule time each week or each month to conduct audits and follow-ups on compliance issues.

Again, the system to develop is the one that meets the organization's needs. Regardless of the system implemented, the basics of the audit process are similar to those traditionally conducted in a health information department.

Creating simple audit tools and reference lists for the most commonly used codes makes auditing easier. In small practices, the actual auditing may need to be delegated to several staff trained in the audit process. The compliance officer should be responsible for training these staff and reviewing auditing practices.

Audits should include billing practices. Activity sheets or encounter forms should be checked against claims submission and reimbursement reports.

One area to pay particular attention to is duplicate billing. Duplicate billing can occur when a group session is run by more than one individual and both individuals submit activity reports for the same service. This problem also can occur when clinicians submit duplicate paperwork to the billing office.

It also is important to review trends identified through the auditing process. Problem areas can be identified that may indicate corrective action, remediation, disciplinary action, system changes, retraining, and further reviews. Making trending reports available to managers provides tools for disciplinary action plans, education and training, and compliance monitoring within a program or department. (See figure 8.2 for an example of a simple trending report.)

Four examples of auditing processes are random one-record audits, electronic claims submission audits, focused reviews of health records, and comprehensive health record reviews.

Random One-Record Audits

A random review of services billed and services documented can be done for each discipline providing care. The number of reviews should be the same for each discipline and is usually calculated by caseload or annual productivity. In a hospital setting, this might be 10 to 20 percent of the person's annual productivity. In an outpatient clinic, the percentage reviewed could be determined by annual productivity, a percentage of the discipline's caseload, or a specific number per quarter (for example, two cases per quarter for each staff).

Automated billing systems can provide a computer printout of services provided to a patient over a specified period of time. This printout then can be checked against the clinical record to ensure that documentation occurred for the specific services provided by the specified individual on the date billed. (See figure 8.3 for a sample billing printout.)

Results of random audits may indicate a more focused review of either an entire record or a particular staff's caseload. (See appendix G for sample audit tools, forms, and worksheets.)

Electronic Claims Submission Audit

A random review of electronic claims submissions should be included as part of the auditing process. This requires a review of diagnostic coding, documentation, CPT coding, and the claim itself before the claim goes out the door. Specific things to review include documentation of the right credentials, length of sessions, content of notes, and the charge sheet sent to the billing office.

Because coding in the behavioral health systems is typically done by clinical staff, special attention should be given to documentation of diagnoses and the coding of these diagnoses. Particular attention also should also be given to physician use of evaluation and management (E/M) **codes.** Problems typically occur with the coding of follow-ups as first visits and meeting the criteria for psychotherapy visits. (See chapter 5 for further details on E/M coding in the behavioral health setting.)

Figure 8.2. Sample trending report

Count of Type / Staff #	Activity code error	Billed w/FKA note	Billed, no note	Client billed w/o service	Day treatment double bill	Incorrect client code	Missing paperwork	Missing signature, credentials, etc.	No SA authorization	Note misdated	Note not billed	Paperwork misfiled	Progress note does not match interventions	Services w/o treatment plan	Tx Plan not found in chart	Grand Total
1558			2													2
1564	1										2					3
1574			1			2										3
1575						1										1
1617			3													3
1643														1		1
1726											1					1
1810										1						1
1813			1	1				10								12
1819											2					2
1883				1							1					2
1918			1													1
1925			4				1								1	6
1989										1						1
2018			1										1			2
2043	1		2								1					4
2046										1						1
2050								1								1
2066	1															1
2071			3			1										4
2117			1													1
2165														1		1
2186	1		1													2
2221			1													1
2232				9												9
2238	1		2					1			1					5
2267										2						2
2275										1						1
2282	1	1	8					1		2	16					29
2290											3					3
99999												1				1
Grand Total	6	1	31	9	2	3	1	4	10	8	27	1	1	2	1	107

Compliance Errors Found in Audits 10/01/02–12/31/02 — Type of Error

Figure 8.3. Sample billing printout

DATE OF AUDIT: _____ AUDIT COMPLETED BY: _____

Insurance	Active	CURRENT DIAGNOSIS
115 MEDICARE PART "B" CLAIMS DEPARTMENT	Y	296.34—MAJ DEPRES, RECRNT–PSYCHOS
121 MEDICAID (ADULTS)	Y	301.60—DEPENDENT PERSONALITY
001 SELF-PAY	Y	317.00—MILD MR

DOS	SERVICE	SERVICE PROVIDED BY	ORIGINAL CHARGE	CPT CODE	INSURANCE COMPANY BILLED	SUPPORTING DOCUMENTATION IN PLACE
7/1/2004	5010–PSYCH REHABILITATION	LOCATION #1	100.00	X0343	INS: 121—MEDICAID (ADULTS)	
7/2/2004	5010–PSYCH REHABILITATION	LOCATION #1	150.00	X0343	INS: 121—MEDICAID (ADULTS)	
7/3/2004	4400–MED ADMINISTRATION	LOCATION #2	30.00	90782	INS: 115—MEDICARE PART "B" CLA	
7/3/2004	5010–PSYCH REHABILITATION	LOCATION #1	25.00	X0343	INS: 121—MEDICAID (ADULTS)	
7/3/2004	2100–CASE MGT CLT F-F	LOCATION #3	86.00	X0137	INS: 121—MEDICAID (ADULTS)	
7/5/2004	5010–PSYCH REHABILITATION	LOCATION #1	150.00	X0343	INS: 121—MEDICAID (ADULTS)	
7/8/2004	5010–PSYCH REHABILITATION	LOCATION #1	150.00	X0343	INS: 121—MEDICAID (ADULTS)	
7/9/2004	5010–PSYCH REHABILITATION	LOCATION #1	150.00	X0343	INS: 121—MEDICAID (ADULTS)	
7/9/2004	2100–CASE MGT CLT F-F	LOCATION #4	43.00	X0137	INS: 121—MEDICAID (ADULTS)	
7/10/2004	5010–PSYCH REHABILITATION	LOCATION #1	150.00	X0343	INS: 121—MEDICAID (ADULTS)	
7/11/2004	5010–PSYCH REHABILITATION	LOCATION #1	150.00	X0343	INS: 121—MEDICAID (ADULTS)	
7/12/2004	5010–PSYCH REHABILITATION	LOCATION #1	150.00	X0343	INS: 121—MEDICAID (ADULTS)	
7/15/2004	5010–PSYCH REHABILITATION	LOCATION #1	150.00	X0343	INS: 121—MEDICAID (ADULTS)	
7/16/2004	4400–MED ADMINISTRATION	LOCATION #2	30.00	90782	INS: 115—MEDICARE PART "B" CLA	
7/16/2004	5010–PSYCH REHABILITATION	LOCATION #1	150.00	X0343	INS: 121—MEDICAID (ADULTS)	
7/16/2004	2100–CASE MGT CLT F-F	LOCATION #3	86.00	X0137	INS: 121—MEDICAID (ADULTS)	
7/17/2004	5010–PSYCH REHABILITATION	LOCATION #1	150.00	X0343	INS: 121—MEDICAID (ADULTS)	
7/18/2004	5010–PSYCH REHABILITATION	LOCATION #1	150.00	X0343	INS: 121—MEDICAID (ADULTS)	
7/19/2004	5010–PSYCH REHABILITATION	LOCATION #1	150.00	X0343	INS: 121—MEDICAID (ADULTS)	
7/22/2004	5010–PSYCH REHABILITATION	LOCATION #1	150.00	X0343	INS: 121—MEDICAID (ADULTS)	

Focused Reviews

Focused reviews of health records are generally conducted on specific activities or trends identified. Again, the focus could be on issues identified on the OIG's work plan (that is, E/M coding and documentation, or partial hospitalizations), trends identified through the internal audit process, or staff reporting of potential risk areas. Areas of potential risk include assessments, physician services, medication monitoring follow-ups by nonphysician staff, per diem programs, and documentation of **case management** services.

Unless the OIG removes partial hospitalizations from its work plan, partial programs should be a major focus for behavioral healthcare organizations. It is recommended that organizations audit 100 percent of their Medicare partial hospitalizations to ensure that all required documentation is in the record and that the day charges agree with the documentation. In an outpatient organization providing a day program or residential services, focused reviews should be similar to those described for partial hospitalizations. The OIG tends to focus on per diem services that have a variety of services bundled as part of the reimbursement package. Moreover, there is concern about medical necessity for these types of programs.

Comprehensive Health Record Reviews

Complete record reviews will be an important part of many HIM departments' chart audits. These reviews include all the components required by the Joint Commission on Accreditation of Healthcare Organizations (JCAHO), the Commission on Accreditation of Rehabilitation Facilities (CARF), or other accrediting or licensing bodies (H&P within 24 hours, lab work, physician orders, and so on). (Appendix G contains a sample audit form from a state Medicaid office on page 424.)

It is important to remember to use the higher standard for guidelines when creating audit worksheets and review processes. In many states, the Medicaid program has more stringent documentation requirements than licensing or accreditation; therefore, auditing tools and processes should focus on these requirements. Some organizations conduct internal reviews consisting of two audit worksheets used simultaneously (for example, compliance audit and state Medicaid audit worksheet). Other organizations conduct separate reviews assigned to different review departments. Organizations that have limited resources usually look at combining the elements of both in one tool and one process.

Compliance Plans and Programs

Each provider must design a compliance plan that fits its size and needs. This is particularly true for behavioral healthcare organizations, which not only vary in size but also often have extremely limited resources. The compliance plan is actually the framework or structure of the organization's compliance program. It should give a complete synopsis or overview of each of the compliance program's components, describe how compliance efforts will be carried out, and communicate the organization's commitment to prevent and detect fraud and abuse. (See sample compliance plans in appendix H.)

Because the overall design of a compliance program is developed in accordance with the organization's resources, the best approach is to start by:

1. Drafting the basic policies and procedures required in a compliance program

2. Developing and implementing auditing and monitoring procedures

3. Commencing staff training

To design the above, individuals responsible for the compliance program need to have a clear understanding of what is required.

The OIG provides guidance on exactly what needs to be in a compliance program. It has recommended that healthcare providers include the following elements in their compliance programs (U.S. Government Printing Office 1998). Each of these components must be evident in the organization's compliance program not only in writing, but also in practice.

Oversight

A specific individual, usually called the compliance officer, must be assigned oversight of the organization's compliance program. This responsibility involves not only creating policies and implementing activities, but also ensuring the organization's commitment to the program's goals. The organizational structure of the healthcare provider should enable the compliance officer to act independently of operational and program areas. Indeed, it is recommended that he or she report to the board of trustees or some other member of the executive staff not responsible for these areas. This individual should also have unimpeded access to legal council. Clearly defined policies detailing oversight of the compliance program should be in place, and the job description for the compliance officer must clearly specify the responsibilities and authority of the position. These responsibilities include:

- Overseeing and monitoring implementation of the compliance program

- Reporting regularly to the governing body, CEO, and compliance committee on the progress of the compliance program and establishing methods to improve the organization's efficiency and quality of services while reducing the potential for fraud and abuse

- Revising the compliance program as changes are needed or when changes in laws and regulations occur

- Developing, providing, or coordinating training programs for all levels of staff on the various elements of compliance

- Ensuring that business associates who provide billing, coding, marketing, and so on are aware of the organization's compliance program

- Communicating with the human resources department to ensure that the National Practitioner Data Bank and Cumulative Sanction Reports are checked for all employees and independent contractors

- Periodically reviewing departments for compliance

- Investigating matters pertaining to compliance and responding to reports of problems or potential violations

- Communicating to managers and employees the need to report suspected fraud and abuse, ensuring them that they can do so without fear of retaliation

The organization's policies should prohibit any individual who has been involved in a healthcare offense from having any direct responsibility of a compliance program (U.S. Government Printing Office 1998, 8996). Moreover, oversight should be set up in a manner that empowers staff to report deficiencies without fear of retaliation. Protocols that govern the responsibilities of a compliance task force or committee should be established, and the group should meet at least quarterly to review progress of the compliance program.

This compliance committee should include the compliance officer, representatives from accounting and billing, program staff (that is nursing, medical staff, social worker, and so on), the HIM manager, and any senior executive who can commit resources. The individuals selected must have integrity, honesty, and commitment to compliance as well as be knowledgeable in the operational aspects of the organization and regulations. The committee would be responsible for reviewing the program's activities, including reviewing trends, prioritizing risks, making recommendations for changes to the program, and committing resources to remedy deficiencies. Individuals responsible for oversight must develop processes to update the organization with regulatory information. However this is done, the organization must indicate how management staff in specific areas of responsibility are made aware of regulatory changes, how the changes are interpreted, and their impact on the staff and the organization.

Policies and Procedures Defining Standards and Best Practices

The healthcare organization should have policies in place that define standards and best practices. (See appendix I for sample policies and procedures.) First and foremost are written standards of conduct. Although each discipline with the organization has its own professional standards of conduct, organizations should have written standards of conduct that affect all employees. These standards should include the organization's commitment to comply with all federal and state standards as well as clearly define the ethical behavior expected of staff. They should be written to reflect the organization's mission, principles, and ethical requirements (which should include prohibiting incentives for upcoding). Individual policies and procedures or protocols should be written and specify areas of potential risk. Along with staff training, they should ensure provider compliance and prevent problems in some of the following areas (U.S. Government Printing Office 1998, 8990):

- Billing for items or services not actually received (for example, bill indicates that 30 minutes of case management was provided on a specific date, but patient denies this and there is no documentation to support the bill)

- Providing services that are not medically necessary (for example, billing occurred for one hour of psychotherapy, but no diagnosis, order, or treatment plan supports the need for psychotherapy)

- Upcoding (for example, billing occurs for 60 minutes of individual counseling when client actually received 60 minutes of group counseling, which is reimbursed at a lower level than individual counseling)

- Billing for outpatient services given in connection with hospital stays, extended care stays, or bundled with other services (for example, this could be considered upcoding, duplicate billing, or unbundling)

- Duplicate billing (for example, billing for the same service twice as a result of submission of duplicate billing documentation, data-entry error, or two provider staff seeing the client at the same time for the same service when billing should occur only once)

- Filing of false cost reports (for example, Part A providers who either inappropriately shift costs to cost centers below reimbursement caps and then shift non-Medicare-related costs to a Medicare cost center or inappropriately reimburse for operating costs)

- Unbundling (for example, billing separately for services that are part of a package, such as per diem rates for specific programs)

- Billing for discharge in lieu of transfer (Per Medicare regulations, when a PPS hospital transfers a patient to another PPS hospital, only the hospital to which the patient is transferred can charge the full DRG. The transferring hospital should only charge Medicare a per diem amount.)

- Failure to refund any credit balances

- Incentives that violate the antikickback statutes

- Financial arrangements among business partners, staff, and the organization

- Patient dumping, which requires all Medicare participating hospitals to at least assess the person presenting for treatment and stabilize the patient prior to transfer to another facility

- Insufficient, incomplete, or missing documentation of services

Written Policies and Procedures for Billing, Claims Submission, Claims Remediation, and Paybacks

Policies and procedures should be written in accordance with current federal and state statutes and regulations for billing and reimbursements and should include mechanisms for communication of these rules between billing and clinical staff (U.S. Government Printing Office 1998).

In settings where claims are submitted after medical record audit, policies should indicate claim submission only when appropriate documentation supporting the claim has been complete. Traditionally in many freestanding outpatient clinics, claims submission occurs prior to record review. In the latter case, policy should indicate mechanisms for correcting any deficiencies in documentation as well as in the coding.

Billing policies should emphasize that the diagnosis and procedures billed must coincide with those documented in the medical record. There should be written policies on proper coding procedures, including how software systems identify services that may not be billed separately and how the billing department reviews these procedures. Lastly, a written process should be in place for informing the appropriate government authority and/or payer of overpayments or incorrectly submitted claims.

Written Documentation Standards

Although healthcare providers have documentation requirements, the requirements often are not clearly defined in written protocols. Organizations should have written standards for all disciplines and ancillary services that address timely, accurate, complete, and legible documentation as defined by government and regulatory agencies. The standards should emphasize that documentation has to support the medical necessity of services provided and that the information contained in progress notes must match the interventions described in the treatment plan or doctor's orders.

Moreover, specific documentation requirements from accreditation organizations must be clearly defined in documentation procedures and routinely communicated to staff. Further, standards should emphasize the importance of an "exact match" of date, service, signature, and credential.

Contracts and Referrals

The healthcare organization should have written policies ensuring that contracts and referrals comply with antikickback statutes and self-referral laws.

Records Policies and Procedures

In addition to policies and procedures governing the creation, storage, retrieval, retention, and destruction of clinical records, organizations must have policies that address claims documentation and compliance program auditing and monitor staff training, complaints, and self-disclosures. The latter can be included either in a policy for administrative documentation or as a part of the compliance program policies. (Figure 8.4 shows a sample audit and monitoring policy.)

Figure 8.4. Sample Audit and Monitoring Policy

Audit and Monitoring

Purpose: To ensure an effective audit and monitoring process has been established for billing and documentation procedures.

Policy: In order to ensure compliance with billing and documentation procedures, a Kent Center Compliance Task Force will be established. Members of this task force/committee will include:

  VP Operations
  Director QI/HI
  Accounting Manager
  Billing Coordinator
  HI Supervisor
  Outcome Specialist
  Director of Training
  VP's of Clinical Services
  CEO (ex-officio)

These individuals will meet at least quarterly to perform the following:

- Review and develop The Kent Center's Compliance and Audit Program (KCCP).
- Review existing policies and procedures in relation to compliance.
- Review results of billing and documentation audits conducted for the purpose of determining compliance.
- Review trends identified through the audit and monitoring process.
- Provide recommendations for changes necessary to improve compliance.

Procedure:

1. Each quarter a billing/audit report will be forwarded to the Compliance Officer from the computer department.
2. The Compliance Officer will routinely select at least 15–20 cases monthly in which billing has occurred. This random sampling will include cases from different programs and different staff.
3. The designated staff will audit the records selected using compliance audit criteria (see attached).
4. Results of the random audit will be entered on the billing/audit report. If there are issues of non-compliance in either billing or documentation, an audit worksheet (see attached) will be forwarded to the appropriate program manager with copies maintained by the Compliance Officer.
5. Corrective action, as stated in the Corrective Action Plan, must occur immediately. (See Corrective Action Plan)
6. The QI staff will prepare a Corrective Action Worksheet (see attached) each month, which identifies the cases referred back to programs for either billing or documentation issues.
7. The Compliance Task Force will review the Corrective Action Reports to determine if there are specific areas of concern that need to be addressed further with staff.
8. A copy of the task force/committees findings, recommendations, and action taken is forwarded to the CEO

Other Policies and Procedures

The healthcare organization should develop a policy that establishes a process by which employees are encouraged to report suspected fraud and abuse without fear of retribution. The policy should specify who to report potential violations to, the information needed, the anonymous hotline number, and the name of the person to contact in the event the staff member reporting a compliance issue becomes the object of retaliation or harassment. Additionally, the organization should have a policy that ensures staff protection from retaliation or harassment. Finally, the organization should develop a policy for self-reporting violations and refunding payments in the event a violation occurs. Disciplinary policies must be fair and consistent and include specific corrective action plans.

Managers and staff should make copies of the disciplinary policies available for easy reference and program personnel training. (See sample policies and procedures in figures 8.5 and 8.6.)

Figure 8.5. Employee Reporting on Non-Compliance Policy

Employee Reporting of Non-Compliance with Professional Practice Standards

Purpose: To establish a process by which employees may report any suspected areas of fraud and abuse to Center administration without fear of retribution.

Policy: Kent Center staff are encouraged and expected to report any concerns/issues of compliance with professional practice standards to Center administration. The Center has established a protected line (extension #444 at 738-1338) which employees may report concerns noting the specifics stated below. Employees reporting potential problems are assured that there will be no retribution for asking questions or reporting possible improper conduct.

Procedure:

1. If an employee encounters a situation, which he/she believes violates the Center's Code of Conduct or professional practice standards, the employee should contact his/her supervisor or an EMT member immediately. An employee also has the option of calling the dedicated line (number above) to report the concern. All reports of potential violations must be noted on the compliance reporting log (see attached) and forwarded to the Director of QI/HI.

2. When reporting a potential violation the following information must be given:
    *   Brief description of the violation being reported, stating specifics.
    *   Date of the potential violation.
    *   Individual(s) involved at the time of the violation.

3. Any inconsistencies in billing or documentation will be reported to the Directors of QI/VP Operations for further investigation. Any inconsistencies in clinical practice standards will be reported to the Director of QI, who will investigate the situation further.

4. All employees are expected to fully cooperate with any investigation undertaken.

5. In the event an employee believes he/she has been subjected to retaliation or harassment as a result of his/her reporting, he/she should contact the Director of Human Resources immediately. The Director of Human Resources will then conduct an internal investigation and report findings to both the individual filing the complaint and the President/CEO.

6. If the Director of Human Resources findings indicate retaliation or harassment has occurred, appropriate disciplinary action of individual(s) involved in these activities will occur immediately.

Figure 8.6. Self-Reporting of Violations Policy

THE KENT CENTER
Self-Reporting of Violations

Purpose: To establish a process that addresses potential violations and reports any violations of laws or regulations to the appropriate government agencies.

Policy: The Kent Center will report any violations of law or regulation to the appropriate government agency(ies) and make any refund for prior payments that are necessary.

Procedure:

1. Anyone with knowledge of a potential violation of law or regulation that may require return of any prior payments should forward to the Director of QI and/or VP Operations all information related to the potential violation. This information should be specific and include: the type of problem, date and place of occurrence, type of activity, and dollar amount involved.

2. The Director of QI and/or VP Operations will collect, assemble, and assess all information relating to the potential violation to determine whether a violation occurred.

3. If a violation did occur, the Director of QI and/or VP Operations will determine whether the violation falls within the scope of an on-going investigation and will notify the CEO and Executive Management Team.
    a. If it is determined the violation does not appear to be within the scope of an on-going investigation, the CEO or designee will report the violation to the government agency and authorize payment of any amount due as a result of the violation.
    b. If it is determined the violation falls within the scope of an on-going investigation, outside legal counsel may be sought. Legal Counsel would present to the government agency pertinent information concerning the violation. This information would be provided, without any payment, in anticipation that any payment would be included in negotiations regarding the resolution of the investigation.

Training and Education

Training staff in the components of compliance and their responsibilities to ensure compliance is critical to the success of the organization's compliance program. All employees should be made aware of compliance policies as well as staff ethical and legal responsibilities. Training should be provided for all new employees early in the employment period. If cultural issues exist in the organization, training should be provided in appropriate languages to ensure that staff members are aware of standards of conduct and reporting procedures.

Compliance training should include training on statutes, regulations, private-payer rules, ethics, trends, potential risks, fraud and abuse laws, coding requirements, claims submission, and marketing practices. As applicable to their job responsibilities, executive management, managers, supervisors, and all other staff should also receive training in the following topics (U.S. Government Printing Office 1998, 8994):

- Government and private-payer reimbursement principles
- Prohibitions on paying or receiving remuneration for referrals
- Proper confirmation of diagnoses
- Submission of claims for a physician when service is given by a nonphysician
- A form for a physician being signed without physician approval
- Alterations to the medical record
- Medications or procedures prescribed without proper authorization
- Proper documentation of services given
- Proper DRG coding
- Duty to report misconduct
- Privacy rules of the Health Insurance Portability and Accountability Act (HIPAA)

Periodically, all staff, clinical and nonclinical, should receive compliance training informing them of updates, trends, and risks. The OIG recommends that participation in training programs be made a condition of employment and that failure to comply with training should result in disciplinary action. Because elements of the compliance program are used in the evaluation of staff performance, training should be ongoing. Supervisory personnel must require strict compliance with policies and procedures as a condition of employment and take appropriate disciplinary action up to, and including, termination when policies are not followed.

A trainer in compliance issues could be an individual from within the organization who has expertise in or knowledge of compliance issues or an outside consultant. If an outside consultant is used, he or she should have experience in working with or providing training in behavioral healthcare organizations. All training provided must be documented with the date, the names of trainers and attendees, and a brief outline of the training content. The OIG also recommends providing professional education courses (for example, coding courses) to appropriate staff, as needed.

Communication Methods and Tools

The compliance officer who has direct access to the organization's governing body is responsible for coordinating and communicating compliance activities. This communication should flow to both the CEO and the staff involved in providing both clinical and administrative services. Because the compliance officer is responsible for designing, implementing, and monitoring the compliance program, he or she should be provided sufficient funding and staff to perform these responsibilities. The compliance officer's has the authority to review all documents relevant to compliance activities, including patient records, billing records, marketing records, arrangements/ contracts with independent contractors, suppliers, and so on.

Open lines of communication need to exist between the compliance officer and all staff in order to encourage reporting of potential fraud and abuse issues. Systems should be in place that enable staff to report concerns in such a way that their reports cannot be diverted by supervisors or other personnel. Moreover, staff should be given written confidentiality and nonretaliation policies (discussed earlier).

The OIG encourages the development of procedures that enable staff to seek clarification of questions on policies and procedures from the compliance officer or a member of the compliance committee. All questions and responses should be dated and documented and the results shared with staff to either clarify the issue or update a policy and procedure. The OIG encourages the use of hotlines, e-mail, memos, or newsletters to exchange information with staff. The hotline telephone number should be posted in common work areas. The compliance officer should keep a log documenting who calls, the nature of the investigation, and the results. Information from this log should be included in reports to the governing body, the CEO, and the compliance committee. Moreover, procedures should specify that although confidentiality is always foremost, there may be a point when the person's identity will be either known or have to be revealed in cases where government authorities become involved.

The compliance officer will need to work closely with legal counsel should claims of fraud and abuse be made by employees who participated in illegal conduct. As mentioned previously, the compliance committee assists not only in providing oversight, but also in refining processes and communicating progress to organization staff. Some of the activities the compliance committee is involved in reviewing and communicating to staff are (U.S. Government Printing Office 1998, 8993):

- Analysis of the organization's environment in relation to compliance with regulatory requirements

- Necessary changes in existing policies and procedures

- Systems developed to carry out the organization's policies and procedures

- Strategies for promoting compliance with programs and detecting potential violations

- Systems for responding to complaints

Internal Audits and Controls

Ongoing evaluation of any process is critical. The OIG believes that "an effective program monitors its own plan implementation and reports results to the CEO" (U.S. Government Printing Office 1998, 8997–8998). This review determines whether the elements of the plan are accomplishing its purposes and whether departments are in compliance with the compliance program's objectives. This review should be done at least once a year and conducted at each site location. This type of review can include questionnaires or interviews with staff to determine if further distribution or review of program standards is necessary (U.S. Government Printing Office 1998, 8996). Another mechanism for internal monitoring is to perform a trend analysis of positive and negative findings over a given period of time as a result of financial and medical record reviews.

Such reports should include areas of suspected noncompliance as well as results from ongoing monitoring. Audits should be focused on the areas identified in the OIG Special Fraud Alerts and Initiatives and on areas the organization has identified as potential risks.

Individuals conducting audits should be familiar with federal and state statutes and payer rules and regulations. When an organization begins monitoring, it may need to establish baselines against which significant deviation would trigger an investigation. If deviation is a result of improper procedures, steps must be taken immediately to correct the problem. Any overpayment discovered as a result of an investigation should be promptly returned to the payer with appropriate documentation and an explanation of why the refund occurred. An annual written report of compliance activities should identify areas where corrective action is needed and recommendations for the next year's compliance activities. (Figure 8.7 shows a sample compliance audit report.)

Finally, the compliance officer should keep a file of all inquiries made to CMS along with documentation of oral and written responses to questions. This file could be vital in proving the organization's attempt to maintain compliance.

Enforcement and Follow-Up

Effective compliance programs should include guidance on disciplinary action procedures for individuals who have failed to follow the organization's policies and procedures or have engaged in wrongdoing. The OIG believes that compliance programs should include written policy establishing the degrees of disciplinary action that may be followed (for example oral warnings, suspension of privileges, terminations, financial penalties, and whether the action was negligent, reckless, or in error). Some disciplinary action can be handled by an immediate supervisor; other times, senior management may be responsible. All disciplinary action must be made in a fair and equitable manner. All levels of employees are subject to the same disciplinary action for similar offenses, including managers, supervisors, the CEO, and medical staff. Staff should be given written documents explaining the range of disciplinary standards for improper conduct.

Problem Resolution and Corrective Action

When there is a report of suspected noncompliance, it is necessary to investigate the alleged concern immediately to determine whether a "material violation" of the law or a requirement of the compliance program has occurred. When noncompliance has occurred, immediate steps must be taken to correct the problem. Such steps could include reporting to law enforcement authorities or the government. When a potential problem has been identified, billing should be stopped immediately and a supervisor notified of the situation. A corrective action plan must be put into place, and any overpayment made to the payer.

If, internally, the organization identifies overpayments or problems with claims submission, they should be reported to the compliance officer who then would look for trends that identify a systems issue or staff non-compliance. The nature of the problem identified will determine the type of corrective action and whether the organization's legal counsel needs to be involved. At a minimum, investigations will include review of relevant documents (medical records, claims submission, coding, and so on) and interviews with appropriate staff.

Records must be maintained describing the nature of the alleged violation, the investigation process, notes, documents, results of the investigation, and any disciplinary action taken. Follow-up reviews will be necessary to determine whether the problem still exists and whether it extends into other areas. If the integrity of the investigation is considered at stake, the employees under investigation should be removed from their current work assignments until the investigation is completed. Documents should be secured to avoid any possible damage or tampering. Disciplinary action should be imposed promptly and according to the organization's policies.

If reporting to the federal government is determined to be necessary, that reporting must occur within 60 days after "credible evidence of a violation" has been confirmed (U.S. Government Printing Office 1998, 8997–8998). Prompt reporting will be considered favorable

Figure 8.7. Sample Compliance Audit Report

The Kent Center Report of Compliance Errors					
Compliance Errors 7/01/03–4/30/04			**Compliance Errors 7/01/02–6/30/03**		
Count of Type of error			Count of Type of error		
Type of error	**Total**	**%**	Type of error	**Total**	**%**
Activity code error	1	2%	Activity code error	67	18%
Billed, no note	11	17%	Billed w/ FKA note	1	0%
Clt billed w/o service	2	3%	Billed, no note	67	18%
Data Entry	4	6%	Clt billed w/o service	11	3%
Double billed	2	3%	Data Entry	10	3%
Incomplete documentation	5	8%	Day Tx double bill	4	1%
Incorrect Clt code billed	1	2%	Double billed	17	5%
Log not submitted	1	2%	Incomplete documentation	2	1%
Missing Paperwork	5	8%	Incorrect Clt code billed	4	1%
Missing signature, credentials, etc.	3	5%	Incorrect dx or code	3	1%
Note Found	3	5%	Missing Paperwork	16	4%
Note misdated	3	5%	Missing signature, credentials, etc.	14	4%
Note not billed	1	2%	No SA Authorization	10	3%
Progress note does not match interventions	3	5%	Note found	7	2%
Services w/o enrollment	7	11%	Note misdated	29	8%
Services w/o tx plan	13	20%	Note not billed	51	14%
Grand Total	**65**		Paperwork misfiled	1	0%
			Progress note does not match interventions	10	3%
Some charts have multiple errors.			Services w/o tx plan	40	11%
			Tx Plan not found in chart	2	1%
			Grand Total	**366**	

Charts found to contain errors has decreased by 27%.

when determining administrative sanctions in the event the organization becomes the target of the OIG investigation. All relevant evidence of alleged violations should be provided to the government.

The "OIG hopes that a voluntarily created compliance program will enable organizations to meet their goals, improve the quality of patient care, and substantially reduce fraud, waste, and abuse as well as the cost of healthcare to federal, state, and private health insurers" (U.S. Government Printing Office 1998, 8998).

Challenges in Measuring Compliance Program Effectiveness

As mentioned previously, measuring the effectiveness of a compliance program is an ongoing process. Compliance activities are labor-intense and costly, to say the least; therefore, every effort should be made to ensure commitment to the compliance program throughout the organization. Mechanisms should be developed to share audit findings with appropriate managers and staff.

Unfortunately, compliance concerns are not fully understood until billing and reimbursement stops. When billing stops, staff usually take notice of deficiencies. Perhaps the most difficult challenge is helping staff, particularly physicians and social workers, to understand the impact of their errors and that the effectiveness of compliance efforts is everyone's business. Organizations may decide to link billing or payback issues to budget reviews. As departments meet to discuss monthly or quarterly budget reviews, figures of lost billing or paybacks can be deducted from their bottom line.

Another challenge is communicating and training staff in compliance updates and changes to policy. The larger the organization, the more difficult the challenge. Effective communication involves contacting all staff affected by the changes in a timely manner through memos and/or e-mails, bulletin board announcements, and/or workshops. Timely follow-up to identified problems and implementation of immediate corrective action also can be a challenge. Executive management and supervisory staff must understand the need to expedite follow-up and corrective action plans. Although ongoing training in these areas is helpful, performance evaluations that identify managerial accountability in compliance emphasize supervisory responsibility to compliance.

Health Insurance Portability and Privacy Act Privacy

In addition to the components of corporate compliance, HIM professionals must be aware of the components of the Health Insurance Portability and Privacy Act (HIPAA) privacy rule. (See chapter 9 for a detailed discussion of confidentiality, privacy, and security.)

Privacy Compliance Programs

On April 14, 2003, the HIPAA **privacy rule** (45 CFR 160-164) went into effect and healthcare organizations needed to have mechanisms in place to ensure compliance with the HIPAA regulations. At the very least, the organization should conduct random reviews of policy and procedures, areas identified as risks in the organization's privacy/security assessments, and incident report trends.

The **privacy officer** should be included in the review of all incidents identified as potential breaches of confidentiality as well as privacy complaints filed with the organization. This can be accomplished by including the privacy officer in the follow-up to the organization's incident reporting and complaint procedures. A careful review of these potential breaches could raise compliance issues and trends that require remediation and possibly further training in privacy practices. Random checks of access to information, distribution of privacy notices, fax procedures, release of information practices, and accounting of disclosures also may identify other compliance problems.

Compliance with privacy practices can be conducted in a variety of ways, including:

- Review fax logs with training sheets, authorizations, and progress notes to ensure that only individuals authorized to fax personal health information (PHI) have been faxing information, that authorizations were received, that the faxing procedures were followed, and that notes were written for any emergency documentation.

- Conduct random reviews of automated reports of users accessing information and/or making data modifications. Compare access and modification rights with security access and minimum necessary protocols.

- Utilize a simple survey tool to question staff on various privacy practices to determine if polices and procedures are working and if staff are actually following them.

- Review release of information practices to determine if compliance issues exist.

Special Considerations about Compliance in Mental Health and Substance Abuse

Some areas of compliance in mental health and substance abuse require special attention. The nature of the type of services provided, and the fact that documentation of patient complaints and responses to treatment are not as "black and white" as physical health, makes coding a real challenge. In addition, most coding is done by clinical staff who are untrained in coding guidelines and, for the most part, use whatever code "looks like a match." It is important to keep in mind that mental health staff are trained in using the DSM IV and have little or no knowledge of ICD-9-CM coding from which reimbursement is made.

Often ICD-9-CM and CPT codes are assigned by billing staff, which, in most outpatient settings, means someone not trained in coding practices.

Health information chart analysis and discharge audits are critical to detecting compliance problems. These audits can be conducted in a variety of ways. HIM staff responsible for chart review prior to billing or after discharge often detect documentation errors or omissions. Specific examples of common coding problems detected within a psychiatric hospital include the following (Diniz, 2004):

- Example 1: Final Diagnosis: MD's final diagnosis on Discharge Face Sheet is Dementia NOS with behavioral disturbances. However, there is no ICD-9-CM or DSM-IV narrative or code that exists for this diagnosis. Code 294.10 or 294.11 is assigned when an additional diagnosis (for example, Alzheimer's, Parkinson's, so forth) exists to describe the cause of the dementia. There is no cause so the code for the above diagnosis is simply 294.8. If, and only if, there is documentation throughout the progress notes that the patient was being treated for severe behavioral disturbances and disturbances of conduct throughout their stay would 312.9 be assigned to Axis I.

- The physician's final diagnosis is bipolar disorder, depressed, in remission. However, the patient was in the hospital for almost a year. The definition of principal diagnosis in the UHDDS coding guidelines is "the condition established after study to be chiefly responsible for occasioning the patient's admission to the hospital for care." After further clarification, the physician changed the severity of the illness to severe.

- Abbreviations are frequently found on discharge face sheets, encounter forms, initial evaluations, and notes. What really is BPD or MDD? The official abbreviation for borderline personality disorder is BPD, but in the case the physician was referring to, it was used to indicate bipolar disorder. As far as MDD (major depressive disorder), is it single, recurrent, severe, are there psychotic features? Unfortunately, it is rare for physicians or clinicians to document the severity of disorders at the time of discharge or throughout the patient's stay. They are unaware of the effect this has on coding assignment.

Yet another problem that occurs more frequently in an outpatient setting, particularly one that either provides both mental health and substance abuse services or specializes in co-occurring disorders, is the proper assignment of principal diagnosis. If a patient is being treated for both major depression and alcohol abuse, the appropriate assignment of the principal diagnosis is necessary for reimbursement to occur. For example, if the service provided was substance abuse counseling, reimbursement often will not occur when the diagnosis is major depression. The same is true if billing occurred for psychotherapy and the bill was submitted under alcohol abuse. This can be particularly problematic because clinicians and software systems are unaware of the issue.

However, the biggest challenge is that of the documentation meeting reimbursement criteria. Few staff members in the mental health or substance abuse settings have received documentation training related to required standards. This is an enormous challenge for healthcare organizations, particularly the small providers with limited training resources. Collaborative efforts with payers and other providers help educate clinical staff, but this is not sufficient to meet the needs of most behavioral healthcare organizations. Perhaps academic institutions should pay closer attention to this training need because it affects successful employment for their graduates. In the meantime, internal training in documentation must be ongoing and required of all staff.

Conclusion

The basic components of compliance apply to all healthcare settings; however, implementation varies by type of organization. Inpatient organizations typically initiate audits and controls prior to submitting a bill whereas many outpatient organizations conduct retrospective reviews. Because the latter requires payback of any omissions or errors, organizations must focus heavily on training clinical, coding, and billing staff to ensure compliance with standards and procedures.

Unless outpatient services are a component of a hospital or a larger corporate entity with resources devoted to compliance, implementing a compliance program can be extremely difficult. Traditionally, outpatient mental health and substance abuse organizations have little or no funding available for extensive compliance activities. As mentioned previously, the design of an organization's compliance program should be developed in accordance with available resources and compliance needs. Most organizations have an idea where they are most vulnerable and often start with a few audits a month, which can validate concerns and identify other problems that exist.

References and Bibliography

Centers for Medicare and Medicaid Services (CMS). 2004. Available on-line at http://www.cms.hhs.gov/.

Diniz, Deborah, RHIT. 2004. Personal correspondence regarding coding problem scenarios.

The Kent Center for Human & Organizational Development November 2001. The Kent Center Orientation Module. Warwick, Rhode Island.

Medicare glossary. 2004. Available on-line at http://www.medicare.gov/Glossary/Search.asp.

Office of Inspector General. 2004. Available on-line at http://oig.hhs.gov/.

U.S. Government Printing Office. June 8, 2004. Federal Register 69(110): 32012–32031. (Full text included in appendix E.2.)

U.S. Government Printing Office. February 23, 1998. Federal Register 63(35): 8987–8998. (Full text included in appendix E.1.)

Chapter 9

Confidentiality, Privacy, and Security of Protected Health Information

Pamela T. Haines, RHIA, and RoseAnn Webb, RHIA, LHRM

The confidentiality, privacy, and security of personal health information (PHI) is a necessary foundation for the delivery of high-quality healthcare. The entire healthcare system is built on the willingness of individuals to reveal the personal details of their lives to their healthcare providers. Because of their professional qualifications, for the past seventy-five years health information management (HIM) administrators and technicians have been entrusted with the management and oversight of PHI use and disclosure, including writing the policies and procedures that govern use and disclosure. With the advent of the Health Insurance Portability and Accountability Act (HIPAA) privacy and security rules, much of what has been best practice among HIM managers throughout the healthcare industry is now federal law. Thus, it is all the more necessary that HIM managers understand the governing laws and the current systems and processes related to PHI in their healthcare organizations, including administrative uses and disclosures that pertain to billing, quality improvement, research, and so forth.

No less now than in the past, PHI is created primarily for the medical record for use in the provision of high-quality healthcare. In the behavioral healthcare setting, especially, the most intimate details of an individual's life and experiences are commonly revealed and documented in the health record. For this reason, mental health records have long been regarded as highly sensitive and, therefore, more protected by law in most states; substance abuse records have been even more protected by federal law.

This chapter discusses many aspects of PHI confidentiality, privacy, and security in the behavioral healthcare setting from the provider's perspective. Because the HIPAA privacy rule now governs PHI use and disclosure throughout the healthcare industry, numerous references to the federal regulations, along with the recently promulgated federal security rule and the federal regulations governing substance abuse records, are included throughout this chapter.

Definitions of Key Terms

A discussion of the confidentiality, privacy, and security of protected health information involves a number of key terms that surface again and again. The following terms are defined specifically as they apply to PHI.

- Confidentiality: Within the context of PHI, confidentiality has been defined as "a legal and ethical concept that establishes the healthcare provider's responsibility for protecting health records and other personal and private information from unauthorized use and disclosure" (LaTour and Eichenwald 2002, 719).

- **Covered entity** (CE): A healthcare provider that transmits any health information in electronic form in connection with a transaction covered by 45 CFR, 160.103 (HHS 2000, §164:103). This definition also applies to any person or organization that furnishes, bills, or is paid for medical or health services in the normal course of business. Health plans and healthcare clearinghouses also are CEs.

- Organized healthcare arrangement: This term refers to (1) a clinically integrated care setting in which individuals typically receive healthcare from more than one provider and (2) an organized system of healthcare in which more than one CE participates and the participating CEs hold themselves out to the public as participating in a joint arrangement and participate in certain joint activities (45 CFR, §164.501). For example, the relationship of independent contracted physicians on staff at a behavioral healthcare facility would be regarded as an organized healthcare arrangement.

- Privacy: Being away from public view, secluded (*Webster's* 1996, 1071), or the right of every individual to be left alone.

- Protected health information (PHI): Individually identifiable health information, including demographic information collected from an individual. This information is protected by the HIPAA privacy rule if it relates to the past, present, or future physical or mental health or condition of an individual; the provision of healthcare to the individual; or the past, present, or future payment for the provision of healthcare to an individual and that identifies the individual or with respect to which there is reasonable basis to believe it can be used to identify the individual (45 CFR, §160.103).

- **Security:** Within the context of PHI, security is defined as "the physical safety of facilities and equipment protected from theft, damage, or unauthorized access; it also includes protection of data, information and [electronic] information networks from loss and damage, as well as unauthorized access and alteration" (LaTour and Eichenwald 2002, 746).

- Workforce: Employees, volunteers, trainees, and other persons whose conduct in the performance of work for a CE is under the direct control of such entity, whether or not they are paid by the CE (45 CFR, §160.103).

Moral and Ethical Background

The importance of adhering to moral and ethical principles is instilled in HIM professionals during their training. HIM professionals become aware of their professional obligations to the myriad entities with which they have day-to-day contact on the job.

AHIMA Code of Ethics

The American Health Information Management Association (AHIMA) Code of Ethics iterates the ethical principle of PHI confidentiality and privacy. (See figure 9.1.) Affirmed by all HIM professionals, the AHIMA Code of Ethics has been revised four times since it was first adopted in 1957. The most recent revision by the House of Delegates in 2004 sets forth the obligation of its members to maintain and promote principles and values that "put service and the health and welfare of persons before self-interest" and every version has addressed the HIM professionals' obligation to "preserve, protect and secure personal health information in any form or

Figure 9.1. AHIMA Code of Ethics 2004

The following ethical principles are based on the core values of the American Health Information Management Association and apply to all health information management professionals. Health information management professionals:

I. Advocate, uphold, and defend the individual's right to privacy and the doctrine of confidentiality in the use and disclosure of information.

II. Put service and the health and welfare of persons before self-interest and conduct themselves in the practice of the profession so as to bring honor to themselves, their peers, and to the health information management profession.

III. Preserve, protect, and secure personal health information in any form or medium and hold in the highest regard the contents of the records and other information of a confidential nature, taking into account the applicable statutes and regulations.

IV. Refuse to participate in or conceal unethical practices or procedures.

V. Advance health information management knowledge and practice through continuing education, research, publications, and presentations.

VI. Recruit and mentor students, peers and colleagues to develop and strengthen professional workforce.

VII. Represent the profession accurately to the public.

VIII. Perform honorably health information management association responsibilities, either appointed or elected, and preserve the confidentiality of any privileged information made known in any official capacity.

IX. State truthfully and accurately their credentials, professional education, and experiences.

X. Facilitate interdisciplinary collaboration in situations supporting health information practice.

XI. Respect the inherent dignity and worth of every person.

Revised and adopted by AHIMA House of Delegates July 1, 2004.

medium and hold in the highest regard the contents of the record and other information of a confidential nature, taking into account the applicable statutes and regulations."

Professional Obligations

HIM professionals have obligations to their employers and to the public as well as to themselves, their peers, and their professional community. These obligations are many and varied.

Obligations to the Employer

Whether working as directors of HIM departments or privacy officers, and in the areas of quality management, compliance, risk management, and so on, HIM professionals have an obligation to their employer to emulate high moral and ethical standards in all they see, hear, and do in accordance with their professional pledge. This includes demonstrating loyalty; protecting committee deliberations; complying with all laws, regulations, and policies that govern the health information system in all formats; recognizing both the authority and power associated with job responsibilities; and accepting compensation only in relationship to work responsibilities (LaTour and Eichenwald 2002, 296).

Obligations to the Public

HIM professionals have an obligation to the public to support and uphold their sound ethical standards of practice, including advocating change when patterns or system problems are not in the best interests of patients. Both AHIMA and its individual members are in a professional position to lend their expertise and ethical values to HIM-related issues across the healthcare industry, including government agencies, departments, and sectors of congress. Their recommendations and/or decisions should always be supported with reliable and valid data. In addition, HIM professionals are obligated to educate the public on their privacy rights as delineated in the privacy rule and other pertinent legislation.

Obligations to Self, Peers, and Professional Community

HIM professionals are obligated to strive for professional excellence through self-assessment and continuing education. Moreover, they should be honest about their degrees, credentials, and work experience. The level of expertise among peers varies, and they should display a readiness to support one another and their professional community association in their common responsibility as leaders in the field of HIM. HIM professionals also have an obligation to become involved in supporting and mentoring HIM students.

Ethical Decision Making

Employers, the public, and the professional community all expect HIM professionals to display ethical and moral principles. They also expect HIM professionals to demonstrate ethical decision making as they contribute to the improvement of healthcare through high-quality information. As stated in *Health Information Management,* ethical decision making should not be based solely on personal moral values or perspectives because not everyone shares the same moral values or perspectives. When one individual sees only one solution to a problem and others have a different solution, ethics (which in healthcare is a decision-making process that requires everyone with competing perspectives and obligations to consider the concerns of other people who have an interest in a common problem) can help in making the appropriate decision (LaTour and Eichenwald 2002, 223, 724–25).

Key Responsibilities of HIM Professionals

The key responsibilities and roles of HIM professionals are derived from their educational background in:

- The basic principles of diseases
- Standardized data sets and coding
- Medical terminology and transcription
- Anatomy and physiology
- Data quality and performance improvement
- Healthcare delivery systems
- Statistics and research
- Finance, medical billing, and reimbursement systems
- Information systems, applications, and technology
- The ethical and legal aspects of HIM

Their specialized professional education prepares HIM professionals to be responsible leaders in managing PHI, protecting the rights of clients to privacy; promoting the confidentiality of PHI and data security; fostering interdisciplinary cooperation and collaboration to ensure that PHI is kept confidential and secure at all times across the entire organization; and training the workforce in the policies and procedures that support the privacy, confidentiality, and security of PHI.

Further, the specialized professional experience of HIM professionals prepares them to be responsible leaders in writing and implementing the policies and procedures required by the HIPAA privacy and security rules, as well as in training the workforce in those same policies and procedures.

Access to and Use of Documentation

In daily practice in behavioral healthcare settings, HIM professionals must endeavor to ensure that medical records and all other forms of PHI are maintained as required by law and generally accepted professional practice. Documentation must not only be accurate, complete, and timely, but also accessible for use in accordance with the need-to-know and minimum necessary principles and applicable law.

Disclosure of Protected Health Information

The inappropriate disclosure of PHI can have serious discriminatory effects for behavioral health clients well beyond their physical health, including loss of job, alienation of family and friends, loss of health insurance, and public humiliation. Thus, HIM professionals have an obligation to apply themselves to the study of both federal and state laws governing the confidentiality of PHI to ensure that privacy and confidentiality are maintained throughout the **release of information** (ROI) process.

Likewise, HIM managers must ensure that throughout the organization PHI is disclosed only as permitted by law. In particular, they should see that all those directly involved in the release of PHI clearly understand their responsibility to act in accordance with the approved policies and procedures and know whom to call when situations arise that they do not have the expertise to resolve.

Protection of Privacy, Maintenance of Confidentiality

HIM professionals in behavioral healthcare settings have always been advocates for their clients' rights to expect their medical records and other PHI to be kept private, including their right to expect that their PHI will be kept confidential by their healthcare provider in accordance with the law. To ensure that **privacy** and **confidentiality** are maintained, controls must be in place throughout the healthcare organization. Because of their professional expertise in this area, HIM managers generally write the organization's policies and procedures that address protection of client privacy and uphold confidentiality.

Protection of Data Security

The confidentiality, privacy, and security of health information and data are inseparable. PHI cannot be kept confidential (as well as accurate, complete, and available for legitimate users) if it is not secure from theft, alteration, loss, damage, unlawful destruction, and unauthorized **access** and use. Thus, security is essential for maintaining the confidentiality of PHI, and information security policies and procedures must always support the policies and procedures that address the confidentiality of PHI regarding access, use, and disclosure in whatever format. Consequently, privacy officers and HIM managers should work closely with the organization's information security officer to ensure that the confidentiality of PHI in electronic systems is maintained in accordance with applicable federal and state laws.

Emergence of E-Health Care

The healthcare industry is being transformed by the emergence of the e-health record. Although its many benefits (in particular, its simultaneous accessibility to multiple users) is lauded, it should not be forgotten that the potential for wrongful disclosure is expanding right along with the enhanced capability of disseminating information and creating local, state, and national databases for healthcare and other related purposes.

In their many roles in behavioral healthcare settings, HIM professionals also have a responsibility in this new era of e-HIM™ to uphold and advance the confidentiality and security of electronic health records no less than in the paper environment. This requires communication of the laws governing PHI confidentiality, privacy, and security with various stakeholders within and outside the organization and promoting responsible decisions in conformity with applicable laws. It also requires increased collaboration with the information technology department to ensure that the transmission of PHI does not compromise the confidentiality, privacy and security requirements of the HIPAA privacy and security rules; 42 CFR, Part 2 (if applicable); and state law.

Management of Sensitive Health Information

HIM professionals in behavioral healthcare settings typically manage the health information of psychiatric and/or drug and alcohol abuse clients whose PHI is governed by more protective federal and/or state laws than the HIPAA privacy rule. As indicated earlier, inappropriate use and disclosure of this highly confidential PHI can result in damaging consequences to a client. Thus, HIM managers have all the more reason to ensure that the confidentiality and security practices of their facilities are in accordance with these more protective laws.

Some clients are even more vulnerable to violations of their privacy rights than others. Such individuals include well-known personalities who are subject to public scrutiny or employees, friends, and family members who may be subject to the curiosity of their coworkers or relatives. The policies and procedures that address internal access and use of PHI in these cases may apply additional restrictions to ensure that the privacy rights of these clients are not violated because of the healthcare organization's failure to recognize their particular circumstances and needs.

The privacy rule also gives clients the right to request restrictions on uses and disclosures of their PHI for treatment, payment, and healthcare operations. However, the organization is not required to agree to the restriction (164.522), as long as it is not contrary to prevailing law. More is said on this subject later in this chapter.

Use and Disclosure of Protected Health Information

HIM managers who are usually responsible for their organization's HIM policies and procedures commonly address the various aspects of use and disclosure of PHI. The term *use* generally refers to internal access for a particular and legitimate purpose. The purpose of the access and use should be in accordance with the individual's job requirements and the organization's policies and procedures. The term *disclosure* refers to the ROI to an external entity and should be authorized by the client or, otherwise, in accordance with applicable law. Blanket use and disclosure of the entire client record is prohibited when less information would be sufficient to meet the need. This concept will be further explained throughout the chapter.

Laws and Regulations Governing PHI Disclosure

Mental health, HIV-AIDS, and substance abuse PHI is specifically regulated by both federal and state laws governing the use and disclosure of medical records and related PHI. Thus, in the development of policies and procedures, HIM managers in behavioral healthcare organizations must ensure that, in carrying out their responsibilities, all members of the workforce:

- Understand their obligations related to the confidentiality, privacy, and security of sensitive PHI

- Are not left to individual interpretation of the laws and regulations that could jeopardize the privacy rights of clients and expose the organization to liability for failure to provide appropriate guidelines on protecting those rights

Laws Regulating Alcohol and Drug Abuse Client Information

In June 2004, the Substance Abuse and Mental Health Services Administration (SAMHSA) Center for Substance Abuse Treatment issued a document entitled "The Confidentiality of Alcohol and Drug Abuse Patient Records Regulation and the HIPAA Privacy Rule: Implications for Alcohol and Substance Abuse Programs" (HHS 2004). The document outlines the principle preemptive aspects of 42 CFR, Part 2, over the HIPAA Privacy Rule and should prove helpful to substance abuse healthcare providers and recipients of substance abuse patient information from substance abuse providers. The entire document may be accessed on the SAMHSA Web page (http://www.samhsa.gov/index.aspx).

HIPAA Privacy Rule

HIPAA provided for the enactment of regulations to protect the privacy of PHI. Subsequently, four years later, the HIPAA Standards for the Privacy of Individually Identifiable Health Information (45 CFR Part 160 and Subparts A and E of Part 164), also called the privacy rule, was signed into law by President Clinton and published in the *Federal Register* on December 28, 2000, by the Department of Health and Human Services (HHS). Under President Bush, the privacy rule became effective on April 14, 2001, with certain modifications adopted and published on August 14, 2002.

The **privacy rule** has three major purposes:

- To protect and enhance the rights of patients by providing them access to their health information and controlling inappropriate use of that information

- To improve the quality of healthcare in the United States by restoring trust in the healthcare system among patients, healthcare professionals, and the multitude of organizations and individuals committed to the delivery of care

- To improve the efficiency and effectiveness of healthcare delivery by creating a national framework for health privacy protection that builds on efforts by states, health systems, and individual organizations

The Office of Civil Rights (OCR) has been charged with oversight of the implementation of the privacy rule. Because of numerous questions received by the OCR and in order to facilitate understanding of the rule, a brief guidance followed by frequently asked questions (FAQs) for particular segments of the rule was published on December 3, 2002. In addition, as new FAQs arise, they will be made available on the OCR's Web page (www.hhs.gov/ocr/hipaa). Nevertheless, for a full understanding of both patient and provider rights and responsibilities under the rule, it is important to check with the rule itself.

Since the implementation date of the HIPAA privacy rule requirements on April 14, 2003, clients receiving mental health and/or substance abuse services also should be informed of their privacy rights by the healthcare organization where they receive their services through a Notice of Privacy Practices (NPP), which is discussed later in this chapter.

The Privacy Act of 1974

The **Privacy Act of 1974** prohibits disclosures of records contained in a system of records maintained by a federal agency (or its contractors) without the written request or consent of the individuals to whom the records pertain. This general rule is subject to various statutory exceptions. In addition to the disclosures explicitly permitted in the statute, the privacy act permits agencies to disclose information for other purposes compatible with the purpose for which the information was collected by identifying the disclosure as a "routine use" and publishing notice of it in the *Federal Register*. The act applies to all federal agencies and contractors that operate privacy act systems of records on behalf of federal agencies.

Some federal agencies and contractors of federal agencies that are CEs under the privacy rules are subject to the privacy act. These entities must comply with all applicable federal statutes and regulations. For example, if the privacy rule permits a disclosure, but the disclosure is not permitted under the privacy act, the federal agency may not make the disclosure. If, however, the privacy act allows a disclosure, but the privacy rule prohibits it, the federal agency will have to apply its discretion in a way that complies with the privacy rule, which means not making the particular disclosure (HHS 2000).

Laws Regulating Alcohol and Drug Abuse Client Information

The federal law governing the confidentiality of alcohol and drug abuse patient records statute, section 543 of the Public Health Service Act, 42 U.S.C.290dd-2, and its implementing regulation, 42 CFR, Part 2, establish confidentiality requirements for patient records maintained by any federally assisted alcohol and/or drug abuse program or personnel who provide alcohol or drug abuse treatment, diagnosis, or referral for treatment. It is important to keep in mind that the term *federally assisted* includes federally conducted or funded programs, federally licensed or certified programs, and programs that are tax exempt or receive Medicare and/or Medicaid payment for services provided. However, certain exceptions apply to records held by the Veterans Administration and the Armed Forces (Subpart B, 2.12[c]).

The privacy rule permits a healthcare provider to disclose information in a number of instances that are prohibited under 42 CFR, Part 2. However, because almost all privacy rule disclosures are permitted and not mandatory, there is generally no conflict with the substance abuse regulations. Thus, a provider that falls under the alcohol and drug abuse regulations would not be in violation of the privacy rule because of a failure to disclose information and would be, in fact, required to adhere to the more protective regulations. It also should be kept in mind that the 42 CFR, Part 2, regulations apply to only federally assisted programs, as described above.

Medicare and Medicaid

The Centers for Medicare and Medicaid Services (CMS) manages two federal health plans: Medicare and Medicaid. Special provisions apply to the maintenance of clinical records of mental health hospitals that are engaged primarily in providing psychiatric services for the diagnosis and treatment of mentally ill persons. These hospitals must meet the special provisions of the Medicare *Conditions of Participation* and Conditions for Coverage in order to participate in the Medicare program.

The confidentiality, privacy, and security of disclosures to Medicare and Medicaid for purposes of treatment and payment may be governed by more restrictive state law than the privacy rule. The federal law governing the PHI of clients in a drug and alcohol abuse program prohibits disclosure of PHI to Medicare and Medicaid without client authorization. (See figure 9.2 for a sample authorization form.)

In the communication and electronic transmission of Medicare and Medicaid claims, behavioral healthcare providers must ensure that the privacy and security requirements of the HIPAA privacy rule, security rule, and the electronic transactions and code sets (TCS) rule, parts 160 and 162, are followed. (It should be noted that CMS has issued a statement permitting healthcare providers to continue to transmit data that do not meet the TCS requirements for electronic transmission until further notice.)

Figure 9.2.   Authorization to disclose PHI

Authorization to Disclose Protected Health Information
(Optional: Name of Organization, Address, Phone and Fax Numbers)

I, _____ Date of Birth_____ Phone #_____
　　　　　(Name of Client)

Authorize: _____ to disclose to: _____
　　　　　(Name of organization　　　　　　　　　　　　　　(Name of person, agency, or organization
　　　　　disclosing information)　　　　　　　　　　　　　　to receive my information)

Address: _____
　　　　　(Address of person, agency, or organization to receive my information)

The following information (Check whatever you want disclosed):

___ Admission Note　　　___ Psychosocial Assessment　　　___ Treatment Plan　　　___ Progress Notes

___ Lab Results　　　___ UDS Results　　　___ Continuing Care Plan
　　　　　　　　　　　　　　　　　　　　　　　and Discharge Summary

___ List Other: _____

Purpose of this disclosure: _____
　　　　　　　　　　　　　　　　(Be as clear and specific as possible)

I understand that my health records and related information are protected under the HIPAA Privacy Rule (federal law 45 CFR, Part 160 & 164) and also may be protected under the federal law governing the Confidentiality of Alcohol and Drug Abuse Patient Records (42 CFR, Part 2) and more protective state law. I understand that my information may not be disclosed without my written authorization unless otherwise provided for in these regulations and laws. I also understand that I may revoke this authorization in writing at any time except to the extent that action has been taken in reliance on it and that in any event this authorization expires automatically as follows:

_____
(Specify the date, event, or condition upon which this authorization expires.)

I understand that generally [insert name of provider] may not condition my treatment on whether I sign an authorization form, but that in certain limited circumstances, I may be denied treatment if I do not sign this form.

Client Signature: _____ Date:_____

Legally authorized representative: _____ Date:_____

Authority to act: _____

Witness:_____

Concerning the question of the need for a business associate agreement (BAA) or an authorization from clients for disclosures for purposes of survey and certification by state survey agencies, the Director for Survey and Certification Group at the Center for Medicaid and State Operations states in a letter dated March 14, 2003, that neither a BAA nor an authorization is required to the extent that a law requires the production of the information for health oversight activities. At the same time, the health oversight agency must limit its uses and disclosures of the PHI it receives to the minimum necessary to accomplish the treatment program's regulatory purpose and may not use the PHI to investigate the individual whose records it has obtained.

Regarding behavioral healthcare organizations that are regulated by 42 CFR, Part 2, Section 2.53, also states that client authorization is not required for Medicare and Medicaid audit and evaluation purposes for the reasons described above.

Research and Institutional Review Boards

Behavioral health medical records are needed to conduct clinical research and study client outcomes for improving client care. Federal law details research protocols; in particular, the privacy rule requirements apply regardless of the research's funding source. Behavioral healthcare organizations must obtain documented approval from their institutional review board (IRB), or privacy board, of a waiver of the authorization of individuals, in whole or in part, that is required by law to use and disclose PHI for purposes of research. The 45 CFR, §164.512(i), standard for uses and disclosure for research purposes should be reviewed carefully as well as other state and/or federal laws governing the use of PHI for research.

The federal drug and alcohol confidentiality law also addresses the confidentiality of research subjects and protects their names and other identifying information. It also references other laws that protect the person engaged in the research from being compelled to disclose any client-identifying information. In this regard, one exception pertains to methadone maintenance programs. If a court order issued under 42 CFR, Part 2, Subpart E, of the drug and alcohol confidentiality law is issued, the research privilege may not be invoked as a defense to a subsequent subpoena.

State Laws and Regulations

The standards and implementation specifications adopted in the privacy rule preempt contrary state law. However, according to the Preamble to the Privacy Rule published in December 2000, the Secretary of the Department of Health and Human Services ruled that three types of state laws that are *more stringent* than the federal requirements take precedence over the Privacy Rule (HHS 2000):

- state laws that are necessary for certain purposes set forth in the Privacy Rule
- state laws that the Secretary determines address controlled substances
- state laws relating to the privacy of individually identifiable health information

Moreover, certain areas of state law (generally relating to public health and oversight of health plans) are explicitly carved out of the general rule of preemption and addressed separately.

For behavioral healthcare organizations that also are regulated by the federal law governing substance abuse records, 42 CFR, Part 2, preempts state law unless it is more restrictive or permitted by this same federal law.

Accreditation Standards

Behavioral healthcare organizations may seek accreditation from accrediting bodies such as the Joint Commission on Accreditation of Healthcare Organizations (JCAHO) and the Commission on Accreditation of Rehabilitation Facilities (CARF).

JCAHO has developed standards to promote the safety and quality of care of the public in all types of healthcare organizations. More information on JCAHO may be found on its Web site at www.jcaho.org. CARF focuses on the areas of the medical and vocational rehabilitation fields to promote high-quality services for people with disabilities and others in need of rehabilitation services. More information on CARF may be found on its Web site at www.carf.org.

These and other accrediting bodies base their accreditation on a comprehensive survey process involving measurement of the healthcare organization's performance compared to predefined standards they have developed. They publish manuals that are updated on an annual basis and include standards that address the confidentiality, privacy, and security of medical records and PHI that support the federal and state laws.

HIM managers in behavioral healthcare settings must be familiar with the standards of their accrediting body and ensure that the confidentiality requirements are appropriately addressed in policies and procedures and reflected in daily practice throughout the organization.

Standards of Practice

Throughout the healthcare industry, HIM managers have promoted the confidentiality and security of medical records and tracked PHI use and disclosure for many years in accordance with federal and state laws and as a matter of professional practice and accountability. In fact, many of the privacy rule standards that protect PHI have been operational in behavioral healthcare organizations under other federal and state laws that already protect mental health and substance abuse PHI through more stringent regulations and statutes. Likewise, HIM professionals have promoted the AHIMA Code of Ethics and other reasonable standards of practice because of the ramifications of discriminatory actions taken against clients with mental health and/or substance abuse problems. Most likely, new standards of practice also will be developed as implementation of the federal laws proceeds in the months and years ahead.

Although the education and experience of HIM professionals is very valuable to the healthcare organization, appropriately addressing these various laws can become very complex. For this reason, many behavioral healthcare organizations retain legal counsel to assist their HIM director with sorting through the vast amount of HIPAA information; 42 CFR, Part 2, and state law and with identifying the appropriate course of action in these cases when laws seem to conflict or their application is unclear.

Uses and Disclosures for Treatment, Payment, and Healthcare Operations

The privacy rule differentiates between obtaining consent to use PHI to treat the client (including use and disclosure of PHI to obtain payment and for healthcare operations, commonly called TPO) and obtaining consent to disclose PHI for other purposes. Obtaining consent for TPO is permitted, but not required by the privacy rule. However, it may still be required by other federal or state law or by the healthcare provider. Disclosure generally refers to the release of information to an entity external to the healthcare organization and requires an authorization.

Required Authorization to Disclose PHI

Consent to disclose PHI is called **authorization** in the privacy rule. An authorization must be obtained from the client for disclosure of health information to external entities such as attorneys, family members, and so on. The rule does not require authorization from the client for use and disclosure of PHI for purposes of treatment, payment (including billing third-party payers), and healthcare operations (164.506[a] and [b]). However, state law for mental health providers may require an authorization for these purposes and the federal law governing programs that deliver substance abuse treatment services does require client authorization to disclose PHI for purposes of TPO.

If the healthcare provider seeks a client authorization, a copy of the signed authorization must be provided to the client. Clients also must be informed of the potential for their information to be redisclosed by the recipient of the PHI and no longer protected by the privacy rule. However, 42 CFR, Part 2, requires a specific statement on the prohibition of redisclosure to accompany every release made with or without the substance abuse client's authorization (§2.31). This requirement is more protective of the client's privacy and thus prevails over the privacy rule. Likewise, when state law is more protective of redisclosure of psychiatric records, it preempts the privacy rule.

Healthcare providers are *not* required to use and/or disclose PHI just because an authorization meets the requirements of the law; blanket authorizations for disclosure are discouraged in accordance with the need-to-know and minimum necessary principles. On the other hand, providers are not held accountable for disclosures in good faith that are based on a valid authorization that meets the requirements of applicable law. A healthcare provider is prohibited from disclosing PHI based on an authorization that is defective (45 CFR, 164.508), and a patient may revoke an authorization in writing at any time, except to the extent that action already has been taken in reliance on it. Signed authorization forms must be documented and retained as long as the record is maintained or at least for six years. (Additional details on the content of authorizations may be found in 45 CFR, 164.508, of the privacy rule and 45 CFR, Part 2, §2.31.)

Care should be taken to verify the identity of those to whom PHI is to be released before it is disclosed. This should be done whether the disclosure is based on an authorization or one of the permitted disclosures in accordance with applicable law. According to the privacy rule, incidental uses and disclosures that occur along with an otherwise authorized or permitted use or disclosure must be limited (164. 530 [c]).

Authorization and Mental Healthcare Providers

The privacy rule specifically states that an authorization is *required* for disclosures of psychotherapy notes, even for TPO purposes. In addition, without authorization, mental healthcare providers also are prohibited from disclosing PHI for TPO and other purposes that involve an external entity when it is prohibited by state law.

Authorization and Substance Abuse Healthcare Providers

The federal law governing the confidentiality of alcohol and drug abuse clients requires that client authorization be obtained before disclosing PHI to any other entity that is not specifically permitted by these regulations. It is noteworthy that 42 CFR, Part 2, does not permit authorized disclosures that would be self-incriminating, except when clients have been referred for services by the courts (42 CFR, Part 2, §2.33 and §2.35). Figure 9.3 delineates the circumstances when information may be disclosed *without* authorization as long as the privacy rule and state law permit the disclosure. The HIM manager would do well to read the full text in 42 CFR, Part 2.

The federal regulations on the confidentiality of alcohol and drug abuse clients do not apply to the Veterans Administration under 38 U.S.C. 4132, but do apply to the Armed Forces under certain conditions (42 CFR §2.12[c][1] and [2]). They also apply to recipients of the information; recipients are prohibited from redisclosing the information they have received under an authorization for a program to disclose the information to the recipient (§2,12[d]). This is in contrast to the privacy rule, which requires the CE to inform patients that their information is no longer protected after it has been disclosed. Because it is more protective, 42 CFR, Part 2, supercedes the privacy rule.

One of the most difficult situations to deal with that illustrates the extent of the privacy afforded clients in a substance abuse program occurs when state law generally permits—or even requires—disclosure in response to a subpoena or court order. "More than any other situation governed by the [substance abuse] regulations, those involving subpoenas, warrants and court

Figure 9.3. Disclosure and alcohol and drug abuse treatment programs

Alcohol and drug treatment programs that are regulated under 42 CFR, Part 2, may only disclose protected health information *without* authorization in the following circumstances:

- Communication within and between a program and with an entity having direct administrative control over the program and its personnel who need the information in connection with their duties that arise out of the provision of services provided (Subpart B, §2.12[c][3])

- Communication between a program and a business associate/qualified service organization §2.12(c)(4)

- Limited information to law enforcement and the courts when a client has committed a crime on program property or against program staff (§2.12[c][5])

- Limited information to report suspected child abuse and neglect(§2.12[c][6])

- For medical emergency to medical personnel Subpart D, §2.51)

- For research activities (Subpart D, §2.52)

- For program audit and evaluation activities (§2.53)

- Upon a court order following the special 42 CFR, Part 2, "good cause" hearing (Subpart E, §2.61 and §2.63) (Note: Other than for purposes of criminal investigation or prosecution, anyone having a legally recognized interest in a disclosure may apply for a hearing [§2.64].)

- Situations in which certain entities apply for the "good cause" hearing to criminally investigate or prosecute a client (§2.65) or the program (§2.66)

orders are best handled by attorneys" when a valid authorization cannot be obtained (LAC 2003, 54–55). With the exception of a court order following a "good cause" hearing to which all parties have been notified to appear, including the provider, 42 CFR, Part 2, §2.31, requires an authorization for the provider to respond to the subpoena, warrant, or court order that meets the requirements of the regulations. Even in the "good cause" hearing, when a judge finds the reasons for the disclosure to be extremely serious, "there are general limits under 42 CFR, Part 2, on the scope of disclosure that a court may authorize. . . . Disclosure must be limited to the information essential to fulfill the purpose of the order, and it must be restricted to those persons who need the information for that purpose. In all other situations, not even a court can order disclosure of confidential communications . . ." (LAC 2003, 52–53; 42 CFR, Part 2, § 2.63).

To summarize, HIM managers in substance abuse programs must ensure that the organization's workforce understands that with the exception of defined instances in the law, communication of PHI without an authorization is prohibited. Without authorization, as stated in 42 CFR, Part 2, §2.13,2.31,2.61ff, disclosure in response to a subpoena or court order or to law enforcement with a search or arrest warrant is prohibited, with only a few exceptions. State laws that are less protective also are preempted.

Minors Seeking Mental Health and/or Substance Abuse Services

Some states permit minors to admit themselves into mental health treatment facilities without parental consent; they also permit minors to authorize disclosure of PHI. Likewise, according to 42 CFR, Part 2, Subpart B, 2.14, if state law permits minors to seek admission for services in a substance abuse program without parental consent, unless the minor lacks the capacity to make rational choice, only the minor can authorize disclosure of his or her PHI, including the disclosure of information to parents.

Content of an Authorization and Other Details

The privacy rule is very detailed regarding the content of an authorization; six core elements are required to disclose PHI, plus certain required statements. (See figure 9.4.) Compound authorizations that allow for disclosure to more than one entity are permitted under certain conditions

Figure 9.4.   Content of an authorization

According to the privacy rule (164.508), the general requirements of an authorization are:
- The name or other specific identification of the person(s) or class of persons authorized to make the requested disclosure
- The name of other specific identification of the person(s) or class of persons to whom the provider may make the requested disclosure
- The description of the information to be disclosed that describes the information in a specific and meaningful way
- A description of the purpose for which the requested information will be used
- An expiration date or event that relates to the requested disclosure
- The signature of the client and date

In addition, the authorization must include statements that inform the client of the following:
- The client's right to revoke the authorization in writing and either the exceptions to the right to revoke the authorization or a reference to the exceptions in the notice of privacy practices
- The ability or inability to condition treatment, payment, or enrollment or eligibility for benefits on whether the client signs an authorization
- The consequences to the client of a refusal to sign the authorization when treatment, enrollment, or eligibility for benefits can be conditioned on signing an authorization form
- The potential for information disclosed under the authorization to be redisclosed by the recipient and no longer be protected

Note: In the case of clients receiving substance abuse services, redisclosure is not permitted and the notification of this must accompany the information disclosed to the recipient. Many programs stamp each page with the notification required by 42 CFR, Part 2, Subpart C, 2.32.

(45 CFR, §164.508). Mental health and substance abuse treatment providers may have to meet additional requirements to ensure that their authorization forms are valid under state law when state law is more protective of client privacy rights. The federal regulations governing the use and disclosure of alcohol and drug abuse PHI are very similar to the six core elements in the privacy rule; these may be found in 42 CFR, Part 2, §2.31 and §2.35. It is imperative that authorization forms be carefully designed to meet the requirements of the federal and state laws that apply, keeping in mind that requirements that are more protective of the client's privacy will prevail. Like the NPP, authorization forms must be written in plain language.

State law may provide further details regarding completion of authorization forms for clients receiving mental health or substance abuse services who, for one reason or another, are unable or prohibited from authorizing disclosures.

Generally, state law regulates who has legal authority to authorize disclosures when clients:

- Are minors
- Have been admitted involuntarily
- Have been declared legally incompetent
- Have a court-appointed guardian

When Disclosure Is Required or Permitted without Authorization

There are only two instances when disclosure is required by the privacy rule, regardless of whether there is an authorization:

- To the patient upon request (with the exception of a few instances delineated in 164.524)
- To the secretary of HHS with regard to a complaint of a violation of the privacy rule (160.310)

The privacy rule defines in detail the *permitted* uses and disclosures *without* authorization in 160.506, 160.510, 160.512, and 160.514. The most frequent purpose for which disclosures are permitted without authorization is for TPO. The privacy rule also permits disclosure for certain other major public or national priorities. It is important to note the use of the words *may* and *permitted* throughout the privacy rule. Their use indicates that the healthcare provider must determine whether the information should be used and/or disclosed. As said above, HIM managers of mental health services need to check their state laws to determine whether they are permitted to disclose PHI for TPO and any other purposes permitted by the privacy rule without authorization. Healthcare providers of alcohol and/or drug abuse services are prohibited from disclosing PHI without authorization, except in a few defined circumstances delineated in figure 9.3.

HIM managers must be knowledgeable of the details of the applicable federal and state laws that impact use and disclosure of PHI and educate their healthcare organizations regarding these laws that have not been abrogated by the HIPAA privacy rule.

When the Opportunity to Agree or Object Is Required

The HIPAA privacy rule requires providers to give their clients the opportunity to prohibit or restrict certain uses and disclosures that are permitted without their authorization by the privacy rule; the words *certain* and *permitted* without authorization should be kept in mind. Details on these certain, permitted uses and disclosures are found in 164.510 of the privacy rule and should be read carefully. Generally, they relate to the facility directory; emergency circumstances; a family member, other relative, or close personal friend involved in the client's care or payment for care; notification of the client's location, general condition, or death; and disaster relief situations. There also are directives related to the above limited uses and disclosures when the client is present at the disclosure and when he or she is not present.

Again, HIM professionals must be aware of and apply any more restrictive state or federal laws (such as 42 CFR, Part 2) that prohibit any or all of the HIPAA-permitted uses and disclosures without authorization, especially when the client is not present. Simply giving the client an opportunity to agree or object may not be an option.

When Authorization and an Opportunity to Agree or Object Is Not Required

According to the privacy rule, a healthcare provider may use or disclose PHI without an authorization and without giving the individual an opportunity to agree or object to the extent that such use and disclosure is required by law and as long as it complies with, and is limited to, the relevant requirements of the law. The privacy rule permits a number of disclosures that may be required by a state or federal law. The details regarding permitted disclosures are found in section 164.512.

However, mental health and substance abuse providers must follow state laws and 42 CFR, Part 2, requirements, which may limit or prohibit permitted uses and disclosures. As indicated earlier, it is necessary to look closely at the laws that govern and determine which law takes precedence. Generally, the more restrictive laws protecting the privacy rights of the client prevail.

Deidentified Health Information

Health information that does not identify a client, and which there is no reason to believe could be used to identify a client, is not PHI. Likewise, individual client health information that has been **deidentified**, and for which there is no reason to believe that it can be used to reidentify a client, is not PHI according to the privacy rule. The rule lists the individual identifiers that must be removed from client information in order to render it unidentifiable. It should be noted that the privacy rule lists the client medical record number as PHI, as well as telephone numbers, e-mail addresses, account numbers, certificate/license numbers, and full-face photographic images. The entire section of 45 CFR, 164.514, should be reviewed because it lists more than twenty individual identifiers as PHI.

Restrictions to Access and Use of PHI

As stated above, with few exceptions, clients have the right to access their entire medical record and other PHI in a designated record set (164.524). Any other federal or state laws that restrict client access must be reviewed to determine whether they still have legal validity based on the above standard of the privacy rule. For other requesters of PHI, the type of information disclosed, whether permitted with or without authorization, should be based on the minimum necessary and need-to-know principles referred to earlier. In other words, the question is: What is needed to carry out the purpose for the request? What is needed is what should be disclosed, whether for use by a member of the provider's workforce to carry out his or her duties or for an external requester who has presented an authorization signed by the client.

All requests for disclosure should be reviewed for proper authorization on an individual basis in accordance with the above principles. The entire medical record should not be used or disclosed routinely, except when specifically justified as the amount that is reasonably necessary for the purpose of the use or disclosure.

The healthcare organization should develop policies and procedures that identify both routine and recurring uses and disclosures of PHI, and nonroutine uses and disclosures.

In summation, the minimum necessary and need-to-know principles should be applied in a reasonable way, including when PHI is requested from and by other healthcare providers. Also, the additional details of the privacy rule (164.514), any applicable state laws, and 42 CFR, Part 2 (especially 2.12ff) should be reviewed to ensure that the practices of the organization are in accordance with the applicable laws related to PHI access, use, and disclosure.

Notice of Privacy Practices, and Client Rights and Provider Responsibilities

The HIPAA privacy rule established a right for patients to receive adequate notice of how their healthcare providers use and disclose PHI. Patients also are to be informed of their privacy rights and the provider's obligations to protect the privacy of their health information.

The directives of the privacy rule are very detailed regarding the presentation and content of the notice. The NPP is to be organized and written in plain language to serve the needs of the reader. The more transparent and understandable the notice is, the more confidence the public will have in the provider's commitment to protect patient privacy.

The NNP must be tailored to the type of services provided. When writing their NNPs, HIM professionals in mental health facilities must keep more restrictive state regulations in mind. Likewise, organizations providing substance abuse referrals, diagnosis, and/or treatment must ensure that their NPPs also conform to the federal regulations that protect the health information of alcohol and drug abuse clients (42 CFR, Part 2, §2.22.) and any more protective state laws.

When drafting an NPP, it is necessary to consider the patients' right to access, restrict access and use, amend, obtain a copy of their information in a designated record set, and receive an accounting of disclosures. Further details on these client rights should be carefully reviewed in the privacy rule (164.522, 164.524, and 164.526).

Likewise, the provider's related rights and responsibilities must be delineated. The NPP must include the name or title and telephone number of the person or office of the provider the patient can contact for further information related to the notice and with which he or she can file a complaint regarding privacy violations. The notice must include a brief description of how patients may complain. All healthcare providers must inform clients in the notice of how they can complain to the secretary of HHS if they believe their rights have been violated and must provide the secretary's address, phone number, and Web page address.

The NPP must be revised to reflect changes in policies and procedures and practices. If the provider has informed its clients in the NPP that it reserves the right to change its privacy practices at any time, the changes may be made effective for PHI that was created or received prior to the effective date of the revision. If the provider has not reserved the right to change its privacy practices in the NPP, it may not implement the changes prior to the effective date of the revised NPP.

An NPP cannot be drafted without reading this part of the rule. The FAQs related to the NPP published on December 3, 2002, by the OCR also should be read to understand what is and is not expected by the OCR at www.hhs.gov/ocr/hipaa/assist.html.

A sample NPP that would be of assistance to substance abuse treatment organizations is provided in figure 9.5. However, 45 CFR, Part 164.520, of the privacy rule and 42 CFR, Part 2, 2.22, also should be read.

Whatever the type of services provided, the privacy officer (discussed in a later section) must keep in mind that the law that is more protective of clients' rights almost always prevails and should be reflected in the NPP.

Disclosures to Affiliated CEs and Organized Healthcare Arrangements

The designation *affiliated covered entity* (ACE) in the privacy rule (164.504) allows legally separate covered entities (for example, a health plan and healthcare provider and/or a clearinghouse) that are under common ownership or control to use and disclose PHI with other CEs as long as they observe the standards that relate to them. The designation of an ACE must be documented and the documentation maintained in accordance with §164.530(j) of the privacy rule. The 42 CFR, Part 2, §2.12(c)(3), also appears to envision at least one aspect of the privacy rule concept of an ACE regarding communication between a treatment program and an organization having direct administrative control over the program.

An organized healthcare arrangement (OHCA) is another type of legal designation permitted in a clinically integrated healthcare setting where patients typically receive healthcare from more than one provider. In behavioral healthcare, a prime example would be contracted medical and clinical staff. Additional examples of OHCAs may be found in §164.501 of the privacy rule.

It should be noted that the ACE and OHCA designations allow multiple providers in a clinically integrated healthcare setting to distribute the same NPP previously discussed and operate under the same authorization forms as long as those involved in the affiliation or arrangement comply with the privacy rule requirements for members of the workforce (45 CFR, 160.103, and 45 CFR, 164.501 and 164.504).

Disclosures to Business Associates and Qualified Service Organizations

The privacy rule permits a healthcare provider to disclose PHI to a **business associate** (BA) in instances where a person or company performs a service or functions for, or on behalf of, the provider other than in the capacity of a member of the provider's workforce (164.103). The BAA allows the provider and the BA to communicate and exchange PHI with each other without an authorization from the provider's patient. In behavioral healthcare, a BAA would be used in administrative services that could be outsourced, such as transcription, coding, legal, actuarial, consulting, and claims processing. The section in the privacy rule (§164.504[e]) on implementation specifications for a BAA should be read in its entirety. It also is important to keep in mind that few BAs perform exactly the same services for the behavioral healthcare provider, so BAAs are not exactly alike.

When substance abuse programs are considering whether to enter into a BAA with an external entity that provides services to, or on behalf of, the treatment program, it is *essential*

Figure 9.5. Sample patient notice

SAMPLE PATIENT NOTICE

THIS NOTICE DESCRIBES HOW MEDICAL AND DRUG- AND ALCOHOL-RELATED INFORMATION ABOUT YOU MAY BE USED AND DISCLOSED AND HOW YOU CAN GET ACCESS TO THIS INFORMATION. PLEASE REVIEW IT CAREFULLY.

General Information

Information regarding your health care, including payment for health care, is protected by two federal laws: the Health Insurance Portability and Accountability Act of 1996 ("HIPAA"), 42 U.S.C. § 1320d et seq., 45 C.F.R. Parts 160 & 164, and the Confidentiality Law, 42 U.S.C. § 290dd-2, 42 C.F.R. Part 2. Under these laws, Green Valley Recovery Center (Green Valley) may not say to a person outside Green Valley that you attend the program, nor may Green Valley disclose any information identifying you as an alcohol or drug abuser, or disclose any other protected information except as permitted by federal law.

Green Valley must obtain your written consent before it can disclose information about you for payment purposes. For example, Green Valley must obtain your written consent before it can disclose information to your health insurer in order to be paid for services. Generally, you must also sign a written consent before Green Valley can share information for treatment purposes or for health care operations. However, federal law permits Green Valley to disclose information *without* your written permission:

1. Pursuant to an agreement with a qualified service organization/business associate;
2. For research, audit, or evaluations;
3. To report a crime committed on Green Valley's premises or against Green Valley personnel;
4. To medical personnel in a medical emergency;
5. To appropriate authorities to report suspected child abuse or neglect;
6. As allowed by a court order.

[Insert more stringent protections provided by State law, if any]

For example, Green Valley can disclose information without your consent to obtain legal or financial services, or to another medical facility to provide health care to you, as long as there is a qualified service organization/business associate agreement in place.

Before Green Valley can use or disclose any information about your health in a manner which is not described above, it must first obtain your specific written consent allowing it to make the disclosure. Any such written consent may be revoked by you in writing.

Your Rights

Under HIPAA you have the right to request restrictions on certain uses and disclosures of your health information. Green Valley is not required to agree to any restrictions you request, but if it does agree, then it is bound by that agreement and may not use or disclose any information that you have restricted except as necessary in a medical emergency.

You have the right to request that we communicate with you by alternative means or at an alternative location. Green Valley will accommodate such requests that are reasonable and will not request an explanation from you. Under HIPAA you also have the right to inspect and copy your own health information maintained by Green Valley, except to the extent that the information contains psychotherapy notes or information compiled for use in a civil, criminal or administrative proceeding or in other limited circumstances.

Under HIPAA you also have the right, with some exceptions, to amend health care information maintained in Green Valley's records, and to request and receive an accounting of disclosures of your health related information made by Green Valley during the six years prior to your request. You also have the right to receive a paper copy of this notice.

Green Valley's Duties

Green Valley is required by law to maintain the privacy of your health information and to provide you with notice of its legal duties and privacy practices with respect to your health information. Green Valley is required by law to abide by the terms of this notice. Green Valley reserves the right to change the terms of this notice and to make new notice provisions effective for all protected health information it maintains. *[Insert description of how the covered entity will provide individuals with a revised notice.]*

Complaints and Reporting Violations

You may complain to Green Valley and the Secretary of the United States Department of Health and Human Services if you believe that your privacy rights have been violated under HIPAA. *[Insert description of how a complaint is filed with the covered entity.]* You will not be retaliated against for filing such a complaint.

Violation of the Confidentiality Law by a program is a crime. Suspected violations of the Confidentiality Law may be reported to the United States Attorney in the district where the violation occurs.

Contact

For further information, contact [insert name or title and telephone number of person or office to contact for further information.]

Effective Date

[Insert date on which notice became effective; cannot be earlier than date on which notice was printed or published.]

Acknowledgement

I hereby acknowledge that I received a copy of this notice.

Dated: _____

(Signature of patient)

---

to first ascertain whether such an agreement is permissible under 42 CFR, Part 2, §2.11 and §2.12. More often than not, substance abuse treatment providers will need to combine the BAA with the qualified service organization agreement (QSOA) of 42 CFR, Part 2, and keep in mind that this agreement will set the parameters for the BAA aspects. Additionally, it should be noted that substance abuse programs are prohibited from entering into a QSOA with other substance abuse programs. Finally, it is worth noting that a substance abuse program could enter into a QSOA with an inpatient mental health provider, for example, but may not need a BAA for this CE because the privacy rule permits disclosures for TPO.

Rediscloser of PHI by the BA to an agent or subcontractor is not permitted in a QSOA/BAA; an authorization from the client is required and the BA is obligated to maintain a record and report to the CE any unauthorized disclosure. The 42 CFR, Part 2, rediscloser-prohibited disclaimer is required on any information disclosed to the QSO/BA, as stated above.

A sample QSOA/BAA is offered in figure 9.6 for providers of substance abuse services under 42 CFR, Part 2.

Accounting and Tracking Disclosures

Clients have a right to receive an accounting of the disclosures of their PHI made by their behavioral healthcare provider during the six years prior to the date on which the accounting is requested, except for disclosures to carry out TPO, disclosures to the client, and certain other instances delineated in the privacy rule. An accounting is not required for any disclosures before April 14, 2003. Section 164.528 of the privacy rule should be read in its entirety for implementation specifications related to the accounting of disclosures.

Suffice it to note here that the privacy rule describes the content of the accounting in great detail in section 164.528. The provider must act on the client's request for the accounting within 60 days of receiving the written request. An extension of thirty days is permitted when the provider is unable to furnish the accounting within the sixty days, but the patient must be informed in writing of the reasons for the delay and the date when the accounting will be provided (164.528[c]). Moreover, there are instances in which a client's right to an accounting of certain disclosures may be suspended temporarily, for example, in certain instances of disclosures to a health oversight agency or law enforcement (164.512[d] or [f] and 164.528[a][2]).

Billing for an Accounting of Disclosures

A healthcare provider is permitted to charge the client for an accounting of disclosures. However, the first accounting in any twelve-month period must be provided to clients at no cost; subsequently, a reasonable cost-based fee may be imposed for each additional request within the same twelve-month period provided the client is informed in advance of the fee and given the opportunity to withdraw or modify the request for a subsequent accounting.

Ownership and Control of the Health Record

It is generally accepted that the medical record is the physical property of the healthcare provider or institution that maintains it and is a business record of the same entity. In many states, legislation addresses the right of ownership. However, the medical record is an unusual type of property because the client has a personal interest in, and a right to access, his or her record and, to a certain extent, to control record access, use, and disclosure. The HIM manager should be prepared to advise clients on their rights and the provider's right of ownership of the business record.

Figure 9.6. Sample QSOA/BAA

**SAMPLE QUALIFIED SERVICE ORGANIZATION/BUSINESS ASSOCIATE AGREEMENT
(QSO/BA AGREEMENT)**

XYZ Service Center ("the Center") and the

_____

(Name of the alcohol/drug program)

(the "Program") hereby enter into an agreement whereby the Center agrees to provide

_____

(Nature of services to be provided to the program)

Furthermore, the Center:

(1) acknowledges that in receiving, transmitting, transporting, storing, processing, or otherwise dealing with any information received from the Program identifying or otherwise relating to the patients in the Program ("protected information"), it is fully bound by the provisions of the federal regulations governing the Confidentiality of Alcohol and Drug Abuse Patient Records, 42 C.F.R. Part 2; and the Health Insurance Portability and Accountability Act (HIPAA), 45 C.F.R. Parts 142, 160, 162 and 164, and may not use or disclose the information except as permitted or required by this Agreement or by law;

(2) agrees to resist any efforts in judicial proceedings to obtain access to the protected information except as expressly provided for in the regulations governing the Confidentiality of Alcohol and Drug Abuse Patient Records, 42 C.F.R. Part 2.

(3) agrees to use appropriate safeguards (*can define with more specificity*) to prevent the unauthorized use or disclosure of the protected information;

(4) agrees to report to the Program any use or disclosure of the protected information not provided for by this Agreement of which it becomes aware (*insert negotiated time & manner terms*);

(5) *[agrees to ensure that any agent, including a subcontractor, to whom the Center provides the protected information received from the Program, or created or received by the Center on behalf of the Program, agrees to the same restrictions and conditions that apply through this agreement to the Center with respect to such information;]**

(6) agrees to provide access to the protected information at the request of the Program, or to an individual as directed by the Program, in order to meet the requirements of 45 C.F.R. §164.524 which provides patients with the right to access and copy their own protected information (*insert negotiated time & manner terms*);

(7) agrees to make any amendments to the protected information as directed or agreed to by the program pursuant to 45 C.F.R. § 164.526 (*insert negotiated time & manner terms*);

(8) agrees to make available its internal practices, books, and records, including policies and procedures, relating to the use and disclosure of protected information received from the Program, or created or received by the Center on behalf of the Program, to the Program or to the Secretary of the Department of Health and Human Services for purposes of the Secretary determining the Program's compliance with HIPAA (*insert negotiated time & manner terms*);

(9) *[agrees to document disclosures of protected information, and information related to such disclosures, as would be required for the Program to respond to a request by an individual for an accounting of disclosures in accordance with 45 C.F.R. § 164.528 (insert negotiated time & manner terms);]**

(10) agrees to provide the Program or an individual information in accordance with paragraph (9) of this agreement to permit the Program to respond to a request by an individual for an accounting of disclosures in accordance with 45 C.F.R. § 164.528 (*insert negotiated time & manner terms*);

Termination

(1) The program may terminate this agreement if it determines that the Center has violated any material term;

(2) Upon termination of this agreement for any reason, the Center shall return or destroy all protected information received from the Program, or created or received by the Center on behalf of the Program. This provision shall apply to protected information that is in the possession of subcontractors or agents of the Center. The Center shall retain no copies of the protected information.

(3) In the event that the Center determines that returning or destroying the protected information is infeasible, the Center shall notify the Program of the conditions that make return or destruction infeasible (*insert negotiated time & manner terms*).

Upon notification that the return or destruction of the protected information is infeasible, the Center shall extend the protections of this Agreement to such protected information and limit further uses and disclosures of the information to those purposes that make the return or destruction infeasible, as long as the Center maintains the information.

Executed this _____ day of _____, 200_____.

President   Program Director
XYZ Service Center   [Name of the Program]
[address]   [address]

*Although HIPAA requires these paragraphs to be included in Business Associate agreements, 42 C.F.R. § 2.11 requires qualified service organizations to abide by the federal drug and alcohol regulations which prohibit such organizations from redisclosing any patient identifying information even to an agent or subcontractor. Legal Action Center has asked HHS for an opinion on this issue.

© Legal Action Center. 2004

State Legislation and Record Retention

The health record is maintained primarily for the delivery of healthcare to a particular individual, but it also has several other purposes. State governments, especially, have regulatory involvement in healthcare systems through state-owned and operated facilities, the funding of medical education and teaching hospitals, the certification of healthcare organizations according to the *Conditions of Participation,* the maintenance of public health departments, and the licensing of healthcare organizations and health occupations. Thus, states regulate retention of the medical record to ensure that it is available for all of the above needs for a certain period of time. HIM managers should refer to state law for specific information related to record retention for their particular behavioral healthcare organization.

State law may specifically prohibit maintaining original medical records outside the healthcare organization that owns the records. In any case, stringent policies and procedures on records management should address such things as employees potentially taking original paper records or copies to their homes where it is more difficult, if not impossible, to monitor confidentiality, access, and use or, in the case of original records, whether they have been subject to alteration, tampering, or destruction.

In many states, the state HIM association affiliated with AHIMA has developed a handbook to assist HIM managers in accepted professional HIM standards of practices related to the use and disclosure of the medical record and PHI in accordance with state law.

HIPAA Privacy Rule Administrative Requirements

The privacy rule contains a number of administrative requirements for healthcare providers. They include:

- Personnel designations

- Policies and procedures related to implementation of the privacy rule, including appropriate administrative, technical, and physical safeguards to protect the privacy of PHI

- Workforce training in the policies and procedures of the CE

- A process for receiving and responding to complaints

- **Sanctions** for violations of the privacy rule and related policies and procedures

Section 164.530 of the privacy rule regarding the administrative requirements should be read in its entirety.

Designation of Privacy Officer and Contact Person or Office

Like all HIPAA privacy rule CEs, behavioral healthcare organizations must document designation of a privacy officer. This individual "is responsible for the development and implementation of the policies and procedures of the entity" that relate to the requirements of section 164.530(a). This section should be read in its entirety to get the full picture of the privacy officer's responsibilities. HIM professionals are generally well qualified to take on the privacy officer role because of their education and experience; in fact, in many healthcare organizations, the HIM director is also the privacy officer.

A contact person or office responsible for receiving complaints by both clients and other persons and for providing further information related to the policies and procedures and the NPP also must be designated and the designation documented (164.530[a]). Many organizations designate the privacy officer as the contact person for practical purposes. (See figure 9.7 for a sample job description.) Likewise, all complaints and their disposition (if any) must be documented. All of this information must be retained for at least six years (164.530[j]).

Figure 9.7. AHIMA Sample Privacy Officer Job Description

Position Title: (Chief) Privacy Officer

Immediate Supervisor: Chief Executive Officer, Senior Executive, or Health Information Management (HIM) Department Head

General Purpose: The privacy officer oversees all ongoing activities related to the development, implementation, maintenance of, and adherence to the organization's policies and procedures covering the privacy of, and access to, patient health information in compliance with federal and state laws and the healthcare organization's information privacy practices.

Responsibilities:

- Provides development guidance and assists in the identification, implementation, and maintenance of organization information privacy policies and procedures in coordination with organization management and administration, the Privacy Oversight Committee, and legal counsel.
- Works with organization senior management and corporate compliance officer to establish an organization-wide Privacy Oversight Committee.
- Serves in a leadership role for the Privacy Oversight Committee's activities.
- Performs initial and periodic information privacy risk assessments and conducts related ongoing compliance monitoring activities in coordination with the entity's other compliance and operational assessment functions.
- Works with legal counsel and management, key departments, and committees to ensure the organization has and maintains appropriate privacy and confidentiality consent, authorization forms, and information notices and materials reflecting current organization and legal practices and requirements.
- Oversees, directs, delivers, or ensures delivery of initial and privacy training and orientation to all employees, volunteers, medical and professional staff, contractors, alliances, business associates, and other appropriate third parties.
- Participates in the development, implementation, and ongoing compliance monitoring of all trading partner and business associate agreements, to ensure all privacy concerns, requirements, and responsibilities are addressed.
- Establishes with management and operations a mechanism to track access to protected health information, within the purview of the organization and as required by law and to allow qualified individuals to review or receive a report on such activity.
- Works cooperatively with the HIM Director and other applicable organization units in overseeing patient rights to inspect, amend, and restrict access to protected health information when appropriate.
- Establishes and administers a process for receiving, documenting, tracking, investigating, and taking action on all complaints concerning the organization's privacy policies and procedures in coordination and collaboration with other similar functions and, when necessary, legal counsel.
- Ensures compliance with privacy practices and consistent application of sanctions for failure to comply with privacy policies for all individuals in the organization's workforce, extended workforce, and for all business associates, in cooperation with Human Resources, the information security officer, administration, and legal counsel as applicable.
- Initiates, facilitates, and promotes activities to foster information privacy awareness within the organization and related entities.
- Serves as a member of, or liaison to, the organization's IRB or Privacy Committee, should one exist. Also serves as the information privacy liaison for users of clinical and administrative systems.
- Reviews all system-related information security plans throughout the organization's network to ensure alignment between security and privacy practices, and acts as a liaison to the information systems department.
- Works with all organization personnel involved with any aspect of release of protected health information, to ensure full coordination and cooperation under the organization's policies and procedures and legal requirements
- Maintains current knowledge of applicable federal and state privacy laws and accreditation standards, and monitors advancements in information privacy technologies to ensure organizational adaptation and compliance.
- Serves as information privacy consultant to the organization for all departments and appropriate entities.
- Cooperates with the Office of Civil Rights, other legal entities, and organization officers in any compliance reviews or investigations.
- Works with organization administration, legal counsel, and other related parties to represent the organization's information privacy interests with external parties (state or local government bodies) who undertake to adopt or amend privacy legislation, regulation, or standard.

Qualifications:

- Certification as an RHIA or RHIT with education and experience relative to the size and scope of the organization.
- Knowledge and experience in information privacy laws, access, release of information, and release control technologies.
- Knowledge in and the ability to apply the principles of HIM, project management, and change management.
- Demonstrated organization, facilitation, communication, and presentation skills.

This description is intended to serve as a scalable framework for organizations in development of a position description for the privacy officer.

Note: The title for this position will vary from organization to organization, and may not be the primary title of the individual serving in the position. "Chief" would most likely refer to very large integrated delivery systems. The term "privacy officer" is specifically mention in the HIPAA Privacy Regulation. The supervisor for this position will vary depending on the institution and its size. Since many of the functions are already inherent in the Health Information or Medical Records Department or function, many organizations may elect to keep this function in that department. The "Privacy Oversight Committee" described here is a recommendation of AHIMA, and should not be considered the same as the "Privacy Committee" described in the HIPAA privacy regulation. A privacy oversight committee could include representation from the organization's senior administration, in addition to departments and individuals who can lend an organization-wide perspective to privacy implementation and compliance. Not all organizations will have an Institutional Review Board (IRB) or Privacy Committee for oversight of research activities. However, should such bodies be present or require establishment under HIPAA or other federal or state requirements, the privacy officer will need to work with this group(s) to ensure authorizations and awareness are established where needed or required.

Source: American Health Information Management Association. 2001. Sample Position Description: (Chief) privacy officer. *Journal of the American Health Information Management Association* 72(6): 37–38.

Privacy Rule Policies and Procedures

A list of privacy rule policies and procedures is provided in figure 9.8. As appropriate and necessary, behavioral healthcare organizations must change their policies and procedures when there are changes in the law or in their privacy practices.

Privacy Safeguards

Privacy officers must ensure that PHI is reasonably protected in whatever format it is maintained from intentional and unintentional uses and disclosures that violate the privacy rule and any other applicable federal and/or state laws governing its confidentiality. These protections must include administrative, physical, and technical safeguards (164.530[c]).

Administrative Safeguards

Administrative safeguards include the above policies and procedures, sanctions, and guidelines related to access and use and the implementation of physical and technical safeguards to protect

Figure 9.8. Privacy rule and related policies and procedures list

- On client authorization for the use of PHI and (Privacy Rule 164.506)
- Client right to revoke authorization (164.508)
- On obtaining and responding to authorizations to use and disclose PHI, including, but not limited to minimum necessary and verification requirements (164.508)
- Use and disclosure of PHI for facility directory—if permitted by applicable law (164.510)
- Use and disclosure of PHI to persons involved in the client's care, as permitted by applicable law
- Legal guardians and other personal representatives
- Use and disclosure of PHI without client authorization (164.512)
- Deidentifying and reidentifying PHI (164.514)
- Business Associates and Qualified Service Organizations and Agreements (45 CFR, Part 164.504 and 42 CFR, Part 2, 2.11)
- Notice of Privacy Practices
- Organized health care arrangements [contracted staff, etc.] (164.501)
- Marketing and PHI (164.514)
- Fundraising and PHI (164.514)
- Establishment and maintenance of the Notice of Privacy Practices (164.520)
- Client right to request restrictions on use and disclosure of PHI (164.522)
- Client right to access, read, and obtain a copy of their PHI in the designated record set (164.524)
- Reports of Child Abuse and Neglect and Abuse of Elderly and Disabled in accordance with applicable law
- Research (164.512)
- Psychotherapy notes (164.501)
- On administrative, technical, and physical safeguards of PHI (164.530(c))
- Client right to amend PHI in the designated record set (164.526)
- Client right to an accounting of disclosures of PHI without authorization (164.528)
- Designation of privacy officer (164.530(a))
- How to respond to subpoenas, court orders, warrants, and law enforcement
- Medical emergencies and crimes on property
- Training of all members of the workforce (164.530(b))
- How to file a complaint, facility contact person or office (164.530(a) and (d)), and information on how to complain to the Office of Civil Rights
- Sanctions for violations of confidentiality and privacy (164.530(e))
- Mitigation of harmful effects of violations (164.530(f))

Note: This list may not be comprehensive for an organization's specific needs related to the Privacy Rule and other applicable law.

PHI. Members of the workforce should be reminded the PHI should not be discussed in public places where conversations might be overheard by passersby or displayed on laptops. Staff who use electronic devices such as laptops, notebooks, Palm Pilots, and personal organizers that may store PHI must be informed and held accountable for appropriate usage of these devices.

Physical Safeguards

Physical safeguards include secure file room maintenance, offices and cabinets where individually identifiable health information in various formats is created and/or used. Likewise, electronic workstations should be made secure. Buildings, file cabinets, and server rooms must have physical safeguards to protect PHI from theft, damage, fire, and other environmental or natural disasters.

Technical Safeguards

Reasonable technical safeguards should be in place to control access to PHI, such as log-ins, passwords, PKI keys, and firewalls. All electronic transmissions must meet the technical stipulations for protecting PHI required by the privacy rule, the security rule, and the rule for electronic transactions and code sets. Appropriate technical safeguards (for example, encryption and virtual private networks [VPNs]) also must be in place before PHI is sent through e-mail. Web sites must be secured via passwords, log-ins, and so on. Regular backups in electronic systems should be scheduled to ensure that information is not lost because of technical failures.

The privacy officer and the security officer (discussed below) must work together to ensure consistency in the implementation of the privacy and security rules and workforce training.

Privacy Training

All members of the workforce are to be trained in the policies and procedures of the organization that relate to the confidentiality and privacy of PHI within a reasonable time after their hire. Members of the workforce include employees, volunteers, trainees, and other persons whose conduct in the performance of work for the provider is under the direct control of the provider, whether or not they are paid by the provider (164.503). Contracted physicians and other staff in an OHCA with a behavioral healthcare organization also must be given appropriate training in the facility's policies and procedures as well as pertinent updates.

Appropriate training should enable members of the workforce to carry out their particular responsibilities in accordance with the law (164.530[b]). For example, clinical and medical staff will need more extensive training related to PHI confidentiality, privacy, and security than housekeeping staff; the billing department will need specific additional training for communication with health plans and clearinghouses; and so on. Privacy training should integrate the other federal and/or state laws that pertain to the CE; otherwise, staff may be uncertain of their responsibilities or unintentionally violate applicable law. Additionally, the workforce must be given training updates when there are changes in the policies and procedures related to PHI use and disclosure. (See figure 9.9 for a list of privacy training topics.)

All training received by the workforce must be documented and maintained for six years (164.530[j]).

Sanctions

Appropriate sanctions must be in place and applied against members of the workforce who violate the policies and procedures related to PHI confidentiality, privacy, and security. However, sanctions are not to be applied to whistleblowers and workforce crime victims as long as the organization's policies and procedures and the requirements of the privacy and security rules are followed (164.530[j]).

Figure 9.9.   Privacy training topics

Privacy training should integrate the Privacy Rule, state law, and, when applicable, the Federal Drug and Alcohol Confidentiality Law. General topics should include, but are not limited to, the following:

- General concepts about the federal and state laws that govern the confidentiality of protected health information and the privacy rights of clients

- Physical security of records and other PHI in file rooms, computers, offices, cabinets and anywhere else they are stored

- Notice of Privacy Practices

- Basic concepts related to maintaining confidentiality of PHI

- Internal access and use of PHI

- Minimum necessary and need to know

- Psychotherapy notes, if applicable

- What constitutes a valid authorization

- Routine disclosures permitted with authorization

- When disclosures are permitted without authorization and what to do

- What to do if law enforcement arrives on the premises with a warrant

- What to do in the event of a crime on property, against staff, or against the program

- Security of PHI

- Sanctions for violations of confidentiality

- How to report breaches of confidentiality

- The contact number of the privacy official for questions related to the confidentiality and privacy aspects of protected health information

Note: Individuals or groups of the workforce will need additional training in accordance with their specific responsibilities and duties.

Complaints to the Covered Entity

Behavioral healthcare providers must have a process in place for clients to make complaints to the CE regarding its policies and procedures that address the requirements of the HIPAA privacy and security regulations. A designated contact person should be given responsibility for receiving complaints and answering questions related to the PNN. All complaints and their disposition (if any) should be documented and the documentation retained for six years from the date it was created or the date it was last in effect, whichever is later (§164.530[d] and (§164.530[j]).

Clients may file a complaint directly with the secretary of HHS in writing, on paper or electronically, within 180 days of when the complainant knew or should have known that the act or omission complained of occurred. Further details on the procedure for filing complaints with HHS may be found in §160.306 of the privacy rule. The NNP should explain to clients how to file complaints with both the healthcare provider and the HHS, as stated above.

The secretary of HHS and the OCR prefer to seek the cooperation of CEs in meeting the requirements of the privacy rule through informal means when they have been found non-compliant and may provide technical assistance to this end. For their part, healthcare providers, upon request from HHS, must provide records, compliance reports, copies of policies and procedures, and other pertinent information related to their practices in accordance with the standards, requirements, and implementation specifications of the privacy rule (§160.306–§160.312).

HIPAA Security Rule Administrative Requirements

Administration of the HIPAA security rule requires the appointment of a security officer and the establishment of policies and procedures. It also involves training for the workforce.

Designation of a Security Officer

Like the privacy rule, the **security rule** requires designation of a **security officer** who is to be responsible for the development and implementation of the policies and procedures related to the security rule (164.308[a][2]).

Policies and Procedures

In writing the security rule policies and procedures, the security officer must take into account the size, complexity, and capability of the organization, its technical infrastructure, its hardware and software security capabilities, the cost of security measures, and the probability and criticality of potential risks to electronic PHI (164.306[b][2]). The policies and procedures must address reasonable administrative, physical, and technical safeguards of PHI and should support the policies and procedures required by the privacy rule. (See figure 9.10 for a list of security rule policies and procedures.)

The security officer must ensure that PHI in electronic systems is protected from unlawful access, destruction, environmental and natural disasters, fire, and theft. There should be an inventory of personal computers and prohibitions on unauthorized removal from the workstations where they were installed. Likewise, there should be an inventory of all other electronic devices. The security officer and the privacy officer must work together to ensure consistency and solidarity among privacy and security rule policies and procedures and in their implementation of workforce training.

Workforce Training

All members of the workforce must be trained in the policies and procedures of the security rule in accordance with their responsibilities. If changes in laws or electronic systems procedures occur, policies and procedures must be updated to reflect the changes and the members of the workforce affected by the change must be trained appropriately. All training received by the workforce must be documented and maintained for six years (164.530[j]).

The compliance date for the security rule is set for no later than April 20, 2005 (164.318[c]).

Sanctions

Appropriate sanctions must be in place and applied against members of the workforce who violate the policies and procedures related to the security of PHI (164.308[a][c]). However, as with the privacy rule, sanctions for violation of the security rule are not to be applied to whistleblowers and workforce crime victims as long as the organization's policies and procedures and the requirements of the security rule are followed.

Conclusion

Protecting the confidentiality, privacy, and security of mental health and substance abuse records, as well as all related PHI, has become a very complicated endeavor in the behavioral healthcare setting. Health information managers, who also may be privacy officers, have significant responsibilities within their healthcare organizations regarding implementation of the

Figure 9.10. Security policies and procedures

Security policies and procedures should include:

- A security management process (164.308(a)(1))
- Assigned security responsibility (security official) (164.308(a)(2))
- Workforce security (164.308(a)(3))
- Information access management (164.308(a)(4))
- Security incident procedures (164.308(a)(6))
- Contingency plan (164.308(a)(7))
- Business associate contracts and other arrangements (164.308(b)(1))
- Facility access controls (164.310(a)(1))
- Workstation use (164.310(b))
- Workstation security (164.310(c))
- Device and media controls (164.310(d)(1))
- Access control (164.312(a)(1))
- Audit control (164.312(b))
- Integrity 164.312(c)(1)
- Person or entity authentication)164.312(d)
- Transmission security 164.312(e)(1)
- Physical security of computers, servers, and other electronic devices
- Use of logins, passwords, encryption, and so forth, for electronic equipment and portable devices
- Backup of electronic tapes, CDs, disks, and so forth
- Secured e-mail and Web sites with the potential to contain PHI

Note: This list may not be all inclusive for a particular behavioral healthcare organization.

various laws regulating use and disclosure of PHI. For this reason, it is imperative that they be familiar with federal and state laws and keep abreast of new legislation in order to carry out the responsibilities entrusted to them.

Because of their daily oversight of PHI use and disclosure in behavioral healthcare organizations, HIM professionals also are well qualified—and should therefore come forward—to take part in the revision and/or development of laws and standards of practice related to the privacy, confidentiality, and security of behavioral healthcare PHI. Their contribution is valuable and necessary (and perhaps sometimes overlooked) within the overall healthcare industry and beyond.

References and Bibliography

Abraham, Prinny Rose. 2001. *Documentation and Reimbursement for Home Care and Hospice Programs.* Chicago: American Health Information Management Association.

American Health Information Management Association. 1998. Code of Ethics. Chicago: AHIMA.

Code of Federal Regulations, Title 42 CFR, Public Health Service, Director for Survey and Certification Group of the Center for Medicaid and State Operations. 2003. Letter of March 14. Available on-line at http://www.cms.hhs.gov/medicaid/survey-cert/sc0315.pdf.

Department of Health and Human Services. 2004. Substance Abuse and Mental Health Services Administration, Center for Substance Abuse Treatment. *The confidentiality of alcohol and drug abuse patient records regulation and the HIPAA Privacy Rule: Implications for alcohol and substance abuse programs.* Available on-line at www.hipaa.samhsa.gov/Part2ComparisonCleared.htm.

Department of Health and Human Services. 2003. Title 42, Public Health, Part 2, *Confidentiality of alcohol and drug abuse patient records.* Available on-line at www.access.gpo.gov/nara/cfr/waisidx_03/42cfr2_03.html.

Department of Health and Human Services. 2000. Privacy Rule Preamble: The Privacy Act of 1974. Available on-line at http://aspe.hhs.gov/admnsimp/.

Health Care Financing Administration, Department of Health and Human Services. 2000 (December). Standards for the Privacy of Individually Identifiable Health Information; Final Rule. 45 CFR, Parts 160 through 164. *Federal Register.* 65(250). Available on-line at www.aspe.hhs.gov/admnsimp.

Health Insurance Portability and Accountability Act of 1996. Public Law 104-191. Available on-line at http://www.hhs.gov/ocr/hipaa/.

Johns, Merida, editor. 2002. *Health Information Management Technology.* Chicago: American Health Information Management Association.

LaTour, Kathleen, and Eichenwald, Shirley, eds. 2002. *Health Information Management.* Chicago: American Health Information Management Association.

Legal Action Center. 2003. *Confidentiality and Communication: A Guide to the Federal Drug and Alcohol Law and HIPAA.* New York City: Legal Action Center.

Webster's new college dictionary, 3rd ed. 1996. New York City: Simon & Schuster, Inc.

Chapter 10

Outcomes Management and Performance Improvement

Tammy Young Lyles, RHIA

Continuous quality improvement (CQI) processes are designed to ensure that all services provided to healthcare consumers meet quality of service standards and outcome expectations. The purpose of implementing quality improvement (QI) processes is to evaluate and improve the services delivered and at the same time improve client outcomes and maintain or increase client satisfaction with services, and to achieve it all effectively and efficiently. Behavioral healthcare organizations develop and implement standards and policies according to many external and internal factors. Though there are more recent definitions, the American Hospital Association (AHA) said it best that QI is "An ongoing, organization-wide framework in which Health Services Organizations and their employees are involved in monitoring and evaluating all aspects of the agency's activities (inputs & processes) and outputs in order to improve them continuously" (AHA 1990).

F. Long (1995) provided a good description of outcomes measurement as follows: "A (health status) measure used in the context of assessing the effects of a (health care) intervention, or lack of intervention, or for measuring the extent to which a desired outcome or end-state is achieved." More simply stated, an **outcome** is a relative, measurable value, something to use to determine if services provided are having an effect (good or bad) on the population being served. By collecting certain information on clients and families receiving services, an organization can review aggregate data to determine the effectiveness (or lack of effectiveness) of services provided.

This chapter focuses on how to plan and measure quality improvement and outcomes management. It describes different performance improvement models and the various resources available to behavioral healthcare organizations that want to initiate a quality improvement program. Finally, the chapter discusses the many different measures that can be used to assess quality improvement program effectiveness.

Quality Improvement and Outcomes Management in Healthcare

Quality assurance (QA) is the process of evaluating service provision. It focuses mostly on clinical structures, processes, and outcomes. QA activities typically involve inspection, usually after the service has occurred, and traditionally have been performed by QA staff, physician advisors, peer review, and various committees. Most QA activities are motivated by regulatory compliance and risk management issues.

Continuous Quality Improvement

Many healthcare organizations have changed to the more proactive approach of CQI instead of QA. The Joint Commission on Accreditation of Healthcare Organizations (JCAHO) defined QI as "a process which de-emphasizes inspection (after the fact) and emphasizes overall improvement by reliable methods to study processes, by removing barriers to cooperation, by taking necessary actions to improve processes, and by fostering a constructive organization-wide commitment to improvement" (1991).

Although this is still an accurate definition, JCAHO standards (2003) define QI as "an approach to a continuous study and improvement of the processes of providing Behavioral Healthcare services to meet the needs of individuals served and others." QA is primarily the "monitoring" of activities, whereas quality improvement or **performance improvement** (PI) assesses the actual process in place and makes recommendations for improvement. Many accrediting bodies still require QA-type processes, along with QI or PI.

CQI focuses on all processes of the organization, not just clinical practices. It involves a gradual progression toward high-quality performance in all areas of the organization. Activities include quality assurance, performance assessment, risk assessment, identification of areas for improvement, comparison to external benchmarks, and attempts to provide better service by continuously monitoring all services provided. CQI activities are performed by everyone in the organization and often involve consumers and other external participants. CQI activities are motivated not only by regulatory compliance, but also by the need to succeed rather than to simply meet minimum regulations.

Developing a CQI Plan

CQI activities are often perceived as extra duty that take staff away from clinical and other direct client care duties. However, CQI is actually a process that helps organizations perform all their services more efficiently and effectively. A CQI plan is a proactive system to identify potential problems before or as they occur and to provide corrective actions concurrently. After implementation, a working CQI plan can help keep the organization competitive in today's healthcare market.

There are many definitions of quality. Behavioral healthcare organizations must determine internal definitions of quality of care and quality of service to use as guidelines for developing an individual CQI Plan. The CQI plan should reflect the healthcare organization's stated mission and strategic plans. These core documents should work together to direct the organization's future. Developing a CQI plan in conjunction with the organization's mission and strategic plan is a current trend among employers demanding that practitioners comply with established policy and procedure and be accountable for treatment provision and expected outcomes. Figure 10.1 lists some basic elements to consider when drafting a CQI Plan.

The Move toward Accreditation

Behavioral healthcare organizations have traditionally been slow to implement QA or CQI activities. Many behavioral healthcare organizations are nonprofit, private, or government organizations and have not responded previously to accreditation agencies such as the JCAHO, the Council on Accreditation (COA), or the Council on Accreditation for Rehabilitation Facilities (CARF). Moreover, they generally have survived on external funding sources such as the United Way, grant monies, and other charitable foundations.

However, with many organizations competing for their dollars, these funding sources are able to select carefully which organizations to support. Funding sources now request documented proof of services provided, self-assessment, and outcomes of service provision. They

Figure 10.1. Elements of a QI plan

A comprehensive QI plan should include or address the following:

- Organizational mission statement
- Goals and objectives
- QI committee activities and responsibilities
- Methods of reviewing/monitoring
- Incident prevention and management
- Record review/clinical review
- Satisfaction
- Community involvement/feedback
- Abuse and neglect reporting
- Performance improvement
- QI deficiencies from external agencies
- Corrective actions
- Internal communication and feedback process
- Confidentiality

primarily want to know what impact service provision has had on consumers or the community. They are no longer satisfied with an organization's simple statements of high-quality care provision. To determine where to spend their dollars, funding sources are using the process of outcomes measurement. An organization that cannot show results is unlikely to receive ongoing funding. If consumers are not showing improvement in functioning or family situations after receiving services, the administration should quickly assess what is happening in the organization. Moreover, today's clients expect healthcare organizations to demonstrate positive results of services provided. Thus, many behavioral healthcare organizations are now seeking accreditation and/or certification from accrediting bodies such as those mentioned above.

Performance Improvement Pioneers

There have been many pioneers in PI efforts. Among the best known are Walter Shewhart, W. Edwards Deming, and Joseph M. Juran.

Shewhart

Walter Shewhart, often referred to as the Grandfather of Total Quality Management, implemented the original ideas of total quality management (TQM). According to SkyMark Corporation, Shewhart preached the importance of adapting management processes to create profitable situations for both businesses and consumers (Skymark 2002). He believed that lack of information (of the processes) could obstruct control and management processes in a productive environment. From this opinion, he developed the PDSA cycle (discussed below) of improving processes, which is still used today.

Deming

W. Edwards Deming also was a pioneer in the field of measuring quality. Deming's statistical approach to measuring quality was influential in redeveloping postwar Japan with General Douglas McArthur. In 1999, both Deming and McArthur were noted in the *Los Angeles Times* as among the fifty people who most influenced business in this century. Deming taught several specific components for organizations to provide high-quality services. Two notable points from his 14 Points for Good Management (The W. Edwards Deming Institute 2000) are:

> Create a constancy of purpose of product and service. Quality comes not from inspection, but from improvement on the production process.

Deming promoted the belief that top leaders of the organization must believe and support the QI process for it to be successful. He further developed his descriptive, enumerative viewpoint of measuring quality and his theory of management after studying under Walter Shewhart.

Deming founded The W. Edwards Deming Institute in 1933 to provide educational services related to his teaching. Four general areas of focus of the institute are:

- Network and support
- Development and outreach
- Educational
- Research

Juran

Joseph M. Juran founded Juran Enterprises, Inc. in 1979 to market his consulting practice on a broader scale. Manufacturing companies were eager to implement QI activities because of increasing competition from Japanese manufacturers. Over time, Juran revised the training services offered to meet the growing needs of businesses, specifically in the field of quality measurement. According to G. Howland Blackiston (1996), former president of Juran Enterprises, Inc., Juran authored many books, including the *Quality Control Handbook* (first released in 1951 and now in its fourth edition), which is still a reference book used by quality managers today.

Performance Improvement Models

Most PI models share several main similarities. Each process begins with identifying an area of concern, assessing steps in the current process, making recommendations for change, and implementing change. The following subsections discuss two such models: the PDSA cycle and the PDCA cycle.

PDSA Cycle

The PDSA (Plan–Do–Study–Act) cycle of quality/performance improvement was developed by Walter Shewhart. His learning and improvement cycle combined creative management thinking with statistical analysis. Shewhart believed that the steps Plan, Do, Study, and Act ultimately lead to total quality improvement. The cycle is based on the idea that constant evaluation of management practices and the willingness of management to make changes are keys to the evolution of any successful organization.

PDCA Cycle

The PDCA (Plan–Do–Check–Act) cycle of quality/performance improvement also was developed by Walter Shewhart, but popularized by Deming in Japan. The method is conceptually simple and easily taught. The PDCA cycle has four basic steps:

1. Plan: Establish goals and objectives. This step involves data collection and analysis to propose a solution for identified issues.

2. Do: The second step tests the proposed solution. This is the implementation stage.

3. Check: Monitor outcomes against desired goals and objectives. Checking monitors the effectiveness of the proposed solution over time.

4. Act: Take appropriate actions, based on findings. This final step formalizes any changes that have proved effective.

Implementation of Performance Improvement

The first step in implementing a PI plan is to research and define expectations for performance. Are best practices published for the services provided? Do any accrediting bodies focus specifically on the area of service provision or type of organization? If so, using these resources will help the organization begin the process of implementing QI activities and developing their own outcome measures.

Although the steps involved can vary greatly based on service provision, most accrediting bodies offering accreditation for behavioral healthcare have specific guidelines for CQI plans and activities. These guidelines can become a valuable teaching tool for healthcare organizations seeking to implement quality practices.

Behavioral healthcare organizations also can look to their state and local mental health agencies and public health and human resources departments for quality guidelines.

Customer Focus

A key component of CQI is customer focus. Does society still reflect the old adage, The customer is always right? Healthcare organizations should continuously focus on customer needs. This obviously includes asking customers what their needs are, comparing the services being provided, and assessing customer satisfaction. Clients, consumers, or patients who receive services are not the only "customers" of behavioral healthcare organizations. Each organization determines specifically who its customers are, but typically customers include:

- Family members: Family members of consumers serve an important role in CQI and outcome management activities in behavioral healthcare organizations. Whether establishing an initial QI plan or revising ongoing outcome measures, organizations should consistently seek the input of family members of consumers. They often provide insight that consumers cannot.

- Local and state departments, such as mental health and human resources.

- Referral sources, including other practitioners, other behavioral healthcare organizations, medical facilities, probation officers, attorneys, and court systems.

- Community advocates, such as associations for the mentally ill, the mentally retarded, substance abuse prevention, domestic violence, and Alcoholics Anonymous.

- Organizational staff, including all staff who interact with the QI or health information management (HIM) departments.

Most accrediting bodies require healthcare organizations to develop some method of obtaining input from all customers or stakeholders. But gathering data is just the beginning. When information is received, it must be evaluated first to determine customer needs and then to assess the organization's services to meet those needs. Finally, changes should be implemented as soon as possible to better meet the needs identified.

Leadership Support

Administrative and supervisory leadership is absolutely necessary in designing, implementing, and maintaining CQI and **outcomes management** activities. Prior to implementing a QI plan, the organization must have a commitment from all management staff, beginning with the executive director. Without leadership support, a CQI plan is difficult to implement and almost impossible to maintain. Administrative (including the **board of directors**) and supervisory leaders must understand and be in agreement with the overall QI process and foresee the positive impact that can be achieved for the organization. Most accrediting bodies require that specific QI information be reported routinely to both the executive director and the board of directors.

Interdisciplinary Involvement

All disciplines of the behavioral healthcare organization must be involved in CQI and outcomes management activities. With the wealth of education, training, and experience throughout the organization, it would be inefficient to have only a few selected persons provide input into the CQI process. Multistaff involvement also increases ownership of organizational issues.

An effective way to utilize all disciplines is through CQI committees. A CQI committee can be directed and managed by specific CQI staff in order to document processes and achievements. However, the committee should reflect the entire organization, with all levels of staff and disciplines participating. Specific subcommittees should be established to address ongoing, categorical issues such as record/documentation reviews; risk assessment; incident reporting; medication management; safety; critical incident review; behavior modification, including physical restraints and seclusion/time-outs; and any others, as needed.

Individuals throughout the organization should be selected based on experience to lead the subcommittees and activities performed. Both administrative and clinical representatives are critical to the success and support of the QI/PI process. Information and documentation then should be reported back to the staff responsible for reporting CQI activities.

Teamwork

An organization with a successful QI program should have a foundation of teamwork. QI committee members, supervisors, and all employees should work together and in the organization's best interests. One major purpose of CQI is to empower all employees with the ability to see things differently, to identify issues or potential problems and to be able (and willing) to present ideas and make suggestions for changes.

The previous practice of QA as a stand-alone process was often viewed as a means of discovering errors and blaming staff. In contrast, CQI is a process of discovering new and better ways to perform services through ongoing efforts across the organization. This mirrors the focus of JCAHO (and other accrediting agencies) away from a punitive culture and toward a quality/safety culture for behavioral healthcare organizations. Staff also achieve a greater understanding of the process by participating in QI activities. Being able to see "the big picture" has proved helpful to many behavioral healthcare staff in their daily duties.

Employee Training

Training the employees of behavioral healthcare organizations is vital for QI and outcomes management processes. As policies and procedures are created and revised to mirror external and internal requirements, employee training becomes an ongoing task. QI staff/QI committee leaders should attempt to routinely attend staff meetings with each treatment program (outpatient, inpatient, day treatment, and so on) if such meetings exist. Designated CQI staff also should work closely with internal training departments. If training departments do not exist, designated QI staff members often serve as trainers in the organizations. If the organization does not have either internal training or a QI department, it should outsource these services. Organizations cannot expect to provide high-quality services and stay competitive in the current healthcare market without investing time and effort in educating employees on the importance of QI functions along with established and revised policies and procedures.

Figures 10.2, 10.3, and 10.4 show simple examples of handouts utilized by QI in staff education sessions. Proper documentation for billing purposes is another good topic for training behavioral healthcare staff.

An excellent opportunity exists for organizations to involve the next generation of professionals by working with interns and students through local universities and colleges. CQI committee meetings should be open to all employees, but a special effort should be made to include any interns or students currently serving the organization, regardless of their field of study.

Figure 10.2. Purposes of the medical record

- To provide a means of communication between all healthcare professionals contributing to the patient's care
- To serve as the basis for planning individual patient care
- To furnish documentary evidence of the course of the patient's illness and treatment during each admission or treatment visit
- To furnish documentary evidence of the course of the patient's illness and treatment to follow-up agencies or facilities to which the patient has been transferred for continued treatment
- To serve as the resource for analysis, study, and evaluation of the quality of care rendered for the patient by quality assessment, quality improvement, and utilization review committees
- To provide documentary evidence for attorneys and court systems of a patient's course of treatment to protect the legal interests of the patient and the organization
- To provide clinical data for use in research and education
- To provide accrediting, licensing, and certifying bodies the assurance that high-quality healthcare is being provided and to accredit, license, and certify the healthcare organization to continue providing services
- To provide information to Medicaid and other third-party payers to facilitate reimbursement

Figure 10.3. Client record reviews

Purpose
Presence of appropriate forms
Completion of forms

Big Picture
Example: Dates match, visitation forms are completed, client name and number are on each document

Consistency (through entire record)
Examples: Personal items brought to organization are returned at discharge
                   Client signatures are on consent/authorization forms

Details (signatures, location, times, daily shift notes, and so on)
Example: Yes _____   No _____
If no, why not? _____ If you mark no, you must answer why not.

Individual Checklist
Each program has its own checklist according to the record format of the program.

Deficiencies must be documented, corrected, and counted for quarterly report.

Ongoing Communication

Ongoing communication of activities, policies, and procedures is essential in maintaining effective CQI and outcomes management practices in any healthcare organization. Each CQI activity should generate a documented feedback loop. For example, a clinical review performed by members of the CQI committee should be documented as a CQI activity. Ideally, a designated employee responsible for CQI would maintain this information. That individual then would report the review findings to the treatment program being reviewed, with a due date for a written response. The program reviewed should respond to the CQI director (or designated employee), acknowledging receipt of the specific report and addressing corrective action plans for any deficiencies or areas of concern noted.

The director of QI or the leader of the QI committee should maintain all reports, reviews, and responses. This allows for an excellent paper trail of QI activities. It is noteworthy to state that all QI information can be legally nondiscoverable when marked accordingly. All QI review activity should be designated as peer review or CQI activity to protect the organization. This can include worksheets, minutes, memos, and any other correspondence specific to QI activities.

Figure 10.4. Consent versus authorization

What's the difference?

Consent

Purpose: To carry out treatment, payment, and healthcare operations

Exceptions: Emergency treatment situations, if required by law to treat an individual (inmates), significant language barriers in an emergency

Authorization

Purpose: To use or disclose protected health information except as otherwise permitted

Inclusion: A consent for uses and disclosures of PHI is required for treatment, payment, and healthcare operations. For use beyond these, a specific authorization is required.

Exceptions: An authorization must be obtained for any use or disclosure of psychotherapy notes except for use by the originator, in training, or to defend a legal action, with oversight by the Agency.

Redisclosure:

Must state that redisclosure will not be made without authorization.

Redisclosure:

Authorization must identify persons or classes of persons to whom entity may make requested use or disclosure.

Conditioning:

Provider may condition treatment on provision of consent.

Conditioning:

A provider may not condition treatment or payment on an authorization except for research-related treatment and when the disclosure is necessary to determine payment of a claim.

Expiration:

None

Expiration:

Date or event that relates to the individual or purpose of use required. Expiration period covered by state standards (Alabama: 1 year from date of signature).

"A covered health care provider must obtain the individual's consent prior to using disclosing protected health information (PHI) to carry out treatment, payment or health care operations. The covered health care provider may, without consent, use or disclose the protected health information IF:

The covered Health care provider:

- has an indirect treatment relationship with the individual (an indirect relationship between a health care provider and an individual in which the provider delivers health care to the individual based on the orders of another health care provider and the health care services, products, diagnoses, or results are typically furnished to the patient through another provider, rather than directly);

- or created or received the PHI in the course of providing health care to an individual who is an inmate;

- in an emergency situation if they get consent as soon as reasonable practical;

- is required by law to treat the individual, and the covered health care provider attempts to obtain such consent but is unable to;

- if they are unable to obtain consent due to substantial barriers to communicating with the individual and consent is clearly inferred."

Source: Volume 65, *Federal Register,* p. 82810, Section 164.506, p. 1449.

When accreditation or licensure agencies or external funding sources request proof of internal review processes, the information is well documented. This process also serves treatment program supervisors with documented evidence of training and education issues reviewed with employees through notation of corrective action plans, which can be used for staff productivity and performance evaluations.

Levels of Responsibility

Although it is ideal to have specific staff responsible for managing, leading, and coordinating CQI activities, each employee of the organization has some level of responsibility in participating in the CQI process. CQI committees and subcommittees direct the organization as an active, ongoing leader of the improvement process.

Implementing a CQI plan leads to the establishment, revision, and implementation of the organization's policies and procedures, strategic planning, and staff training and education. When the system is implemented, all services can become more effective and efficient. Organizing and documenting these activities takes a lot of time, specific focus, and effort, but the rewards can be unlimited to the individual programs as well as the organization. If services are not more effective after a CQI plan is in place, it is much easier to identify the problem areas and develop corrective actions.

Many behavioral healthcare organizations perform CQI activities in their daily operations. A supervisor reviewing a client's record to see what is missing, designing a new form to better capture pertinent data, and sending out a satisfaction survey are all examples of CQI activities. For many organizations, these activities are ongoing and simply need to be documented as CQI. The key is to document processes as they occur, which is easier than attempting to compile information from activities done annually. It is imperative that at least one staff member in each organization be assigned responsibility for coordinating and documenting all CQI information.

Many organizations do not have the financial resources to hire specific CQI staff. CQI is a major component of every healthcare organization, and all organizations should strive to have staff dedicated to the process of managing the CQI activities globally or administratively. Staying current on standards and requirements from all appropriate external agencies can be a full-time position for even the smallest organization. Administration should consider the long-term benefits of hiring CQI staff instead of focusing on the additional salary expense for the organization.

As the quality of services provided throughout the organization improves, and outcome results show proof of the organization's treatment successes, business will increase along with the organization's reputation as a high-quality provider. HIM professionals make excellent candidates for these positions. Their broad knowledge of health information systems, services, documentation requirements, privacy and security issues, and basic adherence to external guidelines allows HIM professionals to coordinate all QI activities effectively and efficiently.

Guidance Resources

Numerous resources are available to behavioral healthcare organizations that need guidance on launching and implementing performance improvement efforts.

Federal Legislation

The Health Insurance Portability and Accountability Act (HIPAA) is a current major focus of federal legislation regarding privacy and security issues. Healthcare organizations deemed as covered entities must be in compliance with the HIPAA guidelines. The HIPAA standards involve several areas of focus, but the primary focus of concern for healthcare organizations is privacy and security. The privacy standards alone are more than 1,500 pages.

Behavioral healthcare organizations must become aware of and maintain compliance with these federal guidelines. There are many exceptions for behavioral healthcare. Stricter guidelines are in place regarding privacy and security based on the nature of the population being served. Ensuring that the organization's practices are in line with HIPAA guidelines often falls to the QI staff. Many organizations retain legal counsel to assist them with sorting through the vast amounts of HIPAA information along with state and local laws concerning privacy, confidentiality, security, and so on. (See chapter 9 for additional information on HIPAA.)

Accrediting Bodies

QI and outcomes management practices were first presented by accrediting bodies of healthcare organizations. (See chapter 7 for a discussion of accrediting bodies.) Initially, behavioral healthcare organizations did not have internal service models or protocols that staff members were expected to follow. Confusing to begin with, these practices are becoming more clearly established. Accreditation agencies now direct healthcare organizations on what to monitor, what activities are required, how to develop internal processes, and so on. Although most accreditation processes are voluntary, there can be financial and legal incentives for organizations to attain accreditation. The most noteworthy advantages of achieving accreditation status are meeting requirements for certain client groups, validating the quality of care provided, and providing a competitive edge against other healthcare organizations.

Additional advantages to accreditation are Medicare and Medicaid reimbursement and meeting requirements for managed care organizations (MCOs) and other third-party payers. Behavioral healthcare organizations can increase their referrals and client caseload by meeting external accreditation guidelines (discussed below).

State and Local Agencies

Each state may have governing state and/or local agencies that certify or extend licensure to behavioral healthcare providers. These agencies establish state or local guidelines and standards of expectations for behavioral healthcare organizations to receive licensure or certification. Organizations frequently report statistical data to these state and local departments.

Managed Care Organizations

MCOs focus on appropriate credentialing of staff providing services, length of treatment, and cost-effectiveness. They often limit the amount of services provided to individuals based on specific criteria for services. The National Committee for Quality Assurance (NCQA) specifically accredits MCOs. The JCAHO also accredits MCOs through application of its standards in the *Comprehensive Accreditation Manual for Managed Behavioral Healthcare.*

Internal and External Benchmarks

A benchmark is a guideline for best practice or service. Healthcare organizations can choose benchmarks based on accreditation agency standards or develop internal benchmarks according to the services being provided. Specialty areas of behavioral healthcare often have difficulty in locating best practice benchmarks for comparison.

Possible resources for benchmarks are discussed in the following subsections.

External Requirements

One role of the organization's CQI staff is to serve as liaison for external accreditation and licensing agencies. Each behavioral healthcare organization must maintain current knowledge of all applicable standards and requirements. Most organizations are required to meet or exceed the standards and requirements of multiple external sources. One organization may be required to meet standards from local and state governing organizations, Medicare *Conditions of Participation,* third-party contractual agreements, and the JCAHO. The simplest way to achieve compliance is to implement the strictest standards that apply to the organization. Having a CQI director allows for close observation of all standards and requirements, along with revisions as they occur. Internal policies and procedures then can be revised accordingly, to be followed by educating and training staff appropriately.

A compilation of on-line databases was printed in the July 2003 *National Council News,* a newsletter of the National Council for Community Behavioral Healthcare. (See figure 10.5 for resources noted for best practices and outcome measures.)

Accreditation Standards

The following organizations issue accreditation standards that behavioral healthcare organizations may use as benchmarks.

Joint Commission on Accreditation of Healthcare Organizations

The Joint Commission on Accreditation of Healthcare Organizations (JCAHO) has been active in behavioral healthcare accreditation since 1969 when it began accrediting organizations providing services for mental retardation and developmentally disabled individuals. In 1972, JCAHO began evaluating and accrediting organizations providing mental health and chemically dependent services. In 2004, JCAHO accredited more than 1,800 behavioral healthcare organizations.

Accreditation is available from JCAHO for several services including addictions, case management, corrections, crisis stabilization, family preservation and wraparound services, forensics, foster care, therapeutic foster care, in-home and on-line services, opioid treatment programs, outpatient, partial hospital, day treatment, adult day care, intensive outpatient (IOP), residential, shelters, and special populations such as children and youth, persons with addictions, persons with disabilities, transitional supervised living, and vocational rehabilitation.

JCAHO standard address the important functions regarding the care of clients and the management of organizations framed as performance objectives that are unlikely to change substantially over time. Standards are developed in consultation with behavioral healthcare experts, providers, measurement experts, clients, and families. In 2000, JCAHO launched an internal review of its standards and requirements for organizations to demonstrate compliance.

JCAHO's internal review led to the 2004 development of the "Shared Visions—New Pathways" process, which shifts the behavioral healthcare organization's focus from survey preparation to safety of client care. By decreasing the overall number of standards and increasing the clarity and relevance of remaining standards, the paperwork and documentation compliance burden is greatly reduced for organizations seeking accreditation.

Organizations perform a Periodic Performance Review (PPR) midway through their accreditation cycle to evaluate their compliance against current standards. Corrective Action Plans (CAP) are then developed based on the areas of noncompliance identified. A new scoring system eliminates the overall score used previously and focuses more on the specific standards needed to achieve and maintain excellent operational systems.

Council on Accreditation for Children and Families Services

The **Council on Accreditation for Children and Families Services** (COA) was founded in 1977 by the Child Welfare League of America (CWLA) and Family Services America (FSA). The COA focuses on best practice standards for services provided to children, youths, and families and accredits organizations throughout the United States and Canada.

According to Chapter 2 of the COA standards manual, Continuous Quality Improvement, each organization is required to demonstrate implementation of a comprehensive CQI plan. As described in Standard G2.1.01, a CQI document or plan should address each of the following (COA 2001, G2.1.01):

- Stakeholder participation
- Long-term planning

Figure 10.5. Resources for best practices and outcome measures

Evidence-Based Mental Health Interventions
The Evaluation Center @ HSRI   www.tecathsri.org
Evidence-based Practices Metabase (EbPMetabase) Version 1.0 is a searchable electronic database containing information about reviews (narrative reviews, systematic reviews, and meta-analyses) that synthesize the evidence on psychosocial interventions for adults with severe mental illness. EbPMetabase can be searched by outcome and disorder. The Evaluation Center @ HSRI is a SAMHSA-funded organization that provides technical assistance to states, public entities within states, and other organizations to improve the evaluation, development, and operation of adult mental health services.
Implementing Evidence-based Mental Health (University of Oxford, Oxford, UK)   www.cebmh.com
This site offers links to journals and databases that contain reviews and studies on evidence-based mental health.
Implementing Evidence-Based Practice Project   www.mentalhealthpractices.org
This site houses information in six evidence-based practices: illness management and recovery, medication management approaches in psychiatry, assertive community treatment, family psychoeducation, supported employment, and co-occurring disorders: integrated dual-diagnosis treatment. Each intervention also provides additional links and resources, training contacts, and articles.
Substance Abuse and Mental Health Services Association (SAMHSA)   www.samhsa.gov
This site is run by the U.S. Department of Health and Human Services and contains information on federally funded grants and mental health and substance abuse developments. This site can be searched to find information on mental health and to learn more about the various initiatives around mental health.
NAMI TRIAD (Treatment Recovery Information and Advocacy Database)   www.nami.org/triadfeature.html
TRIAD is a database available through NAMI (National Association of the Mentally Ill). It plans to include reports on the implementation of evidence-based practices and their outcomes and an interactive guide for consumers and family members on evidence-based treatment for schizophrenia. The TRIAD site also plans to have a national survey regarding consumers' and families' experiences with evidence-based practices, a systematic assessment of discrimination in legislation and newspaper coverage of mental illness across the fifty states, and a national survey of consumer and family member experiences of evidence-based care and outcomes.
Sites Containing Reviews of Interventions for Mental Health and Other Medical Disorders
The Cochrane Collaboration (Based in the UK, but reviews are international) www.update-software.com/cochrane or www.thecochranelibrary.com
The Cochran Library includes several databases containing abstracts, articles, and other information regarding evidence-based health practices. Published on a quarterly basis, its goal is to provide consumers and providers as well as researchers, teachers, and persons at all levels of involvement in healthcare access to an extensive collection of comprehensive and high-quality evidence-based reviews. This database is searchable by keywords of specific interventions or mental illnesses.
The University of York NHS Centre for Reviews and Dissemination (CRD) www.york.ac.uk/inst/crd/index.htm
The CRD contains a number of tools for finding and understanding evidence-based medicine. The site has ten gateways to information on its home page: publications, databases, research, dissemination, about CRD, information and enquiry service, cost-effectiveness information, Cochrane Library training and user group, links, and search. Most useful to finding evidence-based practices are publications, research, and databases.
National Guideline Clearinghouse   www.guideline.gov/resources/guideline_index.aspx
Sponsored by the U.S. Agency for Healthcare Research and Quality, this site allows users to search guidelines for medical interventions. In November 2004, a search for the term *mental health* produced 332 guidelines, whereas the terms *psychiatry* produced 430 guidelines, *psychology* produced 417 guidelines, *depression* produced 256 guidelines, and so on. This database is updated weekly. It should be noted that all the guidelines on this site are not specifically evidence based.

- Short-term planning

- Internal quality monitoring

- Case record review

- Outcomes measurement

- Measurement of consumer satisfaction

- Feedback mechanisms

- Information management

- Corrective action

Specifically required is having a well-defined written process for improving the organization's overall performance and for meeting standards that promote quality outcomes. Standard G2.1.02 in chapter 2 lists additional required elements, including (COA 2001):

- Written description of QI activities

- Assignment of responsibility for coordinating QI activities

- Specific time frames

- Description of stakeholder involvement

- Definitions of methods for monitoring

- Description of reporting processes

- Detail of feedback mechanism and corrective action

- Descriptions of long- and short-term planning

In February 2003, COA conducted a survey of more than 1,000 accredited organizations. Respondents overwhelmingly confirmed that the existing process of accreditation was extremely valuable but needed to be streamlined for content and demonstration of compliance.

To address these concerns, COA assembled a task force of representatives from accredited agencies to work with COA staff to revise and reduce the reaccreditation process for behavioral healthcare agencies. While organizations are still responsible for compliance with all applicable standards, a reaccreditation process, which decreases the paperwork and documentation burden of compliance for organizations previously accredited, has been developed. The number of submitted documents required for compliance has dropped from more than 400 to approximately 40 for reaccreditation visits by COA. This redirected focus reinforces the need for organizations to evaluate themselves continuously and maintain quality service provision at all times. The redesigned reaccreditation process became available for previously accredited organizations in 2004.

Child Welfare League of America

The **Child Welfare League of America** (CWLA) is an association of more than 1,170 public and private nonprofit agencies and organizations across the U.S. and Canada that are devoted to improving life for abused, neglected, and otherwise vulnerable children and young people and their families. It is the nation's oldest and largest membership-based child welfare organization. The CWLA began under the administration of Theodore Roosevelt in 1909 at the White House Conference on the Care of Dependent Children. It also is the oldest and largest publisher of child welfare materials in the world, under its Child & Family Press imprint. CWLA continues to develop standards of excellence and disseminate information through its library and information services (CWLA 2001).

A collaborative agency, the CWLA is committed to providing information on best practices, benchmarking, research information, and general guidelines and education for behavioral healthcare organizations. The CWLA notes the national goals of safety, permanency, and well-being as a framework for its development of an outcome measures system (CWLA 1998).

These national goals were established in response to the congressional directive in section 203 of the Adoption and Safe Families Act of 1997 (ASFA) by a consultation group implemented to guide the development of these core measures. These national outcome measures for state child welfare systems were first published in the *Federal Register* on August 20, 1999.

The CWLA Outcomes 1998 Annual Report initially detailed the guiding principles that led to the choice of these measures and provided further information and examples of specific measures in each of these categories. (See figure 10.6 for examples.) CWLA has continued to address these measures that focus on the well-being of children, youth, and families.

American Osteopathic Association

The **Healthcare Facilities Accreditation Program** (HFAP) of the **American Osteopathic Association** (AOA) is recognized nationally by the federal government, state governments, insurance carriers, and MCOs. The program is one of only two voluntary accreditation programs in the United States authorized by the Centers for Medicare and Medicaid Services (CMS) to survey hospitals under Medicare.

Figure 10.6.   Excerpts from CWLA Outcomes 1998 Annual Report

I.   SAFETY

   1.   To reduce the recurrence of child abuse and/or neglect. An organization providing in home Services might chose an outcome such as, "There will be no re-occurrences of abuse and/or neglect while services are being provided in the family home."

   2.   To reduce the incidence of child abuse and/or neglect in Foster Care. A Foster Care program may collect and measure data of all abuse/neglect incidents occurring to clients currently in Foster Care.

II.   PERMANENCY

   1.   To increase permanency for children in Foster Care. A Foster Care program can review statistics of discharged clients to determine rates of Reunification with biological families, Adoption, and Independence/Emancipation at discharge. Internal benchmarks can be developed, such as "85% of clients successfully discharged from the Foster Care program will be reunited with their Biological Families at discharge."

   2.   To reduce time in foster care to reunification without increasing re-entry. When children are removed from the home, the focus of service delivery should be on safely reunifying the family as soon as possible, when appropriate. Clients returned home too soon may be at risk for re-entry into Out of Home care. A possible Outcome measure could be "Of clients discharged from Out of Home Care, 90% will remain stable in their placed environment at 6 months and 1 year post-discharge."

   3.   To reduce time in Foster Care/Out of Home care to adoption. In some situations, Reunification with biological families is not in the best interest of the client. A goal of service should be to decrease the time a client stays in Out of Home care until a finalized adoption is achieved. A possible outcome measure would be "90% of clients (eligible for and with a Discharge plan of Adoption) admitted to Out of Home care will achieve finalized adoption within 24 months."

III.   WELL-BEING

   Well-being is defined by CWLA as "families having the capacity to provide for their children's needs, children having educational opportunities and achievements appropriate to their abilities, and children receiving physical and mental health services adequate to meet their needs." Measures specific to Well-Being are still being developed at this time. CWLA's plan is to develop a comprehensive framework that will describe the essential components and characteristics of a community-based approach to ensuring every child is healthy, safe and able to reach his or her full potential by making the well-being of children, youth and their families a priority.

Source: American CWLA.

The AOA requires organizations seeking accreditation to follow the Medicare guidelines for QA and PI as published by the Centers for Medicare & Medicaid Services (CMS). According to HFAP's *Accreditation Standards Manual,* a facility's QA/PI program must cover each of the following elements (AOA 2003):

- Development
- Implementing
- Maintaining
- Effective
- Ongoing
- Facilitywide
- Contract services
- Improved outcomes
- Reduction of medical errors

The National Committee for Quality Assurance

The NCQA's accreditation of **managed behavioral healthcare organizations** (MBHOs) rewards organizations that focus on quality, which, in turn, may help improve the nation's healthcare. The NCQA has developed a report card for MBHOs in which they meet quality of care standards.

NCQA MBHO Accreditation Program is designed to:

- Foster accountability among MBHOs for the quality of care and services the members receive

- Provide employers, public purchasers, plans, and consumers with meaningful information regarding MBHOs

- Strengthen MBHO systems for population-based CQI programs

- Encourage effectiveness in the provision of behavioral healthcare by addressing the need for prevention, early intervention, and coordination of behavioral healthcare with medical care

The NCQA approaches accreditation through the complementary strategies of accreditation and PI. The focus is to provide information that enables consumers to make informed healthcare decisions and choices.

Council on Accreditation of Rehabilitation Facilities

CARF is an independent, not-for-profit organization that reviews and grants accreditation services nationally and internationally on request of facilities and individual service programs. The commission approaches accreditation in a consultative process, and assists organizations in improving the quality of services provided, demonstrating value, and meeting internationally recognized organizational and program-specific standards. The mission of CARF is "to promote the quality, value, and optimal outcomes of services through accreditation that centers on enhancing the lives of the persons served" (CARF 2004).

Conditions of Participation

Many organizations have contracts with state departments, Medicaid, third-party payers, and MCOs to provide specific services to consumers. As contracts are developed with these sources, specific requirements should be addressed. Most contracts include details of liability coverage responsibility, staff credentialing requirements, expected services to be provided, reporting processes, confidentiality agreements, and, of course, financial agreements.

MCOs and other third-party payers often have specific guidelines as well. Contracts should be specific to these requirements and updated on a timely basis.

State departments of mental health and mental retardation, Medicaid, and Medicare generally have their own established guidelines and standards by which they expect organizations to practice. These standards should be accessible to behavioral healthcare organizations directly from the individual source.

Outcome Measures

Compiling outcome measures for organizations shows whether high-quality services are being provided and external requirements are being met. (See figure 10.7 for the four basic types of outcome measures.) The data provided through outcome measures are now recognized as being highly useful to:

- Marketing and public relations departments in promoting the organization

- Human resources departments in recruiting and retaining skilled staff and improving staff morale

- The organization in seeking funding for the expansion of or additional service provision

Outcome data are used to assist clinicians in client treatment planning and review, as well as in longitudinal studies to systematically improve the quality of behavioral healthcare throughout the organization.

After many years of QA/QI monitoring, the current consensus is that quality of services can be measured most effectively based on client progress. Many organizations develop quality teams to review and develop outcome measures for the organization. Because most behavioral healthcare organizations are not positioned to have formal QI staff, the quality team may simply be the organization's supervisory staff. QI and outcomes management activities often fall to administrative and program supervisors. When responsibility has been assigned for development of outcome measures, indicators must be defined.

Core Measures

Many accreditation organizations require adherence to some basic or core outcome measures. Core measures are general categories of measurement. (See figure 10.8 for examples of core measures of client services.)

Behavioral healthcare organizations also measure whether service provision adheres to culturally competent practices, state and federal guidelines for permanency planning, expected frequency and length of services, successful completion, and recidivism.

Behavior healthcare organizations must decide what elements are important to monitor, along with the requirements to meet for external sources. Some accreditation organizations require organizations to meet a percentage of their published core measures, along with a number of additional organizationally defined measures. For example, the COA requires any therapeutic foster care program seeking accreditation to have at least one outcome measure that addresses the issue of permanency planning. In other words, each child who enters into a therapeutic foster care program should have a specific, individualized treatment goal regarding where he or she will go after discharge or termination of care. If reunification with the family is a possibility, the child's treatment plan should reflect attempts to work with the family in preparation for his or her discharge. If there is no viable family, other support systems and/or adoption should be pursued.

Figure 10.7. Development of measures

Outcome measures include:

- Specific
- Measurable
- Observable
- Time limited
- Clearly stated
- Achievable

There are four basic types of outcome measures:

1. **Process:** Measures what is done to improve or maintain health (preventive care, counseling to give up unhealthy behaviors, or delivering care that minimizes any deterioration in health). Example: Following completion of program, 80 percent of clients will show improvement in anger management skills as evidenced by pre- and posttest scores.

2. **Accessibility:** Measures how easily and quickly clients can receive services. Examples: Time it takes to get an appointment, time spent in waiting rooms, time it takes for someone to answer the phone, and/or return a call.

3. **Experience:** Measures what the client "experiences" while in care. Example: Eighty percent of clients responding to satisfaction surveys will report services received as good or excellent.

4. **Effectiveness:** Measures effectiveness of services provided or a change in client's status after receiving services. Example: At the time of discharge, 80 percent of clients will have met 80 percent of their identified treatment goals. At six-month follow-up, 90 percent of clients who completed the antismoking class will report continued abstinence from smoking.

For each indicator or measurement chosen, staff must determine what is an acceptable, appropriate, or "quality" outcome. Criteria for each measure must be predetermined. Outcomes must reflect currently acceptable practice and be agreed on by all participating staff. Time frames for review and reporting must be established. When the time frame for data collection is over, a review of the actual outcome compared to the proposed outcome can provide insight into the organization's service provision.

JACHO's ORYX Initiative (discussed in chapter 6) outlined a series of major steps designed to modernize the accreditation process. Standardized core performance measures introduced in 2002 permit comparison of the actual results across hospitals.

As of this writing, the JCAHO does not have core measures specific to behavioral healthcare but does routinely request documented information on client satisfaction, length of treatment, improved functioning after service provision, and so on.

The COA lists the following "domains" of outcome measures for its accredited organizations:

- Change in clinical status
- Change in functional status
- Health, welfare, and safety
- Permanency of life situation

The COA requires specific outcomes measurement for certain populations served. For foster care and adoption programs, the COA requires outcome measurement specific to permanency-of-life situations whereas mental health counseling, day treatment, residential, and substance abuse programs must measure change in clinical status. In child protective services, the COA requires measurement of health, welfare, and safety (COA 2001, G2.7.01).

Figure 10.8. Core measures of client services

- **Appropriateness of service:** Upon any review of records or billing information, it can be determined if the client received services inconsistent with the admitting diagnosis or presenting problem. For example: Has the client received family therapy when the client has no family or support system identified? Is the client being seen weekly/monthly/daily by a psychiatrist when the client is not receiving medications?

- **Necessity of service (medical model):** Often used in hospital settings, the medical model is frequently based on guidelines established by external forces, such as insurers. An example would be if a client expresses suicidal tendencies, close observation or a "closed" facility would be appropriate. If a client is threatening physical harm to others or themselves, physical restraint may be necessary.

- **Availability of services:** Organizations often monitor the availability of their services to determine if they are meeting the needs of their community. Information can be gathered on the number of clients placed on waiting lists or referred to other organizations. This information can help an organization determine whether to expand or limit certain services.

- **Safety:** A review of incident reports, falls, and other safety issues is often performed to determine if the organization is providing a safe environment for service provision.

- **Accessibility:** Many external accrediting bodies require that behavioral healthcare organizations are accessible to the physically handicapped and other individuals. Increasingly, more organizations are required to provide assistance to clients who are hearing and speech impaired, sight impaired, or have cultural and language preferences. A review of resources within an organization can assess the level of accessibility for the population being served.

- **Advocacy:** Some behavioral healthcare organizations work with children in out-of-home placements, such as residential settings, group homes, and foster care. These populations require a great deal of communication with state and local agencies, such as the departments of human resources/welfare. Organizations can play a vital role in long-term planning for clients by working closely with the government agencies involved in the clients' care. There are also national, state, and local advocacy agencies that organizations may affiliate with such as Twelve-Step Groups like Alcoholics Anonymous (AA), Narcotics Anonymous (NA), Gamblers Anonymous (GA), and so on. The National Association for the Mentally Ill (NAMI) is a nonprofit, self-help support and advocacy organization dedicated to achieve equitable services and treatment for the severely mentally ill. NAMI has state and local chapters that work with clients, families, and friends of the mentally ill. Behavioral healthcare organizations can choose to affiliate with many advocacy groups at local, state, and federal levels. QI programs often monitor the amount of contact with advocacy groups for specific populations to assist in determining the continuity and quality of care provided.

- **Effectiveness:** Monitoring the effectiveness of services provided is a commonly used outcome measure. Effectiveness can be measured simply by reviewing success rates such as a client's completion of treatment, ability to return to the home environment (for out-of-home placements), a return to work, school, completion of individual treatment goals, and so on.

- **Efficiency:** Monitoring the efficiency of service provision is a method of reviewing the services that have been provided, compared to the identified needs of the client. Productivity of individual staff can be monitored for number of clients seen, caseloads, and success rates.

- **Continuity:** Many behavioral healthcare organizations provide follow-up or aftercare services to clients after services are completed. Following up with a client in six months or one year after they have completed services can provide valuable information on the continuity of care. Some organizations focus their follow-up on issues identified, but not resolved, level/appropriateness of placement after services, relapse, and so on.

- **Timeliness:** Monitoring the timeliness of services is a fairly simple outcome measure. For example, external guidelines (such as Medicaid and Medicare) require that intakes and treatment plans be completed within a certain time frame to be considered a billable service. An outcome measure can be established to monitor if all initial treatment plans are being done in a timely manner.

- **Cost-effectiveness:** Some organizations choose to monitor overall costs of specific programs. An inpatient substance abuse facility, for example, might calculate the total cost per client, per day to determine the cost-effectiveness of treatment. Managed care organizations (MCOs) and employee assistance programs (EAPs) also calculate total cost per employee to provide information to the client companies that purchase their services. This type of monitor often leads to a reduction in length of stay (for inpatient services) or a reduction in the amount or frequency of sessions/services authorized.

- **Changes in functioning level:** Monitoring changes in the client's level of functioning is a good way to determine if the organization's services provided are having an effect on the client served. One common method of collecting this information is through the use of the GAF (Global Assessment of Functioning) scale, which is shown in figure 10.9. GAF scores are generally recorded at intake through completion of a DSM diagnosis, Axis I-V. Axis V specifically lists the GAF score at the client's admission for services. The GAF score is then updated either quarterly or annually during review/amendment of the client's treatment plan.

- **Compliance with standards/regulations:** Based on findings following an audit or site visit from an external agency, specific reviews can be developed to address any issues identified. For example, if the audit noted that individual treatment plans were not being done in a timely manner, the organization could implement a review process to randomly review a certain percentage of records. The review should focus on comparing the dates of treatment plans to the date of admission/intake, along with the timeliness requirement established by the external agency. If a significant number of cases are found to be delinquent, further training of staff may be necessary. Documentation of reviews, findings, and communications to programs should be maintained, along with any training that occurs. This documentation can be helpful the next time the external agency comes for a visit. The auditors will see that the organization has taken their recommendations seriously.

CARF requires organizations to gather basic information for measuring and managing outcomes. Exact outcome measures are not provided, however; the information gathered must adhere to the following basic principles as outlined in CARF's standards manual (2002). The information gathered must be:

- Relevant to the core values and mission of the healthcare organization
- Linked to benefiting the persons served
- Be of value to stakeholders
- Allow for comparison with internal/historical data and comparable external data, when such are publicly available

Quality Assurance Measures

QA specific measures are designed to assess the quality of service implementation and involve ongoing efforts to determine how close actual service provision is to the service delivery intended (Mordock 2002). QA measures are done routinely to monitor ongoing practices.

Examples of QA measures include:

- One hundred percent of open clinical case records will be reviewed every six months and at closure to monitor documentation compliance.
- Ninety percent of all incoming telephone calls will be answered by the third ring.
- Ninety percent of clients calling for a first appointment will be scheduled within one week of the call.
- Ninety-eight percent of suspected abuse/neglect incidents will be reported in a timely manner to all necessary authorities.
- Ninety-five percent of all requests for client information will be answered within ten working days.

Performance Improvement Measures

PI measures are done routinely to monitor the outcomes of or responses to services provided. Examples of PI measures include:

- Of clients completing satisfaction surveys, 95 percent will rate services received as excellent or good.
- Of referral sources completing satisfaction surveys, 95 percent will rate services provided as excellent or good.
- Ninety percent of children served in therapeutic foster care will remain stabilized in a therapeutic foster home until treatment goals are met and/or the child is moved to a less restrictive environment.
- Eighty-five percent of patient clients will successfully complete treatment as evidenced by recorded progress or resolution of identified treatment goals.
- Clients completing treatment will achieve moderate progress on at least 70 percent of their identified treatment goals by the time of discharge.

Figure 10.9 shows a Global Assessment of Functioning (GAF) scale, a recognized tool for assessing an individual's current level of functioning. By gathering GAF scores periodically throughout service provision, organizations may assess a client's improvement or lack or improvement over time.

Figure 10.9. Global assessment of functioning scale (GAF)

GLOBAL ASSESSMENT OF FUNCTIONING SCALE (GAF)	

Rating: Rate the client's lowest level of functioning in the last week by selecting the lowest range which describes his/her functioning on a hypothetical continuum of mental health illness. For example, a patient whose 'behavior is considerably influenced by delusions' (range 21–30) should be given a rating in that range even though he/she has 'major impairment in several areas' (range 31–40). Use intermediary levels when appropriate (eg., 35, 58, 63). Rate actual functioning independent of whether or not the patient is receiving and may be helped by medication or some other form of treatment. _____

100–91	No symptoms, superior functioning in a wide range of activities, life's problems never seem to get out of hand; is sought out by others because of his/her warmth and integrity.
90–81	Transient symptoms may occur, but good functioning in all areas, interested and involved in a wide range of activities, socially effective, generally satisfied with life, 'everyday' worries that only occasionally get out of hand.
80–71	Minimal symptoms may be present but no more than slight impairment in functioning, varying degrees of 'everyday' worries and problems that sometimes get out of hand.
70–61	Some mild symptoms (e.g., depressive mood and mild insomnia) OR some difficulty in several areas of functioning, but generally functioning fairly well, has some meaningful interpersonal relationships and most untrained people would not consider him/her 'sick'.
60–51	Moderate symptoms OR generally functioning with some difficulty (e.g., few friends, flat affect, depressed mood and pathological self-doubt, euphoric mood and pressured speech, moderately severe antisocial behavior).
50–41	Any serious symptomology or impairment in functioning that most clinicians would think obviously requires treatment or attention (e.g., suicidal preoccupation or gesture, severe obsessional rituals, frequent anxiety attacks, serious antisocial behavior, compulsive drinking).
40–31	Major impairment in several areas, such as work, family relations, judgment, thinking or mood (e.g., depressed, avoids friends, unable to do housework), OR some impairment in reality testing or communication (e.g., speech is at times obscure, illogical or irrelevant), OR single serious suicide attempt.
30–21	Unable to function in almost all areas (e.g., stays in bed all day, no job, no friends) OR behavior is considerably influenced by either delusions or hallucinations OR serious impairment in communication (e.g., sometimes incoherent or unresponsive) or judgment (acts grossly inappropriately).
20–11	Needs some supervision to prevent hurting self and others, or to maintain minimal personal hygiene (e.g., repeated suicide attempts, frequently violent, manic excitement) OR gross impairment in communication (e.g., largely incoherent or mute).
10–1	Needs constant supervision for several days to prevent hurting self or others, and makes no attempt to maintain minimal personal hygiene.

Reprinted with permission from the *Diagnostic and Statistical Manual of Mental Disorders,* Copyright © 2000. American Psychiatric Association.

Organization/Program-Specific Outcome Measures

Most behavioral healthcare organizations have multiple service components. Measures of quality vary from service to service. Outcome or performance measures should be specific to the population being served.

Examples of program-specific outcome measures include:

- Eighty-five percent of clients completing the Domestic Violence Intervention Program will not be court referred back to the program for violent offenses within one year of receiving services.

- Eighty percent of parents participating the Family Attention Deficit Disorder Program will report an increased ability to identify and use family coping skills with their children as a result of services received.

- Eighty percent of children attending substance abuse prevention/education classes will demonstrate an 85 percent increase in knowledge regarding substance abuse prevention as indicated by pre- and posttests.

- Eighty-five percent of clients participating in anger management groups will demonstrate an ability to use positive skills in communication and anger management learned, evidenced by role-play, parental, and teacher reports.

Typical Performance Improvement Projects

Many behavioral healthcare organizations perform PI by focusing efforts on utilization or clinical review, record or administrative review, consumer satisfaction, incident reporting, and, of course, outcome measures. These items are required by most accreditation organizations.

Utilization Management

Utilization management (UM) or utilization review is a process that monitors the appropriateness of service provision through the continuous review of random clinical or service records. Records are reviewed from each service program of the behavioral healthcare organization. A sample of client records for each staff providing services should be reviewed.

Review Criteria

Records are reviewed concurrently and retrospectively to determine whether the services provided are necessary and appropriate and are being rendered in the most appropriate clinical setting. Records are reviewed by preestablished criteria for each program of service. For services to be considered necessary, the professional community must regard them as safe and effective treatment for the problems for which they are sought. In addition, services must be provided at a level of intensity that is consistent with an appropriate focus of treatment. The focus of treatment and the intensity of services are maintained on a continuous basis. Criteria can include:

- Age of clients appropriate for service
- IQ or functional ability to participate in services
- Diagnostic guidelines, both inclusive (client's desire to receive treatment, physical/mental ability to participate, compliance with medication and treatment recommendations) and exclusive (client's lack of participation, active substance abuse, noncompliance with treatment recommendations)
- Discharge indicators (client's lack of minimal progress over a certain time frame, persistent noncompliance with medication or other treatment, need to receive treatment in a different setting)

Figure 10.10 offers a simple method for keeping track of quality improvement in areas identified as needing improvement. Figure 10.11 is a sample QI review form used for clients receiving services in the outpatient setting.

History of Utilization Management

UM began in the acute care hospital setting. Reviews were performed primarily by medical records department staff as a QA practice. The client records were reviewed based on established criteria by external sources such as accreditation agencies and insurers (for example, Blue Cross & Blue Shield, Medicare, and Medicaid). To be an eligible provider of services and to facilitate payment, many insurers required a hospital to agree to allow (or provide) utilization reviews to monitor service provision, continuously evaluating the necessity, appropriateness, quality, and cost-effectiveness of services being provided to their covered members.

Figure 10.10.   QI-identified areas for improvement from external site visits

Standard	First Quarter	Second Quarter	Third Quarter	Fourth Quarter	Total for the Year
Standard 2216 Direct care staff have been trained in safety and crisis intervention.					
Standard 2213 Staff supervision is documented (five elements required).					
Standards 3201.2 and 3408.14 Authorization is received for each release of client information.					
Standard 3512 Restraint debriefings are filed in client records.					
Standard G10.3.05 Staff training on on restraints (four elements) is provided.					
Comments:					

Source: American CWLA.

As health maintenance organizations (HMOs), **preferred provider organizations** (PPOs), and MCOs developed, hospital administrations realized the financial importance of this QA practice and its implications on existing and potential revenue for healthcare. Medical records departments experienced a well-deserved and long overdue recognition for the relevant work they were doing, proving the need for meticulous documentation of services provided.

Record or Administrative Reviews

Review of client records can be performed in all service programs to ensure that all documentation is placed appropriately and completed according to established guidelines. Each program can design a specific format for checking record deficiencies to determine that all documentation is present, complete, and accurate. Record reviews may be done concurrently and at case closure. To ensure objectivity, staff should not review records of cases with which they are involved. Specific checklists should outline required documents for each program's records, including assessments, treatment plans, contact notes, relevant signatures, evidence of case supervision, and treatment plan reviews. Administrative/record review checklists also should document the required time frame for, and the completion of, needed corrections. (See figure 10.12 for an example of a program-specific record review form.)

When the program-specific checklist is established, the review can be done by a variety of staff, including management and support staff. The results of record/administrative reviews also may be used as a management tool to monitor staff adherence to guidelines and clinical standards.

Figure 10.11. Quality improvement review form

| | **Gateway Family Counseling**
Quality Improvement Review Form |

Client Name:	Client #:	DOB:
Admission Date:	Discharge Date:	Program Location: SHL BHM
Reviewer's Name:		Review Date:
Assigned Therapist:		Form Revised: 10/18/04

Item	OK	Deficient	N/A	Reviewer Comments
A. Client Rights/Consents				
1. Fee arrangements documented (LIST insurance, MCD, or private pay & last date verified)				**LIST** _____
2. Consumer Rights forms are signed by client/family (14 yrs old & older must sign for self) (3201)				
3. Application/Consent for Services form signed by client/family (14 yrs old & older must sign for self; under 14 may sign, but also need parent/guardian to sign) (3201)				
4. Consent for Follow-up signed & marked yes or no (3408.15)				
5. Confidentiality forms/Privacy forms signed by client/family (Form must include Privacy at bottom, check for both!)				
6. Advocacy posters posted in program (3201.6)				
7. Special needs identified, addressed (3407.1o, 3407.7b) (linguistics, hearing or sight impaired, mobility) *See Intake Triage, Screening Triage back of right side of record*				
8. Interventions are documented for special accommodations (linguistic, hearing or vision impaired, mobility) (3407.5) *If identified, 'additional comments' page should be used with Intake Triage/Screening Triage documenting accomm made.*				
B. Assessment/Intake				
1. All sections completed (includes: pres problem, mental status, family structure, social Hx, additional Abuse Hx (3407.2h), Prior Tx, Risk, Medical info/Hx, physical health meds (3407.12), tobacco/etoh/drug/disposition)				**LIST GAF score** _____
2. Reviewed and signed by appropriate staff including credentials (3406). Client meets program criteria for admission.				
3. Diagnostic Impression page done by Clinician				
4. Diagnostic Page completed by PhD or MD (3407.3) within 30 days of admit				**List date** _____

(Continued on next page)

Figure 10.11. (Continued)

Item	OK	Deficient	N/A	Reviewer Comments
C. Initial Treatment Planning (30 days or 5 visits) list date of completion				**Date of Completion**_____
1. Goals are individualized to client				
2. All identified issues are addressed (3407.7a)				
3. Interventions address the specified issues noted including external referrals (3407.7c)				
4. Client/family participation is documented				
5. If client notes family/others to be involved in treatment, ROI consent is completed (3407.8)				
6. Estimated length of treatment is documented				
7. Reviewed, signed and dated by appropriate staff, including credentials (3406)				
D. Treatment Plan Review				
1. Completed (minimum) every 90 days (list dates)				**DATE GAF Progress ELOTx**
2. Each is reviewed, signed/approved by appropriate staff including credentials (3406)				
3. Client/family participation is documented (signatures)				
4. All identified issues are addressed (3407.7a)				
5. Medications are reviewed/updated at least quarterly (3407.12) OTC, *agency and non-agency, as well as compliance must be listed*				
6. Collateral sources are involved, as needed				
7. Plan is modified as needed				
E. Service Provision				
1. Documentation that Risks and Benefits of medications prescribed by Gateway were discussed (3104.2)				___ Client has started no new meds in this program ___ No prescribing Physician in program
2. Clients receiving meds are seen by the psychiatrist at least once every 6 months (3104.1)				___ No prescribing Physician in program
3. All services are provided in a timely manner				
4. All services are documented on the CSR				
5. Client signatures on CSR for each service				
6. Timely follow-up w/high-risk clients (non-compliant) (3103) is documented				
7. Long-term cases (>18 months) show documentation of special staffing				

Figure 10.11.   (Continued)

Item	OK	Deficient	N/A	Reviewer Comments
E. Service Provision (Continued)				
8. Contact and general notes are used correctly				
9. Current mental status is completed on each face-to-face session				
10. All documentation guidelines are followed: all entries dated and signed w/credentials, all pages complete, no Liquid Paper, blue ink, faxes, etc. (3406)				
11. Previously noted deficiencies have been corrected				
F. Discharge Summary *(For discharged clients ONLY)*				
1. Discharge Summary is completed within 15 days of discharge or termination of service				
2. Discharge Summary clearly states Aftercare Plan (recommendations, referrals) and is signed and dated by MET (licensed, supervisory staff)				

Notes for reviewers:

Please monitor for any blanks in record. Document any missing or conflicting dates, signatures, lack of credentials, etc.

Watch for inconsistencies in charting, treatment issues, consistency in general.

Anything you mark deficient, please detail so I can write an accurate report back to the program. No one sees these review sheets but QI!

Use this space to list or document any deficiencies or concerns, questions, etc.

List any other issues or concerns:

Figure 10.12. Program-specific record review form

Therapeutic Foster Care Initial Record Review Foster Child					
revised 10/11/04					
CLIENT'S NAME:	Date	Yes	No	NA	Comments
INITIAL PLACEMENT DATE:					
BEEPER SHEET (in protective cover, discard previous)					
CLIENT SERVICE RECORDS CSR (most recent on top)					
PLACEMENT					
Signed placement agreement					
Signed inter-agency agreement					
Placement record					
Pre-placement contacts					
Court orders					
Social Summary from DHR					
Application for admission-TFC					
CONSENTS/AUTHORIZATIONS					
Signed request/consent for services form					
Consumer Rights Information sheet (present)					
Consumer Rights Information sheet SIGNED (client & staff)					
Signed 'Gateway informed consent' form by client (due after 5/00)					
Signed Confidentiality/Privacy form (make sure form includes both!)					
Notification of Restraint practices (completed, signed)					
Authorization for Release of Info (ROI) as needed					
TREATMENT PLANS					
Most current treatment plan review (list date)					
Updated Safety Plan (list date)					
Comprehensive treatment plan due within 30 days of admit					
Initial treatment plan (due within 10 days)					
Initial safety plan					
INTAKE (all due within 10 days)					
Screening Triage					
Initial Client Triage					
Financial info					
Referral					
Presenting Problem					
Mental Status					
Family Structure					
Social History					
Additional Abuse History					
Prior Treatment					
Risk (if you say yes, specific sections below must be completed)					
R/A Suicide/Violence					
R/A Homicide					
R/A Destruction of Property					
R/A Gang					
Medical Information History					
Mental Retardation Status (if needed)					
Medical Hospital/Surgery					
Allergies					
Physical Health Medications					

Figure 10.12.   (Continued)

CLIENT'S NAME:	Date	Yes	No	NA	Comments
INTAKE (Continued)					
Substance Use					
Drug & Alcohol					
Clinical Summary					
Diagnostic Impression					
TFC CLIENT'S NAME:					
MONTHLY SUMMARY (current on top)					
NOTES (includes contact, general group, restraint, amended and Tx Plan review notes)					
All in date order, most recent on top					
BLS billing sheets monthly (filed at the end of each month's notes)					
ISP					
ISP (due every six months) list most recent date					
PSYCHIATRIC (Agency MDs only)					
All notes, evals, reports, updates from Agency MDs					
Diagnosis page (due within 10 days of admit)					
Initial eval (due within 30 days of admit)					
EXTERNAL EVALS/REPORTS					
Psychological reports (due every two years)					
All other externally generated reports					
MEDICAL FORMS					
Medical updates					
Medical Information/History, Med/Hosp/Surgery, Allergies, as updated					
Family Structure, as updated					
PHYSICAL HEALTH MEDICATIONS (minimum update every 6 months)					
Child's physical form (due yearly)					
Vision screening (due yearly)					
Dental screening (due every six months)					
Lead screening (5 yrs old & under)					
Developmental Screening (5 yrs old & under)					
MEDICATION RECORDS					
Date order/most recent on top					
EPSDT (Medicaid Agency Referral Form due yearly)					
SCHOOL					
Current 'blue 'slip (Certificate of Immunization) Check expiration date!					
Report cards (last one for previous year)					
IEP (due yearly) if special Ed. (See beeper sheet Type of Placement)					
Out of County Notification (if needed)					
CORRESPONDENCE					
OTHER					
PROTECTIVE COVER					
Medicaid card					
Social security card					
Birth certificate					
Reviewer:					
Date:					
ADDITIONAL COMMENTS:					
* Staff notified					
* Correction Date					
* Resolved					

Consumer Satisfaction Surveys

Monitoring consumer satisfaction is a widely practiced and ongoing PI activity. In their efforts to improve service provision, behavioral healthcare organizations often solicit feedback from consumers. The client requesting and receiving services is not the behavioral healthcare organization's only consumer. Satisfaction surveys can be given to clients, family members, referral sources, insurance companies, private practitioners, community advocate programs, organizational staff, and so on.

Valuable information can be obtained for program development as well as strategic planning for the entire organization. For reporting purposes, it is best to keep the survey simple, with a limited number of questions. Space should be provided for additional comments and concerns. All surveys should be confidential, but it is acceptable to provide a space for name and contact information for those who wish to provide it.

Satisfaction surveys can be done at different times throughout the course of a client's treatment, quarterly or annually for referral sources, or at other established times throughout the calendar year. The designated QI staff can tabulate results and identify trends in individual programs and across the organization. Reports may be used to address treatment/service issues, customer service, and policy and procedure development and to guide the organization's strategic planning activities.

Figure 10.13 is a sample client satisfaction survey, and figure 10.14 is a sample satisfaction survey for referral sources. Compiling survey results can be done simply. A sample form

Figure 10.13.   Client satisfaction survey

Client Satisfaction Survey

Date: _____

Thank you for the opportunity to provide services to you or your family recently. Please take a few moments to answer the following questions so that we may continue to improve our services. All surveys are confidential.
CIRCLE ONLY ONE ANSWER

	Strongly Agree	Agree	Strongly Disagree	Disagree	Doesn't Apply to Me
1. I am satisfied with the services/help I received.	1	2	3	4	0
2. I am satisfied with the amount of communication I received from (organization) staff.	1	2	3	4	0
3. (Organization) staff were available when I needed them.	1	2	3	4	0
4. I learned new skills that will help me in the future.	1	2	3	4	0
5. I had a chance to express my own ideas and to ask questions.	1	2	3	4	0
6. I was able to help make decisions about what services I received.	1	2	3	4	0
7. Information was reviewed with me about client's rights and responsibilities.	1	2	3	4	0
8. I felt safe during my stay at (organization). (residential, emergency, TFC, TLP, ILP)	1	2	3	4	0
9. My privacy and confidentiality were protected while I received services from (organization).	1	2	3	4	0
10. Rules and guidelines were fair while I received services from (organization).	1	2	3	4	0

Age: _____   Gender: _____   Race/Ethnicity: _____

Comments: Revised Nov 2001

Figure 10.14.   Referral agency satisfaction survey

Referral Agency Satisfaction Survey

Program: _____

Date: _____

Thank you for the opportunity to provide services to your client. Please take a few moments to answer the following questions so that we may continue to improve our services. All surveys are confidential.
CIRCLE ONLY ONE ANSWER

	Agree	Strongly Agree	Disagree	Strongly Disagree	Doesn't Apply to Me
1. The services received were satisfactory.	1	2	3	4	0
2. I received an appropriate amount of communication from (organization) staff.	1	2	3	4	0
3. (Organization) staff was available when needed.	1	2	3	4	0
4. The client learned new skills that will be helpful in the future.	1	2	3	4	0
5. I had the opportunity to participate in treatment planning.	1	2	3	4	0
6. I was able to have input about what services were received.	1	2	3	4	0
7. The client was informed of all rules and guidelines.	1	2	3	4	0
8. (Organization) provided a safe environment for the client. (residential, emergency, TFC, TLP, ILP)	1	2	3	4	0
9. The client's privacy and confidentiality were protected while services were received at (organization).	1	2	3	4	0
10. I would refer another client to (organization).	1	2	3	4	0

Comments:

used for compiling survey results is provided in figure 10.15. Moreover, compiled information can be presented in various ways. The example bar graph in figure 10.16 offers an effective, visual presentation of satisfaction survey results for several programs.

Incident Reports

Reviewing and tabulating data from the organization's incident reporting process is a typical PI activity. Incident reporting has long been considered a QI/PI data collection tool. An incident is any occurrence or happening that is inconsistent with the routine operation of the organization or the routine care of a particular client and/or that has potentially serious medical/legal significance. Examples of incidents that organizations should monitor include medication errors; injury to client, staff, or visitors; runaways; aggressive behavior; refusal to take medications; and physical assaults. Each organization should determine its own areas of risk or concern to be monitored. The person responsible for QI should be involved in the communication loop for all incident reports. (See figure 10.17 for an example incident report.)

Figure 10.15. Satisfaction survey log

SATISFACTION SURVEY LOG PROGRAM: _____				
TOTALS	**1st QTR** Jan, Feb, Mar **Due 4/15**	**2ND QTR** Apr, May, Jun **Due 7/15**	**3RD QTR** Jul, Aug, Sep **Due 10/15**	**4TH QTR** Oct, Nov, Dec **Due 1/15**
# Clients Served				
CLIENTS				
# Client surveys distributed				
# Client surveys returned				
% Rated services excellent % Rated services good				
FAMILY				
# Family surveys distributed				
# Family surveys returned				
% Rated services excellent % Rated service good				
FOSTER FAMILY				
# Foster family surveys distributed				
# Foster family surveys returned				
% Rated services excellent % Rated service good				
REFERRALS				
# Referral agency surveys distributed				
# Referral agency surveys returned				
% Rated services excellent % Rated services good				

Figure 10.16. Satisfaction survey report

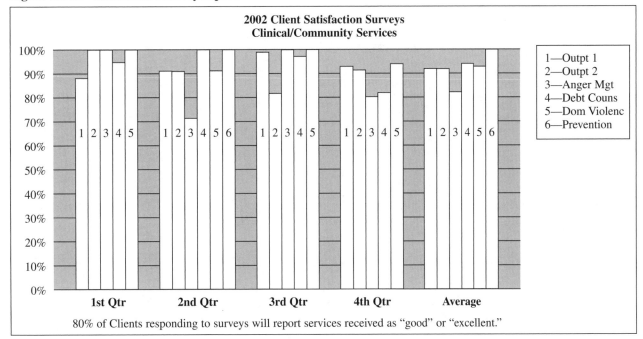

2002 Client Satisfaction Surveys
Clinical/Community Services

1—Outpt 1
2—Outpt 2
3—Anger Mgt
4—Debt Couns
5—Dom Violenc
6—Prevention

1st Qtr   2nd Qtr   3rd Qtr   4th Qtr   Average

80% of Clients responding to surveys will report services received as "good" or "excellent."

Monthly, quarterly, and annual results can be collected and reported to management, executive staff, and board members. Pertinent findings regarding improvement strategies, such as additional staff education, can be implemented as needed. Individual incident reports and compiled results should be maintained separately from client records and considered internal documents. Organizations also may want incident reporting covered by legal counsel as privileged information.

Processes and Reviews

Most accrediting agencies specify the time frames for reviews. If organizations do not have accrediting standards, reviews can occur once or twice a year, or even quarterly. The time frame selected for review should be related to the actual measurement being used and the service components involved. For long-term (one- to two-year) services, an annual review may be sufficient.

Tools and Techniques

Behavioral healthcare organizations should develop review forms and data-capturing methods specific to the service being provided. Sample forms and reports include a form for subcommittee review, specifically to address issues with incident reporting (figure 10.18); an annual policy review form (figure 10.19); and a form on client rights and responsibilities (figure 10.20). Most organizations have some format for presenting rights and responsibilities to clients and families. When signed, these forms also serve as documentation that the information has been provided to the client and/or his or her family.

Documentation Feedback Loop

The documentation feedback loop is essential in CQI activities. As mentioned earlier, accrediting bodies and funding sources want to see documented evidence that organizations are providing high-quality services. Reporting should be distributed not only to the programs

Figure 10.17. Sample incident report form

INCIDENT REPORT	*Circle code that most describes incident or occurrence*	BEHAVIOR REPORT
INCIDENT Codes:		BEHAVIOR Codes:

INCIDENT REPORT
INCIDENT Codes:
01 Medication Error
02 Client Injury
___ Self Injury
___ Accident
03 Physical Assault
___ Client to Client
___ Client to Staff
___ Client to Others
04 Sexual Assault
12 Suicide Attempt
13 Death*
17 Harassment
18 Suspected Abuse/Neglect
19 Illness or Injury of Staff or Visitor
14 Other (must describe)

Circle code that most describes incident or occurrence

BEHAVIOR REPORT
BEHAVIOR Codes:
05 Verbal Assault
06 Runaway
07 Theft
09 Client Aggression
___ Client to Client
___ Client to Staff
___ Client to Others
___ Client to Property
10 Rules Violation
11 Acting Out
15 Refusing Medications
16 Breaking Curfew
14 Other (must describe)

_____ _____
Date & time (am/ pm) of incident   Specific location of incident

_____ _____
Date & time of report   Program enrolled in

Name: _____ Age of Client: _____

Description of incident:_____
_____
_____

Injury? ___Yes ___No   If yes check severity/type of injury:

___ No injury (no pain, no bruising)   ___ MINOR injury (small bruise, no treatment required)

___ Moderate injury (treatment required, x-ray, IV)   ___ MAJOR injury (serious; stitches, Fractures)

If yes, show location of injury on diagram:

Illlustrate on the diagram position or place of injury.

RIS ONLY   Date & time nursing staff notified: _____ Nursing staff signature: _____

Actions/Interventions taken: ___ Verbal de-escalation   ___ Time-out (see page 2)   ___ Removal of client
___ Restraint (see page 2)   ___ Filed police report   ___ Removal of other clients
___ First Aid offered

___ DHR contacted Date _____ Time _____ Person_____

Consequences (describe)_____
_____

Corrective actions: (What steps could have been taken to prevent incident?)
_____

Signature of staff completing report: _____

List all staff involved or witness to incident: _____

Figure 10.17. (Continued)

RESTRAINTS ONLY*

Supervisor/on-call person called? ____ Yes ____ No   Time called _____ a.m./p.m.

Verbal authorization given by _____ Time_____ a.m./p.m.

Describe behavior of child during restraint: _____

_____

Length of time client in restraint: _____ **If more than 15 minutes, Licensed Staff Authorization Required (LPC, LCSW, MD)**

Criteria for release met: ____ Yes ____ No

(Communicating appropriately, calm, no longer combative or threatening, able to discuss situation, etc)

_____   _____
Signature of staff authorizing restraint   Signature of staff observing restraint

Was client left alone at any time? ____ Yes ____ No (detail) _____

Assessment of client following release from restraint: Physical:_____ Emotional: _____

*Restraint Debriefing Form must be completed and placed on client's record

TIME-OUTS ONLY

Personal time-out in room   _____   Length of time client spent in time-out _____

Time-out in seclusion room   _____

Time-out less than 30 minutes   _____

Time-out greater than 30 minutes _____ (detail)_____

_____

Was client left alone at any time?_____

Assessment of client following release from time-out:

Physical: _____   Emotional:_____

Additional Comments: _____

Supervisor actions/comments: Date: _____

_____

Direct staff/clinician actions/comments: Date: _____

_____

Program Director's review: _____ Agree with above actions. Date: _____

Other Actions/comments:_____

_____

QI Received:_____

Executive Director's review: _____ Agree with above actions. Date: _____

Comments: _____

_____

Figure 10.18.   Sample form for a subcommittee review

QUALITY IMPROVEMENT COMMITTEE

Subcommittee Review of Incidents

Based on a review of the submitted incident reports, please answer the following questions:

1.   Was incident due to staff negligence?

2.   Is documentation appropriate and adequate for the incident?

3.   Was incident handled appropriately?

4.   Have appropriate steps been taken (if necessary) to prevent similar incidents from occurring in the future?

(*Please detail any negative responses.)

Other comments/actions/recommendations felt needed by the committee:

_____

_____

_____

_____

_____

_____

_____

_____

_____

_____

PLEASE RETURN FORM TO QI DIRECTOR, ASAP. THANKS!

---

reviewed, but also to appropriate supervisors and the executive director. By establishing an ongoing report practice, organizations can proactively prepare for accreditation site visits or funding source requests and keep current with any areas of concern.

Accreditation reviewers are not interested in seeing storage boxes of data such as record reviews, utilization reviews, and incident reports. Rather, they want to see what has been done with the data collected. The process should show that relevant data were turned into specific reports and given to management across the healthcare organization. Reports provide significant information to help managers make strategic decisions in service planning for the future of their programs as well as the organization. QI committee minutes should reflect the various efforts undertaken to continuously improve quality throughout the organization.

Graphical reports of improvement can be provided for individual programs to show organizationwide results. Basic bar charts can be used to show directors and board members where improvements are being made as well as areas that need attention.

Conclusion

Whether motivated by regulatory or accreditation organizations, funding sources, or internal desires for improvement, all behavioral healthcare organizations should implement continuous quality improvement plans and measure outcomes of service provision. Professionals trained in health information management are often the best candidates to lead the organization's CQI activities.

Figure 10.19. Annual policy review

ANNUAL POLICY REVIEW

STAFF SIGNATURE: _____

PROGRAM: _____ DATE: _____

My signature above denotes that I have attended an annual policy review at (organization). My initials below indicate that I have reviewed each policy.

_____	1.0	Organization mission, philosophy			
_____	4.01	Organizational chart	_____	7.03	Consumer grievance
_____	4.02	Delegation of authority	_____	7.04	Consumer rights handout
_____	4.03	Conflict of interest	_____	7.05	Consumer grievance form
_____	5.0	Quality improvement plan			
			_____	8.01	Client safety & disciplinary standards
_____	6.02	Equal opportunity employment	_____	8.02	Nondiscrimination/cultural diversity
_____	6.04	Harassment	_____	8.03	Reporting of suspected abuse
_____	6.08	Separation	_____	8.11	Electronic communication systems
_____	6.10	General supervision			
_____	6.13	On-the-job injuries	_____	9.03	Confidentiality
_____	6.16	Nonsolicitation	_____	9.04	Confidentiality: AIDS, HIV
_____	6.17	Supervisor–employee relationships	_____	9.05	Confidentiality: Cell phone use
_____	6.22	Organization education presentations & community participation	_____	9.10	Facsimile release of client info
_____	6.26	Grievance process	_____	14.10	Media relations
_____	6.29	Scheduled/unscheduled leave			
_____	6.33	Staff/client personal relationships	_____	15.01	Inclement weather
_____	6.39	Environmental risk	_____	15.05	Safety program
_____	6.42	Catastrophic leave	_____	15.06	Incident/occurrence reporting
_____	6.44	Leave bank			
_____	6.45	FMLA (Family Medical Leave Act)			
_____	6.46	Progressive discipline	_____		Corporate compliance plan
_____	6.47	Administrative leave			
_____	6.50	Employee assistance program			
_____	6.51	Drug testing			
_____	6.32	Credentials			

Revised 1/2002

Figure 10.20. Sample form of client rights and responsibilities

---

(ORGANIZATION)
CONSUMER RIGHTS INFORMATION SHEET

As a consumer of services, you have certain rights guaranteed by the (state) Mental Health Consumers' Rights Act of 1995. Among these are:

THE RIGHT TO:

1. Be treated with dignity and respect in a safe and humane environment, including being free from abuse and neglect or mistreatment
2. Be informed of the need for parental/guardian consent for treatment when considered a minor
3. Participate in service planning for your individual needs
4. Know what services you will receive and how much they will cost
5. Confidentiality of your clinical, medical, and financial information
6. Agree or disagree to participate in research or experimental projects. (ORGANIZATION) DOES NOT ALLOW OR PARTICIPATE IN RESEARCH OR EXPERIMENTAL PROJECTS.
7. Know how to file a complaint/ grievance and get help if you believe that your rights have been violated, including being able to talk to an attorney and/or go to court.
8. Enforce your rights through the court system, if needed.
9. Refuse any mental health services offered unless legally mandated to treatment.
10. Use all the rights of any other citizen of (state).
11. Vote, if of voting age.
12. Be treated in a way that allows you the greatest freedom possible, given your identified needs.
13. If you must be treated in a hospital, you have the right to privacy, food, and shelter and access to dental and medical care, if needed.
14. Be advised when special equipment, such as one-way mirrors in (ORGANIZATION), cameras, or recorders are being used for educational, clinical, and/or safety purposes.

YOUR RESPONSIBILITIES

The freedom to exercise rights comes with the need to accept certain responsibilities. As a consumer of services, you have a responsibility to:

1. Provide complete and accurate information
2. Take an active part in planning and using program services
3. Cooperate with your treatment program, including keeping appointments, attending scheduled activities, and promptly taking care of your financial obligations.
4. Ask questions when you do not understand program instructions.
5. Accept responsibility for the consequences if you refuse services or do not follow program instructions.
6. Follow (ORGANIZATION) rules and regulations, including being considerate and respectful of the rights and property of staff and other clients.
7. Obey the laws that apply to all citizens.

If you have questions about any of your rights, you may ask the intake worker at the time of intake or your individual staff worker at any time during the course of your services. If you think your rights have been violated, you may request, complete, and submit a grievance form and your complaint will be investigated. Each consumer has the right to access outside advocacy programs, without negative consequences. The following are other sources where you may refer questions and complaints:

The Rights Protection and Advocacy Program, Department of Mental Health and Mental Retardation: 1-800-367-0955

Mental Health Consumers of (state): 1-800-000-0000

(State) Alliance for the Mentally Ill: 1-800-000-0000

(State) Disabilities Advocacy Program: 1-800-000-0000

(State) Department of Human Resources: 1-800-000-0000

The above has been reviewed with me, and I have received a copy of the Client Rights and Responsibilities from ORGANIZATION.

Staff: _____

Client: _____ Date: _____

Retain original in client record.

I have also received a copy of Organization's Notice of Privacy Standards.

Client: _____ Date: _____

Revised 10/2002

References and Bibliography

American Health Information Management Association. www.AHIMA.org.

American Hospital Association. 1990. www.hospitalconnect.com.

American Osteopathic Association. www.aoa-net.org.

American Osteopathic Association, Healthcare Facilities Accreditation Program. 2003. Quality Assessment and Performance Improvement (QAPI). In *Requirements for Healthcare Facilities.* Chicago: American Osteopathic Association.

Blackiston, G. Howland. 1996. *A Brief History of Juran Institute: A Barometer of Quality Trends.* Wilton, CT: Juran Institute.

Bowling, A. 1991. *Measuring Health: A Review of Quality of Life Measurement Scales.* Philadelphia, PA: Open University Press.

Child Welfare League of America. www.cwla.org.

Child Welfare League of America. 2001. *Annual Report.* Washington, DC: Child Welfare League of America.

Child Welfare League of America. 1998. *Annual Report.* Washington, DC: Child Welfare League of America.

Christner, Anne Marshall, ed. 1998. *Measuring Outcomes in Children's Services.* Providence, RI: Manisses Communications Groups, Inc.

Council on Accreditation for Children and Family Services. www.coanet.org.

Council on Accreditation for Children and Families Services. 2001. Continuous Quality Improvement. In *Standards and Self-Study Manual,* vol I, 7th ed. New York: Council on Accreditation for Children and Family Services.

Council on Accreditation for Children and Families Services. 2001. *Standards & Self-Study Manual: Private, Not-for-Profit & For-Profit Organizations,* vol. I, 7th ed, version 1-0. New York: COA.

Council on Accreditation of Rehabilitation Facilities. 2004. www.CARF.org.

Council on Accreditation of Rehabilitation Facilities. 2002. Information and outcomes management systems. In *Behavioral Health Standards Manual.* Tucson, AZ: Council on Accreditation of Rehabilitation Facilities.

The 50: People Who Most influenced Business in this Century, *Los Angeles Times,* October 1999.

Joint Commission on Accreditation of Healthcare Organizations. www.JCAHO.org.

Joint Commission on Accreditation of Healthcare Organizations. 2004–2005. *Comprehensive Accreditation Manual for Behavioral Health Care* (CAMBHC). Oakbrook Terrace, IL: JCAHO.

Joint Commission on Accreditation of Healthcare Organizations. 2004. *Shared Visions—New Pathways.* Oakbrook Terrace, IL: JCAHO.

Joint Commission on Accreditation of Healthcare Organizations. 2003. *Comprehensive Accreditation Manual for Behavioral Health Care* (CAMBHC). Oakbrook Terrace, IL: JCAHO.

Joint Commission on Accreditation of Healthcare Organizations. 2000. *Comprehensive Accreditation Manual for Behavioral Health Care* (CAMBHC). Oakbrook Terrace, IL: JCAHO.

Joint Commission on Accreditation of Healthcare Organizations. 1991. *Comprehensive Accreditation Manual for Behavioral Health Care* (CAMBHC). Oakbrook Terrace, IL: JCAHO.

Long, A. F. 1995. Outcomes with audit: A process and outcomes perspective. *Outcomes Briefing* 7(5).

McCullough, C., and B. Schmitt. 1998. *Outcomes in a Managed Care Child Welfare Environment.* Washington, DC: Child Welfare League of America.

Mordock, John B. 2002. *Managing for Outcomes: A Basic Guide to the Evaluation of Best Practices in the Human Services.* Washington, DC: CWLA Press.

National Committee for Quality Assurance. www.ncqa.org.

National Council for Community Behavioral Healthcare. 2003 (July). Finding evidence-based practices: A compilation of online, searchable databases and descriptions of how to use reviews. *National Council News* 26(6).

Royal College of Psychiatrists. 1994. *Psychiatric Instruments and Rating Scales: A Select Bibliography,* 2nd ed. London: Royal College of Psychiatrists.

Shaw, Patricia, et al. 2003. *Quality and Performance Improvement in Healthcare: A Tool for Programmed Learning,* 2nd ed. Chicago: American Health Information Management Association.

W. Edwards Deming Institute. 2000. Accessed on-line at www.deming.org.

Walter Shewhart—The Grandfather of Total Quality Management. SkyMark Corporation. 2002. Accessed on-line at http://www.skymark.com/resources/leaders/shewart.asp.

Wieger, Donald E., and Kenneth B. Solbergh. 2001. *Tracking Mental Health Outcomes.* New York: John Wiley and Sons.

Wilken, D., L. Hallam, and M. Doggett. 1992. *Measures of Need and Outcome for Primary Health Care.* Oxford, Eng.: Oxford University Press.

Additional Resources for Outcome Measures, Performance Indicators, and Benchmarks

The American College of Mental Health Administration (ACMHA)
5 Waterside Place
Pittsburgh PA 15222
(412) 322-3969
www.acmha.org.

The American Psychiatric Association (APA)
1000 Wilson Boulevard
Suite 1825
Arlington VA 22209-3901
(703) 907-7300
apa@psych.org

National Outcomes Management Project: A Benchmarking Collaborative
The Center for Quality Innovations and Research
P.O. Box 198048
Cincinnati, Ohio 45219
(513) 558-2762

Appendix A

Sample Inpatient Forms

Figure A.1. Activity therapy assessment

	4 = Functioning Within Normal Limits	1= Severe Dysfunction
FUNCTIONAL RATING SCALE	3 = Minimal Dysfunction	N/O = Not Observed
Comments Required for rating of 1 or 2	2 = Moderate Dysfunction	

	RATING	COMMENTS
Cognitive Organization		
Attention Span/ Concentration		
Problem Solving/ Judgment		
Direction Following		
Appearance/Hygiene/ Grooming		
Treatment Compliance		
Community Living Skills		

Interests / Hobbies _____

_____

_____

Leisure and Social Functioning _____

_____

_____

Safety Concerns/Special Needs _____

_____

Summary (Assets, Mood, Affect, General Functional Status) _____

_____

_____

_____

_____

Signature: _____   **Date:** _____   **Time**: _____

County of San Diego Health and Human Services Agency MENTAL HEALTH SERVICES San Diego County Psychiatric Hospital **ACTIVITY THERAPY ASSESSMENT** **HHSA:MHS-210 (01-01)**	**Patient Identification**

Figure A.2. Close Observation Record

☐ SUICIDE ☐ ELOPEMENT ☐ CLOSE WATCH ☐ OTHER: _____	

| CODES: ▶ | 1 = Bedroom
2 = Bathroom
3 = Day Room | 4 = Dining Room
5 = Activity Therapy
6 = Hallway | 7 = Courtyard
8 = Therapy Session
9 = Other: _____ | 10 = Other:_____
11 = Other:_____ |

SHIFT		SHIFT		SHIFT	
2330		0730		1530	
2345		0745		1545	
2400		0800		1600	
2415		0815		0615	
2430		0830		0630	
2445		0845		1645	
0100		0900		1700	
0115		0915		1715	
0130		0930		1730	
0145		0945		1745	
0200		1000		1800	
0215		1015		1815	
0230		1030		1830	
0245		1045		1845	
0300		1100		1900	
0315		1115		1915	
0330		1130		1930	
0345		1145		1945	
0400		1200		2000	
0415		1215		2015	
0430		1230		2030	
0445		1245		2045	
0500		1300		2100	
0515		1315		2115	
0530		1330		2130	
0545		1345		2145	
0600		1400		2200	
0615		1415		2215	
0630		1430		2230	
0645		1445		2245	
0700		1500		2300	
0715		1515		2315	

INITIALS	SIGNATURE AND TITLE	INITIALS	SIGNATURE AND TITLE
RN SIGNATURE		DATE	

County of San Diego
Health and Human Services Agency
Mental Health Services
SAN DIEGO COUNTY PSYCHIATRIC HOSPITAL

PATIENT IDENTIFICATION

CLOSE OBSERVATION RECORD

HHSA: MHS-223 (03/01)

Figure A.3. Daily RN assessment/flow sheet

Shift:			Legal Status:					
☐ Day	☐ Evening	☐ Night	☐ Vol.	☐ 5150	☐ Cert	☐ T-Con	☐ P-Con	

LEVEL I

☐ Requires 1:1 or 2:1 supervision	☐ Danger to self
☐ Danger to others	☐ At risk of harm by others

LEVEL II

☐ Requires substantial help with ADL's toileting/meals	☐ Non-ambulatory
☐ Impaired judgment, confusion	☐ Special medical care, e.g., DT risk, seizure precaution, fall risk, frequent V.S., sliding scale insulin. I & O risk of
☐ Psychomotor disturbance, e.g., agitation, pacing	☐ Behavior places patient at risk, e.g., hallucinations, delusion, unusual activities, AWOL attempts
☐ Poor impulse control, e.g., fighting, yelling, screaming, etc. risk of violence	☐ Appointment off unit with staff >2 hrs.
☐ Seclusion/restraint past 24 hrs.	☐ New admission in past 24 hrs.
☐ Close observation (see policy)	

LEVEL III

☐ Administrative stay waiting placement	☐ Minimal assistance with ADL's
☐ Occasional redirection	☐ Contracts for safety

OTHERS

ADL'S	**Nutrition**	**Elimination**	**Pain**
☐ Independent ☐ Needs prompting ☐ Needs assistance ☐ Total care ☐ Refuses	☐ I & O ☐ Eats in cafeteria ☐ %	☐ Needs assistance **Urine:** ☐ Continent ☐ Incontinent **Stools:** ☐ Regular ☐ Loose ☐ Constipated ☐ None	Rating:_____ Location:_____ Meds:_____ ☐ Effective ☐ Not effective ☐ Refused
Admission	**Sleep Patterns**	**Effects of Meds**	**Safety**	**Plan**

Admission	**Sleep Patterns**	**Effects of Meds**	**Safety**	**Plan**
☐ New this shift ☐ In past 24 hours	☐ Naps ☐ C/O Insomnia ☐ Restless/early riser ☐ Hours of sleep this shift	☐ Improving ☐ Not improving ☐ Refusing ☐ Unable to determine	☐ Yes ☐ No contract ☐ Refuses contract	☐ Notify MD ☐ Non-med tx. ☐ Tx problem ☐ Other:_____

*Comments and response:*_____

_____

*Response to treatment and additional observations:*_____

_____

RN Signature:	Date:	Time:

County of San Diego Health and Human Services Agency Mental Health Services SAN DIEGO COUNTY PSYCHIATRIC HOSPITAL **DAILY RN ASSESSMENT/FLOW SHEET** HHSA:MHS-391 (03)	PATIENT IDENTIFICATION:

Figure A.4. Discharge summary outline

<u>**DISCHARGE SUMMARY OUTLINE**</u>

<u>DATE OF ADMISSION:</u>

<u>DATE OF DISCHARGE:</u>

<u>REASON FOR ADMISSION:</u>

<u>MENTAL STATUS EXAM:</u>

<u>ALLERGIES:</u>

<u>MEDICAL ASSESSMENT/PHYSICAL EXAMINATION:</u>

<u>HOSPITAL COURSE:</u>

<u>DIET:</u>

<u>ACTIVITY:</u>

<u>DISCHARGE ARRANGEMENTS:</u>

<u>CONDITION ON DISCHARGE:</u>

<u>LEGAL STATUS:</u>

<u>FUNDS:</u>

<u>PROGNOSIS:</u>

<u>FOLLOW-UP:</u>

<u>CLINICAL IMPRESSION:</u>

<u>DISCHARGE DIAGNOSIS:</u>

Axis   I:
Axis II:
Axis III:
Axis IV:
Axis V: **GAF Current: /Past year:**

<u>MEDICATIONS UPON DISCHARGE:</u>

_____

STAFF PSYCHIATRIST

| County of San Diego County
Health and Human Services Agency
Mental Health Services

SAN DIEGO COUNTY PSYCHIATRIC HOSPITAL

DISCHARGE SUMMARY

HHSA:MHS-202 (09/00) | Patient name:

MR#:   Unit:

D.O.B.   Date: |

Figure A.5. Discharge/aftercare plan

PATIENT INFORMATION

PATIENT NAME	INSURANCE PROVIDER NAME	SOCIAL SECURITY NUMBER
LEGAL STATUS	DISCHARGE ADDRESS	
DISCHARGE PHONE NUMBER	CITY, STATE, ZIP	

Nature Of Problem/Illness:

☐ Disturbance of mood   ☐ Danger to self   ☐ Inability to care for self   ☐ Substance abuse
☐ Disturbance of thought   ☐ Danger to others   ☐ Other: describe _____

Anticipated short-term recovery goals may include:

☐ Independent Or Supported Living   ☐ Part-Time/Full-Time Employment   ☐ Reestablish Family/Social Relationships
☐ Other _____   ☐ Involvement in Substance Recovery Program   ☐ Initiation or Continuation of Educational Goals

OUTPATIENT INSTRUCTIONS

Follow-Up Appointments/ Referrals: Name of Agency/Address	Time/Date	Phone #
Mental Health: _____	_____	_____
_____	_____	_____
_____	_____	_____
Financial: _____	_____	_____
_____	_____	_____
Medical: _____	_____	_____
_____	_____	_____
_____	_____	_____
_____	_____	_____
Chemical Dependency: _____	_____	_____
_____	_____	_____
Other: _____	_____	_____
_____	_____	_____

☐ Conservator/legal representative notified (prior to discharge). Name: _____

Address: _____ Send Copy: ☐ Yes ☐ No

☐ I agree to designate another person to receive a copy of this plan.

   Name: _____   Address: _____

☐ I decline to designate another person.

☐ The above and attached instructions have been explained to me. I have had an opportunity to ask questions and understand the instructions given to me.

Date: _____   Patient Signature _____   Family Signature _____

Social Worker Signature: _____   RN Signature _____

WHITE – Chart   CANARY – Patient   PINK - Agency

	PATIENT IDENTIFICATION
County Of San Diego Health and Human Services Agency Mental Health Services SAN DIEGO COUNTY PSYCHIATRIC HOSPITAL *DISCHARGE/AFTER CARE PLAN* HHSA:MHS203a (01/02)	

Figure A.5. (Continued)

MEDICATION INSTRUCTIONS

1. Read ALL labels for your medications before preparing to take them each time.
2. Contact your physician, outpatient clinic or pharmacist with medication or side effect questions.
3. Obtain medication refills before your prescriptions run out.
4. Keep a list of your medications and any allergies with you.

ALLERGIES: _____

_____

SAFE AND EFFECTIVE USE OF MEDICATIONS

NURSE/PHARMACIST/PHYSICIAN RESPONSIBILITY	PATIENT RESPONSE
☐ Specific medication instructions given	☐ States purpose, schedule, side effects of medications
☐ Food and drug interaction guide given	☐ Unable to restate instructions but agrees to use instruction sheet.
☐ Side effects of medications identified.	☐ Refuses instructions
☐ Patient belongings returned, including personal meds, if indicated	☐ Refuses medication

MEDICATION	DOSE	INSTRUCTIONS AND DOSAGE SCHEDULES

Other treatment recommendations (for example: dietary, medical, use of medical equipment).

_____

_____

_____

_____

PPD: *(Tuberculosis Skin Test)*

☐ History of positive PPD   Chest X-Ray: ☐ Positive ☐ Negative

PPD Date Given _____ Site _____ Time _____ Initials: _____

PPD Date Read _____ Reading: ☐ Negative. ☐ Positive: (mm)_____ Initials:_____

> **PLACE +PPD**
> **STICKER HERE**

HIU Sends Copies: To: _____

Date Sent:_____ Address:_____

Initials: _____

☐ Discharge Summary   ☐ Social Work Assessment   ☐ Psychiatric Assessment   ☐ Medication Records

☐ History and Physical   ☐ Other:_____

RN Signature: _____   LVN/PT Signature: _____   Discharge Date: _____

WHITE – Chart   CANARY – Patient   PINK - Agency

County Of San Diego
Health and Human Services Agency
Mental Health Services
SAN DIEGO COUNTY PSYCHIATRIC HOSPITAL

PATIENT IDENTIFICATION

DISCHARGE/AFTER CARE PLAN

HHSA:MHS203b (01/02)

277

Figure A.6. EPU nursing screen assessment

| Age: | ☐ Male ☐ Female | Ethnicity: | Interpreter Required? ☐ No ☐ Yes | Language: |

| Mode of Transport: ☐ Self ☐ Ambulance ☐ Police Unit_____ | Others Present: | Legal Status: |

Patient Has (check all that apply):   ☐ Glasses   ☐ Contacts   ☐ Dentures   ☐ Hearing Aid   ☐ Other Aids: _____

CURRENT MEDICATIONS:	Dose	Frequency	Taken As Prescribed?	RECENT ALCOHOL AND/OR DRUG USE *Amount/Day Last Used*		
			☐ Yes ☐ No			
			☐ Yes ☐ No	Odor of ETOH on breath?	☐ Yes	☐ No
			☐ Yes ☐ No	Unusual gait and/or uncoordinated?	☐ Yes	☐ No
			☐ Yes ☐ No	History of: ☐ DT's ☐ Blackouts ☐ Seizures ☐ None		

List Current Medical Problem (including any evident lacerations, abrasions, and/or bruises):_____

List Any Abnormalities With a Short Description:_____

PAIN: ☐ No ☐ Yes   If yes, how bad? _____ (0-10) Where? _____ How long? _____

(If patient rates pain at 4 or above complete Pain Assessment). Pain assessment initiated ☐ Yes ☐ No ☐ N/A

B/P _____ T _____ P _____ R _____	Allergies To Medicine or Foods: ☐ No ☐ Yes **Which Ones?** ___
Pregnant? ☐ No ☐ Yes ☐ Unknown	_____
Last Menses:_____	**Describe Reaction:**_____

Chief Psychiatric Complaint:

Oriented to:	☐ Person	☐ Place	☐ Month	☐ Year	☐ Situations	☐ None
Level of Consciousness:	☐ Alert	☐ Lethargic	☐ Stuporous	☐ Comatose		
Appearance:	☐ Clean	☐ Well-nourished	☐ Malodorous	☐ Disheveled	☐ Malnourished	☐ Reddened eyes
Speech:	☐ Normal	☐ Slurred	☐ Loud	☐ Pressured	☐ Slow	☐ Mute
Thought Process:	☐ Coherent	☐ Tangential	☐ Loose Associations		☐ Incoherent	
Behavior:	☐ Cooperative	☐ Tearful	☐ Threatening	☐ Restless	☐ Agitated	☐ Combative
Affect:	☐ Normal	☐ Bland	☐ Flat	☐ Anxious	☐ Frightened	☐ Angry
	☐ Excited	☐ Sad	☐ Withdrawn	☐ Irritable		

Other Information (Optional):
Visual Hallucinations: ☐ No   ☐ Yes   Content:_____
Auditory Hallucinations: ☐ No   ☐ Yes   Content:_____
Homicidal Ideas: ☐ No   ☐ Yes   Content/Plan:
Current Suicidal Ideas: ☐ No   ☐ Yes   Content/Plan:
Suicide Attempts: ☐ No   ☐ Yes   How/When?
Contracts for Safety: ☐ Yes   ☐ No   Comments:
Psychiatric Acuity: ☐ Non-urgent   ☐ Urgent   ☐ Severe (STAT)
Disposition: ☐ RN   ☐ RNCS   ☐ Social Worker   ☐ Medical M.D.   ☐ Psychiatrist   ☐ Other:
Patient Informed of Disposition? ☐ Yes Understands? ☐ Yes ☐ No Will Comply? ☐ Yes ☐ No Comments:
Signature of Registered Nurse (required):   Date: Time:

Figure A.7. Fall risk assessment

(Add points and note total score on the far right side of the page)		**POINTS**
GENERAL DATA – AGE		
_____ Age 65 –70 (1 point)	_____ 70 or older (2 points)	
HISTORY OF FALLS (in past 6 months)		
_____ 1-2 falls (2 points)	_____ 3 or more falls (8 points)	
MEDICATION/TREATMENTS		
_____ Atypical Antipsychotic (2 points)	_____ Anticonvulsant (2 points)	
_____ Antihypertensive (2 points)	_____ Benzodiazepine (2 points)	
_____ Sedative/Hypnotic (3 points)	_____ Antidepressant (TCA) (2 points	
_____ Antipsychotic (2 points)	_____ Alcohol (2 points)	
_____ Antidressant (SSRI) (2 points)		
MENTAL STATUS Confusion:		
_____ Mild (2 points) _____ Moderate (4 points) _____ Severe (8 points)		
PHYSICAL STATUS		
_____ Altered nutritional status (1 point)	_____ Sensory deficits (3 points)	
_____ Fatigue and weakness (2 points)	_____ Visual impairments (3 points)	
ORTHOSTATIC HYPOTENSION		
_____ Drop in systolic of 20 mmHG or more between lying and standing (2 points)		
_____ Drop in diastolic of 20 mmHG or more between lying and standing (2 points)		
GAIT AND BALANCE Assess patient's gait while: (Give 1 point for each positive)		
_____ Standing in one spot with both feet on the ground for 30 seconds without holding on to something.		
_____ Walking straightforward.	_____ Walking making a turn.	
_____ Balance problems when walking.	_____ Dizziness.	
_____ Decrease in muscle coordination.	_____ Wide base of support.	
_____ Jerking or instability when making turns.	_____ Loss of balance while standing.	
_____ Lurching, swaying or slapping gait (1 point).	_____ Gait pattern changes when walking through doorway.	
_____ Use of assistive device (cane, walker furniture).		
ELIMINATION		
_____ Diarrhea (2 points) _____ Nocturia (2 points) _____ Incontinence (3 points)		
A score of 11 or above – Fall Risk	**TOTAL SCORE**	

PLAN OF ACTION
☐ Treatment Plan ☐ Fall precautions ☐ Level of care
☐ N/A Comments (explain):_____

_____

RN Signature	**Date**	**Time**

County of San Diego
Health and Human Services Agency
Mental Health Services
SAN DIEGO COUNTY PSYCHIATRIC HOSPITAL

Patient Name: _____

MR#: _____ Date:_____

FALL RISK ASSESSMENT

HHSA:MHS-206 (10/02)

Figure A.8.   Nursing admission assessment (sample 1)

ADMISSION DATE:_____	**TIME:**_____

NAME PATIENT PREFERS TO BE CALLED:_____

VITAL SIGNS:
  T   P   R   B/P

HT (inches):_____   WT (#):_____   Sex:_____

Eye Color: _____   Hair Color:_____   Age:_____ years old

TRANSPORT:
☐ Ambulatory
☐ Gurney
☐ Wheel Chair
Other:_____

INITIAL DISCHARGE PLANNING
Name of Support Person(s) (relationship):_____

Home Situation: ☐ Alone   ☐ Family   ☐ B&C   ☐ Homeless   ☐ Friend
            ☐ Other psych facility:_____
            ☐ Other: _____

Discharge Needs: _____

SAFETY:
Were there any Sharps/Medications/Matches/Other Dangerous Items on person or clothing?   ☐ Yes   ☐ No

If yes, list: _____

_____

☐ Hx of AWOL   ☐ DTS   ☐ DTO   Contracts for Safety   ☐ Yes   ☐ No
☐ Yes   ☐ No   Expresses thoughts of hurting someone or has made threats in past month.
☐ Yes   ☐ No   History of violence
☐ Yes   ☐ No   Potential for assault or violence is currently present.

If any of the three (3) above boxes is **Yes**, complete a *Violence Risk Assessment* (HHSA:MHS-220) form

---

ABUSE:
☐ Unknown   ☐ Hx of recent abuse   ☐ Hx of abusing others recently. *If yes on Hx, explain*: _____

_____

ORIENTED TO UNIT:
☐ Room   ☐ Bathroom   ☐ Smoke Time   ☐ Unit Program Schedule   ☐ Seclusion/Restraint
☐ Locker   ☐ Patient Rights   ☐ Telephone Access   ☐ Unit Handout   ☐ Unable to Orient

---

COMMUNICABLE DISEASE (Per Hx or self-report):
☐ Hepatitis   ☐ Pediculosis   ☐ Scabies   ☐ Sexually transmitted diseases
☐ Other: _____   ☐ Unable to Respond   ☐ Unknown

SOCIOCULTURAL FACTORS: Special cultural, spiritual or religious needs
☐ No   ☐ Unable to determine   ☐ Yes   If yes, describe:_____

SIGNATURE:	**DATE:**	**TIME:**
RN		

County of San Diego
Health and Human Services Agency
Mental Health Services
SAN DIEGO COUNTY PSYCHIATRIC HOSPITAL

PATIENT IDENTIFICATION

NURSING ADMISSION ASSESSMENT

HHSA:MHS-389-(06/03) page 1 of 2

Figure A.8. (Continued)

MENTAL STATUS EXAM:

Oriented to:	☐ Person	☐ Place	☐ Month	☐ Year	☐ Situation	☐ None
LOC:	☐ Alert	☐ Lethargic	☐ Confused	☐ Stuporous	☐ Comatose	
Appearance:	☐ Clean	☐ Malodorous	☐ Disheveled			
Speech:	☐ Normal	☐ Slurred	☐ Loud	☐ Pressured	☐ Slow	☐ Mute
Thought process:	☐ Coherent	☐ Tangential	☐ Incoherent	☐ Loose associations		
	☐ Other:_____					
Thought content:	☐ Reality based	☐ Other:_____				
Behavior:	☐ Cooperative	☐ Uncooperative	☐ Tearful	☐ Restless	☐ Threatening	
	☐ Agitated	☐ Combative				
Affect:	☐ Euthymic	☐ Blunted	☐ Flat/Masklike	☐ Anxious	☐ Frightened	☐ Angry
	☐ Elevated	☐ Dysphoric	☐ Withdrawn	☐ Irritable		
Posture/Gait:	☐ Erect	☐ Stooped	☐ Normal	☐ Shuffling	☐ Staggering	

ADDITIONAL COMMENTS: _____

_____

_____

ALLERGIES / INTOLERANCES:
☐ NKA   ☐ Medications: _____   ☐ Food:_____

☐ Other:_____   REACTION:_____

VISION: ☐ Glasses   ☐ Contacts   ☐ Limited vision   ☐ Blind
                ☐ Prosthesis: _____   ☐ No known problem

HEARING: ☐ Uses hearing aid   ☐ No known problem ☐ Other (describe): _____

ORAL HYGIENE: ☐ Good   ☐ Fair   ☐ Poor   **DENTURES:**   ☐ Full   ☐ Uppers   ☐ Lowers
                                                                                ☐ Partial   ☐ None

AMBULATION: ☐ Hx of falls last month   ☐ Over age 65   ☐ Unsteady gait
If any of the 3 boxes is checked, complete a Fall Risk Assessment (HHSA:MHS-220) form

GI Hx: ☐ Unable to assess   Last BM_____   ☐ Hx constipation ☐ Hx Diarrhea
                ☐ Rectal bleeding   ☐ Nausea   ☐ Vomiting   ☐ No known problem
                ☐ Other (describe): _____

GU Hx: ☐ Bladder incontinence   ☐ Prostate problems   If checked, describe when: _____
                ☐ Difficulty urinating ☐ No known problem   ☐ Other (describe): _____

OB/GYN Hx: ☐ Unable to determine   ☐ LMP_____   ☐ Pregnant due date: _____
                ☐ Galactorrhea _____   ☐ Menopause   ☐ Premenstrual syndrome
                ☐ Menstrual difficulties   ☐ Other (describe):_____

SIGNATURE:	**DATE:**	**TIME:**
RN		

County of San Diego
Health and Human Services Agency
Mental Health Services
SAN DIEGO COUNTY PSYCHIATRIC HOSPITAL

PATIENT IDENTIFICATION

NURSING ADMISSION ASSESSMENT

HHSA:MHS-389-(06/03) Page 2 of 2

Figure A.9. Nursing admission assessment (sample 2)

PAST SURGICAL/MEDICAL Hx/CHRONIC CONDITIONS:				
☐ Unable to determine	☐ Osteoporosis	☐ Cancer	☐ Seizures	☐ HIV
☐ No known surgeries	☐ Diabetes	☐ COPD	☐ Arthritis	☐ CVA
☐ No known medical Hx	☐ Renal failure	☐ Thyroid	☐ Back surgery	☐ Coronary artery disease
☐ Hx of head injury	☐ Other (describe)_____			

PREVIOUS HOSPITALIZATION PAST 30 DAYS:
☐ No   ☐ Unknown   ☐ Yes Reason (in patient's words): _____

NUTRITIONAL STATUS: ☐ Normal Weight   ☐ Overweight   ☐ Underweight
Likes:_____ Dislikes:_____
          NUTRITIONAL PATIENT REPORT: ☐ **Poor appetite > 1 week**   ☐ **Weight loss > 10 pounds in 1 month**
☐ Refuses to eat because:_____ ☐ Chewing or swallowing difficulties related to: _____
☐ No known problems   ☐ Other (describe):_____ ☐ Dietitian notified

RESPIRATORY STATUS: ☐ Normal   ☐ Wheezes   ☐ SOB   ☐ Coughing   ☐ Sneezing
RESPIRATORY Hx: ☐ Unknown   ☐ Asthma   ☐ Emphysema ☐ Other (describe):_____
TOBACCO: ☐ Never smoked   ☐ Still smokes ☐ Years smoked:_____   Packs/day:_____
Wants to quit: ☐ No   ☐ Yes   ☐ Quit
CARDIAC Hx: ☐ Palpitations   ☐ Unknown   ☐ Hypertension   ☐ Angina   ☐ Other (describe): _____

EDUCATIONAL ABILITY: Understands verbal direction: ☐ Yes   ☐ No
Reads English   ☐ Yes   ☐ No   Speaks English ☐ Yes   ☐ No   Motivated to learn: ☐ Yes   ☐ No
Learns best by ☐ Reading   ☐ Videos   ☐ Groups   ☐ 1:1 sessions   ☐ Other (describe): _____
Learning needs: ☐ About Mental disorder:_____ ☐ About Physical Health Problem: _____
☐ Medications/Drug/Alcohol dependency   ☐ Coping skills   ☐ Grief and loss   ☐ Diet   ☐ Self-Care
☐ Leisure Activities   ☐ STD prevention   ☐ Self help groups   ☐ Relapse Prevention   ☐ ADL's
☐ Other (describe): _____

PAIN ASSESSMENT: Intensity: Pain rating scale (patient selects 0-10) _____   **OR** Wong-Baker faces scale (patient
selects 0,2,4,6,8,10) _____   If pain rating 4 or above on rating scale, complete a Pain Assessment (HHSA:MHS-207) form
Plan: ☐ Notify physician   ☐ Pain medication, as ordered   ☐ Non-medication treatments
          ☐ Patient refuses interventions   ☐ Initiate treatment plan   ☐ Other:_____

SCALP: ☐ Good hygiene   ☐ Poor hygiene   ☐ Scaly   ☐ Head Lice
SKIN COLOR: ☐ Normal   ☐ Flushed   ☐ Jaundice   ☐ Mottled ☐ Pale   ☐ Cyanotic
SKIN TEMP: ☐ Normal   ☐ Cool   ☐ Hot   ☐ Moist   ☐ Other (describe): _____

MARK ON BODY DIAGRAM ANY ABNORMALITIES OBSERVED WITH A SHORT DESCRIPTION:

          ☐ **Dressed**   ☐ **Undressed**

MUSCULO-SKELETAL SYSTEM	SITES	SIZE	*DESCRIPTION*
SCAR (S)			
TATTOO (S)			
WOUNDS/SKIN TEARS/LACERATIONS			
LICE/SCABIES			
BRUISES			
ACNE			
OTHER			

SIGNATURE: **RN**	**DATE:**	**TIME:**

County of San Diego
Health and Human Services Agency
Mental Health Services
SAN DIEGO COUNTY PSYCHIATRIC HOSPITAL

PATIENT IDENTIFICATION

NURSING ADMISSION ASSESSMENT

HHSA: MHS-390 (06/03)

Figure A.10. Psychiatric assessment

This is a psychiatric assessment billed as an MMD provided on site for _____ minutes.

<u>PRESENTING PROBLEM:</u>

      IDENTIFYING DATA/CHIEF COMPLAINT

      HISTORY OF PRESENT ILLNESS

<u>CURRENT NEEDS</u>

      PAST PSYCHIATRIC HISTORY

<u>DRUG/ALCOHOL HISTORY</u>

      MEDICAL HISTORY

      SOCIAL HISTORY

      CULTURAL & RELIGIOUS ISSUES

      INSURANCE STATUS

      VITAL SIGNS:
         Blood pressure: _____ Temperature:_____ Pulse rate: _____ Respiratory rate: _____ Pain (0-10):____

<u>MENTAL STATUS EXAMINATION:</u>

<u>DIAGNOSIS:</u>

      Axis I:
      Axis II:
      Axis III:
      Axis IV:
      Axis V: GAF Current: Past year:

<u>CURRENT POTENTIAL FOR HARM:</u>

<u>INTERPRETIVE SUMMARY:</u>

_____
                     STAFF PSYCHIATRIST

County of San Diego **Health and Human Services Agency** Mental Health Services SAN DIEGO COUNTY PSYCHIATRIC HOSPITAL PSYCHIATRIC ASSESSMENT HHSA:MHS-204 (01/02)	Patient Name: MR#: Unit: D.O.B.: Date

Figure A.11.   Restraint or seclusion assessment

PRECIPITATING EVENT: Behaviors leading to restraint or seclusion:	Nursing Staff Prompts: *(Check all when completed)*
_____ _____ _____ _____ _____ _____	☐ 1:1 initiated by Charge Nurse ☐ MD evaluation within one (1) hour ☐ Clothing search complete ☐ Denial of Rights Form complete ☐ Order obtained every 4 hours ☐ Add to Treatment Plan *(CRU only)*

Clinical interventions used prior to restraint or seclusion: (*check all that apply*)

☐   **Medication Intervention**   ☐   **De-escalation**   ☐   **Voluntary Time Out**

☐ **Threat Reduction** *(for fear)*
  ☐   Mirror person as far as eye contact
  ☐   Give reassurance of safety
  ☐   No touching without permission
  ☐   Stand with arms at side, palms facing forward
  ☐   Calm, confident vocal tone
  ☐   Slow gestures
  ☐   Use rule of five *(no more than 5 words-each word 5 letters or less)*

☐   **Control** *(for frustration)*
  ☐   Maintain eye contact
  ☐   Assess origin/cause of frustration
  ☐   Stand with palms facing down
  ☐   Speak in confident manner
  ☐   Moderate tone of voice
  ☐   Use rule of five

☐ **Detachment** *(for manipulation)*
  ☐   No direct eye contact
  ☐   Speak in firm voice
  ☐   Turn at an angled position
  ☐   Use rule of five
  ☐   Act in a disengaged manner

☐ **Consequation** *(for intimidation)*
  ☐   Use rule of five
  ☐   Confident posture
  ☐   Maintain direct eye contact
  ☐   Don't threaten or argue
  ☐   Identify consequences

Patient's response to above interventions: _____
_____

(circle one below)

Less restrictive interventions have been attempted unsuccessfully and **seclusion/restraint/ambulatory restraint** is necessary to prevent the followings: ☐ Harm to self   ☐ Harm to others

The patient was given the following explanation of reason for seclusion or restraint:_____
_____

Patient grants permission to notify family of Seclusion or Restraint   ☐Yes (if yes document in Progress Notes)
                                                                                                        ☐No

☐ Signed consent for involvement of interested party obtained

(If yes, name of person contacted)_____

Release criteria: ☐ Contracts for Safety   ☐ Reduced Agitation/Impulsively
                                     ☐ No longer danger to self and/or others

Explain: _____

RN Signature _____   **Date**_____   **Time:**_____

County of San Diego
Health and Human Services Agency
Mental Health Services
San Diego County Psychiatric Hospital
RESTRAINT OR SECLUSION ASSESSMENT
HHSA:MHS-225 (11/02)

Patient Identification

Figure A.12. Restraint or seclusion flow sheet

TITLE:	<u>RESTRAINT or SECLUSION FLOW SHEET</u>
FORM NUMBER:	<u>HHSA: MHS-226</u>
<u>WHEN</u>	For use of Restraint or Seclusion procedures and ambulatory restraints.
<u>ON WHOM</u>	All patients in seclusion, restraints or ambulatory restraints.
<u>COMPLETED BY</u>	The Flow sheet will be completed by RNs, and LVNs, PTs and/or MHAs.
<u>MODE OF COMPLETION</u>	Handwritten.

<u>FORMAT</u>

Restraint or Seclusion Flow sheet is a preprinted form to include patient's identification, date, shift, time initiated, and initiator RN signature.

The type of Restraint or Seclusion initiated will be checked.

A new form will be used when the first form is completed or when a new date starts.

Signatures and initials of those staff using the form will be placed in the respective boxes.

"Describe Patient Behaviors" Section:
➢ RN's shall document when a patient is placed into seclusion, restraint, or ambulatory restraints and when these measures are renewed, reduced or discontinued.
➢ Additional pertinent information shall be documented here at least once every hour.
➢ Code numbers from the top of the page shall be used, when applicable.
➢ Additional information may be added to the progress notes.
➢ **"Every 15 minutes" Section:**
➢ May be completed by RN's, LVN's, PT's or MHA's.
➢ Add time and initials (end of row).
➢ Check blanks corresponding to each section.
➢ Add code numbers in "brief behavior description" column.
  ▪ **"Every 2 hour" Section:**
➢ May be completed by RN's, LVN's, PT's or MHA's.
➢ Add time and initials (end of row).
➢ Check and complete blanks corresponding to each section.
  ▪ **"Debriefing" Section:**
➢ **Shall be completed by an RN.**
➢ **Add reason for "no" and additional comments as indicated.**
➢ **If there are no additional comments, write N/A in the blanks provided.**

<u>EXCEPTIONS</u>

None.

06/02

(Continued on next page)

Figure A.12. (Continued)

_____ Date_____ Shift _____ Time Initiated	_____
	Initiator RN Signature Date

Check One: ☐ Seclusion   ☐ Restraint   ☐ Ambulatory Restraints

CODES	Document/check each area every **15 MINUTES** or more frequently as needed.	Document/check each area every TWO (2) HOURS or more frequently as needed.

CODES											

(RN's, LVN's, PT's, MHA's

1. Beating on door/wall	6. Standing still
2. Yelling/screaming	7. Walking/pacing
3. Crying/cursing	8. Thrashing/spitting
4. Laughing/singing	9. Quiet
5. Mumbling	10. Disrobing/sexually inappropriate

11. Other:_____

Initials	Signatures

Time	Describe Patient Behaviors (document once every hour)	RN Initials	Time	Continual visual & auditory observation	Patient is breathing without difficulty CIRCULATION CHECKS	Restraints intact, extremities assessed	Brief behavior description (USE CODES)	Offer of foods/fluids	Offer bathroom/bedpan	Range of Motion (10 minutes)	Pulse & B/P Temperature & Respiration Rate	Initials

Debriefing within 24 hours after episode ☐ Yes ☐ No If no, give reason_____

Comments:_____

County of San Diego
Health and Human Services Agency
Mental Health Services
San Diego County Psychiatric Hospital

Patient Identification

RESTRAINT OR SECLUSION FLOW SHEET

HHSA:MHS-226 (06/02)

Figure A.13.   Social work assessment

DOB: _____ **SS#** _____ **Race/Ethnicity:** _____ **Sex:** ☐ M ☐ F

Marital Status: ☐ Single ☐ Married ☐ Widowed ☐ Separated ☐ Divorced _____ Times Married/Divorced

Legal Status: ☐ Voluntary ☐ 72 Hour Hold ☐ Other _____

Financial Benefits/Insurance: _____ **Payee:** _____

Employment Status: _____ **Vocational History:** _____
_____

Residence: ☐ House ☐ Apartment ☐ Board & Care ☐ Homeless ☐ Other _____

Can patient return? ☐ Yes ☐ No, why not? _____

Family/Social Supports	NAME	RELATIONSHIP	PHONE NUMBER

INTERVIEW WITH PATIENT:

Patient's expectations upon admission and motivation to learn: _____
_____
_____

Patient's description of childhood and history of emotional and behavioral functioning: _____
_____
_____

Educational History (include barriers to learning): _____
_____

Military Service History (include type of discharge): _____

Abuse History (include both patient as victim and as perpetrator): _____
_____

Legal History: _____

Cross Cultural Issues: _____

Religious/ Spiritual Issues: _____

Family History of Mental Illness? _____ Explain: _____
_____

San Diego County
Health and Human Services Agency
Mental Health Services
San Diego County Psychiatric Hospital

SOCIAL WORK ASSESSMENT

HHSA:MHS-209 (5/03) pg 1 of 2

PATIENT NAME: _____

Medical Record #: _____

(Continued on next page)

Figure A.13. (Continued)

MENTAL/BEHAVIORAL STATUS: *(circle appropriate description)*					
General appearance: neat	appropriate	inappropriate	disheveled	unkempt	
Attitude: relaxed	cooperative	guarded	demanding	hostile	abusive
Motor activity: relaxed	anxious	agitated	retarded	catatonic	
Affect: appropriate	broad	flattened	inappropriate	tearful	labile
Mood: angry			apathetic		anxious euphoric
irritable			euthymic		depressed
Speech: clear	pressured	loud	incoherent	mute	rapid
Orientation: time	person	place	situation		
Associations: normal	loose	tangential	bizarre		
Thought content: appropriate	delusional	paranoid	grandiose		
Hallucinations: none	auditory	visual	olfactory	tactile	

Memory:

Long-term	good	fair	poor	impaired	grossly confused
Short-term	good	fair	poor	impaired	grossly confused
Judgment:	good	fair	poor	nil	
Insight:	good	fair	poor	nil	
Suicide potential:	none	ideation	has plan	attempted in past	immediate intent

PAIN ASSESSMENT= RATING (Scale of 0-10):_____ **Name of Doctor Notified:**_____

PRIOR PSYCHIATRIC TREATMENT:☐ None☐ Inpatient☐ Outpatient☐ Day Treatment☐ **Long** Term Care

What has worked best? _____

_____

History of self harm/suicidality: _____

_____

History of harm to others: _____

_____

DRUG/ALCOHOL HISTORY: ☐ Yes ☐ No   Age began:_____ Drug(s) of choice:_____

Treatment History (including periods of sobriety: _____

_____

Patient's perceptions of consequences of abuse: _____

_____

DISCHARGE/AFTERCARE PLANS: _____

_____

_____

Signature: _____LCSW Date: _____   Time:_____

San Diego County	
Health and Human Services Agency	**PATIENT NAME:**_____
Mental Health Services	
San Diego County Psychiatric Hospital	
SOCIAL WORK ASSESSMENT	**Medical Record #:**_____

HHSA:MHS-209 (5/03) pg 2 of 2

Figure A.14.   Treatment plan/problem sheet

MEDICAL CONDITION/MANIFESTED BY: PROBLEM#:_____

_____

_____

If pain is present, identify type: ☐ Acute (relatively brief that subsides as healing takes place

                                     ☐ Chronic Nonmalignant (duration of six (6) months or longer, due to
                                       non-life threatening causes, has not responded to current treatment methods,
                                       may continue for rest of life)

                                     ☐ Other (describe)_____

DISCHARGE GOALS:

     ☐ Patient will participate actively in treatment.

     ☐ Patient will express interest in continuing compliance with treatment.

Pain

     ☐ Patient's pain rating intensity will be within patient's comfort zone.

     ☐ Patient and/or family verbalize measures that provide pain relief, identify plan and resources for
        follow-up care.

OBJECTIVES:

		Time Frame	Date
Date		(within days)	Achieved

MEDICAL CONDITION WITH PAIN

_____κ   _____   _____

Patient will take medication(s) as prescribed and identify reason for
taking, side effects and benefits. Patient will verbalize learning regarding
self-care, pain rating that is satisfactory for comfort and function, and
non-drug treatments treatment for pain management. Patient will express
his/her feelings about pain and/for medical condition.
Patient's pain will be at a satisfactory level for comfort and function.

_____κ Patient will (specify behaviors)_____   _____   _____

			Responsible	
Date		Frequency	Staff	Discipline

_____κ **Physician:**   _____   _____   _____
      Medical Condition with Pain

      Refer patient to specialty clinic, if indicated.

      Prescribe medication(s).

      Adjust patient's pain medication schedule to around the
      clock if indicated.

      Other_____

County of San Diego Health and Human Services Agency Mental Health Services SAN DIEGO COUNTY PSYCHIATRIC HOSPITAL	PATIENT IDENTIFICATION
TREATMENT PLAN, PROBLEM SHEET	
HHSA:MHS 216 (5/03) page 1 of 2	

(Continued on next page)

Figure A.14.   (Continued)

INTERVENTIONS: *(continued)*

	Frequency	Responsible Staff	Discipline
Date			

_____ ☐ **Nursing:**   _____ _____ _____
Medical Condition with Pain

Provide opportunities for expression of feelings regarding
disorder and self-management of same.

Document treatment and response of patient.

Administer and monitor medication(s) and treatments per physician's
order. (Monitor and document patient's response using
pain rating scale and level of comfort statements/behaviors.)

Instruct patient to report medication side effects or other adverse
reactions to medication and non-drug treatments.

Complete pain assessment when indicated

Instruct patient to report effectiveness of pain management treatment.

Educate patient/family about medical condition and pain and use of
helpful descriptors such as pain rating scale, quality, location, duration of pain.

Instruct patient to ask staff for help with pain management.

_____ ☐ **Other:**   _____ _____ _____

_____

_____

_____ ☐ **Groups:**   _____ _____ _____
Medical Condition with Pain
Other_____
Other_____

Teach patient/families about non-drug pain management
activities, such as relaxation, distraction, and pressure points.

Assist patients to practice non-drug pain management techniques and
to select those most useful to use again.

Give patient educational materials to help in retention of learning
and practice of pain relief techniques after discharge.

Signatures	Date	Signatures	Date

County of San Diego Health and Human Services Agency Mental Health Services SAN DIEGO COUNTY PSYCHIATRIC HOSPITAL	PATIENT IDENTIFICATION
TREATMENT PLAN, PROBLEM SHEET	
HHSA:MHS 216 (5/03) page 2 of 2	

Appendix B

Sample Outpatient Forms

Figure B.1.   Abnormal involuntary movement scale

Complete Examination Procedure **MOVEMENT RATINGS**: Rate highest severity observed. Rate movements that occur upon activation one *less* than those observed spontaneously.	Code: 0 = None 1 = Minimal, may be extreme normal 2 = Mild 3 = Moderate 4 = Severe	
Muscles of Facial Expression	Date:	Date:
e.g., movements of forehead, eyebrows, periorbital area, cheeks;	(Circle one)	(Circle one)
include frowning, blinking, smiling, grimacing	0 1 2 3 4	0 1 2 3 4
Lips and Perioral Area e.g., puckering, pouting, smacking	0 1 2 3 4	0 1 2 3 4
Jaw e.g., biting, clenching, chewing, mouth opening, lateral movement	0 1 2 3 4	0 1 2 3 4
Tongue Rate only increase in movement both in and out of mouth, inability to sustain movement	0 1 2 3 4	0 1 2 3 4
Upper (arms, wrists, hands, fingers) Include choric movements, (i.e., slow, irregular, complex, serpentine). Do not include tremor (i.e., repetitive regular, rhythmic).	0 1 2 3 4	0 1 2 3 4
Lower (*legs, knees, ankles, toes*) e.g. lateral knee movement, foot tapping, heel dropping, foot squirming, inversion and eversion of foot	0 1 2 3 4	0 1 2 3 4
Neck, shoulder, hips e.g., rocking, twisting, squirming, pelvic gyrations	0 1 2 3 4	0 1 2 3 4
Severity of abnormal movements	0 1 2 3 4	0 1 2 3 4
Incapacitation due to abnormal movements	0 1 2 3 4	0 1 2 3 4
Patients awareness of abnormal movements Rate only client's report	No Awareness 0 Aware, No Distress 1 Aware, Mild Distress 2 Aware, Moderate distress 3 Aware, severe distress 4	No Awareness 0 Aware, No Distress 1 Aware, Mild Distress 2 Aware, Moderate distress 3 Aware, severe distress 4
Current problems with teeth and/or dentures	No 0 Yes 1	No 0 Yes 1
Does client usually wear dentures?	No 0 Yes 1	No 0 Yes 1

Total:_____   Total:_____

Staff Signature:_____   Date:_____

Staff Signature:_____   Date:_____

County of San Diego Health and Human Services Agency Mental Health Services **ABNORMAL INVOLUNTARY MOVEMENT SCALE (AIMS)** HHSA:MHS-914 (6/2003)	**Client:** _____ **MR/Client ID #:**_____ **Program:**_____

Figure B.2. Authorization to use or disclose

COUNTY OF SAN DIEGO

AUTHORIZATION TO USE OR DISCLOSE PROTECTED HEALTH INFORMATION

I hereby authorize use or disclosure of the named individual's health information as described below.

	DATE:

PATIENT/RESIDENT/CLIENT		
LAST NAME:	FIRST NAME:	MIDDLE INITIAL:
ADDRESS	CITY/STATE:	ZIP CODE:
TELEPHONE NUMBER:	SSN:	DATE OF BIRTH:
AKA'S:		

THE FOLLOWING INDIVIDUAL OR ORGANIZATION IS AUTHORIZED TO MAKE THE DISCLOSURE.		
LAST NAME OR ENTITY:	FIRST NAME:	MIDDLE INITIAL:
ADDRESS	CITY/STATE:	ZIP CODE:
TELEPHONE NUMBER:	DATE:	

THIS INFORMATION MAY BE DISCLOSED TO AND USED BY THE FOLLOWING INDIVIDUAL OR ORGANIZATION.		
LAST NAME OR ENTITY:	FIRST NAME:	MIDDLE INITIAL:
ADDRESS	CITY/STATE:	ZIP CODE:
TELEPHONE NUMBER:	DATE:	
TREATMENT DATES:	PURPOSE OF REQUEST: ☐ AT THE REQUEST OF THE INDIVIDUAL.	

THE FOLLOWING INFORMATION IS TO BE DISCLOSED: (PLEASE CHECK)

☐ History and Physical Examination
☐ Discharge Summary
☐ Progress Notes
☐ Medication Records
☐ Interpretation of images: x-rays, sonograms, etc.
☐ Laboratory Results
☐ Dental Records
☐ Psychiatric Records
☐ HIV/AIDS blood test results; any/all references to those results

☐ Physician Orders
☐ Pharmacy Records
☐ Immunization Records
☐ Nursing Notes
☐ Billing Records
☐ Drug/Alcohol Rehabilitation Records
☐ Complete Record
☐ Other *(Provide description)* _____

County of San Diego
Health and Human Services Agency
Mental Health Services

**AUTHORIZATION TO USE OR DISCLOSE
PROTECTED HEALTH INFORMATION**

23-07 HHSA (04/03)

Client: _____

Record Number: _____

Program: _____

(Continued on next page)

Figure B.2. (Continued)

Sensitive Information: I understand that the information in my record may include information relating to sexually transmitted diseases, acquired immunodeficiency syndrome (AIDS), or infection with the Human Immunodeficiency Virus (HIV). It may also include information about behavioral or mental health services or treatment for alcohol and drug abuse.
Right to Revoke: I understand that I have the right to revoke this authorization at any time. I understand if I revoke this authorization I must do so in writing. I understand that the revocation will not apply to information that has already been released based on this authorization.
Expiration: Unless otherwise revoked, this authorization will expire on the following date, event, or condition: _____   If I do not specify an expiration date, event or condition, this authorization will expire in one (1) calendar year from the date it was signed.
Redisclosure: If I have authorized the disclosure of my health information to someone who is not legally required to keep it confidential, I understand it may be redisclosed and no longer protected. California law generally prohibits recipients of my health information from redisclosing such information except with my written authorization or as specifically required or permitted by law.
Other Rights: I understand that authorizing the disclosure of this health information is voluntary. I can refuse to sign this authorization. I do not need to sign this form to assure treatment. However, if this authorization is needed for participation in a research study, my enrollment in the research study may be denied.   I understand that I may inspect or obtain a copy of the information to be used or disclosed, as provided in 45 Code of Federal Regulations section164.524.   I have right to receive a copy of this authorization. I would like a copy of this authorization.   ☐ Yes   ☐ No

SIGNATURE OF INDIVIDUAL OR LEGAL REPRESENTATIVE	
SIGNATURE:	DATE:
IF SIGNED BY LEGAL REPRESENTATIVE, RELATIONSHIP OF INDIVIDUAL:	

FOR OFFICE USE

VALIDATION	
SIGNATURE OF STAFF PERSON VALIDATING IDENTIFICATION:	DATE:
SIGNATURE OF HEALTH CARE PROVIDER:*	DATE:

* Health care provider approving client access to own records

---

County of San Diego
Health and Human Services Agency
Mental Health Services

**AUTHORIZATION TO USE OR DISCLOSE
PROTECTED HEALTH INFORMATION**
23-07 HHSA (04/03)

Client: _____

Record Number: _____

Program: _____

Figure B.3. Client plan

Care Coordinator: _____   Annual Review Date _____

Goal: _____

Barriers, behaviors, symptoms or obstacles that might jeopardize achieving of goal: _____

Client strengths and abilities to apply toward goal: _____

Objectives (measurable, achievable, time limited, include date:)	Interventions (include frequency, duration)	Person (s) responsible	Date objective completed

I participated in the development of this plan and received a copy:

Client signature: _____   Staff signature: _____   Co-signature (if required): _____
Date: _____   Date: _____   Date: _____

Client Plan Update   Client Plan Update
Client signature: _____   Staff signature: _____   Co-signature (if required): _____
Date: _____   Date: _____   Date: _____

Client: _____

MR/Client ID #: _____

Program: _____

County of San Diego
Health and Human Services Agency
Mental Health Services

CLIENT PLAN

HHSA:MHS-975 (6/2003)

Figure B.4. Demographic/registration report

```
        Report MHS 140
        Run Date: 9-OCT-2002
    Page: 1
```

****
****

CONSUMER INFORMATION

Name:	Justin Thyme	Number	1	Birth date	20-Sep-1990	Age	12
Address	123 SAM ST	SSN	999-99-9991	Sex	M		
	SAN DIEGO, CA 92107	Other ID #:	456789	Language	Mien		
Phone	(619) 555-1212	Marital:	Married	Education:	Grade 11		
Staff:	FEELGOOD, IWANNA (000)	Disability:	None	Ethnicity: White	Origin: Hispanic		
Aliases: JOE B. SHMOE, JONNIE SMITH, DANNY JONES					Hispanic		
RP Owes:	$0.00	Medicaid	Y11999:	Last Eligibility: 1/2000			

Insurance: MEDICARE PT A PRIMARY BC (9997), MEDICARE PT B PRIMARY-TO (9999), PRINCIPAL FINANCIAL GROUP (45) PACIFIC CARE (256)

SIGNIFICANT OTHERS

Name:	Relation	Home Phone	Work Phone	Address	Emergency
Thyme Sr, Justin	Father	(619) 555-1212	(760) 333-3333	555 SE ANZA ST, apt. 23-c, San Diego, CA 92123	X
Blow, Joe	Other	( ) -	(619) 123-4567 x8910		
Thyme, Siesta	Stepmother	(619) 853-1515	(760) 222-4444	1130 S NERD DR, APT 111, SAN DIEGO, CA 92111	

****
****

CLINICAL HISTORY

RU	Opening	Closing	Primary Diagnosis	Clinician	Physician	Total Units	Last Service	Legal Status	Legal Conser
------OPEN EPISODES--									
UBH	22-JUN-2002		295.70	STAFF, GENERAL		7	21-AUG-2002	W5150	UNKN(
TEST - IP	6-JUN-2001					4			
------CLOSED EPISODES--									
UBH	18-JUN-2002	19-JUN-2002	296.50	SHUMAN, JUDY		1	19-JUN-2002	W6000	UNKN(
EPU-OP -ADLT	7-DEC-2001	7-DEC-2001	296.20			0		W6000	PAREN

```
            ************************
            Confidential Information
            ************************
```

Figure B.5. Episode face sheet

```
              EPISODE FACE SHEET

REPORT MHS800
CLIENT NUMBER:                    REPORTING UNIT:
ADMISSION DATE:                   DISCHARGE DATE:
*********************************************************************************

NAME:                  ADDRESS:
MED REC#:              MEDICAID/LAST ELIGIBILITY:
DOB:          AGE:            SEX:
SSN:          MARITAL:        PHONE:
ETHNICITY:    LANGUAGE:       HISPANIC ORIGIN:
EDUCATION:                    DISABILITY:
SOURCE OF INCOME:            TYPE OF EMPLOYMENT:
*********************************************************************************

PERSON TO NOTIFY IN CASE OF EMERGENCY:
 NAME:                  RELATIONSHIP
 ADDRESS:
 NAME:                  RELATIONSHIP:
 ADDRESS:
 HOME PHONE:            WORK PHONE:
*********************************************************************************

CLINICAL HISTORY

REFERRAL FROM:         ADMISSION DATE:        ADMIT TIME:
DISCHARGE DATE:        DISCHARGE TIME:
CLIENT LOCATION:       EFFECTIVE:
BROUGHT FROM:          BROUGHT BY:
SCHOOL NAME:           SCHOOL DISTRICT:


EPISODE STATUS (OPEN)

PRIMARY AXIS I:
SECONDARY AXIS I:
AXIS II:
AXIS III:
AXIS IV:
AXIS V:          PAST
                 CURRENT
                 OPENING GAF

CLINICIAN ID:
PSYCHIATRIST:
LEGAL CONSENT:
LEGAL ENTRY:
LEGAL EXIT:
RELIGION:
REASON FOR DISCHARGE:
LEGAL EXIT:


Referral 1:            Referral 2:


Referral 3:


***********************
Confidential Information
***********************
```

Figure B.6.   Expedited assessment

Date/ Hr: Min	Location / Service	Notes		
		Expedited Assessment:		
		Presenting Problem:		
		Current Medication		
		Current Substance Abuse		
		MSE:		
		Diagnosis		
		Impairment/Disability Use DSM-IV Codes. Indicate (P) – Primary and (S) – Secondary	Enter P in front of Primary	Diagnostic Code
		Axis I:		
		Axis I:		
		Axis I:		
		Axis II:		
		Axis II:		
		Axis III: Relevant Medical Conditions:		
		Axis IV: Psychosocial and Environmental Problems:		
		Axis V: Current GAF: **Highest in Past Year:**		
		Current Potential for Harm:		
		Interpretive Summary:		

County of San Diego
Health and Human Services Agency
Mental Health Services

EXPEDITED ASSESSMENT

Client:_____

MR/Client ID #:_____

Program:_____

Figure B.7.   Informed consent for use of psychotropic medications

INFORMED CONSENT FOR THE USE OF PSYCHOTROPIC MEDICATION

Client Information and Consent (Please read this form carefully and completely)

- You have the right to be informed; be given information about your care and to ask questions.
- You have the right to accept or reject all or any part of your care plan.
- You have the right to revoke consent verbally or in writing to any member of the treating staff for any reason at any time.
- You have the right to language/interpreting services. Services Requested: ☐ YES   ☐ NO
- You have the right to a copy of this Consent: Copy Requested?   ☐ YES   ☐ NO

Emergency Treatment: In certain emergencies, medication may be given to you when it is impractical to obtain consent. However, once the emergency has passed, medication will continue with your informed consent. *(An emergency is a temporary, sudden marked change requiring action to preserve life or prevent serious bodily harm to client or others).*

Your Physician is prescribing the following psychotropic medication(s) for you:

Medication(s) Name	Medication Info. Sheet Given (check box) ☛
	☐ YES ☐ NO
	☐ YES ☐ NO
	☐ YES ☐ NO
	☐ YES ☐ NO
	☐ YES ☐ NO
	☐ YES ☐ NO

In order to be informed and give consent, your doctor will discuss the following information with you:

Verbal Information Discussed with Client

1.   Nature and seriousness of your mental illness

2.   Reason(s) for medication(s) including the likelihood of improving, or not improving with or without the medication(s)

3.   Reasonable alternative treatments and why doctor is recommending this particular treatment

4.   Type, range of frequency and amount (including PRN orders), method (oral or injection), duration of taking medication(s)

5.   Probable side effects known to commonly occur, and any particular side effects likely to occur with you

6.   Possible additional side effects which may occur when taking medication(s) beyond three months

7.   If prescribed a *conventional/typical or atypical antipsychotic medication,* information will be given to you about **tardive dyskinesia,** a possible side effect caused by *typical/atypical antipsychotic medication.* It is characterized by involuntary movements of the face or mouth and/or hands and feet. These symptoms are potentially irreversible and may appear after medication has been discontinued.

County of San Diego
Health and Human Services Agency
Mental Health Services
**INFORMED CONSENT FOR USE OF
PSYCHOTROPIC MEDICATION
Page 1 of 2**

HHSA:MHS-005 Rev. 10/2004

Client: _____

MR/Client ID#:_____

Program: _____

(Continued on next page)

Figure B.7. (Continued)

Client's Consent:

Based upon the information I have read, discussed and/or reviewed with my doctor:
(check one of the following)

☐ I understand and give consent to the use of the psychotropic medication(s) on page one.

☐ I give verbal consent only; refuse to sign form.

☐ I *do not* approve/consent to the use of the psychotropic medication(s) listed below.

Please list: _____

_____

Signature of Client/Legal Rep./Guardian_____ Date _____

Doctor's Statement:

I have reviewed, discussed and recommend the medication plan (page 1) for above client and:

☐ Client gives consent to take these medications.

☐ Client gives verbal consent, but unwilling or unable to sign.

☐ Emergency. Given medication without consent.

☐ Unable to understand risks and benefits, and therefore cannot consent.

☐ Other Comments: _____

_____

Psychiatrist's Signature _____ Date _____

Printed Name_____

Witness Signature (if applicable): _____ Date _____

County of San Diego
Health and Human Services Agency
Mental Health Services
INFORMED CONSENT FOR USE OF
PSYCHOTROPIC MEDICATION
Page 2 of 2

HHSA:MHS-005 Rev. 10/2004

Client: _____

MR/Client ID#:_____

Program:_____

Figure B.8.   Initial mental health assessment

Assessment Date:_____

PRESENTING PROBLEM: (Identifying Data/Chief Complaint and History of Present Illness. Summarize client's request for services **including client's subjective description of the problem.**   Include precipitating factors, objective impairing behaviors, including experiences and stigma if any and prejudice and client's requests/needs.)

_____
_____
_____
_____
_____
_____
_____
_____
_____
_____
_____
_____

PAST PSYCHIATRIC HISTORY: (Previous mental health treatment; where, when, for how long. Include dates/providers related to any prior psychiatric treatment, history, traumatic and/or significant events, include immigration history, and impact if any).

_____
_____
_____
_____
_____
_____
_____
_____
_____
_____
_____
_____
_____
_____

FAMILY HISTORY - _____
_____
_____
_____

Any family members with a history of any of the following? (Please, check all that apply):

	Depression	Schizophrenia	Bipolar	Substance Abuse	Suicide	Other	Effective Treatments
Parent							
Sibling							
Children							
Aunt/Uncle							
Grandparent							

County of San Diego
Health and Human Services Agency
Mental Health Services

INITIAL MENTAL HEALTH ASSESSMENT

HHSA:MHS-912 (6/2003)

Client:_____

MR/Client ID #:_____

Program:_____

Page 1 of 5

(Continued on next page)

Figure B.8.   (Continued)

CULTURE/FAMILY and RECOVERY POTENTIAL:

Birth place: ( ) San Diego ( ) USA ( ) Other (fill in birth place and year moved to USA):_____

Language of choice for therapy: ☐English   ☐Spanish   ☐Vietnamese   ☐Other(fill in Language)

Ethnicity: ☐ Latino/Hispanic   ☐ African American   ☐ Asian/Pacific Islander (fill in):_____

☐ White   ☐ American Indian   ☐ Other (fill in):_____

Culture specific symptomatology/explanations for behavior (May reference Appendix I of DSM-IV-TR)_____

_____

_____

Family/Community Support System- (Live alone?   Describe it, including alternative relationship support, if any.   Who is supportive? Community groups, e.g. AA/NA)

_____

_____

Socio-Economic Factors: (educational achievement, occupation, income source and level).

_____

_____

Religious/Spiritual Issues: (Is R/S important in your life?   If yes, is it a source of strength in your recovery process? Describe how/who: persons, practices.)

_____

_____

_____

ASSETS/STRENGTHS: (What abilities or skills do you have that you would choose to develop during your recovery? What new ones might you choose to develop?)

_____

_____

_____

MEDICAL HISTORY: (Indicate any significant medical history related to client's current mental health condition, including dates/providers related to prior treatment, as well as client's adjustment to co-occurring disabilities.)

_____

_____

_____

Current Medication(s)	*Dose*	Frequency	Taken as Prescribed?
			☐ YES ☐ NO
			☐ YES ☐ NO
			☐ YES ☐ NO
			☐ YES ☐ NO

ALLERGIES AND ADVERSE MEDICATION REACTIONS:

☐ NKA(s)

☐ Other (s)_____

HEALING AND HEALTH: (Alternative healing practices/beliefs. Apart from mental health professionals, who-- or what-- helps you deal with disability/illness? Describe:)

_____

_____

_____

County of San Diego Health and Human Services Agency Mental Health Services	Client:_____
INITIAL MENTAL HEALTH ASSESSMENT	**MR/Client ID #:**_____
HHSA:MHS-912 (6/2003) Page 2 of 5	**Program:**_____

Figure B.8. (Continued)

NAME OF CURRENT PRIMARY CARE PHYSICIAN:
May we consult? ☐Yes ☐No Date Last Seen: _____ Release of Information Form: ☐Yes ☐No

_____
Name   Address   Phone number (including area code)

CLIENT'S HOSPITAL OF CHOICE:

_____
Name   Address   Phone number (including area code)
SUBSTANCE USE INFORMATION Indicate if no history of use ☐ History unknown ☐

Type:	Date of Last Use	Amount of Last Use	Frequency and Amount of Use	Length of Time Using	Age of First Use
_____	____	____	_____	____	___
_____	____	____	_____	____	___
_____	____	____	_____	____	___
_____	____	____	_____	____	___
_____	____	____	_____	____	___

MENTAL STATUS EXAM:

Level of Consciousness:	☐Alert	☐Lethargic	☐Stuporous			
Orientation:	☐Person	☐Place	Time ☐Day ☐Month ☐Year		☐Current Situation	☐None
Appearance:	☐Clean	☐Well-Nourished	☐Malodorous	☐Disheveled	☐Malnourished	☐Reddened Eyes
Speech:	☐Normal	☐Slurred	☐Loud	☐Pressured	☐Slow	☐Mute
Thought Process:	☐Coherent	☐Tangential	☐Circumstantial	☐Incoherent	☐Loose Association	
Behavior:	☐Cooperative	☐Evasive	☐Uncooperative	☐Threatening	☐Agitated	☐Combative
Affect:	☐Appropriate	☐Blunted	☐Flat	☐Restricted	☐Labile	☐Other
Intellect:	☐Normal	☐Below Normal	☐Paucity of Knowledge	☐Vocabulary Poor	☐Poor Abstraction	☐Uncooperative
Mood:	☐Euthymic	☐Elevated	☐Euphoric	☐Depressed	☐Anxious	☐Irritable
Memory:	☐Normal	☐Poor Recent	☐Poor Remote	☐Inability to Concentrate	☐Confabulation	☐Amnesia
Judgment:	☐Normal	☐Poor	☐Unrealistic	☐Unmotivated	☐Uncertain	
Motor:	☐Normal	☐Decreased	☐Agitated	☐Tremors	☐Tics	☐Repetitive Motions
Insight:	☐Normal	☐Adequate	☐Marginal	☐Poor		

Note: A narrative mental status exam may be done on a progress note, in lieu of above.

County of San Diego
Health and Human Services Agency
Mental Health Services

INITIAL MENTAL HEALTH ASSESSMENT
HHSA:MHS-912 (6/2003)

Client:_____
MR/Client ID #:_____
Program:_____
Page 3 of 5

(Continued on next page)

Figure B.8. (Continued)

Visual Hallucinations:	☐No	☐Yes	Specify:_____
Auditory Hallucinations:	☐No	☐Yes	Specify:_____
Delusions:	☐No	☐Yes	Specify:_____

Other Information (optional):_____

POTENTIAL FOR HARM (Include risk factors, e.g. chronic illness, recent loss of job, age)

Current SI   ☐ No ☐ Yes Specify plan: method, vague, passive, imminent_____
_____
_____

Access to means   ☐ No ☐ Yes Specify_____
Previous Attempts   ☐ No ☐ Yes Specify_____
_____

Client Contract for Safety ☐ No ☐ Yes Specify in Progress Notes_____
Current HI   ☐ No ☐ Yes Specify Plan: vague, intent, with/without means_____
_____
_____

Identified Victim   ☐ No ☐ Yes Name and Contact information_____
_____

                           ☐ No ☐ Yes Tarasoff warning _____
Client No Harm Contract ☐ No ☐ Yes Specify in Progress Notes_____
History of Violence   ☐ No ☐ Yes Specify Type: past, current_____

History of Domestic Violence_____
History of Abuse   ☐ No ☐ Yes Specify Type: past, current_____
_____

Abuse Reported   ☐ No ☐ Yes
Probation Officer Contact Info:

Name   Address   Phone (including Area Code)
CONVICTION OF FELONY AND JAIL TIME ☐ No ☐ Yes
What was the conviction for? Length of jail time?
_____

DSM IV DIAGNOSIS: Impairment/Disability Use DSM-IV-TR Codes. Indicate (P) – Primary and (S) – Secondary	Enter P in front of primary	DIAGNOSTIC CODE
AXIS I		
AXIS I		
AXIS I		
AXIS II		
AXIS III Relevant Medical Conditions:		
AXIS IV Psychosocial and Environmental Problems:		
AXIS V Current GAF: Highest in Past Year:		

County of San Diego
Health and Human Services Agency
Mental Health Services

INITIAL MENTAL HEALTH ASSESSMENT

HHSA:MHS-912 (6/2003)

Client:_____

MR/Client ID #:_____

Program:_____

Page 4 of 5

Figure B.8. (Continued)

INTERPRETIVE SUMMARY: (Justification for diagnosis. Summarize and integrate all information gathered from other sources to render clinical judgments regarding intensity, length of treatment and recommendations for services. Clearly state those emotional or behavioral symptoms that interfere with normal functioning. Include evaluation of client's ability and willingness to solve the clients presenting problem.)

_____
_____
_____
_____
_____
_____
_____
_____
_____
_____
_____
_____
_____
_____

Medical Necessity Met: ☐ Yes ☐ No   NOA Issued: ☐ Yes ☐ No (Medi-Cal Clients only)

REHABILITATION/RECOVERY/RECOMMENDATIONS: _____ (List in-house clinical services as well as names of agencies/clinicians currently being received or recommended.)

1. ☐ Assisted Living Services	7. ☐ Employment Services	13. ☐ RAP Plan
2. ☐ Community Services	8. ☐ Group Therapy	14. ☐ Recovery Programs/Socialization Services
3. ☐ Case Management Services	9. ☐ Housing Services	15. ☐ Substance Abuse
4. ☐ Crisis Residential/Hospitalization	10. ☐ Individual Therapy	16. ☐ Support Group
5. ☐ Day Rehabilitation	11. ☐ Medical Treatment	17. ☐ Other
6. ☐ Education/Support	12. ☐ Medication Management	

Number and explain below:

_____ ☐ Current_____

_____ ☐ Proposed Referral_____

_____ ☐ Current_____

_____ ☐ Proposed Referral_____

_____ ☐ Current_____

_____ ☐ Proposed Referral_____

_____ ☐ Current_____

_____ ☐ Proposed Referral_____

_____ ☐ Current_____

_____ ☐ Proposed Referral_____

Completed by: _____ _____ _____ _____
                        Signature   Title   Date   Time Spent

Co-signature: _____ _____ _____
(if required)   Signature   Title   Date

County of San Diego Health and Human Services Agency Mental Health Services	**Client:**_____
	MR/Client ID #:_____
INITIAL MENTAL HEALTH ASSESSMENT	**Program:**_____
HHSA:MHS-912 (6/2003)	Page 5 of 5

Figure B.9. Lab results

CODES:	(+) = POSITIVE	
	(-) = NEGATIVE	
	NT = NOT TESTED	

TYPE OF TEST	NORMAL RESULTS	RESULTS
AMPHETAMINES	NEGATIVE	
COCAINE	NEGATIVE	
THC	NEGATIVE	
MORPHINE	NEGATIVE	
PCP	NEGATIVE	

DATE:		TIME:			
PERFORMED BY:					
PHYSICIAN'S INITIAL:					

Type of test	Results				
	DATE	TIME	RESULTS	PERFORMED BY	M.D.'S INITIALS
PREGNANCY					
BLOOD GLUCOSE (one step)					
OTHER:					

County of San Diego
Health and Human Services Agency
Mental Health Services

LAB RESULTS
HHSA:MHS-993 (6/2003)

Client: _____

MR/Client ID #: _____

Program: _____

Figure B.10. Medical history questionnaire

Date of last visit to a physician: _____   Purpose of Visit: _____

Doctor's name: _____   Phone #: (_____) _____

Address: _____

Name of current personal Physician: _____

Family History	Name:	Age:	If Deceased, Cause of Death	Age at Death	Has any blood relative ever had:	Encircle No or Yes	Who?
Father					Alcoholism	No Yes	
Mother					Drug Problems	No Yes	
Brother/s					Depression	No Yes	
Or					Mental Problems	No Yes	
Sister/s					Psychiatric Treatment	No Yes	
					Epilepsy	No Yes	
Spouse					Neurological Disorder	No Yes	
Children					Suicidal Attempts	No Yes	
Medical History	Please place a check ✔ in front of any questions you would like to discuss in more detail with the Doctor.						

Have you ever had:	Circle No or Yes	
Rheumatic Fever	No	Yes
Epilepsy	No	Yes
Tuberculosis	No	Yes
Nervousness	No	Yes
Mental Problem	No	Yes
Arthritis	No	Yes
Bone or Joint Disease	No	Yes
Meningitis	No	Yes
Gonorrhea or Syphilis	No	Yes
Jaundice	No	Yes
Thyroid Disease	No	Yes
Diabetes	No	Yes
Cancer	No	Yes
High Blood Pressure	No	Yes
Heart Disease	No	Yes
Asthma	No	Yes
Stroke	No	Yes

When was your last physical Examination? _____

What Medications are you allergic to? _____

Have you ever been hospitalized for any major illness? Specify: _____

_____

When and where you hospitalized: _____

Have you ever had an operation? Type and When: _____

Do you currently have any dental problems? _____

Have you had any complications from a childhood disease? _____

When was your last chest x-ray? _____

When was your last electrocardiogram? _____

What do you weigh now? _____

What was your weight one year ago? _____

What was your maximum weight and date? _____

Has Sleep been a problem? _____

Has sex been a problem? _____

Has there been a change in appetite? _____

What activities do you do for fun? _____

What time do you feel your best? _____

What physical complaints, if any do you have? _____

What medications do you take on a regular basis? _____

_____

Doctor's Notes: _____

_____

_____

County of San Diego
Health and Human Services Agency
Mental Health Services

MEDICAL HISTORY QUESTIONNAIRE

HHSA:MHS-911 (6/2003)

Client: _____

MR/Client ID #: _____

Program: _____

Page 1 of 2

(Continued on next page)

Figure B.10. **(Continued)**

Systems History	Place a check ✔ in front of any questions that you would like to discuss in more detail with the Doctor.
	Have you ever had any of the following problems

	Circle	No	Yes		Circle	No	Yes
Any eye disease injury, impaired sight		No	Yes	Night sweats		No	Yes
Any ear disease, injury, impaired hearing		No	Yes	Shortness of breath		No	Yes
Trouble with nose, sinuses, mouth or throat		No	Yes	Palpitations or fluttering heart		No	Yes
Head injuries		No	Yes	Swelling of hands, feet or ankles		No	Yes
Fainting spells		No	Yes	Back, arm or leg problem		No	Yes
Loss of Consciousness		No	Yes	Varicose veins		No	Yes
Convulsions		No	Yes	Kidney disease or stones		No	Yes
Paralysis		No	Yes	Bladder disease		No	Yes
Dizziness		No	Yes	Albumin, sugar, pus, blood in urine		No	Yes
Frequent or severe headaches		No	Yes	Difficulty in urinating		No	Yes
Depression or anxiety		No	Yes	Abnormal thirst		No	Yes
Difficulty concentrating		No	Yes	Stomach trouble or ulcer		No	Yes
Memory problems		No	Yes	Indigestion		No	Yes
Extreme tiredness or weakness		No	Yes	Appendicitis		No	Yes
Hallucinations		No	Yes	Liver or gallbladder disease		No	Yes
Enlarged glands		No	Yes	Colitis or other bowel disease		No	Yes
Enlarged thyroid or goiter		No	Yes	Hemorrhoids or rectal bleeding		No	Yes
Skin disease		No	Yes	Constipation or diarrhea		No	Yes
Chronic or frequent cough		No	Yes	Crying spells		No	Yes
Chest pain or angina pectoris		No	Yes	Suicidal thoughts		No	Yes
Coughing up blood		No	Yes	Loss of appetite		No	Yes

Habits
Do you smoke: ☐ Tobacco ☐ Cigarettes   How many packs a day_____
Do you drink: ☐ Coffee ☐ Tea ☐ Cola Drinks   How many cups/glasses a day_____
Do you take alcoholic beverages: ☐ Never ☐ Rarely ☐ Moderately ☐ Daily
Has alcohol use been a problem: ☐ Yes ☐ No   Have you ever been treated for alcoholism: ☐ Yes ☐ No
Have you ever taken street drugs: ☐ Yes ☐ No   Which drug/s:_____
  During what Period:_____ How often:_____
  When was the last time that you used any drug:_____
Have you ever been treated for a drug problem: ☐ Yes ☐ No   When:_____

WOMEN ONLY: Menstrual History
Age at onset:_____ Cycle:_____ Days (from start to start)   Date of last period:_____
Duration:_____ Days   Regular: ☐ Yes ☐ No   Pain or Cramps: ☐ Yes ☐ No
How many pregnancies:_____ Miscarriages:_____   Age of youngest living child:_____

Military History   Not Applicable ☐

Branch_____   Rank at Discharge_____
When did you serve?_____ to_____
Type of discharge_____

Signature of Client or Guardian_____

Date Completed:_____   (Optional)

Doctor's Notes and Recommendations:

Physician's Signature & Date Reviewed.

County of San Diego
Health and Human Services Agency
Mental Health Services

MEDICAL HISTORY QUESTIONNAIRE

HHSA:MHS-911 (6/2003)

Client: _____

MR/Client ID #:_____

Program: _____

Page 2 of 2

Figure B.11. Medication management

Client identified self according to Policy and Procedure 05-01-25: ☐ Yes ☐ No ☐ N/A

Medication Name	Strength	Frequency	Quantity	Refill	Indication (check all that apply)*	Change from Previous Visit?	New/ Continuing/ Discontinue
					☐ S ☐ OS ☐ SE	☐ Yes ☐ No	☐ New ☐ Cont. ☐ D/C
					☐ S ☐ OS ☐ SE	☐ Yes ☐ No	☐ New ☐ Cont. ☐ D/C
					☐ S ☐ OS ☐ SE	☐ Yes ☐ No	☐ New ☐ Cont. ☐ D/C
					☐ S ☐ OS ☐ SE	☐ Yes ☐ No	☐ New ☐ Cont. ☐ D/C
					☐ S ☐ OS ☐ SE	☐ Yes ☐ No	☐ New ☐ Cont. ☐ D/C
					☐ S ☐ OS ☐ SE	☐ Yes ☐ No	☐ New ☐ Cont. ☐ D/C
					☐ S ☐ OS ☐ SE	☐ Yes ☐ No	☐ New ☐ Cont. ☐ D/C
					☐ S ☐ OS ☐ SE	☐ Yes ☐ No	☐ New ☐ Cont. ☐ D/C
					☐ S ☐ OS ☐ SE	☐ Yes ☐ No	☐ New ☐ Cont. ☐ D/C
					☐ S ☐ OS ☐ SE	☐ Yes ☐ No	☐ New ☐ Cont. ☐ D/C
					☐ S ☐ OS ☐ SE	☐ Yes ☐ No	☐ New ☐ Cont. ☐ D/C

Generic Equivalent permitted unless otherwise noted.

☐ County Pharmacy

Pharmacy Name: _____ Pharmacy Phone Number: ( ) _____

☐ Mail Out ☐ Fax **Pickup:** ☐ Pharmacy ☐ Clinic **Medi-Cal:** ☐ Yes ☐ No

_____ _____ _____ _____
Date   Signature MD/DO or RN under SNP   CA License No.   Activity Code

_____   _____
Printed Name   DEA Number

*S = Meds Targeted at core symptom OS = Meds targeted at other symptoms SE = Meds for side effects of S or OS

SNP = Standardized Nursing Procedure

County of San Diego Health and Human Services Agency Mental Health Services **MEDICATION MANAGEMENT** **(SCRIPT)** HHSA:MHS-994 (6/2003)	**Client**	**Client:** _____ **MR/Client ID#:** _____ **DOB:** _____ **Address:** _____
	Program	**Program:** _____ **Phone #** _____ **Address:** _____

NCR

Figure B.12. Outpatient discharge summary

Date of Admission: _____   Discharge Date: _____

Diagnosis at Discharge – DSM – IV-TR
Code

Axis I: _____   _____

   _____   _____

Axis II:_____   _____

Axis III:_____   _____

Axis IV:_____   _____

Axis V:_____   _____

* CAUTIONS/DANGERS/ALLERGIES*

_____

Reason for Admission: (Presenting Problem)_____

_____

_____

Reason for Termination: _____

_____

_____

Assessment Results; Course of Treatment and Response to Treatment: _____

_____

_____

_____

_____

_____

_____

_____

_____

_____

_____

_____

_____

_____

_____

_____

_____

_____

_____

_____

_____

_____

_____

_____

County of San Diego
Health and Human Services Agency
Mental Health Services

OUT PATIENT DISCHARGE SUMMARY

HHSA:MHS-920 (6/2003)

Client:_____

MR/Client ID #:_____

Program:_____

Page 1 of 2

Figure B.12. (Continued)

Assessment Results; Course of Treatment and response to treatment – (Continued from front): _____

_____

_____

_____

_____

_____

_____

_____

_____

_____

_____

Treatment Complete   ☐ Yes ☐ No

History or Propensity for Violence, Fire setting, Criminal Activity, Sex Offences, or Suicide Attempts: _____

_____

_____

_____

_____

_____

_____

_____

_____

_____

_____

_____

_____

_____

_____

Discharge Medication: (Name/dose/frequency/amount dispensed)_____

_____

_____

Prognosis: (6 month – 12 month, present level of functioning) _____

_____

_____

Discharge Plan/recommendations/disposition: (Aftercare plan, living arrangements)_____

_____

_____

_____

Referred to:_____ Appointment Date:_____ Time:_____

Signature
Clinician:_____ Discipline:_____ Date: _____

County of San Diego Health and Human Services Agency Mental Health Services **OUT PATIENT DISCHARGE SUMMARY** HHSA:MHS-920 (6/2003)	**Client:**_____ **MR/Client ID #:**_____ **Program:**_____ Page 2 of 2

Figure B.13. Problem list

PROBLEM LIST					
Identification Number					
Medical Record Number					
Last Name		First Name		Middle Initial	
Date of Birth					
PROBLEM NUMBER	DATE ENTERE	LIST SIGNIFICANT ACUTE AND CHRONIC CONDITIONS INCLUDING SURGICAL		PROBLEM RESOLVED	DATE RESOLVED
1					
2					
3					
4					
5					
6					
7					
8					
9					
10					
11					
12					
13					
14					
15					
16					
17					
18					
19					
20					

Figure B.14. Progress note

Date/ Procedure Code	Face to face time/ total time (in minutes) Location *	Notes

＊   NOTE: Services are clinic based unless otherwise noted

County of San Diego
Health and Human Services Agency
Mental Health Services

PROGRESS NOTE

HHSA:MHS-979 (10/9/2002)

Client:_____

MR/Client ID #:_____

Program:_____

Figure B.15.   Recovery/crisis plan

Early warning signs that I need help are:

When I have any of these early warning signs I will:

The resources I have available to me are: (Include telephone numbers)

If I go into crisis I would like ACCESS to:

_____		_____	
Client Signature	Date:	Staff Signature:	Date:

County of San Diego
Health and Human Services Agency
Mental Health Services

RECOVERY/CRISIS PLAN

HHSA:MHS-116 (6/2003)

Client:_____

MR/Client ID #:_____

Program:_____

Figure B.16. Vital signs

Date	Time	Temp.	Pulse	Resp.	Wt.	Ht.	Blood Pressure	Signature & Classification

County of San Diego
Health and Human Services Agency
Mental Health Services

VITAL SIGNS/WEIGHT/HEIGHT RECORD

HHSA:MHS-909 (6/2003)

Client:_____

MR/Client ID #:_____

Program:_____

Appendix C

Standards for the Form and Content of the Behavioral Healthcare Record

Documentation Requirements	Joint Commission on Accreditation of Healthcare Organizations	Medicare *Conditions of Participation* or Other Regulations
The hospital initiates and maintains a health record for every individual assessed or treated.	IM.7.1	
A health record must be maintained for every individual evaluated or treated in the hospital.		482.24
Only authorized individuals make entries in health records.	IM.7.1.1	
Every health record entry is dated, its author identified and, when necessary, authenticated.	IM.7.8	
Hospitals establish policies and mechanisms to ensure that only an author can authenticate his or her entry. Indications of authentication can include written signatures or initials, rubber stamps, or computer "signatures" (or sequence of keys). The medical staff rules and regulations or policies define what entries, if any, by house staff or nonphysicians must be counter-signed by supervising physicians.	Intent of IM.7.8	
All entries must be legible and complete and must be authenticated and dated promptly by the person (identified by name and discipline) who is responsible for ordering, providing, or evaluating the service furnished.		482.24(c)(1)
The author of each entry must be identified and must authenticate his or her entry.		482.24(c)(1)(i)
Authentication may include signatures, written initials, or computer entries.		482.24(c)(1)(ii)
The health record contains sufficient information to identify the client, support the diagnosis, justify the treatment, document the course and results, and promote continuity of care among healthcare providers.	IM.7.2	482.24(c)
To facilitate consistency and continuity in client care, the health record contains very specific data and thorough information, including: • The client's name, address, date of birth, and the name of any legally authorized representative • The legal status of patients receiving mental health services • Emergency care provided to the client prior to arrival, if any • The record and findings of the client's assessment • Conclusions or impressions drawn from the medical history and physical examination • The diagnosis or diagnostic impression • The reasons for admission or treatment • The goals of treatment and the treatment plan *(Continued)*	Intent of IM.7 through IM.7.2	

Documentation Requirements	Joint Commission on Accreditation of Healthcare Organizations	Medicare *Conditions of Participation or Other Regulations*
• Evidence of known advance directives		

- Evidence of known advance directives
- Evidence of informed consent, when required by hospital policy
- Diagnostic and therapeutic orders, if any
- All diagnostic and therapeutic procedures and test results
- All operative and other invasive procedures performed, using acceptable disease and operative terminology that includes etiology, as appropriate
- Progress notes made by the medical staff and other authorized individuals
- All reassessments and any revisions of the treatment plan
- Clinical observations
- The client's response to care
- Consultation reports
- Every medication ordered or prescribed for an inpatient
- Every medication dispensed to an ambulatory client or an inpatient on discharge
- Every dose of medication administered and any adverse drug reaction
- All relevant diagnoses established during the course of care
- Any referrals and communications made to external or internal providers and to community agencies
- Conclusions at termination of hospitalization
- Discharge instructions to the client and family

Clinical resumes and discharge summaries, or a final progress note or transfer summary. A concise clinical resume included in the health record at discharge provides important information to other caregivers and facilitates continuity of care. For patients discharged to ambulatory (outpatient) care, the clinical resume summarizes previous levels of care.

The discharge summary contains the following information:

- The reason for hospitalization
- Significant findings
- Procedures performed and treatment rendered
- The client's condition at discharge
- Instructions to the client and family
- For normal newborns with uncomplicated deliveries, or for patients hospitalized less than 48 hours with only minor problems, a progress note may substitute for the clinical resume.
- The medical staff defines what problems and interventions may be considered minor.
- The progress note may be handwritten. It documents the client's condition at discharge and discharge instructions.
- When a client is transferred within the same organization from one level of care to another and the caregivers change, a transfer summary may be substituted for the clinical resume. A transfer summary briefly describes the client's condition at time of transfer and the reason for the transfer. When the caregivers remain the same, a progress note may suffice.

Documentation Requirements	Joint Commission on Accreditation of Healthcare Organizations	Medicare *Conditions of Participation* or Other Regulations
All records must document the following, as appropriate: • Admitting diagnosis results of all consultative evaluations of the client and appropriate findings by clinical and other staff involved in the care of the client • Documentation of complications, hospital-acquired infections, and unfavorable reactions to drugs and anesthesia		482.24(c)(2)(ii) 482.24(c)(2)(iii) 482.24(c)(2)(iv)
The client's history and physical examination, nursing assessment, and other screening assessments are completed within 24 hours of admission as an inpatient.	PE. 1.7.1	
When a history and physical examination have been performed within 30 days before admission, a durable, legible copy of this report may be used in the client's record, provided any changes that may have occurred are recorded in the health record at the time of admission.	PE.1.7.1.1	
Before surgery, the client's physical examination and medical history, any indicated diagnostic tests, and a preoperative diagnosis are completed and recorded in the client's record.	PE.1.8	
There must be a complete history and physical workup in the chart of every client prior to surgery, except in emergencies. When this has been dictated, but not yet recorded in the client's chart, there must be a statement to the effect and an admission note in the chart by the practitioner who admitted the client.		482.5 l(b)(l)
A physical examination and medical history are to be done no more than 7 days before or 48 hours after an admission for each client by a doctor of medicine or osteopathy or, for patients admitted only for oromaxillofacial surgery, by an oromaxillofacial surgeon who has been granted such privileges by the medical staff in accordance with state law.		482.24(c)(2)(i) 482.22(c)(5)
Plans of care are developed and documented in the client's health record before the operative or other procedure is performed.	TX.5.3	
The hospital must ensure that the nursing staff develops and keeps current a nursing care plan for each client.		482.23(b)(4)
All records must document all practitioners' orders.		482.24(c)(2)(vi)
All orders for drugs and biologicals must be in writing and signed by the practitioner or practitioners responsible for the care of the client.		482.23(c)(2)
Verbal orders of authorized individuals are accepted and transcribed by qualified personnel who are identified by title or category in the medical staff rules and regulations.	IM.7.7	
When telephone or verbal orders must be used, they must be: • Accepted only by personnel authorized to do so by the medical staff policies and procedures, consistent with federal and state law • Signed or initialed by the prescribing practitioner as soon as possible • Used infrequently		482.23(c)(2)(i) 482.23(c)(2)(ii) 482.23(c)(2)(iii)

Documentation Requirements	Joint Commission on Accreditation of Healthcare Organizations	Medicare *Conditions of Participation* or Other Regulations

Restraint and seclusion documentation and reporting varies by state. California's documentation is listed here as an example of general requirements. Further, more specific requirements for specific populations, such as children in group homes, follow:
 	
(a) Care provided to a client in restraint or seclusion shall be documented in the client record.
  (1) The policies and procedures of the mental health rehabilitation center shall describe the manner in which this documentation shall be entered in the client record.
  (2) Notations, check marks, and flow charts are allowable if the chart provides opportunity for narrative descriptions by staff, when appropriate, and when sufficient to provide the necessary information.
(b) The documentation shall include, but not be limited to, all of the following:
  (1) Clinical condition, circulation, condition of limbs, and attention to hydration, elimination, and nutrition needs.
  (2) Behavior assessments
  (3) Justification for continued use of restraint or seclusion, the types of behaviors that would facilitate release, and evidence that this information was communicated to the client along with his or her response, if any.
  (4) Time placed in and time removed from restraint or seclusion.
  (5) 15-minute observations and assessments
  (6) When face-to-face interaction does not occur, documentation of the reason why that interaction was inappropriate or unnecessary and what alternative means were used to determine the client was not in distress.
(c) Quarterly, any facility that uses restraint or seclusion shall report to the local mental health director or designee, who shall transmit copies to the Department, all of the following:
  (1) The number of restraint or seclusion incidents, or both.
  (2) The number of restraint or seclusion incidents according to age, sex, race, and primary diagnosis.
  (3) The client's age shall be classified as one of the following:
    (A) Age 18 to 64 years, inclusive, and
    (B) Age 65 and over.
    (C) Facilities that use restraint or seclusion, or both, shall have written policies and procedures concerning their use. These policies shall include the standards and procedures for all of the following:
      (i) Placement of a person in restraint or seclusion, including a list of less restrictive alternatives, the situations in which the use of restraint or seclusion is to be considered and the physician(s) and psychologist(s) who can order its use.
      (ii) Assessment and release, including guidelines for duration of use or specific behavioral criteria for release.
      (iii) Provision of nursing care and medical care, including the administration of medication.
  (4) Procedures for advocate notification regarding any client restrained or secluded for more than eight
  (8) hours.   *(Continued)*
		CA Code of Regulations Title 9. Division 1 DMH Chapter 3.5 784.38

Documentation Requirements	Joint Commission on Accreditation of Healthcare Organizations	Medicare *Conditions of Participation* or Other Regulations
(5) Provision of staff training. (d) Facilities that use restraint or seclusion shall implement an oversight process to ensure that all incidents of seclusion and restraint are reviewed and that any incidents or patterns of use that do not comply with the mental health rehabilitation centers' policies and procedures or other clinical or legal standards are investigated. This oversight process shall ensure that appropriate policies and procedures are developed and implemented, including training of staff. Consumer input into the oversight process shall be incorporated.		Title 9 Ca 784.38
Restraint and Seclusion Reporting: Child in Group Home **§ 84061.Reporting Requirements.** (a) The licensee shall ensure that the child's authorized representative is notified no later than the next working day if the following circumstances have occurred without the authorized representative's participation: (3) Each time the child has been placed in a manual restraint, to be reported as required in Sections 84805 (b) Incident reports must include the following: (1) When the incident report is used to report the use of manual restraints, the report must include the following: (A) Date and time of the other manual restraints involving the same child in the past 24 hours. (B) A description of the child's behavior that required the use of manual restrains and description of the precipitating factors that led to the intervention. (C) Description of what manual restraints were used and how long the child was restrained. (D) Description of what nonphysical interventions were utilized prior to the restraint; explanation of why more restrictive interventions were necessary. (E) Description of injuries sustained by the child or facility personnel. What type of medical treatment was sought, and where was child taken? Explanation if medical treatment was sought for injuries. (F) Name(s) of facility personnel who provided the manual restraint. (G) Name(s) of facility personnel who witnessed the child's behavior and the restraint. (H) The child's verbal response and physical appearance, including a description of any injuries at the completion of the restraint. (I) If it is determined by the post incident review, as required in Section 84806, that facility personnel did not attempt to prevent the manual restraint, a description of what action should have been taken by facility personnel to prevent the manual restraint incident. What corrective action will be taken or not taken, and why? (c) When the incident report is used to report a runaway situation, the report must include the following: (A) If a manual restraint was used, and if it is determined by the post incident review, as required in Section 84806, that facility personnel did not attempt to prevent the manual restraint, a description of what action should have been taken by facility personnel to prevent the manual restraint incident. What corrective action will be taken or not taken, and why?		Cal Title 9 84061

Documentation Requirements	Joint Commission on Accreditation of Healthcare Organizations	Medicare *Conditions of Participation or Other Regulations*
Treatment and Care Plans		
Antipsychotic Medication Consent Include: Description of medicine, date, patient signature, psychiatrist signature and date, witness signature and date if client refuses to sign, indicate target signs and symptoms, client right to refuse medication, advisement that in an emergency physician may order client be given antipsychotic medication without their consent. Advisement that client may withdraw consent at any time by telling any staff member of their decision, alternatives to using medication, consequences of not taking medication.		

Outpatient
 	
All information submitted must be legible and document for each date of service, the following information:
    Name of client
    Name and professional license of provider (MD, PhD, LCSW)
    Date of service
    Use of nonstandardized medical abbreviations is not acceptable.
    Time spent in psychotherapy encounter must be included.
		Medicare Billing Guide

What Is Not Covered by Medicare Teaching grooming skills, monitoring activities of daily living, recreational therapy (such as dance, art, play), social interaction, or educational activities. Psychotherapy services are not covered for profound mental retardation.		Medicare Billing Guide
Psychiatric Diagnostic Interview (CPT Code 90801, 90620) Includes history, mental status, or disposition. It may also include communication with the family or other sources, ordering and medical interpretation of laboratory or other medical diagnostic studies. In certain circumstances, other informants will be seen in lieu of the client. The medical record must indicate that the client has a psychiatric illness and/or is demonstrating emotional or behavioral symptoms sufficient to interfere with normal functioning. The medical records must also reflect the elicitation of a complete medical, including past, family, social, and psychiatric history; establishment of tentative diagnosis; and evaluation of the client's ability and willingness to work to solve the client's mental health problem. This includes a complete mental status examination but does not include psychiatric treatment.		Medicare Billing Guide
The psychiatric diagnostic interview will be covered by Medicare once, at the time of the initial evaluation of an illness or suspected illness. Subsequent coverage of this service can be allowed when reported again for the same client if a new episode of illness occurs or after a hiatus from treatment of six months or longer. It may also be utilized on the initial admission to inpatient status after a six-month hiatus in treatment or readmission to inpatient status due to complications of the underlying condition. For interactive psychiatric diagnostic interview examinations, the medical records must also indicate that the person being evaluated does not have the ability to interact through normal verbal communicative channels.		Medicare Billing Guide

Documentation Requirements	Joint Commission on Accreditation of Healthcare Organizations	Medicare *Conditions of Participation* or Other Regulations
Individual Psychotherapy Indicate in note: Type of psychotherapy provided (insight-oriented, behavior modifying and/or supportive vs. interactive), the place of service (office vs. inpatient), the face-to-face time spent with the client providing psychotherapy, and the provision of medical evaluation and management services, if any, that are provided on the same date of service as psychotherapy.		Medicare Billing Guide
Collateral		
Family counseling under Medicare is only covered when the primary purpose of such counseling is the treatment of the client's condition. Medicare will cover family counseling when: • Observing the client's interaction with family members; assessing the capability of the family members in aiding the management of the client. • Assisting the family members in aiding the management of the client. • The beneficiary is withdrawn and uncommunicative. The family is counseled on management of the client's condition, which does not include counseling for treatment of a family member's problem.		
Documentation must explain the exact purpose for performing the service and specifically state how that purpose relates to the client's condition.		Medicare Billing Guide
Group Psychotherapy A form of treatment into which a distinct group of patients is guided by a psychotherapist for the purpose of helping one another effect personality change. Documentation must indicate that the client has a psychiatric illness and/or is demonstrating emotional or behavioral symptoms sufficient to interfere with normal functioning. For interactive psychotherapy, the records must also indicate that the person being evaluated does not have the ability to interact through normal verbal communication channels.		Medicare Billing Guide
Outpatient Progress Notes (Therapeutic Summary) Each visit: What happened during the therapy in relation to the initial findings? What therapeutic interventions were used? What progress is made toward the treatment goal? Are any new obstacles to treatment discovered? Are there any revisions to the diagnosis or therapeutic plan? Have any referrals been made for other therapy? Have any consultations been made to obtain additional diagnosis or treatment recommendations? **Time Spent in Encounter** Cognitive skills, such as behavior modification, insight and supportive interactions, and discussion of reality were applied to produce therapeutic change. For interactive psychotherapy, the record must indicate that the person being evaluated does not have the ability to interact through normal verbal communication channels.		Medicare Billing Guide

Documentation Requirements	Joint Commission on Accreditation of Healthcare Organizations	Medicare *Conditions of Participation* or Other Regulations
Concomitant Physiological Disease If the client has a medical condition likely to affect the mental condition, such as mild dementia of Alzheimer's type or symptomatic hypothythroidism, the initial diagnostic assessment should address the need for or results of a medical evaluation. The medical evaluation documentation will be used by NHIC to assess whether the psychological services are potentially effective.		Medicare Billing Guide
Psychoactive Medications Documentation should include a statement about the potential benefit of psychoactive drug therapy. It also must reflect an evaluation of the client's signs and symptoms, the response to the medication, consideration of drug interactions, adverse drug effects, and changes in pharmacologic regiments. Documentation must show that the service billed was reasonable and medically necessary for the billed diagnosis.		Medicare Billing Guide
Narcosynthesis (Administration of sedative or tranquilizer drugs to relax the client and remove inhibitions for discussion of subjects difficult for the client to discuss freely when in fully conscious state) Document medical necessity of the procedure, specific pharmacological agent, dosage administered, and whether the technique was effective or noneffective.		Medicare Billing Guide
Medical Necessity Each entry into the medical record must be able to "stand alone." In other words, it must support the fact that the level of service billed was rendered and the provider of the service is licensed to perform that service. Documentation must substantiate the level of service billed.		Medicare Billing Guide
Medical Necessity If progress toward the treatment goal is unclear, as measured by a change in functional impairment or development, a consultation will be considered medically necessary unless the documents justify it is reasonable.		Medicare Billing Guide
Medical Necessity Psychiatric services rendered over a prolonged period of time may be subject to medical necessity justification; for example, additional documentation may be requested, indicating necessity for continued treatments.		Medicare Billing Guide
Medical Necessity In all instances where prolonged or lengthy sessions of psychotherapy are provided, medical necessity documentation must be indicated in the client's medical records. The documentation must also support the necessity for performance of the service and indicate the length of time spent in actual psychotherapy.		Medicare Billing Guide

Documentation Requirements	Joint Commission on Accreditation of Healthcare Organizations	Medicare *Conditions of Participation or Other Regulations*
Medical Necessity The medical record must indicate that the client has a psychiatric illness or is demonstrating emotional behavioral symptoms sufficient enough to interfere with normal functioning and must include the time spent in the psychotherapy encounter and cognitive skills, such as behavior modification, insight, and supportive interactions, and discussion of reality were applied to produce a therapeutic change. For interactive psychotherapy, the medical records must also indicate that the person being evaluated does not have the ability to interact through normal verbal communication channels.		Medicare Billing Guide
The impairment treated should involve a significant area of: • Life functioning for adults or • Development for children		Medicare Billing Guide
Initial Diagnostic Assessment Client subjective complaint or symptoms Objective impairing behaviors Diagnosis as listed in ICD-9-CM codebook coded to the highest level of specificity Note: Use of DSM-IV codes for billing purposes is not recognized. However, notation of DSM-IV codes in the medical record may be useful in review determinations.		Medicare Billing Guide
Treatment goal should focus on stabilizing, reducing, or eliminating the impairment(s) listed. If the goal is only stabilization, not reversal, there must be evidence of significant deterioration immediately prior to therapy.		Medicare Billing Guide
Therapeutic plan should specify the therapeutic intervention(s) to be used. Therapeutic interventions should clearly require the knowledge and skill of the licensed practitioner. Some procedure codes (for example, 90805, 90807, 90809, 90811, 90813, 90815, 90817, 90819, and 90822) are limited to those licensed to provide evaluation and management services. The number of visits required should be estimated. A referral relationship with a physician should be indicated. This relationship should address possible physiological causes for impairments and the possible need for psychoactive medication.		Medicare Billing Guide
Psychological Testing When psychological testing or neurological testing is provided, the medical record must reflect the actual tests performed. In those instances where a report is required due to the unusual testing time, the report must include the actual tests performed and indicate the reason(s) for unusual testing time.		
Electroconvulsive therapy		

Documentation Requirements	Joint Commission on Accreditation of Healthcare Organizations	Medicare *Conditions of Participation* or Other Regulations
Tests, Lab, and X ray Date ordered, transcriber signature and professional designation, date scheduled, date performed, dates of refusal, and signature/class of staff performing test completion or documenting refusal. Document reason for refusal.		
Close Observation Record: Inpatient-SDCPH Record every 15 minutes; checks necessary to maintain safety. Note location of client, specific area of concern (e.g., suicide, elopement, or close watch or other risk). Registered nurse shall sign, date, and review close observation documentation.		
Restraint or Seclusion Assessment: SDCPH Documentation initiated and implemented immediately following any use of seclusion or restraint procedures. Record patient's identification, precipitating event (behavior leading to restraint or seclusion), behavior warranting seclusion or restraint, interventions attempted prior to use of seclusion/restraint, response to interventions, reason for seclusion or restraint or ambulatory restraints, permission to notify family of seclusion or restraint, explanation given to client, and release criteria. Documentation of 1:1; MD evaluation within one hour; clothing search completed; Denial of Rights form completed; order obtained every four hours; Add to Treatment Plan; registered nurse signature, date, and time.		
Restraint or Seclusion Flow Sheet: SDCPH Registered nurse to document when a client is placed into seclusion, restraint, or ambulatory restraints and when these measures are renewed, reduced, or discontinued. Documentation to include: client behaviors (once per hour); every 15 minutes, document time, visual and auditory observation, client breathing without difficulty, circulation checks, restraints intact, extremities assessed, description of behavior. Every two hours or more frequently, as needed, offer of food/fluids, bathroom, bedpan, range of motion for 10 minutes, pulse and blood pressure, temperature, and respiration rate. Debriefing within 24 hours after episode documented.		

Documentation Requirements	Joint Commission on Accreditation of Healthcare Organizations	Medicare *Conditions of Participation* or Other Regulations
Advisement of Client Rights and Responsibilities Rights and responsibilities to include: a. Right to wear own clothing, keep and use personal possessions including toilet articles, and to keep/spend a reasonable sum of his/her own money b. To have access to individual storage space for private use c. To see visitors each day d. To have reasonable access to telephones, both to make and receive confidential calls or to have such call made for one e. To have ready access to letter-writing materials, including stamps, and to mail and receive unopened correspondence f. To refuse shock treatment and any form of convulsive therapy g. To refuse psychosurgery h. To see and receive the services of a client advocate who has no direct or indirect clinical or administrative responsibility for the person i. To request a writ of habeas corpus j. To have reports of pain accepted and acted on by healthcare professionals k. Other rights, as specified by regulation Client acknowledges receipt by signing; individual giving client document also signs. Attempts to give document to client are also documented on the form should they be unable to be advised upon admission.		

Client Responsibilities
 	
1. The client has the responsibility to provide to the best of his/her knowledge, accurate and complete information about:
  a. Present complaints
  b. Past illnesses
  c. Previous hospitalizations
  d. Medications currently being used, or
  e. Prescribed within the last six (6) months, other matters relating to his/her health.
 	
The client is responsible for:
 	
2. Following the treatment plan recommended by the attending psychiatrist and treatment team responsible for his/her care. This may include following the instructions of treatment team members as they implement the plan of care.
 	
3. His/her actions if he/she refuses treatment or does not follow the treatment plan recommendations.
 	
4. Ensuring that the financial obligations of his/her health care are fulfilled as promptly as possible.
 	
5. Following hospital rules and regulations affecting client care, conduct, and safety.
 	
6. Being considerate of the rights of other patients and hospital personnel and for assisting in the control of noise, smoking, and the number of visitors.
 	
7. Being respectful of the property of other persons and the hospital.		

Documentation Requirements	Joint Commission on Accreditation of Healthcare Organizations	Medicare *Conditions of Participation* or Other Regulations
Denial of Client Rights When an order is written by the MD to deny a client one of his/her rights, the denial of the right must be documented in the medical record. Good cause for denial of the right shall also be documented. Restoration of rights shall be documented in the client's treatment record. A monthly report of denial of client rights shall be submitted to the State Dept. of Mental Health. (Each State Department of Health and Human Services and/or Mental Health Authority provides a form for this purpose for uniformity.) (Assumption)		
Detention: 72 Hours When a client is detained on an involuntary basis for psychiatric evaluation, an application for 72-hour detention for evaluation and treatment must be completed by psychiatrist and peace officer. Each State Department of Mental Health or Mental Health Authority has specific forms to be used for this purpose.		
Involuntary Client Advisement Each person admitted for 72-hour evaluation is required to be given specific information orally and in writing about why he/she is being placed in the psychiatric facility, how long he/she may be held, and advising him/her of his/her right to a lawyer and a hearing before a judge if he/she is held for a longer period of time. Each State Department of Mental Health or Mental Health Authority has specific forms to be used for this purpose.		
Notice of Certification When psychiatrist/psychologist alleges that an individual is, as the result of a mental disorder or impairment, a danger to others, to him/herself, or gravely disabled, the client must be so certified in order for the client to continue to be held.		
Client Request for Release As mental health clients are sometimes held involuntarily, there must be in place a mechanism for them to request a hearing/petition for their release. This is referred to as a writ of habeas corpus. They petition the court requesting that a judge determine the appropriateness of their being held against their will. Normally, the court in your jurisdiction determines the content and format of the documents to be used for this purpose. (Assumption)		
Refusal of Treatment Voluntary patients in psychiatric care, just like their counterparts in a medical setting, may request to be released against medical advice. The client must sign a legal form demanding release and acknowledging that he/she understands the terms and responsibilities that may result from the release.		

Documentation Requirements	Joint Commission on Accreditation of Healthcare Organizations	Medicare *Conditions of Participation or Other Regulations*
Signed X-ray reports of all examinations performed shall be made part of the client's hospital record.		482.26(d)
The radiologist or other practitioner who performs radiology services must sign reports of his or her interpretations.		482.26(d)(l)
The health record thoroughly documents operative or other procedures and the use of sedation or anesthesia.	IM.7.3	
A preoperative diagnosis is recorded before surgery by the licensed independent practitioner responsible for the client.	IM.7.3.1	
Operative reports dictated or written immediately after surgery record the name of the primary surgeon and assistants, findings, technical procedures used, specimens removed, and postoperative diagnosis.	IM.7.3.2	
The completed operative report is authenticated by the surgeon and filed in the health record as soon as possible after surgery.	EM.7.3.2.1	
When the operative report is not placed in the health record immediately after surgery, a progress note is entered immediately.	IM.7.3.2.2	
Postoperative documentation records the client's vital signs and level of consciousness; medications (including intravenous fluids), blood, and blood components; any unusual events or postoperative complications; and management of such events.	IM.7.3.3	
Postoperative documentation records the client's discharge from the postsedation or postanesthesia care area by the responsible licensed independent practitioner or according to discharge criteria.	IM.7.3.4.	
Compliance with discharge criteria is fully documented in the client's health record.	IM.7.3.4.1	
Postoperative documentation records the name of the licensed independent practitioner responsible for discharge.	IM.7.3-.5	
An informed consent for surgery shall be part of the client's chart before surgery is performed. It must be dated, timed, and signed by the client and the physician informant.		482.51(b)(2)

Documentation Requirements	Joint Commission on Accreditation of Healthcare Organizations	Medicare *Conditions of Participation or Other Regulations*
An operative report describing the reason for procedure, gross findings, operative procedure (techniques), and tissues removed or altered must be written or dictated immediately following surgery and signed by the surgeon.		482.51(b)(6)
A presedation or preanesthesia assessment is performed for each client before beginning moderate or deep sedation and before anesthesia induction.	TX.2.1	
A preanesthesia evaluation is performed within 48 hours prior to surgery by an individual qualified to administer anesthesia.		482.52(b)(1)
Standards for the Form and Content of the Health Record		
An intraoperative anesthesia record is provided.		482.52(b)(2)
With respect to inpatients, a postanesthesia follow-up report is written within 48 hours after surgery by the individual who administers the anesthesia.		482.52(b)(3)
A. Preanesthesia evaluation is documented by an individual qualified to administer anesthesia and is performed within 48 hours prior to the anesthesia event of surgery.		482.52(b)
The hospital must maintain signed and dated reports of nuclear medicine interpretations, consultations, and procedures.		482.53(d)
The practitioner approved by the medical staff to interpret diagnostic procedures must sign and date the interpretation of these tests.		482.53(d)(2)
When emergency, urgent, or immediate care is provided, the time and means of arrival are also documented in the health record.	IM.7.5	
The health record notes when a client receiving emergency, urgent, or immediate care left against medical advice.	IM.7.5.1	
The health record of a client receiving emergency, urgent, or immediate care notes the conclusions at termination of treatment, including final disposition, condition at discharge, and instructions for follow-up care.	IM.7.5.2	
When authorized by the client or a legally authorized representative, a copy of the emergency services provided is available to the practitioner or medical organization providing follow-up care.	IM.7.5.3	

Appendix D

Principles of Form and Screen Design

Every acute care facility must institute a well-thought-out system for managing its patient care documentation tools. This requirement is the same whether the facility uses paper-based health records, computer-based health records, or a combination of preprinted health record forms, computer-generated reports, and data-entry software. As acute care facilities gradually move toward implementing paperless electronic health record (EHR) systems, the forms design process will evolve to a screen (or view) design process. Although the health record format will change, the principles of effective design and management will still apply.

Principles of Design: All Health Record Formats

- Every form or view should be designed with its end users in mind so that the form or view fulfills its purpose and is easy to complete.

- Every form or view should include completion instructions so that the data collected will be as consistent as possible.

- Every form or view should include a title that clearly represents the form/view's purpose.

- Every form or view should include adequate space provisions for dates, signatures, and other elements of authentication.

- Every form or view should be as simple as possible and still fulfill its purpose.

- Forms and views that include similar information and are utilized by the same users should be combined whenever feasible.

- The elements on each form or view should be arranged logically, and similar information should be grouped together.

- When possible, forms and views should use only standard medical symbols, acronyms, and abbreviations.

- When space limitations make it necessary to use unusual abbreviations and acronyms, a key should be added to the form, or a link to the definition should be made provided in an electronic system.

- Ambiguous abbreviations should never be used on health record forms or views.

Principles of Design: Paper-Based Health Records

- All of the paper-based health record forms used by a facility should follow a similar format. Typically:

  —Forms are 8.5 by 11 inches in size.

  —Forms are one-sided (that is, nothing is printed on the reverse side).

  —Form headings (top or bottom of the page) include the name of the facility and the name of the form, and headings are repeated on every page of multipage forms.

  —Pages of multipage forms are numbered in sequence.

  —A space is left blank at the same position on every page of every form to accommodate a patient identification label. Labels usually include at least the patient's full name, date of birth, and health record number. Some facilities also include the patient's Social Security number, the name of the patient's physician, the date of admission, or other identifying data. Most facilities now use bar codes in their identification systems to streamline access and filing processes.

  —Notations at the bottom of each form are used for version control and usually note the form's title and control number and indicate the date on which the form was last revised.

  —Margins are standardized to accommodate the style of chart holder used in the facility.

  —The same style of type (for example, all capital letters) and type size and font (for example, ten-point Helvetica) are used on every form. Type sizes below eight points are generally considered illegible.

  —Corner marks are placed in the form's top and bottom margins to make document scanning more efficient.

- The Joint Commission on Accreditation of Healthcare Organizations requires hospitals to prohibit the use of the following abbreviations in handwritten health record documentation:

  —U for unit

  —IU and iu

  —QD and qd

  —QOD and qod

  —Zero after the decimal point

  —No zero before the decimal point

  —MS, MSO4, and MgSO4

- Rules should be used to demarcate separate sections of a form or view.

- Care should be taken in using shading to highlight specific areas of a form because information in the shaded sections may become illegible in scanned documents.

- Adequate space should be provided to accommodate the information to be entered by the user (for example, three lines of space should be left blank to allow the user to fill in a mailing address).

- Space-saving devices such as check-off boxes should be used whenever possible.

- The paper used for printing forms should be appropriate to the amount of use the record is likely to receive. Twenty-pound, white stock is generally adequate for use in printers, scanners, and photocopiers. Black ink reproduces more clearly than other colors.

Principles of Design: Electronic Health Records

- Menus and submenus should be provided to make navigation between views easy, and the menus and submenus should be sequenced in a logical order.

- Patient identifiers should be visible on every view to prevent errors in documentation.

- Printability should be considered in the use of color.

- Designs should be attractive, but simple to allow maximum area for data content.

- Data fields should be large enough to accommodate the information to be collected.

- Default values such as the current date and automatic numbering should be used whenever possible to reduce the amount of keyboarding needed.

- Data-editing functions should be protected by password to prevent unauthorized or unintentional alteration.

Principles of Management

- Acute care facilities should establish organizationwide guidelines for the creation and maintenance of the facility's information capture and health record documentation tools.

- Acute care facilities should institute an approval process to control the number of different health record forms and computer views in use.

- The roles and responsibilities of the facility's medical records committee in regard to health record content, format, and vocabulary should be spelled out in the facility's medical staff bylaws or health record policies.

- The roles and responsibilities of the facility's medical records committee in regard to the forms approval process should be spelled out in the facility's medical staff bylaws or health record policies.

- When new or revised paper forms are approved and implemented, the existing stock of out-of-date forms should be retrieved from patient care units and storage and then destroyed.

- Every paper form in use should be assigned a unique number, and a master list of forms that includes their titles, control numbers, and the approval date or the date when the form was last revised should be maintained.

- The collection of health record information should be streamlined to avoid unnecessary duplication of data and data collection efforts.

Sources

Kiger, Linda S. 2002. Information-capture design and principles. In *Health Information Management: Principles and Organization for Health Information Services,* 5th ed. Ed. Margaret A. Skurka. San Francisco: Jossey-Bass.

McCain, Mary Cole. 2002. Paper-based health records. In *Health Information Management: Concepts, Principles, and Practice.* Ed. Kathleen M. LaTour and Shirley Eichenwald. Chicago: American Health Information Management Association.

Appendix E

Federal Register Documents

OIG Compliance Program Guidance for Hospitals

The following document was prepared by the Office of the Inspector General (OIG), in the Department of Health and Human Services. It was originally published by the U.S. Government Printing Office on February 23, 1998 (*Federal Register* 63[35]:8987–8998). This article is available at http://oig.hhs.gov/authorities/docs/cpghosp.pdf.

I. Introduction

The Office of the Inspector General (OIG) of the Department of Health and Human Services (HHS) continues in its efforts to promote voluntarily developed and implemented compliance programs for the health care industry. The following compliance program guidance is intended to assist hospitals and their agents and subproviders (referred to collectively in this document as "hospitals") develop effective internal controls that promote adherence to applicable Federal and State law, and the program requirements of Federal, State, and private health plans. The adoption and implementation of voluntary compliance programs significantly advance the prevention of fraud, abuse, and waste in these health care plans while at the same time furthering the fundamental mission of all hospitals, which is to provide quality care to patients.

Within this document, the OIG intends to provide first, its general views on the value and fundamental principles of hospital compliance programs, and, second, specific elements that each hospital should consider when developing and implementing an effective compliance program. While this document presents basic procedural and structural guidance for designing a compliance program, it is not in itself a compliance program. Rather, it is a set of guidelines for a hospital interested in implementing a compliance program to consider. The recommendations and guidelines provided in this document must be considered depending upon their applicability to each particular hospital.

Fundamentally, compliance efforts are designed to establish a culture within a hospital that promotes prevention, detection, and resolution of instances of conduct that do not conform to Federal and State law, and Federal, State, and private payor health care program requirements, as well as the hospital's ethical and business policies. In practice, the compliance program should effectively articulate and demonstrate the organization's commitment to the compliance process. The existence of benchmarks that demonstrate implementation and achievements are essential to any effective compliance program. Eventually, a compliance program should become part of the fabric of routine hospital operations.

Specifically, compliance programs guide a hospital's governing body (e.g., Boards of Directors or Trustees), Chief Executive Officer (CEO), managers, other employees and physicians, and other health care professionals in the efficient management and operation of a hospital. They are especially critical as an internal control in the reimbursement and payment areas, where claims and billing operations are often the source of fraud and abuse and, therefore, historically have been the focus of government regulation, scrutiny, and sanctions.

It is incumbent upon a hospital's corporate officers and managers to provide ethical leadership to the organization and to assure that adequate systems are in place to facilitate ethical and legal conduct. Indeed, many hospitals and hospital organizations have adopted mission statements articulating their commitment to high ethical standards. A formal compliance program, as an additional element in this process, offers a hospital a further concrete method that may improve quality of care and reduce waste. Compliance programs also provide a central coordinating mechanism for furnishing and disseminating information and guidance on applicable Federal and State statutes, regulations, and other requirements.

Adopting and implementing an effective compliance program requires a substantial commitment of time, energy, and resources by senior management and the hospital's governing body.[1]

Programs hastily constructed and implemented without appropriate ongoing monitoring will likely be ineffective and could result in greater harm or liability to the hospital than no program at all. While it may require significant additional resources or reallocation of existing resources to implement an effective compliance program, the OIG believes that the long-term benefits of implementing the program outweigh the costs.

A. Benefits of a Compliance Program

In addition to fulfilling its legal duty to ensure that it is not submitting false or inaccurate claims to government and private payors, a hospital may gain numerous additional benefits by implementing an effective compliance program. Such programs make good business sense in that they help a hospital fulfill its fundamental caregiving mission to patients and the community, and assist hospitals in identifying weaknesses in internal systems and management.

Other important potential benefits include the ability to:

- Concretely demonstrate to employees and the community at large the hospital's strong commitment to honest and responsible provider and corporate conduct;

- Provide a more accurate view of employee and contractor behavior relating to fraud and abuse;

- Identify and prevent criminal and unethical conduct;

- Tailor a compliance program to a hospital's specific needs;

- Improve the quality of patient care;

- Create a centralized source for distributing information on health care statutes, regulations, and other program directives related to fraud and abuse and related issues;

- Develop a methodology that encourages employees to report potential problems;

- Develop procedures that allow the prompt, thorough investigation of alleged misconduct by corporate officers, managers, employees, independent contractors, physicians, other health care professionals and consultants;

- Initiate immediate and appropriate corrective action; and

- Through early detection and reporting, minimize the loss to the Government from false claims, and thereby reduce the hospital's exposure to civil damages and penalties, criminal sanctions, and administrative remedies, such as program exclusion.[2]

Overall, the OIG believes that an effective compliance program is a sound investment on the part of a hospital.

The OIG recognizes that the implementation of a compliance program may not entirely eliminate fraud, abuse and waste from the hospital system. However, a sincere effort by hospitals to comply with applicable Federal and State standards, as well as the requirements of private health care programs, through the establishment of an effective compliance program, significantly reduces the risk of unlawful or improper conduct.

B. Application of Compliance Program Guidance

There is no single "best" hospital compliance program, given the diversity within the industry. The OIG understands the variances and complexities within the hospital industry and is sensitive to the differences among large urban medical centers, community hospitals, small, rural hospitals, specialty hospitals, and other types of hospital organizations and systems. However, elements of this guidance can be used by all hospitals, regardless of size, location or corporate structure, to establish an effective compliance program. We recognize that some hospitals may not be able to adopt certain elements to the same comprehensive degree that others with more extensive resources may achieve. This guidance represents the OIG's suggestions on how a hospital can best establish internal controls and monitoring to correct and prevent fraudulent activities. By no means should the contents of this guidance be viewed as an exclusive discussion of the advisable elements of a compliance program.

The OIG believes that input and support by representatives of the major hospital trade associations is critical to the development and success of this compliance program guidance. Therefore, in drafting this guidance, the OIG received and considered input from various hospital and medical associations, as well as professional practice organizations. Further, we took into consideration previous OIG publications, such as Special Fraud Alerts and Management Advisory Reports, the recent findings and recommendations in reports issued by OIG's Office of Audit Services and Office of Evaluation and Inspections, as well as the experience of past and recent fraud investigations related to hospitals conducted by OIG's Office of Investigations and the Department of Justice.

As appropriate, this guidance may be modified and expanded as more information and knowledge is obtained by the OIG, and as changes in the law, and in the rules, policies, and procedures of the Federal, State and private health plans occur. The OIG understands that hospitals will need adequate time to react to these modifications and expansions to make any necessary changes to their voluntary compliance programs. We recognize that hospitals are already accountable for complying with an extensive set of statutory and other legal requirements, far more specific and complex than what we have referenced in this document. We also recognize that the development and implementation of compliance programs in hospitals often raise sensitive and complex legal and managerial issues.[3] However, the OIG wishes to offer what it believes is critical guidance for providers who are sincerely attempting to comply with the relevant health care statutes and regulations.

II. Compliance Program Elements

The elements proposed by these guidelines are similar to those of the clinical laboratory model compliance program published by the OIG in February 1997[4] and our corporate integrity agreements.[5] The elements represent a guide—a process that can be used by hospitals, large or small, urban or rural, for-profit or not for-profit. Moreover, the elements can be incorporated into the managerial structure of multi-hospital and integrated delivery systems. As we stated in our clinical laboratory plan, these suggested guidelines can be tailored to fit the needs and financial realities of a particular hospital. The OIG is cognizant that with regard to compliance programs, one model is not suitable to every hospital. Nonetheless, the OIG believes that every hospital, regardless of size or structure, can benefit from the principles espoused in this guidance.

The OIG believes that every effective compliance program must begin with a formal commitment by the hospital's governing body to include *all* of the applicable elements listed below. These elements are based on the seven steps of the Federal Sentencing Guidelines.[6] Further, we believe that every hospital can implement most of our recommended elements that expand upon the seven steps of the Federal Sentencing Guidelines.[7] We recognize that full implementation of all elements may not be immediately feasible for all hospitals. However, as a first step, a good faith and meaningful commitment on the part of the hospital administration, especially the governing body and the CEO, will substantially contribute to a program's successful implementation.

At a minimum, comprehensive compliance programs should include the following seven elements:

1. The development and distribution of written standards of conduct, as well as written policies and procedures that promote the hospital's commitment to compliance (e.g., by including adherence to compliance as an element in evaluating managers and employees) and that address specific areas of potential fraud, such as claims development and submission processes, code gaming, and financial relationships with physicians and other health care professionals;

2. The designation of a chief compliance officer and other appropriate bodies, e.g., a corporate compliance committee, charged with the responsibility of operating and monitoring the compliance program, and who report directly to the CEO and the governing body;

3. The development and implementation of regular, effective education, and training programs for all affected employees;

4. The maintenance of a process, such as a hotline, to receive complaints, and the adoption of procedures to protect the anonymity of complainants and to protect whistleblowers from retaliation;

5. The development of a system to respond to allegations of improper/illegal activities and the enforcement of appropriate disciplinary action against employees who have violated internal compliance policies, applicable statutes, regulations or Federal health care program requirements;

6. The use of audits and/or other evaluation techniques to monitor compliance and assist in the reduction of identified problem area; and

7. The investigation and remediation of identified systemic problems and the development of policies addressing the non-employment or retention of sanctioned individuals.

A. Written Polices and Procedures

Every compliance program should require the development and distribution of written compliance policies that identify specific areas of risk to the hospital. These policies should be developed under the direction and supervision of the chief compliance officer and compliance committee, and, at a minimum, should be provided to all individuals who are affected by the particular policy at issue, including the hospital's agents and independent contractors.

1. Standards of Conduct

Hospitals should develop standards of conduct for all affected employees that include a clearly delineated commitment to compliance by the hospital's senior management[8] and its divisions, including affiliated providers operating under the hospital's control,[9] hospital-based physicians and other health care professionals (e.g., utilization review managers, nurse anesthetists, physician assistants and physical therapists). Standards should articulate the hospital's commitment to comply with all Federal and State standards, with an emphasis on preventing fraud and abuse. They should state the organization's mission, goals, and ethical requirements of compliance and reflect a carefully crafted, clear expression of expectations for all hospital governing body members, officers, managers, employees, physicians, and, where appropriate, contractors and other agents. Standards should be distributed to, and comprehensible by, all employees (e.g., translated into other languages and written at appropriate reading levels, where appropriate). Further, to assist in ensuring that employees continuously meet the expected high standards set forth in the code of conduct, any employee handbook delineating or expanding upon these standards of conduct should be regularly updated as applicable statutes, regulations and Federal health care program requirements are modified.[10]

2. Risk Areas

The OIG believes that a hospital's written policies and procedures should take into consideration the regulatory exposure for each function or department of the hospital. Consequently, we recommend that the individual policies and procedures be coordinated with the appropriate training and educational programs with an emphasis on areas of special concern that have been identified by the OIG through its investigative and audit functions.[11] Some of the special areas of OIG concern include:[12]

- Billing for items or services not actually rendered;[13]
- Providing medically unnecessary services;[14]
- Upcoding;[15]
- "DRG creep;"[16]
- Outpatient services rendered in connection with inpatient stays;[17]
- Teaching physician and resident requirements for teaching hospitals;
- Duplicate billing;[18]
- False cost reports;[19]
- Unbundling;[20]
- Billing for discharge in lieu of transfer;[21]
- Patients' freedom of choice;[22]
- Credit balances—failure to refund;
- Hospital incentives that violate the anti-kickback statute or other similar Federal or State statute or regulation;[23]
- Joint ventures;[24]
- Financial arrangements between hospitals and hospital-based physicians;[25]
- Stark physician self-referral law;
- Knowing failure to provide covered services or necessary care to members of a health maintenance organization; and
- Patient dumping.[26]

Additional risk areas should be assessed as well by hospitals and incorporated into the written policies and procedures and training elements developed as part of their compliance programs.

3. Claim Development and Submission Process

A number of the risk areas identified above, pertaining to the claim development and submission process, have been the subject of administrative proceedings, as well as investigations and prosecutions under the civil False Claims Act and criminal statutes. Settlement of these cases often has required the defendants to execute corporate integrity agreements, in addition to paying significant civil damages and/or criminal fines and penalties. These corporate integrity agreements have provided the OIG with a mechanism to advise hospitals concerning what it feels are acceptable practices to ensure compliance with applicable Federal and State statutes, regulations, and program requirements. The following recommendations include a number of provisions from various corporate integrity agreements. While these recommendations include examples of effective policies, each hospital should develop its own specific policies tailored to fit its individual needs.

With respect to reimbursement claims, a hospital's written policies and procedures should reflect and reinforce current Federal and State statutes and regulations regarding the submission of claims and Medicare cost reports. The policies must create a mechanism for the billing or reimbursement staff to communicate effectively and accurately with the clinical staff. Policies and procedures should:

- Provide for proper and timely documentation of all physician and other professional services prior to billing to ensure that only accurate and properly documented services are billed;

- Emphasize that claims should be submitted only when appropriate documentation supports the claims and only when such documentation is maintained and available for audit and review. The documentation, which may include patient records, should record the length of time spent in conducting the activity leading to the record entry, and the identity of the individual providing the service. The hospital should consult with its medical staff to establish other appropriate documentation guidelines;

- State that, consistent with appropriate guidance from medical staff, physician and hospital records, and medical notes used as a basis for a claim submission should be appropriately organized in a legible form so they can be audited and reviewed;

- Indicate that the diagnosis and procedures reported on the reimbursement claim should be based on the medical record and other documentation, and that the documentation necessary for accurate code assignment should be available to coding staff; and

- Provide that the compensation for billing department coders and billing consultants should not provide any financial incentive to improperly upcode claims.

The written policies and procedures concerning proper coding should reflect the current reimbursement principles set forth in applicable regulations[27] and should be developed in tandem with private payor and organizational standards. Particular attention should be paid to issues of medical necessity, appropriate diagnosis codes, DRG coding, individual Medicare Part B claims (including evaluation and management coding) and the use of patient discharge codes.[28]

a. Outpatient services rendered in connection with an inpatient stay: Hospitals should implement measures designed to demonstrate their good faith efforts to comply with the Medicare billing rules for outpatient services rendered in connection with an inpatient stay. Although not a guard against intentional wrongdoing, the adoption of the following measures are advisable:

- Installing and maintaining computer software that will identify those outpatient services that may not be billed separately from an inpatient stay; or

- Implementing a periodic manual review to determine the appropriateness of billing each outpatient service claim, to be conducted by one or more appropriately trained individuals familiar with applicable billing rules; or

- With regard to each inpatient stay, scrutinizing the propriety of any potential bills for outpatient services rendered to that patient at the hospital, within the applicable time period. In addition to the presubmission undertakings described above, the hospital may implement a postsubmission testing process, as follows:

- Implement and maintain a periodic postsubmission random testing process that examines or re-examines previously submitted claims for accuracy;

- Inform the fiscal intermediary and any other appropriate government fiscal agents of the hospital's testing process; and

- Advise the fiscal intermediary and any other appropriate government fiscal agents in accordance with current regulations or program instructions with respect to return of overpayments of any incorrectly submitted or paid claims and, if the claim has already been paid, promptly reimburse the fiscal intermediary and the beneficiary for the amount of the claim paid by the government payor and any applicable deductibles or copayments, as appropriate.

b. Submission of claims for laboratory services: A hospital's policies should take reasonable steps to ensure that all claims for clinical and diagnostic laboratory testing services are accurate and correctly identify the services ordered by the physician (or other authorized requestor) and performed by the laboratory. The hospital's written policies and procedures should require, at a minimum,[29] that:

- The hospital bills for laboratory services only after they are performed;

- The hospital bills only for medically necessary services;

- The hospital bills only for those tests actually ordered by a physician and provided by the hospital laboratory;

- The CPT or HCPCS code used by the billing staff accurately describes the service that was ordered by the physician and performed by the hospital laboratory;

- The coding staff: (1) Only submit diagnostic information obtained from qualified personnel; and (2) contact the appropriate personnel to obtain diagnostic information in the event that the individual who ordered the test has failed to provide such information; and

- Where diagnostic information is obtained from a physician or the physician's staff after receipt of the specimen and request for services, the receipt of such information is documented and maintained.

c. Physicians at teaching hospitals: Hospitals should ensure the following with respect to all claims submitted on behalf of teaching physicians:

- Only services actually provided may be billed;

- Every physician who provides or supervises the provision of services to a patient should be responsible for the correct documentation of the services that were rendered;

- The appropriate documentation must be placed in the patient record and signed by the physician who provided or supervised the provision of services to the patient;

- Every physician is responsible for assuring that in cases where that physician provides evaluation and management (E&M) services, a patient's medical record includes appropriate documentation of the applicable key components of the E&M service provided or supervised by the physician (e.g., patient history, physician examination, and medical decision making), as well as documentation to adequately reflect the procedure or portion of the service performed by the physician; and

- Every physician should document his or her presence during the key portion of any service or procedure for which payment is sought.

d. Cost reports: With regard to cost report issues, the written policies should include procedures that seek to ensure full compliance with applicable statutes, regulations and program requirements and private payor plans. Among other things, the hospital's procedures should ensure that:

- Costs are not claimed unless based on appropriate and accurate documentation;

- Allocations of costs to various cost centers are accurately made and supportable by verifiable and auditable data;

- Unallowable costs are not claimed for reimbursement;

- Accounts containing both allowable and unallowable costs are analyzed to determine the unallowable amount that should not be claimed for reimbursement;

- Costs are properly classified;

- Fiscal intermediary prior year audit adjustments are implemented and are either not claimed for reimbursement or claimed for reimbursement and clearly identified as protested amounts on the cost report;

- All related parties are identified on Form 339 submitted with the cost report and all related party charges are reduced to cost;

- Requests for exceptions to TEFRA (Tax Equity and Fiscal Responsibility Act of 1982) limits and the Routine Cost Limits are properly documented and supported by verifiable and auditable data;

- The hospital's procedures for reporting of bad debts on the cost report are in accordance with Federal statutes, regulations, guidelines, and policies;

- Allocations from a hospital chain's home office cost statement to individual hospital cost reports are accurately made and supportable by verifiable and auditable data; and

- Procedures are in place and documented for notifying promptly the Medicare fiscal intermediary (or any other applicable payor, e.g., TRICARE (formerly CHAMPUS) and Medicaid) of errors discovered after the submission of the hospital cost report, and where applicable, after the submission of a hospital chain's home office cost statement.

With regard to bad debts claimed on the Medicare cost report, see also section six, below, on Bad Debts.

4. Medical Necessity—Reasonable and Necessary Services

A hospital's compliance program should provide that claims should only be submitted for services that the hospital has reason to believe are medically necessary and that were ordered by a physician[30] or other appropriately licensed individual.

As a preliminary matter, the OIG recognizes that licensed health care professionals must be able to order any services that are appropriate for the treatment of their patients. However,

Medicare and other government and private health care plans will only pay for those services that meet appropriate medical necessity standards (in the case of Medicare, i.e., "reasonable and necessary" services). Providers may not bill for services that do not meet the applicable standards. The hospital is in a unique position to deliver this information to the health care professionals on its staff. Upon request, a hospital should be able to provide documentation, such as patients' medical records and physicians' orders, to support the medical necessity of a service that the hospital has provided. The compliance officer should ensure that a clear, comprehensive summary of the "medical necessity" definitions and rules of the various government and private plans is prepared and disseminated appropriately.

5. Anti-Kickback and Self-Referral Concerns

The hospital should have policies and procedures in place with respect to compliance with Federal and State anti-kickback statutes, as well as the Stark physician self-referral law.[31] Such policies should provide that:

- All of the hospital's contracts and arrangements with referral sources comply with all applicable statutes and regulations;

- The hospital does not submit or cause to be submitted to the Federal health care programs claims for patients who were referred to the hospital pursuant to contracts and financial arrangements that were designed to induce such referrals in violation of the anti-kickback statute, Stark physician self-referral law or similar Federal or State statute or regulation; and

- The hospital does not enter into financial arrangements with hospital-based physicians that are designed to provide inappropriate remuneration to the hospital in return for the physician's ability to provide services to Federal health care program beneficiaries at that hospital.[32]

Further, the policies and procedures should reference the OIG's safe harbor regulations, clarifying those payment practices that would be immune from prosecution under the anti-kickback statute. See 42 CFR 1001.952.

6. Bad Debts

A hospital should develop a mechanism[33] to review, at least annually: (1) whether it is properly reporting bad debts to Medicare; and (2) all Medicare bad debt expenses claimed, to ensure that the hospital's procedures are in accordance with applicable Federal and State statutes, regulations, guidelines and policies. In addition, such a review should ensure that the hospital has appropriate and reasonable mechanisms in place regarding beneficiary deductible or copayment collection efforts and has not claimed as bad debts any routinely waived Medicare copayments and deductibles, which waiver also constitutes a violation of the anti-kickback statute. Further, the hospital may consult with the appropriate fiscal intermediary as to bad debt reporting requirements, if questions arise.

7. Credit Balances

The hospital should institute procedures to provide for the timely and accurate reporting of Medicare and other Federal health care program credit balances. For example, a hospital may redesignate segments of its information system to allow for the segregation of patient accounts reflecting credit balances. The hospital could remove these accounts from the active accounts and place them in a holding account pending the processing of a reimbursement claim to the appropriate program. A hospital's information system should have the ability to print out the individual patient accounts that reflect a credit balance in order to permit simplified tracking of credit balances.

In addition, a hospital should designate at least one person (e.g., in the Patient Accounts Department or reasonable equivalent thereof) as having the responsibility for the tracking, recording, and reporting of credit balances. Further, a comptroller or an accountant in the hospital's Accounting Department (or reasonable equivalent thereof) may review reports of credit balances and reimbursements or adjustments on a monthly basis as an additional safeguard.

8. Retention of Records

Hospital compliance programs should provide for the implementation of a records system. This system should establish policies and procedures regarding the creation, distribution, retention, storage, retrieval, and destruction of documents. The two types of documents developed under this system should include: (1) all records and documentation, e.g., clinical and medical records and claims documentation, required either by Federal or State law for participation in Federal health care programs (e.g., Medicare's conditions of participation requirement that hospital records regarding Medicare claims be retained for a minimum of five years, see 42 CFR 482.24(b)(1) and HCFA (CMS) Hospital Manual section 413(C)(12–91)); and (2) all records necessary to protect the integrity of the hospital's compliance process and confirm the effectiveness of the program, e.g., documentation that employees were adequately trained; reports from the hospital's hotline, including the nature and results of any investigation that was conducted; modifications to the compliance program; self-disclosure; and the results of the hospital's auditing and monitoring efforts.[34]

9. Compliance as an Element of a Performance Plan

Compliance programs should require that the promotion of, and adherence to, the elements of the compliance program be a factor in evaluating the performance of managers and supervisors. They, along with other employees, should be periodically trained in new compliance policies and procedures. In addition, all managers and supervisors involved in the coding, claims, and cost report development and submission processes should:

- Discuss with all supervised employees the compliance policies and legal requirements applicable to their function;

- Inform all supervised personnel that strict compliance with these policies and requirements is a condition of employment; and

- Disclose to all supervised personnel that the hospital will take disciplinary action up to and including termination or revocation of privileges for violation of these policies or requirements.

In addition to making performance of these duties an element in evaluations, the compliance officer or hospital management should include in the hospital's compliance program a policy that managers and supervisors will be sanctioned for failure to instruct adequately their subordinates or for failing to detect noncompliance with applicable policies and legal requirements, where reasonable diligence on the part of the manager or supervisor would have led to the discovery of any problems or violations and given the hospital the opportunity to correct them earlier.

B. Designation of a Compliance Officer and a Compliance Committee

1. Compliance Officer

Every hospital should designate a compliance officer to serve as the focal point for compliance activities. This responsibility may be the individual's sole duty or added to other management responsibilities, depending upon the size and resources of the hospital and the complexity of the task. Designating a compliance officer with the appropriate authority is critical to the success of the program, necessitating the appointment of a high-level official in the hospital with direct access to the hospital's governing body and the CEO.[35] The officer should have sufficient funding and staff to perform his or her responsibilities fully. Coordination and communication are the key functions of the compliance officer with regard to planning, implementing, and monitoring the compliance program.

The compliance officer's primary responsibilities should include:

- Overseeing and monitoring the implementation of the compliance program;[36]

- Reporting on a regular basis to the hospital's governing body, CEO and compliance committee on the progress of implementation, and assisting these components in establishing methods to improve the hospital's efficiency and quality of services, and to reduce the hospital's vulnerability to fraud, abuse and waste;

- Periodically revising the program in light of changes in the needs of the organization, and in the law and policies and procedures of government and private payor health plans;

- Developing, coordinating, and participating in a multifaceted educational and training program that focuses on the elements of the compliance program, and seeks to ensure that all appropriate employees and management are knowledgeable of, and comply with, pertinent Federal and State standards;

- Ensuring that independent contractors and agents who furnish medical services to the hospital are aware of the requirements of the hospital's compliance program with respect to coding, billing, and marketing, among other things;

- Coordinating personnel issues with the hospital's Human Resources office (or its equivalent) to ensure that the National Practitioner Data Bank and Cumulative Sanction Report[37] have been checked with respect to all employees, medical staff and independent contractors;

- Assisting the hospital's financial management in coordinating internal compliance review and monitoring activities, including annual or periodic reviews of departments;

- Independently investigating and acting on matters related to compliance, including the flexibility to design and coordinate internal investigations (e.g., responding to reports of problems or suspected violations) and any resulting corrective action with all hospital departments, providers and subproviders,[38] agents and, if appropriate, independent contractors; and

- Developing policies and programs that encourage managers and employees to report suspected fraud and other improprieties without fear of retaliation.

The compliance officer must have the authority to review all documents and other information that are relevant to compliance activities, including, but not limited to, patient records, billing records, and records concerning the marketing efforts of the facility and the hospital's arrangements with other parties, including employees, professionals on staff, independent contractors, suppliers, agents, and hospital-based physicians, etc. This policy enables the compliance officer to review contracts and obligations (seeking the advice of legal counsel, where appropriate) that may contain referral and payment issues that could violate the anti-kickback statute, as well as the physician self-referral prohibition and other legal or regulatory requirements.

2. Compliance Committee

The OIG recommends that a compliance committee be established to advise the compliance officer and assist in the implementation of the compliance program.[39] The committee's functions should include:

- Analyzing the organization's industry environment, the legal requirements with which it must comply, and specific risk areas;

- Assessing existing policies and procedures that address these areas for possible incorporation into the compliance program;

- Working with appropriate hospital departments to develop standards of conduct and policies and procedures to promote compliance with the institution's program;

- Recommending and monitoring, in conjunction with the relevant departments, the development of internal systems and controls to carry out the organization's standards, policies and procedures as part of its daily operations;

- Determining the appropriate strategy/approach to promote compliance with the program and detection of any potential violations, such as through hotlines and other fraud reporting mechanisms; and

- Developing a system to solicit, evaluate and respond to complaints and problems.

The committee may also address other functions as the compliance concept becomes part of the overall hospital operating structure and daily routine.

C. Conducting Effective Training and Education

The proper education and training of corporate officers, managers, employees, physicians, and other health care professionals, and the continual retraining of current personnel at all levels, are significant elements of an effective compliance program. As part of their compliance programs, hospitals should require personnel to attend specific training on a periodic basis, including appropriate training in Federal and State statutes, regulations, and guidelines, and the policies of private payors, and training in corporate ethics, which emphasizes the organization's commitment to compliance with these legal requirements and policies.

These training programs should include sessions highlighting the organization's compliance program, summarizing fraud and abuse laws, coding requirements, claim development and submission processes, and marketing practices that reflect current legal and program standards. The organization must take steps to communicate effectively its standards and procedures to all affected employees, physicians, independent contractors, and other significant agents, e.g., by requiring participation in training programs and disseminating publications that explain in a practical manner specific requirements.[40] Managers of specific departments or groups can assist in identifying areas that require training and in carrying out such training. Training instructors may come from outside or inside the organization. New employees should be targeted for training early in their employment.[41] Any formal training undertaken by the hospital as part of the compliance program should be documented by the compliance officer.

A variety of teaching methods, such as interactive training, and training in several different languages, particularly where a hospital has a culturally diverse staff, should be implemented so that all affected employees are knowledgeable of the institution's standards of conduct and procedures for alerting senior management to problems and concerns. Targeted training should be provided to corporate officers, managers and other employees whose actions affect the accuracy of the claims submitted to the Government, such as employees involved in the coding, billing, cost reporting and marketing processes. Given the complexity and interdependent relationships of many departments, proper coordination and supervision of this process by the compliance officer is important. In addition to specific training in the risk areas identified in section II.A.2, above, primary training to appropriate corporate officers, managers and other hospital staff should include such topics as:

- Government and private payor reimbursement principles;

- General prohibitions on paying or receiving remuneration to induce referrals;

- Proper confirmation of diagnoses;

- Submitting a claim for physician services when rendered by a nonphysician (i.e., the "incident to" rule and the physician physical presence requirement);

- Signing a form for a physician without the physician's authorization;

- Alterations to medical records;

- Prescribing medications and procedures without proper authorization;

- Proper documentation of services rendered; and

- Duty to report misconduct.

Clarifying and emphasizing these areas of concern through training and educational programs are particularly relevant to a hospital's marketing and financial personnel, in that the pressure to meet business goals may render these employees vulnerable to engaging in prohibited practices.

The OIG suggests that all relevant levels of personnel be made part of various educational and training programs of the hospital. Employees should be required to have a minimum number of educational hours per year, as appropriate, as part of their employment responsibilities.[42] For example, for certain employees involved in the billing and coding functions, periodic training in proper DRG coding and documentation of medical records should be required.[43] In hospitals with high employee turnover, periodic training updates are critical.

The OIG recommends that attendance and participation in training programs be made a condition of continued employment and that failure to comply with training requirements should result in disciplinary action, including possible termination, when such failure is serious. Adherence to the provisions of the compliance program, such as training requirements, should be a factor in the annual evaluation of each employee.[44] The hospital should retain adequate records of its training of employees, including attendance logs and material distributed at training sessions.

Finally, the OIG recommends that hospital compliance programs address the need for periodic professional education courses that may be required by statute and regulation for certain hospital personnel.

D. Developing Effective Lines of Communication

1. Access to the Compliance Officer

An open line of communication between the compliance officer and hospital personnel is equally important to the successful implementation of a compliance program and the reduction of any potential for fraud, abuse and waste. Written confidentiality and nonretaliation policies should be developed and distributed to all employees to encourage communication and the reporting of incidents of potential fraud.[45] The compliance committee should also develop several independent reporting paths for an employee to report fraud, waste, or abuse so that such reports cannot be diverted by supervisors or other personnel.

The OIG encourages the establishment of a procedure so that hospital personnel may seek clarification from the compliance officer or members of the compliance committee in the event of any confusion or question with regard to a hospital policy or procedure. Questions and responses should be documented and dated and, if appropriate, shared with other staff so that standards, policies and procedures can be updated and improved to reflect any necessary changes or clarifications. The compliance officer may want to solicit employee input in developing these communication and reporting systems.

2. Hotlines and Other Forms of Communication

The OIG encourages the use of hotlines (including anonymous hotlines), e-mails, written memoranda, newsletters, and other forms of information exchange to maintain these open lines of communication. If the hospital establishes a hotline, the telephone number should be made readily available to all employees and independent contractors, possibly by conspicuously posting the telephone number in common work areas.[46] Employees should be permitted to report matters on an anonymous basis. Matters reported through the hotline or other communication sources that suggest substantial violations of compliance policies, regulations, or statutes should be documented and investigated promptly to determine their veracity. A log should be maintained by the compliance officer that records such calls, including the nature of any investigation and its results. Such information should be included in reports to the governing body, the CEO and compliance committee. Further, while the hospital should always strive to maintain the confidentiality of an employee's identity, it should also explicitly communicate that there may be a point where the individual's identity may become known or may have to be revealed in certain instances when governmental authorities become involved.

The OIG recognizes that assertions of fraud and abuse by employees who may have participated in illegal conduct or committed other malfeasance raise numerous complex legal and management issues that should be examined on a case-by-case basis. The compliance officer should work closely with legal counsel, who can provide guidance regarding such issues.

E. Enforcing Standards Through Well-Publicized Disciplinary Guidelines

1. Discipline Policy and Actions

An effective compliance program should include guidance regarding disciplinary action for corporate officers, managers, employees, physicians, and other health care professionals who have failed to comply with the hospital's standards of conduct, policies and procedures, or Federal and State laws, or those who have otherwise engaged in wrongdoing, which have the potential to impair the hospital's status as a reliable, honest and trustworthy health care provider.

The OIG believes that the compliance program should include a written policy statement setting forth the degrees of disciplinary actions that may be imposed upon corporate officers, managers, employees, physicians, and other health care professionals for failing to comply with the hospital's standards and policies and applicable statutes and regulations. Intentional or reckless noncompliance should subject transgressors to significant sanctions. Such sanctions could range from oral warnings to suspension, privilege revocation (subject to any applicable peer review procedures), termination or financial penalties, as appropriate. The written standards of conduct should elaborate on the procedures for handling disciplinary problems and those who will be responsible for taking appropriate action. Some disciplinary actions can be handled by department managers, while others may have to be resolved by a senior hospital administrator. Disciplinary action may be appropriate where a responsible employee's failure to detect a violation is attributable to his or her negligence or reckless conduct. Personnel should be advised by the hospital that disciplinary action will be taken on a fair and equitable basis. Managers and supervisors should be made aware that they have a responsibility to discipline employees in an appropriate and consistent manner.

It is vital to publish and disseminate the range of disciplinary standards for improper conduct and to educate officers and other hospital staff regarding these standards. The consequences of noncompliance should be consistently applied and enforced, in order for the disciplinary policy to have the required deterrent effect. All levels of employees should be subject to the same disciplinary action for the commission of similar offenses. The commitment to compliance applies to all personnel levels within a hospital. The OIG believes that corporate officers, managers, supervisors, medical staff and other health care professionals should be held accountable for failing to comply with, or for the foreseeable failure of their subordinates to adhere to, the applicable standards, laws, and procedures.

2. New Employee Policy

For all new employees who have discretionary authority to make decisions that may involve compliance with the law or compliance oversight, hospitals should conduct a reasonable and prudent background investigation, including a reference check, as part of every such employment application.[47] The application should specifically require the applicant to disclose any criminal conviction, as defined by 42 U.S.C. 1320a–7(i), or exclusion action. Pursuant to the compliance program, hospital policies should prohibit the employment of individuals who have been recently convicted of a criminal offense related to health care or who are listed as debarred, excluded or otherwise ineligible for participation in Federal health care programs (as defined in 42 U.S.C. 1320a–7b(f)).[48] In addition, pending the resolution of any criminal charges or proposed debarment or exclusion, the OIG recommends that such individuals should be removed from direct responsibility for or involvement in any Federal health care program.[49] With regard to current employees or independent contractors, if resolution of the matter results in conviction, debarment or exclusion, the hospital should terminate its employment or other contract arrangement with the individual or contractor.

F. Auditing and Monitoring

An ongoing evaluation process is critical to a successful compliance program. The OIG believes that an effective program should incorporate thorough monitoring of its implementation and regular reporting to senior hospital or corporate officers.[50] Compliance reports created by this ongoing monitoring, including reports of suspected noncompliance, should be maintained by the compliance officer and shared with the hospital's senior management and the compliance committee.

Although many monitoring techniques are available, one effective tool to promote and ensure compliance is the performance of regular, periodic compliance audits by internal or external auditors who have expertise in Federal and State health care statutes, regulations and Federal health care program requirements. The audits should focus on the hospital's programs or divisions, including external relationships with third-party contractors, specifically those with substantive exposure to government enforcement actions. At a minimum, these audits should be designed to address the hospital's compliance with laws governing kickback arrangements, the physician self-referral prohibition, CPT/HCPSC ICD–9 coding, claim development and submission, reimbursement, cost reporting and marketing. In addition, the audits and reviews should inquire into the hospital's compliance with specific rules and polices that have been the focus of particular attention on the part of the Medicare fiscal intermediaries or carriers, and law enforcement, as evidenced by OIG Special Fraud Alerts, OIG audits and evaluations, and law enforcement's initiatives. See section II.A.2, *supra.* In addition, the hospital should focus on any areas of concern that have been identified by any entity, i.e., Federal, State, or internally, specific to the individual hospital.

Monitoring techniques may include sampling protocols that permit the compliance officer to identify and review variations from an established baseline.[51] Significant variations from the baseline should trigger a reasonable inquiry to determine the cause of the deviation. If the inquiry determines that the deviation occurred for legitimate, explainable reasons, the compliance officer, hospital administrator or manager may want to limit any corrective action or take no action. If it is determined that the deviation was caused by improper procedures, misunderstanding of rules, including fraud and systemic problems, the hospital should take prompt steps to correct the problem. Any overpayments discovered as a result of such deviations should be returned promptly to the affected payor, with appropriate documentation and a thorough explanation of the reason for the refund.[52]

Monitoring techniques may also include a review of any reserves the hospital has established for payments that it may owe to Medicare, Medicaid, TRICARE or other Federal health care programs. Any reserves discovered that include funds that should have been paid to

Medicare or another government program should be paid promptly, regardless of whether demand has been made for such payment.

An effective compliance program should also incorporate periodic (at least annual) reviews of whether the program's compliance elements have been satisfied, e.g., whether there has been appropriate dissemination of the program's standards, training, ongoing educational programs and disciplinary actions, among others. This process will verify actual conformance by all departments with the compliance program. Such reviews could support a determination that appropriate records have been created and maintained to document the implementation of an effective program. However, when monitoring discloses that deviations were not detected in a timely manner due to program deficiencies, appropriate modifications must be implemented. Such evaluations, when developed with the support of management, can help ensure compliance with the hospital's policies and procedures.

As part of the review process, the compliance officer or reviewers should consider techniques such as:

- On-site visits;

- Interviews with personnel involved in management, operations, coding, claim development and submission, patient care, and other related activities;

- Questionnaires developed to solicit impressions of a broad cross-section of the hospital's employees and staff;

- Reviews of medical and financial records and other source documents that support claims for reimbursement and Medicare cost reports;

- Reviews of written materials and documentation prepared by the different divisions of a hospital; and

- Trend analysis, or longitudinal studies, that seek deviations, positive or negative, in specific areas over a given period.

The reviewers should:

- Be independent of physicians and line management;

- Have access to existing audit and health care resources, relevant personnel and all relevant areas of operation;

- Present written evaluative reports on compliance activities to the CEO, governing body and members of the compliance committee on a regular basis, but no less than annually; and

- Specifically identify areas where corrective actions are needed.

With these reports, hospital management can take whatever steps are necessary to correct past problems and prevent them from reoccurring. In certain cases, subsequent reviews or studies would be advisable to ensure that the recommended corrective actions have been implemented successfully.

The hospital should document its efforts to comply with applicable statutes, regulations and Federal health care program requirements. For example, where a hospital, in its efforts to comply with a particular statute, regulation or program requirement, requests advice from a government agency (including a Medicare fiscal intermediary or carrier) charged with administering a Federal health care program, the hospital should document and retain a record of the request and any written or oral response. This step is extremely important if the hospital intends to rely on that response to guide it in future decisions, actions or claim reimbursement requests or appeals. Maintaining a log of oral inquiries between the hospital and third parties represents an additional basis for establishing documentation on which the organization may rely to demonstrate attempts at compliance. Records should be maintained demonstrating reasonable reliance and due diligence in developing procedures that implement such advice.

G. Responding to Detected Offenses and Developing Corrective Action Initiatives

1. Violations and Investigations

Violations of a hospital's compliance program, failures to comply with applicable Federal or State law, and other types of misconduct threaten a hospital's status as a reliable, honest and trustworthy provider capable of participating in Federal health care programs. Detected but uncorrected misconduct can seriously endanger the mission, reputation, and legal status of the hospital. Consequently, upon reports or reasonable indications of suspected noncompliance, it is important that the chief compliance officer or other management officials initiate prompt steps to investigate the conduct in question to determine whether a material violation of applicable law or the requirements of the compliance program has occurred, and if so, take steps to correct the problem.[53] As appropriate, such steps may include an immediate referral to criminal and/or civil law enforcement authorities, a corrective action plan,[54] a report to the Government,[55] and the submission of any overpayments, if applicable.

Where potential fraud or False Claims Act liability is not involved, the OIG recognizes that HCFA (CMS) regulations and contractor guidelines already include procedures for returning overpayments to the Government as they are discovered. However, even if the overpayment detection and return process is working and is being monitored by the hospital's audit or coding divisions, the OIG still believes that the compliance officer needs to be made aware of these overpayments, violations or deviations and look for trends or patterns that may demonstrate a systemic problem.

Depending upon the nature of the alleged violations, an internal investigation will probably include interviews and a review of relevant documents. Some hospitals should consider engaging outside counsel, auditors, or health care experts to assist in an investigation. Records of the investigation should contain documentation of the alleged violation, a description of the investigative process, copies of interview notes and key documents, a log of the witnesses interviewed and the documents reviewed, the results of the investigation, e.g., any disciplinary action taken, and the corrective action implemented. While any action taken as the result of an investigation will necessarily vary depending upon the hospital and the situation, hospitals should strive for some consistency by utilizing sound practices and disciplinary protocols. Further, after a reasonable period, the compliance officer should review the circumstances that formed the basis for the investigation to determine whether similar problems have been uncovered.

If an investigation of an alleged violation is undertaken and the compliance officer believes the integrity of the investigation may be at stake because of the presence of employees under investigation, those subjects should be removed from their current work activity until the investigation is completed (unless an internal or Government-led undercover operation is in effect). In addition, the compliance officer should take appropriate steps to secure or prevent the destruction of documents or other evidence relevant to the investigation. If the hospital determines that disciplinary action is warranted, if should be prompt and imposed in accordance with the hospital's written standards of disciplinary action.

2. Reporting

If the compliance officer, compliance committee or management official discovers credible evidence of misconduct from any source and, after a reasonable inquiry, has reason to believe that the misconduct may violate criminal, civil, or administrative law, then the hospital promptly should report the existence of misconduct to the appropriate governmental authority[56] within a reasonable period, but not more than sixty (60) days[57] after determining that there is credible evidence of a violation.[58] Prompt reporting will demonstrate the hospital's good faith and willingness to work with governmental authorities to correct and remedy the problem. In addition, reporting such conduct will be considered a mitigating factor by the OIG in determining administrative sanctions (e.g., penalties, assessments, and exclusion), if the reporting provider becomes the target of an OIG investigation.[59]

When reporting misconduct to the Government, a hospital should provide all evidence relevant to the alleged violation of applicable Federal or State law(s) and potential cost impact. The compliance officer, under advice of counsel, and with guidance from the governmental authorities, could be requested to continue to investigate the reported violation. Once the investigation is completed, the compliance officer should be required to notify the appropriate governmental authority of the outcome of the investigation, including a description of the impact of the alleged violation on the operation of the applicable health care programs or their beneficiaries. If the investigation ultimately reveals that criminal or civil violations have occurred, the appropriate Federal and State officials[60] should be notified immediately.

As previously stated, the hospital should take appropriate corrective action, including prompt identification and restitution of any overpayment to the affected payor and the imposition of proper disciplinary action. Failure to repay overpayments within a reasonable period of time could be interpreted as an intentional attempt to conceal the overpayment from the Government, thereby establishing an independent basis for a criminal violation with respect to the hospital, as well as any individuals who may have been involved.[61] For this reason, hospital compliance programs should emphasize that overpayment obtained from Medicare or other Federal health care programs should be promptly returned to the payor that made the erroneous payment.[62]

III. Conclusion

Through this document, the OIG has attempted to provide a foundation to the process necessary to develop an effective and cost-efficient hospital compliance program. As previously stated, however, each program must be tailored to fit the needs and resources of an individual hospital, depending upon its particular corporate structure, mission, and employee composition. The statutes, regulations and guidelines of the Federal and State health insurance programs, as well as the policies and procedures of the private health plans, should be integrated into every hospital's compliance program.

The OIG recognizes that the health care industry in this country, which reaches millions of beneficiaries and expends about a trillion dollars, is constantly evolving. However, the time is right for hospitals to implement a strong voluntary compliance program concept in health care. As stated throughout this guidance, compliance is a dynamic process that helps to ensure that hospitals and other health care providers are better able to fulfill their commitment to ethical behavior, as well as meet the changes and challenges being imposed upon them by Congress and private insurers. Ultimately, it is the OIG's hope that a voluntarily created compliance program will enable hospitals to meet their goals, improve the quality of patient care, and substantially reduce fraud, waste and abuse, as well as the cost of health care to Federal, State and private health insurers.

Footnotes

1. Indeed, recent case law suggests that the failure of a corporate Director to attempt in good faith to institute a compliance program in certain situations may be a breach of a Director's fiduciary obligations. See, e.g., *In re Caremark International Inc. Derivative Litigation*, 698 A.2d 959 (Ct. Chanc. Del. 1996).

2. The OIG, for example, will consider the existence of an *effective* compliance program that pre-dated any Governmental investigation when addressing the appropriateness of administrative penalties. Further, the False Claims Act, 31 U.S.C. 3729–3733, provides that a person who has violated the Act, but who voluntarily discloses the violation to the Government, in certain circumstances will be subject to not less than double, as opposed to treble, damages. See 31 U.S.C. 3729(a).

3. Nothing stated herein should be substituted for, or used in lieu of, competent legal advice from counsel.

4. See 62 FR 9435, March 3, 1997.

5. Corporate integrity agreements are executed as part of a civil settlement between the health care provider and the Government to resolve a case arising under the False Claims Act (FCA), including the *qui tam* provisions of the FCA, based on allegations of health care fraud or abuse. These OIG-imposed programs are in effect for a period of three to five years and require many of the elements included in this compliance guidance.

6. See United States Sentencing Commission Guidelines, *Guidelines Manual,* 8A1.2, comment. (n.3(k)).

7. Current HCFA (CMS) reimbursement principles provide that certain of the costs associated with the creation of a voluntarily established compliance program may be allowable costs on certain types of hospitals' cost reports. These allowable costs, of course, must at a minimum be *reasonable* and related to patient care. See generally 42 U.S.C. 1395x(v)(1)(A) (definition of reasonable cost); 42 CFR 413.9(a) and (b)(2) (costs related to patient care). In contrast, however, costs specifically associated with the implementation of a corporate integrity agreement in response to a Government investigation resulting in a civil or criminal judgment or settlement are unallowable, and are also made specifically and expressly unallowable in corporate integrity agreements and civil fraud settlements.

8. The OIG strongly encourages high-level involvement by the hospital's governing body, chief executive officer, chief operating officer, general counsel, and chief financial officer, as well as other medical personnel, as appropriate, in the development of standards of conduct. Such involvement should help communicate a strong and explicit statement of compliance goals and standards.

9. E.g., skilled nursing facilities, home health agencies, psychiatric units, rehabilitation units, outpatient clinics, clinical laboratories, dialysis facilities.

10. The OIG recognizes that not all standards, policies and procedures need to be communicated to all employees. However, the OIG believes that the bulk of the standards that relate to complying with fraud and abuse laws and other ethical areas should be addressed and made part of all affected employees' training. The hospital must appropriately decide which additional educational programs should be limited to the different levels of employees, based on job functions and areas of responsibility.

11. The OIG periodically issues Special Fraud Alerts setting forth activities believed to raise legal and enforcement issues. Hospital compliance programs should require that the legal staff, chief compliance officer, or other appropriate personnel, carefully consider any and all Special Fraud Alerts issued by the OIG that relate to hospitals. Moreover, the compliance programs should address the ramifications of failing to cease and correct any conduct criticized in such a Special Fraud Alert, if applicable to hospitals, or to take reasonable action to prevent such conduct from reoccurring in the future. If appropriate, a hospital should take the steps described in Section G regarding investigations, reporting and correction of identified problems.

12. The OIG's work plan is currently available on the Internet at http://www.dhhs.gov/progorg/oig.

13. Billing for services not actually rendered involves submitting a claim that represents that the provider performed a service all or part of which was simply not performed. This form of billing fraud occurs in many health care entities, including hospitals and nursing homes, and represents a significant part of the OIG's investigative caseload.

14. A claim requesting payment for medically unnecessary services intentionally seeks reimbursement for a service that is not warranted by the patient's current and documented medical condition. See 42 U.S.C. 1395y(a)(1)(A) ("no payment may be made under part A or part B for any expenses incurred for items or services which . . . are not reasonable and necessary for the diagnosis or treatment of illness or injury or to improve the functioning of the malformed body member"). On every HCFA (CMS) claim form, a physician must certify that the services were medically necessary for the health of the beneficiary.

15. "Upcoding" reflects the practice of using a billing code that provides a higher payment rate than the billing code that actually reflects the service furnished to the patient. Upcoding has been a major focus of the OIG's enforcement efforts. In fact, the Health Insurance Portability and Accountability Act of 1996 added another civil monetary penalty to the OIG's sanction authorities for upcoding violations. See 42 U.S.C. 1320a–7a(a)(1)(A).

16. Like upcoding, "DRG creep" is the practice of billing using a Diagnosis Related Group (DRG) code that provides a higher payment rate than the DRG code that accurately reflects the service furnished to the patient.

17. Hospitals that submit claims for non-physician outpatient services that were already included in the hospital's inpatient payment under the Prospective Payment System (PPS) are in effect submitting duplicate claims.

18. Duplicate billing occurs when the hospital submits more than one claim for the same service or the bill is submitted to more than one primary payor at the same time. Although duplicate billing can occur due to simple error, systematic or repeated double billing may be viewed as a false claim, particularly if any overpayment is not promptly refunded.

19. As another example of health care fraud, the submission of false costs reports is usually limited to certain Part A providers, such as hospitals, skilled nursing facilities, and home health agencies, which are reimbursed in part on the basis of their self-reported operating costs. An OIG audit report on the misuse of fringe benefits and general and administrative costs identified millions of dollars in unallowable costs that resulted from providers' lack of internal controls over costs included in their Medicare cost reports. In addition, the OIG is aware of practices in which hospitals inappropriately shift certain costs to cost centers that are below their reimbursement cap and shift non-Medicare related costs to Medicare cost centers.

20. "Unbundling" is the practice of submitting bills piecemeal or in fragmented fashion to maximize the reimbursement for various tests or procedures that are required to be billed together and therefore at a reduced cost.

21. Under the Medicare regulations, when a prospective payment system (PPS) hospital transfers a patient to another PPS hospital, only the hospital to which the patient was transferred may charge the full DRG; the transferring hospital should charge Medicare only a per diem amount.

22. This area of concern is particularly important for hospital discharge planners referring patients to home health agencies, DME suppliers or long term care and rehabilitation providers.

23. Excessive payment for medical directorships, free or below market rents, or fees for administrative services, interest-free loans and excessive payment for intangible assets in physician practice acquisitions are examples of arrangements that may run afoul of the anti-kickback statute. See 42 U.S.C. 1320a–7b(b) and 59 FR 65372 (12/19/94).

24. Equally troubling to the OIG is the proliferation of business arrangements that may violate the anti-kickback statute. Such arrangements are generally established between those in a position to refer business, such as physicians, and those providing items or services for which a Federal health care program pays. Sometimes established as "joint ventures," these arrangements may take a variety of forms. The OIG currently has a number of investigations and audits underway that focus on such areas of concern.

25. Another OIG concern with respect to the anti-kickback statute is hospital financial arrangements with hospital-based physicians that compensate physicians for less than the fair market value of services they provide to hospitals or require physicians to pay more than market value for services provided by the hospital. See OIG Management Advisory Report: "Financial Arrangements Between Hospitals and Hospital-Based Physicians." OEI–09–89–0030, October 1991. Examples of such arrangements that may violate the anti-kickback statute are token or no payment for Part A supervision and management services; requirements to donate equipment to hospitals; and excessive charges for billing services.

26. The patient anti-dumping statute, 42 U.S.C. 1395dd, requires that all Medicare participating hospitals with an emergency department: (1) Provide for an appropriate medical screening examination to determine whether or not an individual requesting such examination has an emergency medical condition; and (2) if the person has such a condition, (a) stabilize that condition; or (b) appropriately transfer the patient to another hospital.

27. The official coding guidelines are promulgated by HCFA (CMS), the National Center for Health Statistics, the American Medical Association and the American Health Information Management Association. See International Classification of Diseases, 9th Revision, Clinical Modification (ICD9–CM); 1998 Health Care Financing Administration Common Procedure Coding System (HCPCS); and Physicians' Current Procedural Terminology (CPT).

28. The failure of hospital staff to: (i) document items and services rendered; and (ii) properly submit them for reimbursement is a major area of potential fraud and abuse in Federal health care programs. The OIG has undertaken numerous audits, investigations, inspections and national enforcement initiatives aimed at reducing potential and actual fraud, abuse, and waste. Recent OIG audit reports, which have focused on

issues such as hospital patient transfers incorrectly paid as discharges, and hospitals' general and administrative costs, continue to reveal abusive, wasteful or fraudulent behavior by some hospitals. Our inspection report entitled "Financial Arrangements between Hospitals and Hospital-Based Physicians," see fn. 25, *supra,* and our Special Fraud Alerts on Hospital Incentives to Physicians and Joint Venture Arrangements, further illustrate how certain business practices may result in fraudulent and abusive behavior.

29. The OIG's February 1997 Model Compliance Plan for Clinical Laboratories provides more specific and detailed information than is contained in this section, and hospitals that have clinical laboratories should extract the relevant guidance from both documents.

30. For Medicare reimbursement purposes, a physician is defined as: (1) a doctor of medicine or osteopathy; (2) a doctor of dental surgery or of dental medicine; (3) a podiatrist; (4) an optometrist; and (5) a chiropractor, all of whom must be appropriately licensed by the state. 42 U.S.C. 1395x(r).

31. Towards this end, the hospital's in-house counsel or compliance officer should, inter alia, obtain copies of all OIG regulations, special fraud alerts and advisory opinions concerning the anti-kickback statute, Civil Monetary Penalties Law (CMPL) and Stark physician self-referral law (the fraud alerts and anti-kickback or CMPL advisory opinions are published on HHS OIG's home page on the Internet), and ensure that the hospital's policies reflect the guidance provided by the OIG.

32. See fn. 25, *supra.*

33. E.g., assigning in-house counsel or contracting with an independent professional organization, such as an accounting, law, or consulting firm.

34. The creation and retention of such documents and reports may raise a variety of legal issues, such as patient privacy and confidentiality. These issues are best discussed with legal counsel.

35. The OIG believes that there is some risk to establishing an independent compliance function if that function is subordinance to the hospital's general counsel, or comptroller or similar hospital financial officer. Free standing compliance functions help to ensure independent and objective legal reviews and financial analyses of the institution's compliance efforts and activities. By separating the compliance function from the key management positions of general counsel or chief hospital financial officer (where the size and structure of the hospital make this a feasible option), a system of checks and balances is established to more effectively achieve the goals of the compliance program.

36. For multi-hospital organizations, the OIG encourages coordination with each hospital owned by the corporation or foundation through the use of a headquarter's compliance officer, communicating with parallel positions in each facility, or regional office, as appropriate.

37. The Cumulative Sanction Report is an OIG-produced report available on the Internet at http://www.dhhs.gov/progorg/oig. It is updated on a regular basis to reflect the status of health care providers who have been excluded from participation in the Medicare and Medicaid programs. In addition, the General Services Administration maintains a monthly listing of debarred contractors on the Internet at http://www.arnet.gov/epls. Also, once the data base established by the Health Care Fraud and Abuse Data Collection Act of 1996 is fully operational, the hospital should regularly request information from this data bank as part of its employee screening process.

38. E.g., skilled nursing facilities and home health agencies.

39. The compliance committee benefits from having the perspectives of individuals with varying responsibilities in the organization, such as operations, finance, audit, human resources, utilization review, social work, discharge planning, medicine, coding, and legal, as well as employees and managers of key operating units.

40. Some publications, such as OIG's Management Advisory Report entitled "Financial Arrangements between Hospitals and Hospital-Based Physicians," Special Fraud Alerts, audit and inspection reports, and advisory opinions, as well as the annual OIG work plan, are readily available from the OIG and could be the basis for standards, educational courses and programs for appropriate hospital employees.

41. Certain positions, such as those involving the coding of medical services, create a greater organizational legal exposure, and therefore require specialized training. One recommendation would be for a hospital to attempt to fill such positions with individuals who have the appropriate educational background and training.

42. Currently, the OIG is monitoring approximately 165 corporate integrity agreements that require many of these training elements. The OIG usually requires a minimum of one to three hours annually for basic training in compliance areas. More is required for speciality fields such as billing and coding.

43. Accurate coding depends upon the quality and completeness of the physician's documentation. Therefore, the OIG believes that active staff physician participation in educational programs focusing on coding and documentation should be emphasized by the hospital.

44. In addition, where feasible, the OIG believes that a hospital's outside contractors, including physician corporations, should be afforded the opportunity to participate in, or develop their own, compliance training and educational programs, which complement the hospital's standards of conduct, compliance requirements, and other rules and regulations.

45. The OIG believes that whistleblowers should be protected against retaliation, a concept embodied in the provisions of the False Claims Act. In many cases, employees sue their employers under the False Claims Act's *qui tam* provisions out of frustration because of the company's failure to take action when a questionable, fraudulent or abusive situation was brought to the attention of senior corporate officials.

46. Hospitals should also post in a prominent, available area the HHS OIG Hotline telephone number, 1–800–HHS–TIPS (447–8477), in addition to any company hotline number that may be posted.

47. See fn. 37, *supra.*

48. Likewise, hospital compliance programs should establish standards prohibiting the execution of contracts with companies that have been recently convicted of a criminal offense related to health care or that are listed by a Federal agency as debarred, excluded, or otherwise ineligible for participation in Federal health care programs.

49. Prospective employees who have been officially reinstated into the Medicare and Medicaid programs by the OIG may be considered for employment upon proof of such reinstatement.

50. Even when a hospital is owned by a larger corporate entity, the regular auditing and monitoring of the compliance activities of an individual hospital must be a key feature in any annual review. Appropriate reports on audit findings should be periodically provided and explained to a parent organization's senior staff and officers.

51. The OIG recommends that when a compliance program is established in a hospital, the compliance officer, with the assistance of department managers, should take a "snapshot" of their operations from a compliance perspective. This assessment can be undertaken by outside consultants, law or accounting firms, or internal staff with authoritative knowledge of health care compliance requirements. This "snapshot," often used as part of benchmarking analyses, becomes a baseline for the compliance officer and other managers to judge the hospital's progress in reducing or eliminating potential areas of vulnerability. For example, it has been suggested that a baseline level include the frequency and percentile levels of various diagnosis codes and the increased billing of complications and co-morbidities.

52. In addition, when appropriate, as referenced in section G.2 reports of fraud or systemic problems should also be made to the appropriate governmental authority.

53. Instances of noncompliance must be determined on a case-by-case basis. The existence, or amount, of a *monetary* loss to a health care program is not solely determinative of whether or not the conduct should be investigated and reported to governmental authorities. In fact, there may be instances where there is no monetary loss at all, but corrective action and reporting are still necessary to protect the integrity of the applicable program and its beneficiaries.

54. Advice from the hospital's in-house counsel or an outside law firm may be sought to determine the extent of the hospital's liability and to plan the appropriate course of action.

55. The OIG currently maintains a voluntary disclosure program that encourages providers to report suspected fraud. The concept of voluntary self-disclosure is premised on a recognition that the Government alone cannot protect the integrity of the Medicare and other Federal health care programs. Health care providers must be willing to police themselves, correct underlying problems and work with the Government to resolve these matters. The OIG's voluntary self-disclosure program has four prerequisites: (1) the disclosure must be on behalf of an entity and not an individual; (2) the disclosure must be truly voluntary (i.e., no pending proceeding or investigation); (3) the entity must disclose the nature of the wrongdoing and the harm to the Federal programs; and (4) the entity must not be the subject of a bankruptcy proceeding before or after the self-disclosure.

56. I.e., Federal and/or State law enforcement having jurisdiction over such matter. Such governmental authority would include DOJ and OIG with respect to Medicare and Medicaid violations giving rise to causes of actions under various criminal, civil and administrative false claims statutes.

57. To qualify for the "not less than double damages" provision of the False Claims Act, the report must be provided to the Government within thirty (30) days after the date when the hospital first obtained the information. 31 U.S.C. 3729(a).

58. The OIG believes that some violations may be so serious that they warrant immediate notification to governmental authorities, prior to, or simultaneous with, commencing an internal investigation, e.g., if the conduct: (1) is a clear violation of criminal law; (2) has a significant adverse effect on the quality of care provided to program beneficiaries (in addition to any other legal obligations regarding quality of care); or (3) indicates evidence of a systemic failure to comply with applicable laws, an existing corporate integrity agreement, or other standards of conduct, regardless of the financial impact on Federal health care programs.

59. The OIG has published criteria setting forth those factors that the OIG takes into consideration in determining whether it is appropriate to exclude a health care provider from program participation pursuant to 42 U.S.C. 1320a–7(b)(7) for violations of various fraud and abuse laws. See 62 FR 67392, December 24, 1997.

60. Appropriate Federal and State authorities include the Criminal and Civil Divisions of the Department of Justice, the U.S. Attorney in the hospital's district, and the investigative arms for the agencies administering the affected Federal or State health care programs, such as the State Medicaid Fraud Control Unit, the Defense Criminal Investigative Service, and the Offices of Inspector General of the Department of Health and Human Services, the Department of Veterans Affairs, and the Office of Personnel Management (which administers the Federal Employee Health Benefits Program).

61. See 42 U.S.C. 1320a–7b(a)(3).

62. Normal repayment channels as described in HCFA's (CMS's) manuals and guidances are the appropriate vehicle for repaying identified overpayments. Hospitals should consult with its fiscal intermediary or HCFA for any further guidance regarding these repayment channels. Interest will be assessed, when appropriate. See 42 CFR 405.376.

Federal Register Documents

OIG Draft Supplemental Compliance Program Guidance for Hospitals

The following document was prepared by the Office of Inspector General (OIG), in the Department of Health and Human Services. It was originally published by the U.S. Government Printing Office on June 8, 2004 (Federal Register 69[110]: 32012–32031). This article is available at http://oig.hhs.gov/authorities/docs/04/060804hospitaldraftsuppCPGFR.pdf.

Background

Several years ago, the OIG embarked on a major initiative to engage the private health care community in preventing the submission of erroneous claims and in combating fraud and abuse in the Federal health care programs through voluntary compliance efforts. In the last several years, the OIG has developed a series of compliance program guidances (CPGs) directed at the following segments of the health care industry: hospitals; clinical laboratories; home health agencies; third-party billing companies; the durable medical equipment, prosthetics, orthotics, and supply industry; hospices; Medicare+Choice organizations; nursing facilities; physicians; ambulance suppliers; and pharmaceutical manufacturers. CPGs are intended to encourage the development and use of internal controls to monitor adherence to applicable statutes, regulations, and program requirements. The suggestions made in these CPGs are not mandatory, and the CPGs should not be viewed as exhaustive discussions of beneficial compliance practices or relevant risk areas. Copies of these CPGs can be found on the OIG webpage at http://oig.hhs.gov.

Supplementing the Compliance Program Guidance for Hospitals

The OIG originally published a CPG for the hospital industry on February 23, 1998.[1] Since that time, there have been significant changes in the way hospitals deliver, and are reimbursed for, health care services. In response to these developments, on June 18, 2002, the OIG published a notice in the **Federal Register** titled "Solicitation of Information and Recommendations for Revising the Compliance Program Guidance for the Hospital Industry."[2] The OIG received 11 comments from various interested parties. In light of the public comments and our consideration of the issues, we have decided to supplement, rather than revise, the 1998 guidance.

Many public commenters sought guidance on the application of specific Medicare rules and regulations related to payment and coverage, an area beyond the scope of this OIG guidance.

Hospitals with questions about the interpretation or application of payment and coverage rules or regulations should contact their Fiscal Intermediaries (FIs) or the national Centers for Medicare and Medicaid Services (CMS) office, as appropriate.

To ensure full and meaningful input from the industry, we are publishing this supplemental CPG in draft form with a 45-day comment period. We will then review the comments and publish a final supplemental CPG.

Draft Supplemental Compliance Program Guidance for Hospitals

I. Introduction

Continuing its efforts to promote voluntary compliance programs for the health care industry, the Office of Inspector General (OIG) of the Department of Health and Human Services (the Department) publishes this Supplemental Compliance Program Guidance for Hospitals.[3] This document supplements, rather than replaces, the OIG's 1998 CPG for the hospital industry, 63 FR 8987 (February 23, 1998), which addressed the fundamentals of establishing an effective compliance program.[4] Neither this supplemental CPG, nor the original 1998 CPG, is a model compliance program. Rather, collectively the two documents offer a set of guidelines that hospitals should consider when developing and implementing a new compliance program or evaluating an existing one.

We are mindful that many hospitals have already devoted substantial time and resources to compliance efforts. We believe that those efforts demonstrate the industry's good faith commitment to ensuring and promoting integrity. For those hospitals with existing compliance programs, this document may serve as a benchmark or comparison against which to measure ongoing efforts and as a roadmap for updating or refining their compliance plans.

In crafting this CPG, we considered, among other things, the public comments received in response to the solicitation notice published in the **Federal Register,**[5] as well as relevant OIG and Centers for Medicare & Medicaid Services (CMS) statutory and regulatory authorities (including the Federal anti-kickback statute, together with the safe harbor regulations and preambles,[6] and CMS transmittals and program memoranda); other OIG guidance (such as OIG advisory opinions, Special Fraud Alerts, bulletins, and other guidance); experience gained from investigations conducted by the OIG's Office of Investigations, the Department of Justice, and the State Medicaid Fraud Units; and relevant reports issued by the OIG's Office of Audit Services and Office of Evaluation and Inspections.[7] We also consulted generally with CMS, the Department's Office for Civil Rights, and the Department of Justice.

A. Benefits of a Compliance Program

A successful compliance program addresses the public and private sectors' mutual goals of reducing fraud and abuse; enhancing health care providers' operations; improving the quality of health care services; and reducing the overall cost of health care services. Attaining these goals benefits the hospital industry, the government, and patients alike. Compliance programs help hospitals fulfill their legal duty to refrain from submitting false or inaccurate claims or cost information to the Federal health care programs[8] or engaging in other illegal practices. A hospital may gain important additional benefits by voluntarily implementing a compliance program, including:

- Demonstrating the hospital's commitment to honest and responsible corporate conduct;

- Increasing the likelihood of preventing, identifying, and correcting unlawful and unethical behavior at an early stage;

- Encouraging employees to report potential problems to allow for appropriate internal inquiry and corrective action; and

- Through early detection and reporting, minimizing any financial loss to government and taxpayers, as well as any corresponding financial loss to the hospital.

The OIG recognizes that implementation of a compliance program may not entirely eliminate improper or unethical conduct from the operations of health care providers. However, an effective compliance program demonstrates a hospital's good faith effort to comply with applicable statutes, regulations, and other Federal health care program requirements and may significantly reduce the risk of unlawful conduct and corresponding sanctions.

B. Application of Compliance Program Guidance

Given the diversity of the hospital industry, there is no single "best" hospital compliance program. The OIG recognizes the complexities of the hospital industry and the differences among hospitals and hospital systems. Some hospital entities are small and may have limited resources to devote to compliance measures; others are affiliated with well-established, large, multi-facility organizations with a widely dispersed work force and significant resources to devote to compliance.

Accordingly, this supplemental CPG is not intended to be one-size-fits-all guidance. Rather, the OIG strongly encourages hospitals to identify and focus their compliance efforts on those areas of potential concern or risk that are most relevant to their individual organizations. Compliance measures adopted by a hospital to address identified risk areas should be tailored to fit the unique environment of the organization (including its structure, operations, resources, and prior enforcement experience). In short, the OIG recommends that each hospital adapt the objectives and principles underlying this guidance to its own particular circumstances.

In section II below, titled "Fraud and Abuse Risk Areas," we present several fraud and abuse risk areas that are particularly relevant to the hospital industry. Each hospital should carefully examine these risk areas and identify those that potentially impact the hospital. Next, in section III, "Hospital Compliance Program Effectiveness," we offer recommendations for assessing and improving an existing compliance program to better address identified risk areas. Finally, in section IV, "Self-Reporting," we set forth the actions hospitals should take if they discover credible evidence of misconduct.

II. Fraud and Abuse Risk Areas

This section is intended to help hospitals identify areas of their operations that present a potential risk of liability under several key Federal fraud and abuse statutes and regulations. This section focuses on areas that are currently of concern to the enforcement community and is not intended to address all potential risk areas for hospitals. Importantly, the identification of a particular practice or activity in this section is not intended to imply that the practice or activity is necessarily illegal in all circumstances or that it may not have a valid or lawful purpose underlying it.

This section addresses the following areas of significant concern for hospitals: (A) Submission of accurate claims and information; (B) the referral statutes; (C) payments to reduce or limit services; (D) the Emergency Medical Treatment and Labor Act (EMTALA); (E) substandard care; (F) relationships with Federal health care program beneficiaries; (G) HIPAA Privacy and Security Rules; and (H) billing Medicare or Medicaid substantially in excess of usual charges. In addition, a final section (I) addresses several areas of general interest that, while not necessarily matters of significant risk, have been of continuing interest to the hospital community. This guidance does not create any new law or legal obligations, and the discussions in this guidance are not intended to present detailed or comprehensive summaries of lawful and unlawful activity. Nor is this guidance intended as a substitute for consultation with CMS or a hospital's

Fiscal Intermediary (FI) with respect to the application and interpretation of Medicare payment and coverage provisions, which are subject to change. Rather, this guidance should be used as a starting point for a hospital's legal review of its particular practices and for development or refinement of policies and procedures to reduce or eliminate potential risk.

A. Submission of Accurate Claims and Information

Perhaps the single biggest risk area for hospitals is the preparation and submission of claims or other requests for payment from the Federal health care programs. It is axiomatic that all claims and requests for reimbursement from the Federal health care programs—and all documentation supporting such claims or requests—must be complete and accurate and must reflect reasonable and necessary services ordered by an appropriately licensed medical professional who is a participating provider in the health care program from which the individual or entity is seeking reimbursement. Hospitals must disclose and return any overpayments that result from mistaken or erroneous claims.[9] Moreover, the knowing submission of a false, fraudulent, or misleading statement or claim is actionable. A hospital may be liable under the False Claims Act[10] or other statutes imposing sanctions for the submission of false claims or statements, including liability for civil monetary penalties or exclusion.[11] Underlying assumptions used in connection with claims submission should be reasoned, consistent, and appropriately documented, and hospitals should retain all relevant records reflecting their efforts to comply with Federal health care program requirements.

Common and longstanding risks associated with claims preparation and submission include inaccurate or incorrect coding, upcoding, unbundling of services, billing for medically unnecessary services or other services not covered by the relevant health care program, billing for services not provided, duplicate billing, insufficient documentation, and false or fraudulent cost reports. While hospitals should continue to be vigilant with respect to these important risk areas, we believe these risk areas are relatively well understood in the industry and, therefore, they are not generally addressed in this section.[12] Rather, the following discussion highlights evolving risks or risks that appear to the OIG to be under-appreciated by the industry. The risks are grouped under the following topics: Outpatient procedure coding; admissions and discharges; supplemental payment considerations; and use of information technology. By necessity, this discussion is illustrative, not exhaustive, of risks associated with the submission of claims or other information. In all cases, hospitals should consult the applicable laws, rules, and regulations.

1. Outpatient Procedure Coding

The implementation of Medicare's Hospital Outpatient Prospective Payment System (OPPS)[13] increased the importance of accurate procedure coding for hospital outpatient services. Previously, hospital coding concerns mainly consisted of ensuring accurate ICD–9–CM diagnosis and procedure coding for reimbursement under the inpatient prospective payment system (PPS). Hospitals reported procedure codes for outpatient services, but were reimbursed for outpatient services based on their charges for services. With OPPS, procedure codes effectively became the basis for Medicare reimbursement. Under OPPS, each reported procedure code is assigned to a corresponding Ambulatory Payment Classification (APC) code. Hospitals are then reimbursed a predetermined amount for each APC, irrespective of the specific level of resources used to furnish the service. In implementing OPPS, CMS developed new rules governing the use of procedure code modifiers for outpatient coding.[14] Because incorrect procedure coding may lead to overpayments and subject a hospital to liability for the submission of false claims, hospitals need to pay close attention to coder training and qualifications.

Hospitals should also review their outpatient documentation practices to ensure that claims are based on complete medical records and that the medical record supports the level of service claimed. Under OPPS, hospitals must generally include on a single claim all services provided to the same patient on the same day. Coding from incomplete medical records may create problems in complying with this claim submission requirement. Moreover, submitting claims for services that are not supported by the medical record may also result in the submission of improper claims.

In addition to the coding risk areas noted above and in the 1998 hospital CPG, other specific risk areas associated with incorrect outpatient procedure coding include the following:

- *Billing on an outpatient basis for "inpatient-only" procedures*—CMS has identified several procedures for which reimbursement is typically allowed only if the service is performed in an inpatient setting.[15]

- *Submitting claims for medically unnecessary services by failing to follow the FI's local medical review policies*—Each FI publishes local medical review policies (LMRPs) that identify certain procedures that may only be rendered when specific conditions are present. In addition to relying on a physician's sound clinical judgment with respect to the appropriateness of a proposed course of treatment, hospitals should regularly review and become familiar with their individual FI's LMRPs. LMRPs should be incorporated into a hospital's regular coding and billing operations.[16]

- *Submitting duplicate claims or otherwise not following the National Correct Coding Initiative guidelines*—CMS developed the National Correct Coding Initiative (NCCI) to promote correct coding methodologies. NCCI identifies certain codes that should not be used together because they are either mutually exclusive or one is a component of another. If a hospital uses code pairs that are listed in the NCCI and those codes are not detected by the editing routines in the hospital's billing system, the hospital may submit duplicate or unbundled claims. Intentional manipulation of code assignments to maximize payments and avoid NCCI edits constitutes fraud. Unintentional misapplication of the NCCI coding and billing guidelines may also give rise to overpayments or civil liability for hospitals that have developed a pattern of inappropriate billing. To minimize risk, hospitals should ensure that their coding software includes up-to-date NCCI edit files.[17]

- *Submitting incorrect claims for ancillary services because of outdated Charge Description Masters*—Charge Description Masters (CDMs) list all of the hospital's charges for items and services and include the underlying procedure codes necessary to bill for those items and services. Outdated CDMs create significant compliance risk for hospitals. Because the Healthcare Common Procedure Coding System (HCPCS) codes and APCs are updated regularly, hospitals should pay particular attention to the task of updating the CDM to ensure the assignment of correct codes to outpatient claims. This should include timely updates, proper use of modifiers, and correct associations between procedure codes and revenue codes.[18]

- *Circumventing the multiple procedure discounting rules*—A surgical procedure performed in connection with another surgical procedure may be discounted. However, certain surgical procedures are designated as nondiscounted, even when performed with another surgical procedure. Hospitals should ensure that the procedure codes selected represent the actual services provided, irrespective of the discounting status. They should also review the annual OPPS rule update to understand more fully CMS's multiple procedure discounting rule.[19]

- *Failing to follow CMS instructions regarding the selection of proper evaluation and management codes*—Hospitals should take steps to ensure that the evaluation and management (E/M) codes that are used to describe medical services provided to patients follow published CMS guidelines.[20]

- *Improperly billing for observation services*—In certain circumstances, Medicare provides a separate APC payment for observation services for patients with diagnoses of chest pain, asthma, or congestive heart failure. Claims for these observation services must correctly reflect the diagnosis and meet certain other requirements. Billing for observation services in situations that do not satisfy the requirements is inappropriate and may result in hospital liability. Hospitals should develop, and become familiar with, CMS's detailed policies for the submission of claims for observation services.[21]

2. Admissions and Discharges

Often, the status of patients at the time of admission or discharge significantly influences the amount and method of reimbursement hospitals receive. Therefore, hospitals have a duty to ensure that admission and discharge policies are updated and reflect current CMS rules. Risk areas with respect to the admission and discharge processes include the following:

- *Failure to follow the "same-day rule"*—OPPS rules require hospitals to include on the same claim all OPPS services provided at the same hospital, to the same patient, on the same day, unless certain conditions are met. Hospitals should review internal billing systems and procedures to ensure that they are not submitting multiple claims for OPPS services delivered to the same patient on the same day.[22]

- *Abuse of partial hospitalization payments*—Under OPPS, Medicare provides a per diem payment for specific hospital services rendered to behavioral and mental health patients on a partial hospitalization basis. Examples of improper billing under the partial hospitalization program include, without limitation: reducing the range of services offered; withholding services that are medically appropriate; billing for services not covered; and billing for services without a certificate of medical necessity.[23]

- *Same-day discharges and readmissions*—Same-day discharges and readmissions may indicate premature discharges, medically unnecessary readmissions, or incorrect discharge coding. Hospitals should have procedures in place to review discharges and admissions carefully to ensure that they reflect prudent clinical decision-making and are properly coded.[24]

- *Violation of Medicare's post-acute care transfer policy*—The post-acute care transfer policy provides that, for certain designated DRGs, a hospital will receive a per diem transfer payment, rather than the full DRG payment, if the patient is discharged to certain postacute care settings.[25] There are currently 29 DRGs that are subject to CMS's postacute care transfer policy; however, CMS may revise the list of designated DRGs periodically.[26] To avoid improperly billing for discharges, hospitals should pay particular attention to CMS's post-acute care transfer policy and keep an accurate list of all designated DRGs subject to that policy.

- *Improper churning of patients by long-term care hospitals co-located in acute care hospitals*—Long term care hospitals that are co-located within acute care hospitals may qualify for PPS-exempt status if certain regulatory requirements are satisfied.[27] Hospitals should not engage in the practice of churning, or inappropriately transferring, patients between the host hospital and the hospital-within-a-hospital.

3. Supplemental Payment Considerations

Under the Medicare program, in certain limited situations, hospitals may claim payments in addition to, or in some cases in lieu of, the normal reimbursement available to hospitals under the regular payment systems. Eligibility for these payments depends on compliance with specific criteria. Hospitals that claim supplemental payments improperly are liable for fines and penalties under Federal law. Examples of specific risks that hospitals should address include the following:

- *Improper reporting of the costs of "pass-through" items*—"Pass-through" items are certain items of new technology and drugs for which Medicare will reimburse the hospital based on costs during a limited transitional period.[28]

- *Abuse of DRG outlier payments*—Recent investigations revealed substantial abuse of outlier payments by hospitals with Medicare patients. Hospital management, compliance staff, and counsel should familiarize themselves with CMS's new outlier rules and requirements intended to curb abuses.[29]

- *Improper claims for incorrectly designated "provider-based" entities*—Certain hospital-affiliated entities and clinics can be designated as "provider based," which allows for a higher level of reimbursement for certain services.[30] Hospitals should take steps to ensure that facilities or organizations are only designated as provider-based if they satisfy the criteria set forth in the regulations.

- *Improper claims for clinical trials*—Since September 2000, Medicare has covered items and services furnished during certain clinical trials, as long as those items and services would typically be covered for Medicare beneficiaries, but for the fact that they are provided in an experimental or clinical trial setting. Hospitals that participate in clinical trials should review the requirements for submitting claims for patients participating in clinical trials.[31]

- *Improper claims for organ acquisition costs*–Hospitals that are approved transplantation centers may receive reimbursement on a reasonable cost basis to cover the costs of acquisition of certain organs.[32] Organ acquisition costs are only reimbursable if a hospital satisfies several requirements, such as having adequate cost information, supporting documentation, and supporting medical records.[33] Hospitals must also ensure that expenses not related to organ acquisition, such as transplant and posttransplant activities and costs from other cost centers, are not included in the hospital's organ acquisition costs.[34]

- *Improper claims for cardiac rehabilitation services*—Medicare covers reasonable and necessary cardiac rehabilitation services under the hospital "incident-to" benefit, which requires that the services of nonphysician personnel be furnished under a physician's direct supervision. In addition to satisfying the supervision requirement, hospitals must ensure that cardiac rehabilitation services are reasonable and necessary.[35]

- *Failure to follow Medicare rules regarding payment for costs related to educational activities*[36]—Hospitals should pay particular attention to these rules when implementing dental or other education programs, particularly those not historically operated at the hospital.

4. Use of Information Technology

The implementation of the OPPS increased the need for hospitals to pay particular attention to their computerized billing, coding, and information systems. Billing and coding under the OPPS is more data intensive than billing and coding under the inpatient PPS. When the OPPS began, many hospitals' existing systems were unable to accommodate the new requirements and required adjustments.

As the health care industry moves forward, hospitals will increasingly rely on information technology. For example, HIPAA Privacy and Security Rules (discussed below in section II.G), electronic claims submission[37], electronic prescribing, networked information sharing among providers, and systems for the tracking and reduction of medical errors, among others, will require hospitals to depend more on information technologies. Information technology presents new opportunities to advance health care efficiency, but also new challenges to ensuring the accuracy of claims and the information used to generate claims. It is often difficult for purchasers of computer systems and software to know exactly how the system operates and generates information.

Prudent hospitals will take steps to ensure that they thoroughly assess all new computer systems and software that impact coding, billing, or the generation or transmission of information related to the Federal health care programs or their beneficiaries.

B. The Referral Statutes: The Physician Self-Referral Law (the "Stark" Law) and the Federal Anti-Kickback Statute

1. The Physician Self-Referral Law

From a hospital compliance perspective, the physician self-referral law (section 1877 of the Social Security Act (Act), commonly known as the "Stark" law) should be viewed as a threshold statute. Simply put, hospitals face significant financial exposure unless their financial relationships with referring physicians fit squarely in statutory or regulatory exceptions to the statute. The statute prohibits hospitals from submitting—and Medicare from paying—any claim for a "designated health service" (DHS) if the referral of the DHS comes from a physician with whom the hospital has a prohibited financial relationship.[38] This is true even if the prohibited financial relationship is the result of inadvertence or error. In addition, hospitals and physicians that knowingly violate the statute may be subject to civil monetary penalties and exclusion from the Federal health care programs. Under certain circumstances, a knowing violation of the Stark law may also give rise to liability under the False Claims Act. Because all inpatient and outpatient hospital services (including services furnished directly by a hospital or by others "under arrangements" with a hospital) are DHS under the statute[39], hospitals must diligently review all financial relationships with referring physicians for compliance with the Stark law.

For purposes of analyzing a financial relationship under the Stark law, the following three-part inquiry is useful:

- Is there a *referral* from a *physician* for a *designated health service?* If not, then there is no Stark law issue (although other fraud and abuse authorities, such as the anti-kickback statute, may be implicated). If the answer is "yes," the next inquiry is:

- Does the physician (or an immediate family member) have a *financial relationship* with the entity furnishing the DHS (*e.g.,* the hospital)? Again, if the answer is no, the Stark law is not implicated. However, if the answer is "yes," the third inquiry is:

- Does the financial relationship fit in an *exception?* If not, the statute has been violated.

Detailed definitions of the highlighted terms (and others) are set forth in regulations at 42 CFR 411.351 through 411.361 (substantial additional explanatory material appears in the regulatory preambles to the final regulations: 66 FR 856 (January 4, 2001); 69 FR 16054 (March 26, 2004); and 69 FR 17933 (April 6, 2004)). Importantly, a financial relationship can be almost any kind of direct or indirect ownership or investment relationship (*e.g.,* stock ownership, a partnership interest, or secured debt) or direct or indirect compensation arrangement, whether in cash or in-kind (*e.g.,* a rental contract, personal services contract, salary, gift, or gratuity), between a referring physician (or immediate family member) and a hospital. Moreover, the financial relationship need not relate to the provision of DHS (*e.g.,* a joint venture between a hospital and a physician to operate a hospice would create an indirect compensation relationship between the hospital and the physician for Stark law purposes).

The statutory and regulatory exceptions are the key to compliance with the Stark law. Any financial relationship between the hospital and a physician who refers to the hospital must fit in an exception. Exceptions exist in the statute and regulations for many common types of business arrangements. To fit in an exception, an arrangement must squarely meet all of the conditions set forth in the exception. Importantly, it is the actual relationship between the parties, and not merely the paperwork, that must fit in an exception. Unlike the anti-kickback safe harbors, which are voluntary, fitting in an exception is mandatory under the Stark law.

Compliance with a Stark law exception does not immunize an arrangement under the anti-kickback statute. Rather, the Stark law sets a minimum standard for arrangements between physicians and hospitals. Even if a hospital-physician relationship qualifies for a Stark law exception, it should still be reviewed for compliance with the anti-kickback statute. The anti-kickback statute is discussed in greater detail in the next subsection.

Because of the significant exposure for hospitals under the Stark law, we recommend that hospitals implement systems to ensure that all conditions in the exceptions upon which they rely are fully satisfied. For example, many of the exceptions, such as the rental and personal services exceptions, require signed, written agreements with physicians. We are aware of numerous instances in which hospitals failed to maintain these signed written agreements, often inadvertently (*e.g.,* a holdover lease without a written lease amendment; a physician hired as an independent contractor for a short-term project without a signed agreement). To avoid a large overpayment, hospitals should ensure frequent and thorough review of their contracting and leasing processes. The final regulations contain a new limited exception for certain inadvertent, temporary instances of noncompliance with another exception. This exception may only be used on an occasional basis. Hospitals should be mindful that this exception is not a substitute for vigilant contracting and leasing oversight. In addition, hospitals should review the new reporting requirements at 42 CFR 411.361, which generally require hospitals to retain records that the hospitals know or should know about in the course of prudently conducting business. Hospitals should ensure that they have policies and procedures in place to address these requirements.

In addition, because many exceptions to the Stark law require fair market value compensation for items or services actually needed and rendered, hospitals should have appropriate processes for making and documenting reasonable, consistent, and objective determinations of fair market value and for ensuring that needed items and services are furnished or rendered. Other areas that may require careful monitoring include, without limitation, tracking the total value of non-monetary compensation provided annually to each referring physician, tracking the provision and value of medical staff incidental benefits, and monitoring the provision of professional courtesy.[40] As discussed further in the anti-kickback section below, hospitals should exercise care when recruiting physicians. Importantly, while the final regulations contain a limited exception for certain joint recruiting by hospitals and existing group practices, the exception strictly forbids the use of income guarantees that shift group practice overhead or expenses to the hospital or any payment structure that otherwise transfers remuneration to the group practice.

Further information about the Stark law and applicable regulations can be found on CMS's webpage at *http://cms.gov/medlearn/refphys.asp.* Information regarding CMS's Stark advisory opinion process can be found at *http://cms.gov/physicians/aop/default.asp.*

2. The Federal Anti-Kickback Statute

Hospitals should also be aware of the Federal anti-kickback statute, section 1128B(b) of the Act, and the constraints it places on business arrangements related directly or indirectly to items or services reimbursable by any Federal health care program, including, but not limited to, Medicare and Medicaid. The anti-kickback statute prohibits in the health care industry some practices that are common in other business sectors, such as offering gifts to reward past or potential new referrals.

The anti-kickback statute is a criminal prohibition against payments (in any form, whether the payments are direct or indirect) made purposefully to induce or reward the referral or generation of Federal health care program business. The anti-kickback statute addresses not only the offer or payment of anything of value for patient referrals, but also the offer or payment of anything of value in return for purchasing, leasing, ordering, or arranging for or recommending the purchase, lease, or ordering of any item or service reimbursable in whole or in part by a Federal health care program. The statute extends equally to the solicitation or acceptance of remuneration for referrals or the generation of other business payable by a Federal health care program. Liability under the anti-kickback statute is determined separately for each party involved. In addition to criminal penalties, violators may be subject to civil monetary penalties and exclusion from the Federal health care programs. Hospitals should also be mindful that compliance with the anti-kickback statute is a condition of payment under Medicare and other Federal health care programs. See, *e.g.,* Medicare Federal Health Care Provider/Supplier Application, CMS Form 855A, Certification Statement at section 15, paragraph A.3, available on CMS's webpage at *http://www.cms.gov/providers/enrollment/forms/.* As such, liability may arise under the False Claims Act where the anti-kickback statute violation results in the submission of a claim for payment under a Federal health care program.

Although liability under the anti-kickback statute ultimately turns on a party's intent, it is possible to identify arrangements or practices that may present a significant potential for abuse. For purposes of analyzing an arrangement or practice under the anti-kickback statute, the following two inquiries are useful:

- Does the hospital have any remunerative relationship between itself (or its affiliates or representatives) and persons or entities in a position to generate Federal health care program business for the hospital (or its affiliates) directly or indirectly? Persons or entities in a position to generate Federal health care program business for a hospital include, for example, physicians and other health care professionals, ambulance companies, clinics, hospices, home health agencies, nursing facilities, and other hospitals.

- With respect to any remunerative relationship so identified, could one purpose of the remuneration be to induce or reward the referral or recommendation of business payable in whole or in part by a Federal health care program? Importantly, under the anti-kickback statute, neither a legitimate business purpose for the arrangement, nor a fair market value payment, will legitimize a payment if there is also an illegal purpose (*i.e.,* inducing Federal health care program business).

Although any arrangement satisfying both tests implicates the anti-kickback statute and requires careful scrutiny by a hospital, the courts have identified several potentially aggravating considerations that can be useful in identifying arrangements at greatest risk of prosecution. In particular, hospitals should ask the following questions, among others, about any potentially problematic arrangements or practices they identify:

- Does the arrangement or practice have a potential to interfere with, or skew, clinical decision-making?

- Does the arrangement or practice have a potential to increase costs to Federal health care programs, beneficiaries, or enrollees?

- Does the arrangement or practice have a potential to increase the risk of overutilization or inappropriate utilization?

- Does the arrangement or practice raise patient safety or quality of care concerns?

Hospitals that have identified potentially problematic arrangements or practices can take a number of steps to reduce or eliminate the risk of an anti-kickback violation. Detailed guidance relating to a number of specific practices is available from several sources. Most importantly, the anti-kickback statute and the corresponding regulations establish a number of "safe harbors" for common business arrangements. The following safe harbors are of most relevance to hospitals:

- Investment interests safe harbor, 42 CFR 1001.952(a);

- Space rental safe harbor, 42 CFR 1001.952(b);

- Equipment rental safe harbor, 42 CFR 1001.952(c);

- Personal services and management contracts safe harbor, 42 CFR 1001.952(d);

- Sale of practice safe harbor, 42 CFR 1001.952(e);

- Referral services safe harbor, 42 CFR 1001.952(f);

- Discount safe harbor, 42 CFR 1001.952(h);

- Employment safe harbor, 42 CFR 1001.952(i);

- Group purchasing organizations safe harbor, 42 CFR 1001.952(j);

- Waiver of beneficiary coinsurance and deductible amounts safe harbor, 42 CFR 1001.952(k);

- Practitioner recruitment safe harbor, 42 CFR 1001.952(n);

- Obstetrical malpractice insurance subsidies safe harbor, 42 CFR 1001.952(o);

- Cooperative hospital services organizations safe harbor, 42 CFR 1001.952(q);

- Ambulatory surgical centers safe harbor, 42 CFR 1001.952(r);

- Ambulance replenishing safe harbor, 42 CFR 1001.952(v); and

- Safe harbors for certain managed care and risk sharing arrangements, 42 CFR 1001.952(m), (t), and (u).[41]

Safe harbor protection requires strict compliance with all applicable conditions set out in the relevant safe harbor.[42] Although compliance with a safe harbor is voluntary and failure to comply with a safe harbor does not mean an arrangement is illegal per se, we recommend that hospitals structure arrangements to fit in a safe harbor whenever possible. Arrangements that do not fit in a safe harbor must be evaluated on a case-by-case basis.

Other available guidance includes special fraud alerts and advisory bulletins issued by the OIG identifying and discussing particular practices or issues of concern and OIG advisory opinions issued to specific parties about their particular business arrangements.[43] A hospital concerned about an existing or proposed arrangement may request a binding OIG advisory opinion regarding whether the arrangement violates the Federal anti-kickback statute or other OIG fraud and abuse authorities, using the procedures set out at 42 CFR part 1008. The safe harbor regulations (and accompanying **Federal Register** preambles), fraud alerts and bulletins, advisory opinions (and instructions for obtaining them, including a list of frequently asked questions), and other guidance are available on the OIG webpage at *http:/oig.hhs.gov.*

The following discussion highlights several known areas of potential risk under the anti-kickback statute. The propriety of any particular arrangement can only be determined after a detailed examination of the attendant facts and circumstances. The identification of a given practice or activity as "suspect" or as an area of "risk" does not mean it is necessarily illegal or unlawful, or that it cannot be properly structured to fit in a safe harbor; nor does it mean that the practice or activity is not beneficial from a clinical, cost, or other perspective. Rather, the areas identified below are areas of activity that have a potential for abuse and that should receive close scrutiny from hospitals. The discussion highlights potential risks under the anti-kickback statute arising from hospitals' relationships in the following five categories: (a) joint ventures; (b) compensation arrangements with physicians; (c) relationships with other health care entities; (d) recruitment arrangements; (e) discounts; (f) medical staff credentialing; and (g) malpractice insurance subsidies. (In addition, the kickback risks associated with gainsharing arrangements are discussed below in section II.C of this guidance).

Physicians are the primary referral source for hospitals, and, therefore, most of the discussion below focuses on hospitals' relationships with physicians. Notwithstanding, hospitals also receive referrals from other health care professionals, including physician assistants and nurse practitioners, and from other providers and suppliers (such as ambulance companies, clinics, hospices, home health agencies, nursing facilities, and other hospitals). Therefore, in addition to reviewing their relationships with physicians, hospitals should also review their relationships with non-physician referral sources to ensure that the relationships do not violate the anti-kickback statute. The principles described in the following discussions can be used to assess the risk associated with relationships with both physician and non-physician referral sources.

a. Joint Ventures: The OIG has a long-standing concern about joint venture arrangements between those in a position to refer or generate Federal health care program business and those providing items or services reimbursable by Federal health care programs.[44] In the context of joint ventures, our chief concern is that remuneration from a joint venture might be a disguised payment for past or future referrals to the venture or to one or more of its participants. Such remuneration may take a variety of forms, including dividends, profit distributions, or, with respect to contractual joint ventures, the economic benefit received under the terms of the operative contracts.

When scrutinizing joint ventures under the anti-kickback statute, hospitals should examine the following factors, among others:

- *The manner in which joint venture participants are selected and retained.* If participants are selected or retained in a manner that takes into account, directly or indirectly, the value or volume of referrals, the joint venture is suspect. The existence of one or more of the following indicators suggests that there might be an improper nexus between the selection or retention of participants and the value or volume of their referrals:

  —a substantial number of participants are in a position to make or influence referrals to the venture, other participants, or both;

  —participants that are expected to make a large number of referrals are offered a greater or more favorable investment or business opportunity in the joint venture than those anticipated to make fewer referrals;

  —participants are actively encouraged or required to make referrals to the joint venture;

  —participants are encouraged or required to divest their ownership interest if they fail to sustain an "acceptable" level of referrals;

  —the venture (or its participants) tracks its sources of referrals and distributes this information to the participants; or

  —the investment interests are nontransferable or subject to transfer restrictions related to referrals.

- *The manner in which the joint venture is structured.* The structure of the joint venture is suspect if a participant is already engaged in the line of business to be conducted by the joint venture, and that participant will own all or most of the equipment, provide or perform all or most of the items or services, or take responsibility for all or most of the day-to-day operations. With this kind of structure, the co-participant's primary contribution is typically as a captive referral base.

- *The manner in which the investments are financed and profits are distributed.* The existence of one or more of the following indicators suggests that the joint venture may be a vehicle to disguise referrals:

  —participants are offered investment shares for a nominal or no capital contribution;

  —the amount of capital that participants invest is disproportionately small, and the returns on the investment are disproportionately large, when compared to a typical investment in a new business enterprise;

—participants are permitted to borrow their capital investments from another participant or from the joint venture, and to pay back the loan through deductions from profit distributions, thus eliminating even the need to contribute cash;

—participants are paid extraordinary returns on the investment in comparison with the risk involved; or

—a substantial portion of the gross revenues of the venture are derived from participant-driven referrals.

In light of the obvious risk inherent in joint ventures, whenever possible, hospitals should structure joint ventures to fit squarely in one of the following safe harbors for investment interests:

- The "small entity" investment safe harbor, 42 CFR 1001.952(a)(2), which applies to returns on investments as long as no more than 40 percent of the investment interests are held by investors who are in a position to make or influence referrals to, furnish items or services to, or otherwise generate business for the venture (interested investors), no more than 40 percent of revenues come from referrals or business otherwise generated from investors, and all other conditions are satisfied;[45]

- The safe harbor for investment interests in an entity located in an underserved area, 42 CFR 1001.952(a)(3), which applies to ventures located in medically underserved areas (as defined in regulations issued by the Department and set forth at 42 CFR part 51c), as long as no more than 50 percent of the investment interests are held by interested investors and all other conditions are satisfied; or

- The hospital-physician ambulatory surgical center (ASC) safe harbor, 42 CFR 1001.952(r)(4). This safe harbor only protects investments in Medicare-certified ASCs owned by hospitals and certain qualifying physicians. Importantly, it does not protect investments by hospitals and physicians in non-ASC clinical joint ventures, including, for example, cardiac catheterization or vascular labs, oncology centers, and dialysis facilities. Investors in such clinical ventures should look to other safe harbors and to the factors noted above.

These safe harbors protect remuneration in the form of returns on investment interests (*i.e.,* money paid by an entity to its owners or investors as dividends, profit distributions, or the like). However, they do not protect payments made by participating investors to a venture or payments made by the venture to other parties, such as vendors, contractors, or employees (although in some cases these arrangements may fit in other safe harbors).

As we originally observed in our 1989 Special Fraud Alert on Joint Venture Arrangements,[46] joint ventures may take a variety of forms, including a contractual arrangement between two or more parties to cooperate in a common and distinct enterprise providing items or services, thereby creating a "contractual joint venture." We elaborated more fully on contractual joint ventures in our 2003 Special Advisory Bulletin on Contractual Joint Ventures.[47] Contractual joint ventures pose the same kinds of risks as equity joint ventures and should be analyzed similarly. Factors to consider include, for example, whether the hospital is expanding into a new line of business created predominately or exclusively to serve the hospital's existing patient base, whether a would-be competitor of the new line of business is providing all or most of the key services, and whether the hospital assumes little or no bona fide business risk. An example of a potentially problematic contractual joint venture would be a hospital contracting with an existing durable medical equipment (DME) supplier to operate the hospital's newly formed DME subsidiary (with its own DME supplier number) on essentially a turnkey basis, with the hospital primarily furnishing referrals and assuming little or no business risk.[48]

Hospitals should be aware that, for reasons described in our 2003 Special Advisory Bulletin on Contractual Joint Ventures,[49] safe harbor protection may not be available for contractual joint ventures, and attempts to carve out separate contracts and qualify each separately for safe harbor protection may be ineffectual and leave the parties at risk under the statute.[50]

If a hospital is planning to participate, directly or indirectly, in a joint venture involving referring physicians and the venture does not qualify for safe harbor protection, the hospital should scrutinize the venture with care, taking into account the factors noted above, and consider obtaining advice from an experienced attorney. At a minimum, to reduce (but not necessarily eliminate) the risk of abuse, hospitals should consider (i) barring physicians employed by the hospital or its affiliates from referring to the joint venture; (ii) taking steps to ensure that medical staff and other affiliated physicians are not encouraged in any manner to refer to the joint venture; (iii) notifying physicians annually in writing of the preceding policy; (iv) refraining from tracking in any manner the volume of referrals attributable to particular referrals sources; (v) ensuring that no physician compensation is tied in any manner to the volume or value of referrals to, or other business generated for, the venture; (vi) disclosing all financial interests to patients;[51] and (vii) requiring that other participants in the joint venture adopt similar steps.

b. Compensation Arrangements With Physicians: Hospitals enter into a variety of compensation arrangements with physicians whereby physicians provide items or services to, or on behalf of, the hospital. Conversely, in some arrangements, hospitals provide items or services to physicians. Examples of these compensation arrangements include, without limitation, medical director agreements; personal or management services agreements; space or equipment leases; and agreements for the provision of billing, nursing, or other staff services. Although many compensation arrangements are legitimate business arrangements, compensation arrangements may violate the anti-kickback statute if one purpose of the arrangement is to compensate physicians for past or future referrals.[52]

The general rule of thumb is that any remuneration flowing between hospitals and physicians should be at fair market value for actual and necessary items furnished or services rendered based upon an arm's-length transaction and should not take into account, directly or indirectly, the value or volume of any past or future referrals or other business generated between the parties. Arrangements under which hospitals provide physicians with items or services for free or less than fair market value, relieve physicians of financial obligations they would otherwise incur, or inflate compensation paid to physicians for items or services pose significant risk. In such circumstances, an inference arises that the remuneration may be in exchange for generating business.

In particular, hospitals should review their physician compensation arrangements and carefully assess the risk of fraud and abuse using the following factors, among others:

- Are the items and services obtained from a physician legitimate, commercially reasonable, and necessary to achieve a legitimate business purpose of the hospital (apart from obtaining referrals)? Assuming that the hospital needs the items and services, does the hospital have multiple arrangements with different physicians, so that in the aggregate the items or services provided by all physicians exceed the hospital's actual needs (apart from generating business)?

- Does the compensation represent fair market value in an arm's-length transaction for the items and services? Could the hospital obtain the services from a non-referral source at a cheaper rate or under more favorable terms? Does the remuneration take into account, directly or indirectly, the value or volume of any past or future referrals or other business generated between the parties? Is the compensation tied, directly or indirectly, to Federal health care program reimbursement?

- Is the determination of fair market value based upon a reasonable methodology that is uniformly applied and properly documented? If fair market value is based on comparables, the hospital should ensure that the comparison entities are *not* actual or potential referral sources, so that the market rate for the services is not distorted.

- Is the compensation commensurate with the fair market value of a physician with the skill level and experience reasonably necessary to perform the contracted services?

- Were the physicians selected to participate in the arrangement in whole or in part because of their past or anticipated referrals?

- Is the arrangement properly and fully documented in writing? Are the physicians documenting the services they provide? Is the hospital monitoring the services?

- In the case of physicians staffing hospital outpatient departments, are safeguards in place to ensure that the physicians do not use hospital outpatient space, equipment, or personnel to conduct their private practice and that they bill the appropriate site-of-service modifier?

Whenever possible, hospitals should structure their compensation arrangements with physicians to fit in a safe harbor. Potentially applicable are the space rental safe harbor, 42 CFR 1001.952(b), the equipment rental safe harbor, 42 CFR 1001.952(c), the personal services and management contracts safe harbor, 42 CFR 1001.952(d), the sale of practice safe harbor, 42 CFR 1001.952(e), the referral services safe harbor, 42 CFR 1001.952(f), the employee safe harbor, 42 CFR 1001.952(i), the practitioner recruitment safe harbor, 42 CFR 1001.952(n), and the obstetrical malpractice insurance subsidies safe harbor, 42 CFR 1001.952(o). An arrangement must fit squarely in a safe harbor to be protected. Arrangements that do not fit in a safe harbor should be reviewed in light of the totality of all facts and circumstances. At minimum, hospitals should develop policies and procedures requiring physicians to document, and the hospital to monitor, the services or items provided under compensation arrangements (including, for example, by using written time reports). In some cases, particularly rentals, hospitals should consider obtaining an independent fair market valuation using appropriate health care valuation standards.

Arrangements between hospitals and hospital-based physicians (*e.g.,* anesthesiologists, radiologists, and pathologists) raise some different concerns. In these arrangements, it is typically the hospitals making referrals to the physicians, rather than the physicians making referrals to the hospitals. Such arrangements may violate the anti-kickback statute if the arrangements: (i) Compensate physicians for less than the fair market value of goods or services provided by the physicians to the hospitals; or (ii) require physicians to pay more than the fair market value for services provided by the hospitals.[53] We are aware that hospitals have long provided for the delivery of certain hospital-based physician services through the grant of a contract to a physician or physician group akin to a franchise, which shifts management, staffing, and other administrative functions, and in some cases limited clinical duties, to physicians at no cost to the hospitals. Such arrangements are of value to the hospital as well as the physicians, value that may well have nothing to do with the value or volume of referrals flowing from the hospital to the hospital-based physicians. In an appropriate context, an arrangement that requires a hospital-based physician or physician group to perform reasonable administrative or clinical duties directly related to their hospital-based professional services at no charge to the hospital or its patients would not violate the anti-kickback statute. Whether a particular arrangement with hospital-based physicians runs afoul of the anti-kickback statute would depend on the specific facts and circumstances, including the intent of the parties.

c. Relationships With Other Health Care Entities: As addressed in the preceding subsection, hospitals may obtain referrals of Federal health care program business from a variety of health care professionals and entities. In addition, when furnishing inpatient, outpatient, and related services, hospitals often direct or influence referrals for items and services reimbursable by Federal health care programs. For example, hospitals may refer patients to, or order items or services from, home health agencies,[54] skilled nursing facilities, durable medical equipment companies, laboratories, pharmaceutical companies, and other hospitals. In cases where a hospital is the referral source for other providers or suppliers, it would be prudent for the hospital to scrutinize carefully any remuneration flowing to the hospital from the provider or supplier to ensure compliance with the anti-kickback statute, using the principles outlined above. Remuneration may include, for example, free or below-market-value items and services or the relief of a financial obligation.

Hospitals should also review their managed care arrangements to ensure compliance with the anti-kickback statute. Managed care arrangements that do not fit within one of the managed care and risk sharing safe harbors at 42 CFR 1001.952(m), (t), or (u) must be evaluated on a case-by-case basis.

d. Recruitment Arrangements: Many hospitals provide incentives to recruit a physician or other health care professional to join the hospital's medical staff and provide medical services to the surrounding community. When used to bring needed physicians to an underserved community, these arrangements can benefit patients. However, recruitment arrangements pose substantial fraud and abuse risk.

In most cases, the recruited physician establishes a private practice in the community instead of becoming a hospital employee.[55] Such arrangements potentially implicate the anti-kickback statute if one purpose of the recruitment arrangement is to induce referrals to the recruiting hospital. Safe harbor protection is available for certain recruitment arrangements offered by hospitals to attract primary care physicians and practitioners to health professional shortage areas (HPSAs), as defined in regulations issued by the Department.[56] The scope of this safe harbor is very limited. In particular, the safe harbor does not protect (a) recruitment arrangements in areas that are not designated as HPSAs, (b) recruitment of specialists, or (c) joint recruitment with existing physician practices in the area.

Because of the significant risk of fraud and abuse posed by improper recruitment arrangements, hospitals should scrutinize these arrangements with care. When assessing the degree of risk associated with recruitment arrangements, hospitals should examine the following factors, among others:

- *The size and value of the recruitment benefit.* Does the benefit exceed what is reasonably necessary to attract a qualified physician to the particular community? Has the hospital previously tried and failed to recruit or retain physicians?

- *The duration of payout of the recruitment benefit.* Total benefit payout periods extending longer than three years from the initial recruitment agreement should trigger heightened scrutiny.

- *The practice of the existing physician.* Is the physician a new physician with few or no patients or an established practitioner with a ready stream of referrals? Is the physician relocating from a substantial distance so that referrals are unlikely to follow or is it possible for the physician to bring an established patient base?

- *The need for the recruitment.* Is the recruited physician's specialty necessary to provide adequate access to medically necessary care for patients in the community? Do patients already have reasonable access to comparable services from other providers or practitioners in or near the community? An assessment of community need based wholly or partially on the competitive interests of the recruiting hospital or existing physician practices would subject the recruitment payments to heightened scrutiny under the statute.

Significantly, hospitals should be aware that the practitioner recruitment safe harbor does not protect "joint recruitment" arrangements between hospitals and other entities or individuals, such as solo practitioners, group practices, or managed care organizations, pursuant to which the hospital makes payments directly or indirectly to the other entity or individual. These joint recruitment arrangements present a high risk of fraud and abuse and have been the subject of recent government investigations and prosecutions. These arrangements can easily be used as vehicles to disguise payments from the hospital to an existing referral source—typically an existing physician practice—in exchange for the existing practice's referrals to the hospital. Suspect payments to existing referral sources may include, among other things, income guarantees that shift costs from the existing referral source to the recruited physician and overhead and build-out costs funded for the benefit of the existing referral source. Hospitals should review all "joint recruiting" arrangements to ensure that remuneration does not inure in whole or in part to the benefit of any party other than the recruited physician.

e. Discounts: Public policy favors open and legitimate price competition in health care. Thus, the anti-kickback statute contains an exception for discounts offered to customers that submit claims to the Federal health care programs, if the discounts are properly disclosed and accurately reported.[57] However, to qualify for the exception, the discount must be in the form of a reduction in the price of the good or service based on an arm's-length transaction. In other words, the exception covers only reductions in the product's price. Moreover, the regulation provides that the discount must be given at the time of sale or, in certain cases, set at the time of sale, even if finally determined subsequent to the time of sale (*i.e.,* a rebate).

In conducting business, hospitals sell and purchase items and services reimbursable by Federal health care programs. Therefore, hospitals should thoroughly familiarize themselves with the discount safe harbor at 42 CFR 1001.952(h). In particular, depending on their role in the arrangement, hospitals should pay attention to the discount safe harbor requirements applicable to "buyers," "sellers," or "offerors." Compliance with the safe harbor is determined separately for each party. In general, hospitals should ensure that all discounts—including rebates—are properly disclosed and accurately reflected on hospital cost reports. If a hospital offers a discount on an item or service to a buyer, it should ensure that the discount is properly disclosed on the invoice or other documentation for the item or service.

The discount safe harbor does not protect a discount offered to one payor but not to the Federal health care programs. Accordingly, in negotiating discounts for items and services paid from a hospital's pocket (such as those reimbursed under the Medicare Part A prospective payment system), the hospital should ensure that there is no link or connection, explicit or implicit, between discounts offered or solicited for that business and the hospital's referral of business billable by the seller directly to Medicare or another Federal health care program. For example, a hospital should not engage in "swapping" by accepting from a supplier an unreasonably low price on Part A services that the hospital pays for out of its own pocket in exchange for hospital referrals that are billable by the supplier directly to Part B (*e.g.,* ambulance services). Suspect arrangements include below-cost arrangements or arrangements at prices lower than the prices offered by the supplier to other customers with similar volumes of business, but without Federal health care program referrals.

Hospitals may also receive discounts on items and services purchased through group purchasing organizations (GPOs). Discounts received from a vendor in connection with a GPO to which a hospital belongs should be properly disclosed and accurately reported on the hospital cost reports. Although there is a safe harbor for payments made by a vendor to a GPO as part of an agreement to furnish items or services to a group of individuals or entities, 42 CFR 1001.952(k), the safe harbor does not protect the discount received by the individual or entity.[58]

f. Medical Staff Credentialing: Certain medical staff credentialing practices may implicate the anti-kickback statute. For example, conditioning privileges on a particular number of referrals or requiring the performance of a particular number of procedures, beyond volumes necessary to ensure clinical proficiency, potentially raise substantial risks under the statute. On the other hand, a credentialing policy that categorically refuses privileges to physicians with significant conflicts of interest would not appear to implicate the statute in most situations. Hospitals are advised to examine their credentialing practices to ensure that they do not run afoul of the anti-kickback statute. The OIG has solicited comments about, and is considering, whether further guidance in this area is appropriate.[59]

g. Malpractice Insurance Subsidies: The OIG historically has been concerned that a hospital's subsidy of malpractice insurance premiums for potential referral sources, including hospital medical staff, may be suspect under the anti-kickback statute, because the payments may be used to influence referrals. The OIG has established a safe harbor for medical malpractice premium subsidies provided to obstetrical care practitioners in primary health care shortage areas.[60] Depending on the circumstances, premium support may also be structured to fit in other safe harbors.

We are aware of the current disruption (*i.e.,* dramatic premium increases, insurers' withdrawals from certain markets, and/or sudden termination of coverage based upon factors other than the physicians' claims history) in the medical malpractice liability insurance markets in some States.[61] Notwithstanding, hospitals should review malpractice insurance subsidy arrangements closely to ensure that there is no improper inducement to referral sources. Relevant factors include, without limitation:

- Whether the subsidy is being provided on an interim basis for a fixed period in a State or States experiencing severe access or affordability problems;

- Whether the subsidy is being offered only to current active medical staff (or physicians new to the locality or in practice less than a year, *i.e.,* physicians with no or few established patients);

- Whether the criteria for receiving a subsidy is unrelated to the volume or value of referrals or other business generated by the subsidized physician or his practice;

- Whether physicians receiving subsidies are paying at least as much as they currently pay for malpractice insurance (*i.e.,* are windfalls to physicians avoided);

- Whether physicians are required to perform services or relinquish rights, which have a value equal to the fair market value of the insurance assistance; and

- Whether the insurance is available regardless of the location at which the physician provides services, including, but not limited to, other hospitals.

No one of these factors is determinative, and this list is illustrative, not exhaustive, of potential considerations in connection with the provision of malpractice insurance subsidies. Parties contemplating malpractice subsidy programs that do not fit into one of the safe harbors may want to consider obtaining an advisory opinion. Parties should also be mindful that these subsidy arrangements also implicate the Stark law.

C. Payments To Reduce or Limit Services: Gainsharing Arrangements

The civil monetary penalty set forth in section 1128A(b)(1) of the Act prohibits a hospital from knowingly making a payment directly or indirectly to a physician as an inducement to reduce or limit items or services furnished to Medicare or Medicaid beneficiaries under the physician's direct care.[62] Hospitals that make (and physicians that receive) such payments are liable for civil monetary penalties (CMPs) of up to $2,000 per patient covered by the payments.[63] The statutory proscription is very broad. The payment need not be tied to an actual diminution in care, so long as the hospital knows that the payment may influence the physician to reduce or limit services to his or her patients. There is no requirement that the prohibited payment be tied to a specific patient or to a reduction in medically necessary care. In short, any hospital incentive plan that encourages physicians through payments to reduce or limit clinical services directly or indirectly violates the statute.

We are aware that a number of hospitals are engaged in, or considering entering into, incentive arrangements commonly called "gainsharing." While there is no fixed definition of a "gainsharing" arrangement, the term typically refers to an arrangement in which a hospital gives physicians a percentage share of any reduction in the hospital's costs for patient care attributable in part to the physicians' efforts. We recognize that, properly structured, gainsharing arrangements can serve legitimate business and medical purposes, such as increasing efficiency, reducing waste, and, thereby, potentially increasing a hospital's profitability. However, the plain language of section 1128A(b)(1) of the Act prohibits tying the physicians' compensation for services to reductions or limitations in items or services provided to patients under the physicians' clinical care.[64]

In addition to the CMP risks described above, gainsharing arrangements can also implicate the anti-kickback statute if the cost-savings payments are used to influence referrals. For example, the statute is potentially implicated if a gainsharing arrangement is intended to influence physicians to "cherry pick" healthy patients for the hospital offering gainsharing payments and steer sicker (and more costly) patients to hospitals that do not offer gainsharing payments. Similarly, the statute may be implicated if a hospital offers a cost-sharing program with the intent to foster physician loyalty and attract more referrals. In addition, we have serious concerns about overly broad arrangements under which a physician continues for an extended time to reap the benefits of previously-achieved savings or receives cost-savings payments unrelated to anything done by the physician, whether work, services, or other undertaking (*e.g.*, a change in the way the physician practices).

Wherever possible, hospitals should consider structuring cost-saving arrangements to fit in the personal services safe harbor. However, in many cases, protection under the personal services safe harbor is not available because gainsharing arrangements typically involve a percentage payment (*i.e.*, the aggregate fee will not be set in advance, as required by the safe harbor). Finally, gainsharing arrangements may also implicate the Stark law.

D. Emergency Medical Treatment and Labor Act (EMTALA)

Hospitals should review their obligations under EMTALA (section 1867 of the Act) to evaluate and treat individuals who come to their emergency departments and other facilities. Hospitals should pay particular attention to when an individual must receive a medical screening exam to determine whether that individual is suffering from an emergency medical condition. When such a screening or treatment of an emergency medical condition is required, it cannot be delayed to inquire about an individual's method of payment or insurance status. If the hospital's emergency department (ED) is "on diversion" and an individual comes to the ED for evaluation or treatment of a medical condition, the hospital is required to provide such services despite its diversionary status.

Hospital emergency departments may not transfer an individual with an unstable emergency medical condition unless the benefits of such a transfer outweigh the risks. In such circumstances, the hospital must arrange for a transfer that will minimize the risks to the individual and that has been prearranged with the facility to which the individual is being transferred. Moreover, when a hospital receives a call from another facility requesting that it accept an appropriate transfer of a patient with an emergency, it must accept that patient for transfer if it has specialized capabilities to treat the patient that the transferring hospital does not have and it has the capacity to treat the patient.

A hospital must provide appropriate screening and treatment services within the full capabilities of its staff and facilities. This includes access to specialists who are on call. Thus, hospital policies and procedures should be clear on how to access the full services of the hospital and all staff should understand the hospital's obligations to patients under EMTALA. In particular, on-call physicians need to be educated as to their responsibilities to emergency patients, including the responsibility to accept appropriately transferred patients from other facilities. In addition, all persons working in emergency departments should be periodically trained and reminded of the hospital's EMTALA obligations and hospital policies and procedures designed to ensure that such obligations are met.

For further information about EMTALA, hospitals are directed to: (i) The anti-dumping statute at section 1867 of the Act; (ii) the anti-dumping statute's implementing regulations at 42 CFR part 489; (iii) our 1999 Special Advisory Bulletin on the Patient Anti-Dumping Statute, 64 FR 61353 (November 10, 1999), available on our webpage at *http://oig.hhs.gov/*

fraud/docs/alertsandbulletins/frdump.pdf; and (iv) CMS's EMTALA resource webpage located at *http://www.cms.gov/providers/emtala/emtala.asp.*

E. Substandard Care

The OIG has authority to exclude any individual or entity from participation in Federal health care programs if the individual or entity provides unnecessary items or services (*i.e.,* items or services in excess of the needs of a patient) or substandard items or services (*i.e.,* items or services of a quality which fails to meet professionally recognized standards of health care).[65] Significantly, neither knowledge nor intent is required for exclusion under this provision. The exclusion can be based upon unnecessary or substandard items or services provided to any patient, even if that patient is not a Medicare or Medicaid beneficiary.

We are mindful that the vast majority of hospitals are fully committed to providing quality care to their patients. To achieve their quality-related goals, hospitals should continually measure their performance against comprehensive standards. For example, hospitals should meet all of the Medicare hospital conditions of participation (COP), including without limitation, the COP pertaining to a quality assessment and performance program at 42 CFR 482.21 and the hospital COP pertaining to the medical staff at 42 CFR 482.22. Hospitals that have elected to be reviewed by the Joint Commission on Accreditation of Healthcare Organizations (JCAHO) should maintain their JCAHO accreditation.[66] In addition, hospitals should develop their own quality of care protocols and implement mechanisms for evaluating compliance with those protocols.

Finally, in reviewing the quality of care provided, hospitals must not limit their review to the quality of their nursing and other ancillary services. Instead, hospitals must also take an active part in monitoring the quality of medical services provided at the hospital by appropriately overseeing the credentialing and peer review of their medical staffs.

F. Relationships With Federal Health Care Beneficiaries

Hospitals' relationships with Federal health care beneficiaries may also implicate the fraud and abuse laws. In particular, hospitals should be aware that section 1128A(a)(5) of the Act authorizes the OIG to impose CMPs on hospitals (and others) that offer or transfer remuneration to a Medicare or Medicaid beneficiary that the offeror knows or should know is likely to influence the beneficiary to order or receive items or services from a particular provider, practitioner, or supplier for which payment may be made under the Medicare or Medicaid programs. The definition of "remuneration" expressly includes the offer or transfer of items or services for free or other than fair market value, including the waiver of all or part of a Medicare or Medicaid cost-sharing amount.[67] In other words, hospitals may not offer valuable items or services to Medicare or Medicaid beneficiaries to attract their business. In this regard, hospitals should familiarize themselves with the OIG's August 2002 Special Advisory Bulletin on Offering Gifts and Other Inducements to Beneficiaries.[68]

1. Gifts and Gratuities

Hospitals should scrutinize any offers of gifts or gratuities to beneficiaries for compliance with the CMP provision prohibiting inducements to Medicare and Medicaid beneficiaries. The key inquiry under the CMP is whether the remuneration is something that the hospital knows or should know is likely to influence the beneficiary's selection of a particular provider, practitioner, or supplier for Medicare or Medicaid payable services. As interpreted by the OIG, section 1128A(a)(5) does not apply to the provision of items or services valued at less than $10 per item and $50 per patient in the aggregate on an annual basis.[69] A special exception for incentives to promote the delivery of preventive care services is discussed below at section II.I.2.

2. Cost-Sharing Waivers

In general, hospitals are obligated to collect cost-sharing amounts owed by Federal health care program beneficiaries. Waiving owed amounts may constitute prohibited remuneration to beneficiaries under section 1128A(a)(5) of the Act or the anti-kickback statute. Certain waivers of Part A inpatient cost-sharing amounts may be protected by structuring them to fit in the safe harbor for waivers of beneficiary inpatient coinsurance and deductible amounts at 42 CFR 1001.952(k). In particular, under the safe harbor, waived amounts may not be claimed as bad debt; the waivers must be offered uniformly across the board, without regard to the reason for admission, length of stay, or DRG; and waivers may not be made as part of any agreement with a third-party payer, unless the third-party payer is a Medicare SELECT plan under section 1882(t)(1) of the Act.[70]

In addition, hospitals (and others) may waive cost-sharing amounts on the basis of a beneficiary's financial need, so long as the waiver is not routine, not advertised, and made pursuant to a good faith, individualized assessment of the beneficiary's financial need or after reasonable collection efforts have failed.[71] The OIG recognizes that what constitutes a good faith determination of "financial need" may vary depending on the individual patient's circumstances and that hospitals should have flexibility to take into account relevant variables. These factors may include, for example:

- The local cost of living;

- A patient's income, assets, and expenses;

- A patient's family size; and

- The scope and extent of a patient's medical bills.

Hospitals should use a reasonable set of financial need guidelines that are based on objective criteria and appropriate for the applicable locality. The guidelines should be applied uniformly in all cases. While hospitals have flexibility in making the determination of financial need, we do not believe it is appropriate to apply inflated income guidelines that result in waivers for beneficiaries who are not in genuine financial need. Hospitals should consider that the financial status of a patient may change over time and should recheck a patient's eligibility at reasonable intervals sufficient to ensure that the patient remains in financial need. For example, a patient who obtains outpatient hospital services several times a week would not need to be rechecked every visit. Hospitals should take reasonable measures to document their determinations of Medicare beneficiaries' financial need. We are aware that in some situations patients may be reluctant or unable to provide documentation of their financial status. In those cases, hospitals may be able to use other reasonable methods for determining financial need, including, for example, documented patient interviews or questionnaires.

In sum, hospitals should review their waiver policies to ensure that the policies and the manner in which they are implemented comply with all applicable laws. For more information about cost-sharing waivers, hospitals should review our February 2, 2004 paper on "Hospital Discounts Offered To Patients Who Cannot Afford To Pay Their Hospital Bills," containing a section titled "Reductions or Waivers of Cost-Sharing Amounts for Medicare Beneficiaries Experiencing Financial Hardship" and available on our webpage at *http://oig.hhs.gov/fraud/ docs/alertsandbulletins/2004/FA021904hospitaldiscounts.pdf.*[72]

3. Free Transportation

The plain language of the CMP prohibits offering free transportation to Medicare or Medicaid beneficiaries to influence their selection of a particular provider, practitioner, or supplier. Notwithstanding, hospitals can offer free local transportation of *low* value (*i.e.,* within the $10 per item and $50 annual limits).[73] Luxury and specialized transportation, such as limousines or ambulances, would exceed the low value threshold and are problematic, as are arrangements tied in any manner to the volume or value of referrals and arrangements tied to particularly lucrative treatments or medical conditions. However, we have indicated that we are considering developing a regulatory exception for some complimentary local transportation provided to beneficiaries residing in a hospital's primary service area.[74] Accordingly, until such time as we promulgate a final rule on complimentary local transportation under section 1128A(a)(5) or indicate our intention not to proceed with such rule, we have indicated that we will not impose administrative sanctions for violations of section 1128A(a)(5) of the Act in connection with hospital-based complimentary transportation programs that meet the following conditions:

- The program was in existence prior to August 30, 2002, the date of publication of the Special Advisory Bulletin on Offering Gifts and Other Inducements to Beneficiaries.

- Transportation is offered uniformly and without charge or at reduced charge to all patients of the hospital or hospital-owned ambulatory surgical center (and may also be made available to their families).

- The transportation is only provided to and from the hospital or a hospital-owned ambulatory surgical center and is for the purpose of receiving hospital or ambulatory surgery center services (or, in the case of family members, accompanying or visiting hospital or ambulatory surgical center patients).

- The transportation is provided only within the hospital's or ambulatory surgical center's primary service area.

- The costs of the transportation are not claimed directly or indirectly by any Federal health care program cost report or claim and are not otherwise shifted to any Federal health care program.

- The transportation does not include ambulance transportation.

Other arrangements are subject to a case-by-case review under the statute to ensure that no improper inducement exists.

G. HIPAA Privacy and Security Rules

As of April 14, 2003, all hospitals transmitting electronic transactions to health plans were required to comply with the privacy rules of the Health Insurance Portability and Accountability Act (HIPAA). Generally, the HIPAA privacy rule addresses the use and disclosure of individuals' health information (protected health information or PHI) by hospitals and other covered entities, as well as standards for individuals' privacy rights to understand and control how their health information is used. The privacy rule, 45 CFR parts 160 and 164, and other helpful information about how it applies, including frequently asked questions, can be found on the webpage of the Department's Office for Civil Rights (OCR) at *http://www.hhs.gov/ocr/hipaa/*. Questions about the privacy rule should be submitted to OCR. Hospitals can contact OCR by following the instructions on its webpage, *http:// www.hhs.gov/ocr/contact.html,* or by calling the HIPAA toll-free number, (866) 627-7748.

To ease the burden of complying with the new requirements, the privacy rule gives hospitals and other covered entities flexibility to create their own privacy procedures. Each hospital should make sure that it is compliant with all applicable provisions of the privacy rule, including provisions pertaining to required disclosures (such as required disclosures to the Department when it is undertaking a compliance investigation or review or enforcement action) and that its privacy procedures are tailored to fit its particular size and needs.

The final HIPAA security rule was published in the **Federal Register** on February 20, 2003. It is available on CMS's webpage at *http://www.cms.gov/ hipaa/hipaa2*. The security rule specifies a series of administrative, technical, and physical security procedures for hospitals that are covered entities and other covered entities to use to assure the confidentiality of electronic PHI. Hospitals that are covered entities must be compliant with the security rule by April 20, 2005. The security rule requirements are flexible and scalable, which allows each covered entity to tailor its approach to compliance based on its own unique circumstances. Covered entities can consider their organization and capabilities, as well as costs, in designing their security plans and procedures. Questions about the HIPAA security rules should be submitted to CMS. Hospitals can contact CMS by following the instructions on its webpage, *http://www.cms.gov/hipaa/hipaa2/ contact,* or by calling the HIPAA toll-free number, (866) 627-7748.

H. Billing Medicare or Medicaid Substantially in Excess of Usual Charges

Section 1128(b)(6)(A) of the Act provides for the permissive exclusion from Federal health care programs of any provider or supplier that submits a claim based on costs or charges to the Medicare or Medicaid programs that is "substantially in excess" of its usual charge or cost, unless the Secretary finds there is "good cause" for the higher charge or cost. The exclusion provision does not require a provider to charge everyone the same price; nor does it require a provider to offer Medicare or Medicaid its "best price." However, providers cannot routinely charge Medicare or Medicaid substantially more than they usually charge others. Hospitals have raised concerns regarding the impact of the exclusion authority on hospital services, and the OIG is considering those concerns in the context of the rulemaking process.[75] The OIG's policy regarding application of the exclusion authority to discounts offered to uninsured and underinsured patients is discussed below.

I. Areas of General Interest

Although in most cases the following areas do not pose significant fraud and abuse risk, the OIG has received numerous inquiries from hospitals and others on these topics. Therefore, we offer the following guidance to assist hospitals in their review of these arrangements.

1. Discounts to Uninsured Patients

No OIG authority, including the Federal anti-kickback statute, prohibits or restricts hospitals from offering discounts to uninsured patients who are unable to pay their hospital bills.[76] In addition, the OIG has never excluded or attempted to exclude any provider or supplier for offering discounts to uninsured or underinsured patients under the permissive exclusion authority at section 1128(b)(6)(A) of the Act. However, to provide additional assurance to the industry, the OIG recently proposed regulations that would define key terms in the statute.[77] Among other things, the proposed regulations would make clear that free or substantially reduced charges to uninsured persons would not affect the calculation of a provider's or supplier's "usual" charges, as the term "usual charges" is used in the exclusion provision. The OIG is currently reviewing the public comments to the proposed regulations. Until such time as a final regulation is promulgated or the OIG indicates its intention not to promulgate a final rule, it will continue to be the OIG's enforcement policy that when calculating their "usual charges" for purposes of section 1128(b)(6)(A), individuals and entities do not need to consider free or substantially reduced charges to (i) uninsured patients or (ii) underinsured patients who are self-paying patients for the items or services furnished. In offering such discounts, a hospital should reflect full uniform charges, rather than the discounted amounts, on its Medicare cost report and make the FI aware that it has reported its full charges.[78]

Under CMS rules, Medicare generally reimburses a hospital for a percentage of the "bad debt" of a Medicare beneficiary (*i.e.,* unpaid deductibles or coinsurance) as long as the hospital bills a patient and engages in reasonable, consistent collection efforts.[79] However, as explained in CMS's paper titled "Questions On Charges For The Uninsured," a hospital can forgo any collection effort aimed at a Medicare patient, if the hospital, using its customary methods, can document that the patient is indigent or medically indigent.[80] In addition, if the hospital also determines that no source other than the patient is legally responsible for the unpaid deductibles and coinsurance, the hospital may claim the amounts as Medicare bad debts.

CMS rules provide that a hospital can determine its own individual indigency criteria as long as it applies the criteria to Medicare and non-Medicare patients uniformly. For Medicare patients, however, if a hospital wants to claim Medicare bad debt reimbursement, CMS requires documentation to support the indigency determination. To claim Medicare bad debt reimbursement, the hospital must follow the guidance stated in the Provider Reimbursement Manual.[81] A hospital should examine a patient's total resources, which could include, but are not limited to, an analysis of assets, liabilities, income, expenses, and any extenuating circumstances that would affect the determination. The hospital should document the method by which it determined the indigency and include all backup information to substantiate the determination. In addition, if collection efforts are made, Medicare requires the efforts to be documented in the patient's file with copies of the bill(s), follow-up letters, and reports of telephone and personal contacts. In the case of a dually-eligible patient (*i.e.,* a patient entitled to both Medicare and Medicaid), the hospital must include a denial of payment from the State with the bad debt claim.

2. Preventive Care Services

Hospitals, particularly non-profit hospitals, frequently participate in community-based efforts to deliver preventive care services. The Medicare and Medicaid programs encourage patients to access preventive care services. The prohibition against beneficiary inducements at section 1128A(a)(5) of the Act does not apply to incentives offered to promote the delivery of certain preventive care services, if the programs are structured in accordance with the regulatory requirements at 42 CFR 1003.101. Generally, to fit within the preventive care exception, a service must be a prenatal service or post-natal well-baby visit or a specific clinical service described in the current U.S. Preventive Services Task Force's *Guide to Clinical Preventive Services*[82] that is reimbursed by Medicare or Medicaid. Obtaining the service may not be tied directly or indirectly to the provision of other Medicare or Medicaid services. In addition, the incentives may not be in the form of cash or cash equivalents and may not be disproportionate to the value of the preventive care provided. From an anti-kickback perspective, the chief concern is whether an arrangement to induce patients to obtain preventive care services is intended to induce other business payable by a Federal health care program. Relevant factors in making this evaluation would include, but not be limited to: the nature and scope of the preventive care services; whether the preventive care services are tied directly or indirectly to the provision of other items or services and, if so, the nature and scope of the other services; the basis on which patients are selected to receive the free or discounted services; and whether the patient is able to afford the services.

3. Professional Courtesy

Although historically "professional courtesy" referred to the practice of physicians waiving the entire professional fee for other physicians, the term is variously used in the industry now to describe a range of practices involving free or discounted services (including "insurance only" billing) furnished to physicians and their families and staff. Some hospitals have used the term "professional courtesy" to describe various programs that offer free or discounted hospital services to medical staff, employees, community physicians, and their families and staff. Although many professional courtesy programs are unlikely to pose a significant risk of abuse (and many may be legitimate employee benefits programs eligible for the employee safe harbor), some hospital-sponsored "professional courtesy" programs may implicate the fraud and abuse statutes.

In general, whether a professional courtesy program runs afoul of the anti-kickback statute turns on whether the recipients of the professional courtesy are selected in a manner that takes into account, directly or indirectly, any recipient's ability to refer to, or otherwise generate business for, the hospital. Also relevant is whether the physicians have solicited the professional courtesy in return for referrals. With respect to the Stark law, the key inquiry is whether the arrangement fits in the exception for professional courtesy at 42 CFR 411.357(s). Finally, hospitals should evaluate the method by which the courtesy is granted. For example, "insurance only" billing offered to a Federal program beneficiary potentially implicates the anti-kickback statute, the False Claims Act, and the CMP provision prohibiting inducements to Medicare and Medicaid beneficiaries (discussed in section II.F above). Notably, the Stark law exception for professional courtesy requires that insurers be notified if "professional courtesy" includes "insurance only" billing.

III. Hospital Compliance Program Effectiveness

Hospitals with an organizational culture that values compliance are more likely to have effective compliance programs and thus be better able to prevent, detect, and correct problems. Building and sustaining a successful compliance program rarely follows the same formula from organization to organization. However, such programs generally include: The commitment of the hospital's governance and management at the highest levels; structures and processes that create effective internal controls; and regular self-assessment and enhancement of the existing compliance program. The 1998 CPG provided guidance for hospitals on establishing sound internal controls.[83] This section discusses the important roles of corporate leadership and self-assessment of compliance programs.

A. Code of Conduct

Every effective compliance program necessarily begins with a formal commitment to compliance by the hospital's governing body and senior management. Evidence of that commitment should include active involvement of the organizational leadership, allocation of adequate resources, a reasonable timetable for implementation of the compliance measures, and the identification of a compliance officer and compliance committee vested with sufficient autonomy, authority, and accountability to implement and enforce appropriate compliance measures. A hospital's leadership should foster an organizational culture that values, and even rewards, the prevention, detection, and resolution of problems. Moreover, hospitals' leadership and management should ensure that policies and procedures, including, for example, compensation structures, do not create undue pressure to pursue profit over compliance. In short, the hospital should endeavor to develop a culture that values compliance from the top down and fosters compliance from the bottom up. Such an organizational culture is the foundation of an effective compliance program.

Although a clear statement of detailed and substantive policies and procedures—and the periodic evaluation of their effectiveness—is at the core of a compliance program, the OIG recommends that hospitals also develop a general organizational statement of ethical and compliance principles that will guide the entity's operations. One common expression of this statement of principles is a code of conduct. The code should function in the same fashion as a constitution, *i.e.,* as a document that details the fundamental principles, values, and framework for action within an organization. The code of conduct for a hospital should articulate a commitment to compliance by management, employees, and contractors, and should summarize the broad ethical and legal principles under which the hospital must operate. Unlike the more detailed policies and procedures, the code of conduct should be brief, easily readable, and cover general principles applicable to all members of the organization.

As appropriate, the OIG strongly encourages the participation and involvement of the hospital's board of directors, officers (including the chief executive officer (CEO)), members of senior management, and other personnel from various levels of the organizational structure in the development of all aspects of the compliance program, especially the code of conduct. Management and employee involvement in this process communicates a strong and explicit commitment by management to foster compliance with applicable Federal health care program requirements. It also communicates the need for all managers, employees, contractors, and medical staff members to comply with the organization's code of conduct and policies and procedures.

B. Regular Review of Compliance Program Effectiveness

Hospitals should regularly review the implementation and execution of their compliance program elements. This review should be conducted at least annually and should include an assessment of each of the basic elements individually, as well as the overall success of the program. This review should help the hospital identify any weaknesses in its compliance program and implement appropriate changes.

A common method of assessing compliance program effectiveness is measurement of various outcomes indicators (*e.g.,* billing and coding error rates, identified overpayments, and audit results). However, we have observed that exclusive reliance on these indicators may cause an organization to miss crucial underlying weaknesses. We recommend that hospitals examine program outcomes and assess the underlying structure and process of each compliance program element. We have identified a number of factors that may be useful when evaluating the effectiveness of basic compliance program elements. Hospitals should consider these factors, as well as others, when developing a strategy for assessing their compliance programs. While no one factor is determinative of program effectiveness, the following factors are often observed in effective compliance programs.

1. Designation of a Compliance Officer and Compliance Committee

The compliance department is the backbone of the hospital's compliance program. The compliance department should be led by a well-qualified compliance officer, who is a member of senior management, and should be supported by a compliance committee. The purpose of the compliance department is to implement the hospital's compliance program and to ensure that the hospital complies with all applicable Federal health care program requirements. To ensure that the compliance department is meeting this objective, each hospital should conduct an annual review of its compliance department. Some factors that the organization may wish to consider in its evaluation include the following:

- Does the compliance department have a clear, well-crafted mission?

- Is the compliance department properly organized?

- Does the compliance department have sufficient resources (staff and budget), training, authority, and autonomy to carry out its mission?

- Is the relationship between the compliance function and the general counsel function appropriate to achieve the purpose of each?

- Is there an active compliance committee, comprised of trained representatives of each of the relevant functional departments, as well as senior management?

- Are *ad hoc* groups or task forces assigned to carry out any special missions, such as conducting an investigation or evaluating a proposed enhancement to the compliance program?

- Does the compliance officer have direct access to the governing body, the president or CEO, all senior management, and legal counsel?

- Does the compliance officer have a good working relationship with other key operational areas, such as internal audit, coding, billing, and clinical departments?

- Does the compliance officer make regular reports to the board of directors and other hospital management concerning different aspects of the hospital's compliance program?

2. Development of Compliance Policies and Procedures, Including Standards of Conduct

The purpose of compliance policies and procedures is to establish bright-line rules that help employees carry out their job functions in a manner that ensures compliance with Federal health care program requirements and furthers the mission and objective of the hospital itself. Typically, policies and procedures are written to address identified risk areas for the organization. As hospitals conduct a review of their written policies and procedures, some of the following factors may be considered:

- Are policies and procedures clearly written, relevant to day-to-day responsibilities, readily available to those who need them, and re-evaluated on a regular basis?

- Does the hospital monitor staff compliance with internal policies and procedures?

- Have the standards of conduct been distributed to the Board of Directors, all officers, all managers, employees, contractors, and medical staff?

- Has the hospital developed a risk assessment tool, which is re-evaluated on a regular basis, to assess and identify weaknesses and risks in operations?

- Does the risk assessment tool include an evaluation of Federal health care program requirements, as well as other publications, such as OIG CPGs, Work Plans, Special Advisory Bulletins, and Special Fraud Alerts?

3. Developing Open Lines of Communication

Open communication is essential to maintaining an effective compliance program. The purpose of developing open communication is to increase the hospital's ability to identify and respond to compliance problems. Generally, open communication is a product of organizational culture and internal mechanisms for reporting instances of potential fraud and abuse. When assessing a hospital's ability to communicate potential compliance issues effectively, a hospital may wish to consider the following factors:

- Has the hospital fostered an organizational culture that encourages open communication, without fear of retaliation?

- Has the hospital established an anonymous hotline or other similar mechanism so that staff, contractors, patients, visitors, and medical staff can report potential compliance issues?

- How well is the hotline publicized; how many and what types of calls are received; are calls logged and tracked (to establish possible patterns); and does the caller have some way to be informed of the hospital's actions?

- Are all instances of potential fraud and abuse investigated?

- Are the results of internal investigations shared with the hospital governing body and relevant departments on a regular basis?

- Is the governing body actively engaged in pursuing appropriate remedies to institutional or recurring problems?

- Does the hospital utilize alternative communication methods, such as a periodic newsletter or compliance intranet web site?

4. Appropriate Training and Education

Hospitals that fail to train and educate their staff adequately risk liability for the violation of health care fraud and abuse laws. The purpose of conducting a training and education program is to ensure that each employee, contractor, or any other individual that functions on behalf of the hospital is fully capable of executing his or her role in compliance with rules, regulations, and other standards. In reviewing their training and education programs, hospitals may consider the following factors:

- Does the hospital provide qualified trainers to conduct annual compliance training to its staff, including both general and specific training pertinent to the staff's responsibilities?

- Has the hospital evaluated the content of its training and education program on an annual basis and determined that the subject content is appropriate and sufficient to cover the range of issues confronting its employees?

- Has the hospital kept up-to-date with any changes in Federal health care program requirements and adapted its education and training program accordingly?

- Has the hospital formulated the content of its education and training program to consider results from its audits and investigations; results from previous training and education programs; trends in hotline reports; and OIG, CMS, or other agency guidance or advisories?

- Has the hospital evaluated the appropriateness of its training format by reviewing the length of the training sessions; whether training is delivered via live instructors or via computer-based training programs; the frequency of training sessions; and the need for general and specific training sessions?

- Does the hospital seek feedback after each session to identify shortcomings in the training program, and does it administer post-training testing to ensure attendees understand and retain the subject matter delivered?

- Has the hospital s governing body been provided with appropriate training on fraud and abuse laws?

- Has the hospital documented who has completed the required training?

- Has the hospital assessed whether to impose sanctions for failing to attend training or to offer appropriate incentives for attending training?

5. Internal Monitoring and Auditing

Effective auditing and monitoring plans will help hospitals avoid the submission of incorrect claims to Federal health care program payors. Hospitals should develop detailed annual audit plans designed to minimize the risks associated with improper claims and billing practices. Some factors hospitals may wish to consider include the following:

- Is the audit plan re-evaluated annually, and does it address the proper areas of concern, considering, for example, findings from previous years' audits, risk areas identified as part of the annual risk assessment, and high volume services?

- Does the audit plan include an assessment of billing systems, in addition to claims accuracy, in an effort to identify the root cause of billing errors?

- Is the role of the auditors clearly established and are coding and audit personnel independent and qualified, with the requisite certifications?

- Is the audit department available to conduct unscheduled reviews and does a mechanism exist that allows the compliance department to request additional audits or monitoring should the need arise?

- Has the hospital evaluated the error rates identified in the annual audits?

- If the error rates are not decreasing, has the hospital conducted a further investigation into other aspects of the hospital compliance program in an effort to determine hidden weaknesses and deficiencies?

- Does the audit include a review of all billing documentation, including clinical documentation, in support of the claim?

6. Response to Detected Deficiencies

By consistently responding to detected deficiencies, hospitals can develop effective corrective action plans and prevent further losses to Federal health care programs. Some factors a hospital may wish to consider when evaluating the manner in which it responds to detected deficiencies include the following:

- Has the hospital created a response team, consisting of representatives from the compliance, audit, and any other relevant functional areas, which may be able to evaluate any detected deficiencies quickly?

- Are all matters thoroughly and promptly investigated?

- Are corrective action plans developed that take into account the root causes of each potential violation?

- Are periodic reviews of problem areas conducted to verify that the corrective action that was implemented successfully eliminated existing deficiencies?

- When a detected deficiency results in an identified overpayment to the hospital, are overpayments promptly reported and repaid to the FI?

- If a matter results in a probable violation of law, does the hospital promptly disclose the matter to the appropriate law enforcement agency.[84]

7. Enforcement of Disciplinary Standards

By enforcing disciplinary standards, hospitals help create an organizational culture that emphasizes ethical behavior. Hospitals may consider the following factors when assessing the effectiveness of internal disciplinary efforts:

- Are disciplinary standards well-publicized and readily available to all hospital personnel?

- Are disciplinary standards enforced consistently across the organization?

- Is each instance involving the enforcement of disciplinary standards thoroughly documented?

- Are employees, contractors and medical staff checked routinely (*e.g.,* at least annually) against government sanctions lists, including the OIG's List of Excluded Individuals/Entities (LEIE)[85] and the General Services Administration's Excluded Parties Listing System.

In sum, while no single factor is conclusive of an effective compliance program, the preceding seven areas form a useful starting point for developing and maintaining an effective compliance program.

IV. Self-Reporting

Where the compliance officer, compliance committee, or a member of senior management discovers credible evidence of misconduct from any source and, after a reasonable inquiry, believes that the misconduct may violate criminal, civil, or administrative law, the hospital should promptly report the existence of misconduct to the appropriate Federal and State authorities[86] within a reasonable period, but not more than 60 days,[87] after determining that there is credible evidence of a violation.[88] Prompt voluntary reporting will demonstrate the hospital's good faith and willingness to work with governmental authorities to correct and remedy the problem. In addition, reporting such conduct will be considered a mitigating factor by the OIG in determining administrative sanctions (*e.g.,* penalties, assessments, and exclusion), if the reporting hospital becomes the subject of an OIG investigation.[89] To encourage providers to make voluntary disclosures, the OIG published the Provider Self-Disclosure Protocol.[90]

When reporting to the government, a hospital should provide all information relevant to the alleged violation of applicable Federal or State law(s) and the potential financial or other impact of the alleged violation. The compliance officer, under advice of counsel and with guidance from the governmental authorities, could be requested to continue to investigate the reported violation. Once the investigation is completed, and especially if the investigation ultimately reveals that criminal, civil or administrative violations have occurred, the compliance officer should notify the appropriate governmental authority of the outcome of the investigation, including a description of the impact of the alleged violation on the applicable Federal health care programs or their beneficiaries.

V. Conclusion

In today's environment of increased scrutiny of corporate conduct and increasingly large expenditures for health care, it is imperative for hospitals to establish and maintain effective compliance programs. These programs should foster a culture of compliance that begins at the highest levels and extends throughout the organization. This supplemental CPG is intended as a resource for hospitals to help them operate effective compliance programs that decrease errors, fraud, and abuse and increase compliance with Federal health care program requirements for the benefit of the hospitals and public alike.

Dated: May 20, 2004.

Footnotes

1. *See* 63 FR 8987 (February 23, 1998), available on our webpage at *http://oig.hhs.gov/authorities/docs/cpghosp.pdf.*

2. *See* 67 FR 41433 (June 18, 2002), available on our webpage at *http://oig.hhs.gov/authorities/docs/cpghospitalsolicitationnotice.pdf.*

3. For purposes of convenience in this guidance, we use the term "hospitals" to refer to individual hospitals, multi-hospital systems, health systems that own or operate hospitals, academic medical centers, and any other organization that owns or operates one or more hospitals. Where applicable, the term "hospitals" is also intended to include, without limitation, hospital owners, officers, managers, staff, agents, and sub-providers. This guidance primarily focuses on hospitals reimbursed under the inpatient prospective payment system. While other hospitals should find this CPG useful, we recognize that they may be subject to different laws, rules, and regulations and, accordingly, may have different or additional risk areas and may need to adopt different compliance strategies. We encourage all hospitals to establish and maintain ongoing compliance programs.

4. The 1998 OIG Compliance Guidance for Hospitals is available on our webpage at *http://oig.hhs.gov/authorities/docs/cpghosp.pdf.*

5. *See* 67 FR 41433 (June 18, 2002), "Solicitation of Information and Recommendations for Revising a Compliance Program Guidance for the Hospital Industry," available on our webpage at *http://oig.hhs.gov/authorities/docs/cpghospitalsolicitationnotice.pdf.*

6. *See* 42 U.S.C. 1320a–7b(b). *See also* 42 CFR 1001.952. The safe harbor regulations and preambles are available on our webpage at *http://oig.hhs.gov/fraud/safeharborregulations.html#1.*

7. OIG materials are available on our webpage at *http://oig.hhs.gov.*

8. The term "Federal health care programs," as defined in 42 U.S.C. 1320a–7b(f), includes any plan or program that provides health benefits, whether directly, through insurance, or otherwise, which is funded directly, in whole or in part, by the United States Government (other than the Federal Employees Health

Benefit Plan described at 5 U.S.C. 8901–8914) or any State health plan (*e.g.*, Medicaid or a program receiving funds from block grants for social services or child health services). In this document, the term "Federal health care program requirements" refers to the statutes, regulations, and other rules governing Medicare, Medicaid, and all other Federal health care programs.

9. *See* 42 U.S.C. 1320a-7b(a)(3).

10. The False Claims Act (31 U.S.C. 3729–33), among other things, prohibits knowingly presenting or causing to be presented to the Federal government a false or fraudulent claim for payment or approval, knowingly making or using or causing to be made or used a false record or statement to have a false or fraudulent claim paid or approved by the government, and knowingly making or using or causing to be made or used, a false record or statement to conceal, avoid, or decrease an obligation to pay or transmit money or property to the government. The Act defines "knowing" and "knowingly" to mean that "a person, with respect to the information (1) has actual knowledge of the information; (2) acts in deliberate ignorance of the truth or falsity of the information; or (3) acts in reckless disregard of the truth or falsity of the information, and no proof of specific intent to defraud is required." 31 U.S.C. 3729(b).

11. In some circumstances, inaccurate or incomplete reporting may lead to liability under the Federal anti-kickback statute. In addition, hospitals should be mindful that many states have fraud and abuse statutes—including false claims, anti-kickback, and other statutes—that are not addressed in this guidance.

12. To review the risk areas discussed in the original hospital CPG, *see* 63 FR 8987, 8990 (February 23, 1998), available on our webpage at *http://oig.hhs.gov/authorities/docs/cpghosp.pdf*.

13. Congress enacted the OPPS in section 4523 of the Balanced Budget Act of 1997. OPPS became effective on August 1, 2001. CMS promulgated regulations implementing the OPPS at 42 CFR Part 419. For more information regarding the OPPS, *see http://www.cms.gov/providers/hopps/*.

14. The list of current modifiers is listed in the Current Procedural Terminology (CPT) coding manual. However, hospitals should pay particular attention to CMS transmittals and program memoranda that may introduce new or altered application of modifiers for claims submission and reimbursement purposes. *See* chapter 4, section 20.6 of the Medicare Claims Processing Manual at *http://www.cms.gov/manuals/104_claims/clm104c04.pdf*.

15. The list of "inpatient-only" procedures appears in the annual update to the OPPS rule. For the 2004 final rule, the "inpatient-only" list is found in Addendum E. *See http://www.cms.gov/regulations/hopps/2004f*.

16. A hospital may contact its FI to request a copy of the pertinent LMRPs, or visit CMS's webpage at *http://www.cms.gov/mcd* to search existing local and national policies.

17. More information regarding NCCI can be obtained from CMS's webpage at *http://www.cms.gov/medlearn/ncci.asp*.

18. For information relating to HCPCS code updates, *see http://www.cms.gov/medicare/hcpcs/*. For information relating to annual APC updates, *see http://www.cms.gov/providers/hopps/*.

19. *See http://www.cms.gov/medlearn/refopps.asp*.

20. Section 1848(c)(5) of the Social Security Act (42 U.S.C. 1395w-4(c)(5)) mandated the development of a uniform coding system to describe physician services. E/M documentation guidelines can be accessed at *http://www.cms.gov/medlearn/emdoc.asp*.

21. *See* CMS Program Transmittal A–02–026, available on CMS's webpage at *http://www.cms.gov/manuals/pm_trans/A02026.pdf*.

22. *See* chapter 1, section 50.2 of the Medicare Claims Processing Manual, available on CMS's webpage at *http://www.cms.gov/manuals/104_claims/clm104c01.pdf*.

23. *See* chapter 4, section 260 of the Medicare Claims Processing Manual, available on CMS's webpage at *http://www.cms.gov/manuals/104_claims/clm104c04.pdf*.

24. *See, e.g.,* OIG Audit Report A–03–01–00011, "Review of Medicare Same-Day, Same-Provider Acute Care Readmissions in Pennsylvania During Calendar Year 1998," August 2002, available on our webpage at *http://oig.hhs.gov/oas/reports/region3/30100011.pdf*.

25. *See* 42 CFR 412.4(c). *See, e.g.,* OIG Audit Report A–04–00–01220 "Implementation of Medicare's Post-acute Care Transfer Policy," October 2001, available on our webpage at *http://oig.hhs.gov/oas/reports/region4/40001220.pdf.*

26. The initial 10 designated DRGs were selected by the Secretary, pursuant to section 1886(d)(5)(J) of the Social Security Act (42 U.S.C. 1395ww(d)(5)(J)). With the 2004 fiscal year PPS rule, CMS revised the list of DRGs paid under CMS's post-acute care transfer policy, bringing the total number of designated DRGs to 29. See 68 FR 45346, 45406 (August 1, 2003). *See also* chapter 3, section 40.2.4 of the Medicare Claims Processing Manual, available on CMS's webpage at *http://www.cms.gov/manuals/104_claims/clm104c03.pdf.*

27. *See* 42 CFR 412.22(e).

28. For more information regarding CMS's APC "pass-through" payments, *see http://www.cms.gov/providers/hopps/apc.asp.*

29. *See* 42 CFR 412.84; 68 FR 34493 (June 9, 2003).

30. The criteria for determining whether a facility or organization is provider-based can be found at 42 CFR 413.65. In April 2003, CMS published Transmittal A–03–030, outlining changes to the criteria for provider-based designation. *See http://www.cms.gov/manuals/pm_trans/A03030.pdf.*

31. To view Medicare's National Coverage Decision regarding clinical trials, *see http://www.cms.gov/coverage/8d2.asp.* Specific requirements for submitting claims for reimbursement for clinical trials can be accessed on CMS's webpage at *http://www.cms.gov/coverage/8d4.asp.*

32. *See* 42 CFR 412.2(e)(4), 42 CFR 412.113(d), and 42 CFR 413.203. *See generally* 42 CFR Part 413 (setting forth the principles of reasonable cost reimbursement).

33. *See* Medicare's Provider Reimbursement Manual (PRM), Part I, section 2304 and Part II, section 3610, available on CMS's webpage at *http://www.cms.gov/manuals/cmstoc.asp.*

34. *See* 42 CFR 412.100. *See also,* chapter 3, section 90 of the Medicare Claims Processing Manual, available on CMS's webpage at *http://www.cms.gov/manuals/104_claims/clm104c03.pdf. See, e.g.,* OIG Audit Report A–04–02–02017, "Audit of Medicare Costs for Organ Acquisitions at Tampa General Hospital," April 2003, available on our webpage at *http://oig.hhs.gov/oas/reports/region4/40202017.pdf.*

35. *See* section 35–25 of the Medicare Coverage Issues Manual. *See, e.g.,* OIG Audit Report A–01–03–00516, "Review of Outpatient Cardiac Rehabilitation Services at the Cooley Dickinson Hospital," December 2003, available on our webpage at *http://oig.hhs.gov/oas/reports/region1/10300516.pdf.*

36. Payments for direct graduate medical education (GME) and indirect graduate medical education (IME) costs are in part based upon the number of full-time equivalent (FTE) residents at each hospital and the proportion of time residents spend in training. Hospitals that inappropriately calculate the number of FTE residents risk receiving inappropriate medical education payments. Hospitals should have in place procedures regarding (i) resident rotation monitoring, (ii) resident credentialing, (iii) written agreements with non-hospital providers, and (iv) the approval process for research activities. For more information regarding medical education reimbursement, *see* 42 CFR 413.86 (GME requirements) and 42 CFR 412.105 (IME requirements). *See, e.g.,* OIG Audit Report A–01–01–00547 "Review of Graduate Medical Education Costs Claimed by the Hartford Hospital for Fiscal Year Ending September 30, 1999," October 2003, available on our webpage at *http://oig.hhs.gov/oas/reports/region1/10100547.pdf.*

37. For more information regarding Medicare's Electronic Data Interchange programs, *see http://www.cms.gov/providers/edi/.*

38. The statute also prohibits physicians from referring DHS to entities, including hospitals, with which they have prohibited financial relationships. However, the billing prohibition and nonpayment sanction apply only to the DHS entity (*e.g.,* the hospital). *See* section 1877(a) of the Act. Section 1903(s) of the Act extends the statutory prohibition to Medicaid-covered services.

39. The statute lists ten additional categories of DHS, including, among others, clinical laboratory services, radiology services, and durable medical equipment. *See* section 1877(h)(6) of the Act. Hospitals and health systems that own or operate free-standing DHS entities should be mindful of the ten additional DHS categories.

40. Hospitals affiliated with academic medical centers should be aware that the regulations contain a special exception for certain academic medical center arrangements. *See* 42 CFR 411.353(e). Specialty hospitals should be mindful of certain limitations on new physician-owned specialty hospitals contained in section 507 of the Medicare Prescription Drug, Improvement and Modernization Act of 2003. *See* CMS's One-Time Notification regarding the 18-month moratorium on physician investment in specialty hospitals, CMS Manual System Pub. 100–20 One-Time Notification, Transmittal 26 (March 19, 2004), available on CMS's webpage at *http://www.cms.gov/manuals/pm_trans/R62OTN.pdf.*

41. Importantly, the anti-kickback statute safe harbors are not the same as the Stark law exceptions described above at section II.B.1 of this guidance. An arrangement's compliance with the anti-kickback statute and the Stark law must be evaluated separately.

42. Parties to an arrangement cannot obtain safe harbor protection by entering into a sham contract that complies with the written agreement requirement of a safe harbor and appears, on paper, to meet all of the other safe harbor requirements, but does reflect the actual arrangement between the parties. In other words, in assessing compliance with a safe harbor, the OIG examines not only whether the written contract satisfies all of the safe harbor requirements, but also whether the actual arrangement satisfies the requirements.

43. While informative for guidance purposes, an OIG advisory opinion is binding only with respect to the particular party or parties that requested the opinion. The analyses and conclusions set forth in OIG advisory opinions are very fact-specific. Accordingly, hospitals should be aware that different facts may lead to different results.

44. *See* 1989 Special Fraud Alert on Joint Venture Arrangements, reprinted in the **Federal Register,** 59 FR 65372 (December 19, 1994), and available on our webpage at *http://oig.hhs.gov/fraud/docs/alertsandbulletins/121994.html.*

45. There is also a safe harbor for investment interests in large entities (*i.e.,* entities with over fifty million dollars in assets), 42 CFR 1001.952(a)(1).

46. *See* 1989 Special Fraud Alert on Joint Venture Arrangements, *supra* note 44.

47. This Special Advisory Bulletin is available on our webpage at *http://oig.hhs.gov/fraud/docs/alertsandbulletins/042303SABJointVentures.pdf.*

48. Contractual ventures with existing clinical laboratories and outpatient therapy providers, among others, are also potentially problematic, particularly if the venture is functionally a turnkey operation that enables a hospital to use its captive referrals to expand into a new line of business with little or no contribution of resources or assumption of real risk.

49. *See* 2003 Special Advisory Bulletin on Contractual Joint Ventures, *supra* note 47.

50. The Medicare program permits hospitals to furnish services "under arrangements" with other providers or suppliers. Hospitals frequently furnish services "under arrangements" with an entity owned, in whole or in part, by referring physicians. Standing alone, these "under arrangements" relationships do not fall within the scope of problematic contractual joint ventures described in the Special Fraud Alert; however, these relationships will violate the anti-kickback statute if remuneration is purposefully offered or paid to induce referrals (*e.g.,* paying above-market rates for the services to influence referrals or otherwise tying the arrangements to referrals in any manner). These "under arrangements" relationships should be structured, when possible, to fit within an anti-kickback safe harbor. They must fit within a Stark law exception, even if the service furnished "under arrangements" is not itself a DHS. *See* 66 FR 941–2 (January 4, 2001); 69 FR 16054, 16106 (March 26, 2004).

51. While disclosure to patients does not offer sufficient protection against Federal health care program abuse, effective and meaningful disclosure offers some protection against possible abuses of patient trust.

52. As previously noted, a hospital should ensure that each compensation arrangement with a referring physician fits squarely in a statutory or regulatory exception to the Stark law.

53. Arrangements between hospitals and hospital-based physicians were the topic of a Management Advisory Report (MAR) titled "Financial Arrangements Between Hospitals and Hospital-Based Physicians," OEI–09–89–00330, available on our webpage at *http://oig.hhs.gov/oei/reports/oei-09-89-00330.pdf.*

54. When referring to home health agencies, hospitals must comply with section 1861(ee)(2)(D) and (H) of the Act, requiring that Medicare participating hospitals, as part of the discharge planning process, (i) share with each beneficiary a list of Medicare-certified home health agencies that serve the beneficiary's geographic area and that request to be listed and (ii) identify any home health agency in which the hospital has a disclosable financial interest or that has a financial interest in the hospital.

55. Properly structured, payments to physicians who become hospital employees may be protected by the employee safe harbor at 42 CFR 1001.952(i).

56. *See* 42 CFR 1001.952(n).

57. *See* 42 U.S.C. 1320a–7b(b)(3)(A); 42 CFR 1001.952(h).

58. To preclude improper shifting of discounts, the safe harbor excludes GPOs that wholly own their members or have members that are subsidiaries of the parent company that wholly owns the GPO. Hospitals with affiliated GPOs should be mindful of these limitations.

59. *See* our "Solicitation of New Safe Harbors and Special Fraud Alerts," 67 FR 72894 (December 9, 2002), available on our webpage at *http://oig.hhs.gov/authorities/docs/solicitationannsafeharbor.pdf.*

60. *See* 42 CFR 1001.952(o).

61. *See* OIG letter on hospital corporation's medical malpractice insurance assistance program, available on our webpage at *http://oig.hhs.gov/fraud/docs/alertsandbulletins/MalpracticeProgram.pdf.*

62. The prohibition applies only to reductions or limitations of items or services provided to Medicare and Medicaid fee-for-service beneficiaries. *See* section 1128A(b)(1)(A) of the Act. *See also* our August 19, 1999 letter regarding "Social Security Act sections 1128A(b)(1) and (2) and hospital-physician incentive plans for Medicare or Medicaid beneficiaries enrolled in managed care plans," available on our webpage at *http://oig.hhs.gov/fraud/docs/alertsandbulletins/gsletter.htm.*

63. *See* sections 1128A(b)(1)(B) & (b)(2) of the Act.

64. A detailed discussion of gainsharing can be found in our July 1999 Special Advisory Bulletin titled "Gainsharing Arrangements and CMPs for Hospital Payments to Physicians to Reduce or Limit Services to Beneficiaries," available on our webpage at *http://oig.hhs.gov/fraud/docs/alertsandbulletins/gainsh.htm.*

65. *See* section 1128(b)(6)(B) of the Act, which is available through the Internet at *http://www4.law.cornell.edu/uscode/42/1320a-7.html.*

66. JCAHO's Comprehensive Accreditation Manual for Hospitals is available through the Internet at *http://www.jcrinc.com/subscribers/perspectives.asp?durki=6065 &site=10&return=2815.*

67. *See* section 1128A(i)(6) of the Act.

68. The Special Advisory Bulletin on Offering Gifts and Other Inducements to Beneficiaries, 65 FR 24400, 24411 (April 26, 2000), is available on our webpage at *http://oig.hhs.gov/fraud/docs/alertsandbulletins/SABGiftsandInducements.pdf.*

69. *Ibid.*

70. The OIG has proposed a rule to extend this safe harbor to protect waivers of Part B cost-sharing amounts pursuant to agreements with Medicare SELECT plans. *See* 67 FR 60202 (September 25, 2002), available on our webpage at *http://oig.hhs.gov/fraud/docs/safeharborregulations/MedicareSELECTNPRMFederalRegister.pdf.* However, the OIG is still considering comments on this rule, and it has not been finalized.

71. *See* section 1128A(a)(6)(A) of the Act.

72. *See also* OIG's Special Fraud Alert on Routine Waiver of Copayments or Deductibles Under Medicare Part B, issued May 1991, republished in the **Federal Register** at 59 FR 65373, 65374 (December 19, 1994), and available on our webpage at *http://oig.hhs.gov/fraud/docs/alertsandbulletins/121994.html.*

73. Our position on local transportation of nominal value is more fully set forth in the preamble to the final rule enacting 42 CFR 1003.102(b)(13). *See* 65 FR 24400, 24411 (April 26, 2000).

74. *See supra* note 68.

75. *See* Notice of Proposed Rulemaking regarding "Clarification of Terms and Application of Program Exclusion Authority for Submitting Claims Containing Excessive Charges," 68 FR 53939 (September 15, 2003), available on our webpage at *http://oig.hhs.gov/authorities/docs/FRSIENPRM.pdf.*

76. Discounts offered to underinsured patients potentially raise a more significant concern under the anti-kickback statute, and hospitals should exercise care to ensure that such discounts are not tied directly or indirectly to the furnishing of items or services payable by a Federal health care program. For more information, *see* our February 2, 2004 paper on "Hospital Discounts Offered To Patients Who Cannot Afford To Pay Their Hospital Bills," available on our webpage at *http://oig.hhs.gov/fraud/docs/alertsandbulletins/2004/FA021904 hospitaldiscounts.pdf,* and CMS's paper titled "Questions On Charges For The Uninsured," dated February 17, 2004, and available on CMS's webpage at *http://www.cms.gov/FAQ_Uninsured.pdf.*

77. *See* 68 FR 53939 (September 15, 2003), available on our webpage at *http://oig.hhs.gov/authorities/docs/FRSIENPRM.pdf.*

78. For more information, *see* CMS's paper titled "Questions On Charges For The Uninsured," dated February 17, 2004, and available on CMS's webpage at *http://www.cms.gov/FAQ_Uninsured.pdf.*

79. *See* 42 CFR 413.80 and Medicare's Provider Reimbursement Manual, Part II, chapter 11, section 1102.3.L, available on CMS's webpage at *http://www.cms.gov/manuals/pub152/PUB_15_2.asp.*

80. *See* "Questions On Charges For The Uninsured," dated February 17, 2004 and available on CMS's webpage at *http://www.cms.gov/FAQ_Uninsured.pdf.* In the paper, CMS further explains that hospitals may, but are not required to, determine a patient's indigency using a sliding scale. In this type of arrangement, the provider would agree to deem the patient indigent with respect to a portion of the patient's account (*e.g.,* a flat percentage of the debt based on the patient's income, assets, or the size of the patient's liability relative to their income). In the case of a Medicare patient who is determined to be indigent using this method, the amount the hospital decides, pursuant to its policy, not to collect from the patient can be claimed by the provider as Medicare bad debt. The hospital must, however, engage in a reasonable collection effort to collect the remaining balance. *Ibid.*

81. *See* Medicare's Provider Reimbursement Manual, Part II, chapter 11, section 1102.3.L, available on CMS's webpage at *http://www.cms.gov/manuals/pub152/PUB_15_2.asp.*

82. Available on the Internet at *http://www.ahrq.gov/clinic/cps3dix.htm.*

83. Among other things, the 1998 hospital CPG includes a detailed discussion of the structure and processes that make up the recommended seven elements of a compliance program. The seven basic elements of a compliance program are: designation of a compliance officer and compliance committee; development of compliance policies and procedures, including standards of conduct; development of open lines of communication; appropriate training and education; response to detected offenses; internal monitoring and auditing; and enforcement of disciplinary standards.

84. For more information on when to self-report, *see* section IV, below.

85. *See http://oig.hhs.gov/fraud/exclusions.html.* The OIG also makes available Monthly Supplements for Standard LEIE, which can be compared to existing hospital personnel lists.

86. Appropriate Federal and State authorities include the OIG, CMS, the Criminal and Civil Divisions of the Department of Justice, the U.S. Attorney in relevant districts, the Food and Drug Administration, the Department's Office for Civil Rights, the Federal Trade Commission, the Drug Enforcement Administration, the Federal Bureau of Investigation, and the other investigative arms for the agencies administering the affected Federal or State health care programs, such as the State Medicaid Fraud Control Unit, the Defense Criminal Investigative Service, the Department of Veterans Affairs, the Health Resources and Services Administration, and the Office of Personnel Management (which administers the Federal Employee Health Benefits Program).

87. In contrast, to qualify for the "not less than double damages" provision of the False Claims Act, the provider must provide the report to the government within 30 days after the date when the provider first obtained the information. *See* 31 U.S.C. 3729(a).

88. Some violations may be so serious that they warrant immediate notification to governmental authorities prior to, or simultaneous with, commencing an internal investigation. By way of example, the OIG believes a provider should immediately report misconduct that: (1) Is a clear violation of administrative, civil, or criminal laws; (2) has a significant adverse effect on the quality of care provided to Federal health care program beneficiaries; or (3) indicates evidence of a systemic failure to comply with applicable laws or an existing corporate integrity agreement, regardless of the financial impact on Federal health care programs.

89. The OIG has published criteria setting forth those factors that the OIG takes into consideration in determining whether it is appropriate to exclude an individual or entity from program participation pursuant to 42 U.S.C. 1320a-7(b)(7) for violations of various fraud and abuse laws. *See* 62 FR 67392 (December 24, 1997).

90. *See* 63 FR 58399 (October 30, 1998), available on our webpage at *http://oig.hhs.gov/authorities/docs/ selfdisclosure.pdf.*

Appendix F

AHIMA Practice Briefs

Seven Steps to Corporate Compliance: The HIM Role

Today, healthcare providers in all settings are developing and implementing compliance programs in an effort to ensure ethical business practices in accordance with compliance program guidance from the Department of Health and Human Services Office of the Inspector General (OIG). This is becoming necessary due to the increased severity of penalties established by the Health Insurance Portability and Accountability Act (HIPAA) of 1996 (public law 104–191) and the Balanced Budget Act of 1997 (public law 105–33). By ensuring ethical business practices through compliance programs, healthcare providers are reducing their risk of criminal and civil litigation.

As part of the process that is vital to accurate billing, HIM professionals should be involved in the development of a corporate compliance program. HIM skills that are fundamental to effective compliance include:

- a strong knowledge base and experience in appropriate coding and billing practices

- knowledge of multiple reimbursement systems

- knowledge of multiple regulations, standards, policies, and requirements pertaining to clinical documentation, coding, and billing

- knowledge of multiple third-party payer requirements

- the ability to accurately interpret and implement regulatory standards

- the ability to interpret legal requirements

- an established rapport with physicians and other healthcare practitioners

- strong managerial, leadership, and interpersonal skills

- strong analytical skills

HIM professionals are well suited to guiding the development and implementation of a corporate compliance program based on their skills and experience ensuring compliance within the HIM department. At a minimum, the HIM professional should, as part of the compliance committee, collaborate with other healthcare professionals in the development of the corporate compliance program by participating in the process and by sharing expertise to ensure compliance throughout the organization. Furthermore, partnering with HIM professionals to develop a corporate compliance program can bring improved health record documentation, improved coding accuracy, prevention of billing errors, and provision of a mechanism to identify problem areas.

There are a number of ways for HIM professionals to contribute to the development of their organizations' corporate compliance programs. These contributions revolve around the seven key elements of a corporate compliance program. The key elements, modeled after the Federal Sentencing Guidelines, are incorporated into all of the OIG's current compliance program guidances. They also provide the main structural components to corporate integrity agreements used in Medicare fraud and/or abuse settlements.

The information that follows is only a guide. Tailor each component to meet the internal needs of your facility.

Oversight

The oversight of HIM compliance begins with the corporate compliance officer—a corporate role for which HIM professionals are uniquely qualified to serve, with their management, leadership, communication skills, and knowledge of myriad regulatory and reimbursement requirements. Given that accurate documentation, coding, and billing are imperative to healthcare compliance, the HIM professional's skill set is the perfect match for the position at any organization.

An HIM professional should always serve on the organization's compliance committee (regardless of whether the corporate compliance officer is an HIM professional—it is essential to have the perspective of an HIM department staff member). In addition, there are other key compliance positions for HIM professionals, such as corporate compliance auditor and compliance coding specialist.

Policies and Procedures

The OIG recommends that an organization's policies and procedures address areas of special concern, as identified by the OIG in its Compliance Guidance for Hospitals. Many of these risk areas fall within the realm of HIM, including billing for items or services not rendered, providing medically unnecessary services, upcoding, DRG creep, outpatient services rendered in connection with inpatient stays, unbundling, documentation issues, and billing for discharge in lieu of transfer.

Specific issues to address when creating HIM compliance policies are the education and training requirements for HIM personnel, including billing and coding personnel. HIM policies and procedures should ensure that:

- coding and billing are based on accurate and timely medical record documentation

- all rejected claims pertaining to diagnosis and procedure codes are reviewed

- proper and timely documentation of all physician and other professional services is obtained prior to billing

- compensation for coders and consultants does not provide any financial incentive to improperly coded claims

- a process for pre- and post-submission review is in place

- the proper selection and sequencing of diagnoses occurs

- the correct application of official coding rules and guidelines occurs

- a process for reporting potential/actual violations exists

- a process for identification of coding errors is in place

HIM professionals must actively participate in the development of organizationwide policies and procedures pertaining to accurate, complete, and timely documentation and proper coding practices. This includes documentation and coding policies and procedures that may lie outside the functions of the HIM department (for example, chargemaster maintenance, review of claim rejections due to coding and documentation issues, outpatient registration, and the receipt of documentation from physicians' offices supporting medical necessity of diagnostic tests). It should also include involvement in creating policies and procedures related to the organization's health record retention and maintenance of patient confidentiality, developed in accordance with federal and state requirements.

HIM professionals can use their knowledge of coding and billing requirements and computer systems to recommend system edits and reminders—this will reduce coding and billing errors. They are also an important resource for clarification of coding and documentation protocols and development of tools and processes to promote compliance with those protocols. Furthermore, their knowledge of monitoring processes to ensure HIM compliance with the various regulatory bodies (for example, Medicare, Medicaid, Emergency Medical Treatment and Active Labor Act [EMTALA], and the Joint Commission on Accreditation of Healthcare Organizations [JCAHO]) makes them good candidates to assist in the development and implementation of corrective action plans.

HIM professionals should be key contributors to the development and promotion of the corporate compliance program. Written policies and procedures should reflect current regulatory requirements and guidance from the model compliance programs. Furthermore, the policies and procedures must be appropriately maintained, reviewed, and revised.

Education

One of the key elements in a compliance program is effective education, training, and continual retraining for all employees—at all levels—on applicable local, state, and federal regulations and other payer requirements. Training programs should be detailed and comprehensive, covering general areas of compliance and specific policies and procedures. Even in the absence of specifically delegated compliance duties, HIM expertise is necessary in all aspects of the design, development, and implementation of compliance education.

Design education and training to meet the educational needs of all employees. This may lead to the creation of internal and/or external educational programs. Use educational strategies to ensure that appropriate information is correctly disseminated. Separate the training into two sessions—general and focused—depending on the employees' involvement in various compliance risk areas. Design a general session for all employees, keeping in mind that more focused sessions may be required depending on employee tasks. Develop focused training programs for all employees who participate in high-risk activities, such as coding, billing, and patient confidentiality. Focused training programs should also be developed in response to regulatory changes, identified areas of deficiency, investigative focus, or corrective action plans. The educational structure should include a projected number of minimum education hours per year—designed to appropriately address the needs of different employees.

HIM professionals should provide input and guidance on the content and structure of the general sessions. Factor adherence to provisions of the compliance program into annual employee evaluations. Provide continual involvement in identification, revision, and updating educational sessions and materials. More specifically, HIM professionals should develop and disseminate information about patient confidentiality and record retention policies and procedures.

Get involved in the development and maintenance of an attestation of employee understanding of the material presented. Adequate records of attendance and educational materials should be maintained as well.

Use HIM skills and knowledge to educate physicians and facility staff on coding, documentation, and compliance. HIM professionals are uniquely qualified to develop and implement educational training programs involving HIM and related processes, such as physician and ancillary staff education related to coding and documentation. They should, therefore, be responsible for current and ongoing employee education related to those areas. HIM professionals can assist in identification of areas requiring specific training and in the development and implementation of training in those areas. Make sure to select timely and relevant educational topics assimilated through review of health information processes. Specific focus topics include:

- specific government and private payer reimbursement principles

- appropriate documentation practices

- relationship of coding to documentation

- regulatory rules and requirements pertaining to coding, billing, and documentation

- proper selection and sequencing of diagnoses

- impact of documentation on the clinical, operational, and financial aspects of healthcare delivery

- medical necessity

- chargemaster development and use

- improper alterations to documentation

- confidentiality

- record retention

- physician-specific education related to documentation, coding, and reimbursement rules

- duty to identify and appropriately report misconduct

In light of the government's patient education initiative to help identify and report fraud, HIM professionals must take responsibility for enabling patients to understand health information practices. Teach patients about access to patient records and the relationship of record documentation to the patient billing process. Enhanced patient understanding will help reduce patient dissatisfaction and beneficiary reports of fraud.

HIM professionals need to develop comprehensive education and training for the HIM components of the corporate compliance program. The OIG expects education to cover the applicable statutes, rules, and program instructions.

The education and training policies should include a plan to address the risk areas for fraud, waste, and abuse; the integrity of the patient information system; and the methodology to ensure accuracy of documentation, coding, and billing processes. In addition, education should reflect the current reimbursement principles set forth in applicable statutes and regulations as well as federal, state, and payer healthcare program requirements.

HIM professionals must develop and coordinate compliance education and training programs in a timely manner. Relevant education and training resource materials should be maintained, updated, and made available to all appropriate personnel. Be sure to include resources for current regulations, coding, documentation, and billing.

An essential component of an effective compliance program is one that provides proper education and training for all personnel, including managers, supervisors, employees, and physicians. Include all independent contractors and other external agents as well. Ask these entities to sign an agreement of understanding and compliance with the organization's compliance program as part of their contractual agreement.

Provide all education and training within a structured format that outlines content, audience, and time frames for completion. Implementing an educational program should be an ongoing process that includes the training of new personnel and continuous retraining of current personnel.

Communication

The OIG's Compliance Guidance for Hospitals states, "an open line of communication between the compliance officer and hospital personnel is equally important to the successful implementation of a compliance program and the reduction of any potential for fraud, abuse and waste" (HHS 1998c).

The HIM professional has the ability to effectively communicate a culture of corporate compliance by:

- encouraging communication for reporting incidents of potential fraud through corporate policies addressing confidentiality, anonymity, and nonretaliation

- adequately outlining how potential problems should be reported, according to a specific chain of command

- emphasizing that reporting potential problems is the duty of all employees

- supporting the use of the compliance hotline to report potential problems

- ensuring that employees know how to access the compliance officer to clarify a hospital policy or procedure or to ask a question

- establishing communication through e-mail, memos, newsletters, and suggestion boxes

- thoroughly communicating and conspicuously posting the hotline telephone number

- encouraging employees to ask questions and report possible problems

- presenting compliance material in a nonthreatening manner that does not negatively affect employee morale or relationships with managers

- communicating without patronizing

- building on the idea that healthcare employees are honest and ethical individuals

Collaborate with the business office, chief financial officer, and chief executive officer to develop mechanisms to communicate new or revised regulatory requirements or reimbursement policies in an effective and timely manner to all affected personnel to ensure coding and billing accuracy. Also, establish procedures to obtain clarification from the payer or another official source when questions arise. HIM professionals should serve as the key corporate resource for questions and clarification of health information documentation and coding requirements. Their education, background, and skills related to documentation and coding make them the logical choice to work as or with the corporate compliance officer on communicating corporate compliance to regulations, policies, and guidelines related to documentation and coding.

Disciplinary Policy and Action

According to the OIG, "an effective compliance program should include guidance regarding disciplinary action for corporate officers, managers, employees, physicians, and other healthcare professionals who have failed to comply with the healthcare organization's standards of conduct, policies and procedures, federal, state, or private payer healthcare program requirements, or federal and state laws, or those who have otherwise engaged in wrongdoing, which has the potential to impair the organization's status as a reliable, honest and trustworthy provider. The OIG believes that corporate officers, managers, supervisors, medical staff, and other healthcare professionals should be held accountable for failing to comply with, or for the foreseeable failure of their subordinates to adhere to, the applicable standards, laws, and procedures" (HHS 1998c).

The compliance program should include a written policy statement setting forth the disciplinary actions for corporate officers, managers, employees, physicians, and other healthcare professionals who fail to comply with facility standards and policies, and applicable federal and state statutes and regulations. Disciplinary actions can range from verbal warnings to suspension, revocation of privileges (pursuant to any applicable peer review procedures), termination, or financial penalties.

The written policy should specify the procedures for handling disciplinary problems and identify who will be responsible for taking appropriate action. Some disciplinary actions can be handled by department managers, whereas others may need to be resolved by administration (e.g., issues involving high-level personnel or physicians).

All employees should be subject to the same disciplinary action for committing similar offenses. It is critical to publish the written policy on improper conduct and educate officers, physicians, and employees about compliance. The consequences of noncompliance should be consistently applied and enforced. The commitment to compliance applies to all personnel levels within the organization.

HIM management personnel should collaborate with human resources, the compliance officer, and other department managers to develop policies and procedures to determine disciplinary action for managers, employees, contractors, and physicians who fail to comply with the organization's and state and federal standards. Organizational policies and procedures should cover the processes for imposing disciplinary action, including levels of authority for imposing various types of discipline, proper documentation of offenses and actions taken, protocol for reporting disciplinary actions to the compliance officer, and appropriate follow-up measures.

Ensure that all HIM contractual arrangements require the contractor to comply with the healthcare organization's standards and policies and procedures and all applicable laws and regulations. Contracts should spell out the consequences of noncompliance on the part of the contractor, including immediate termination of the contract if serious noncompliance issues occur. Educate HIM contractors on the organization's standards, policies, and procedures, and procure a signed agreement from the contractor that they will abide by these standards.

HIM staff must be educated on the organization's disciplinary policies in order to fully comprehend the consequences of noncompliance. Apply disciplinary policies consistently and fairly within each manager's area of responsibility and work with human resources, other department managers, and administration to ensure that organizational standards and state and federal laws and regulations are enforced consistently across the organization.

HIM supervisors should know how to provide proper training and oversight for their areas of responsibility, as they can be held accountable for their subordinates' noncompliance. Supervisors should be aware of their responsibilities in disciplining employees appropriately and consistently.

Incorporate the promotion of, and adherence to, the elements of the organization's compliance program into the performance evaluations of HIM managerial and supervisory staff. Evaluate whether fair and consistent disciplinary actions were taken, and whether proper training and guidance was provided to staff members. In addition, incorporate adherence to the compliance program into the performance evaluations of nonsupervisory HIM staff. Just as lack of adherence to the compliance program should have a negative impact on a performance evaluation, demonstrated commitment to the effectiveness of the compliance program (such as successful identification and resolution of a problem or implementation of process improvements to achieve accurate and complete medical record documentation) should have a positive impact.

HIM supervisors should help develop sanctions for physicians who fail to comply with the organization's or federal and state standards. This includes sanctions for failure to comply with documentation completion requirements as stipulated in medical staff bylaws, rules, and regulations. Enforcement should be consistent. Incidents of nonenforcement or inconsistent enforcement should be reported to the compliance officer. Sanctions might include revocation of clinical privileges (for serious violations) or financial penalties. Factor adherence to the applicable elements of the compliance program into the physicians' reappointment credentialing process.

Auditing and Monitoring

Auditing and monitoring an organization's operations are key to ensuring compliance and adherence to their policies and procedures. Auditing and monitoring can also identify areas of potential risk and those areas where additional education is required. All potential areas of risk and those currently identified by the OIG as targets on their work plan should be audited, including:

- DRG miscoding

- miscoded observational stays

- duplicate outpatient billings

- services billed under arrangement

- transfers billed as discharges

- 72-hour window rule

- medical necessity

- PATH

- partial hospitalization

HIM professionals can use their expertise in designing audit protocols and analyzing data to assist other departments in developing auditing and monitoring processes and evaluating the results. The HIM professional may also assist in the actual audits of other departments. HIM professionals also can use their data analysis skills to help administration and/or the corporate compliance officer analyze the findings of audit activities.

The laboratory department is an excellent area for HIM professionals to provide assistance in interpreting medical necessity requirements.

HIM professionals come in contact with information and data that span many areas. A thorough knowledge of the corporate compliance program and accrediting and regulatory requirements will let them be strong members of the organization's auditing and monitoring team. In this role, HIM professionals can help identify problems, develop creative solutions, and perform continuous monitoring.

HIM professionals may also be able to identify problems that others might not be aware of, thanks to their knowledge and exposure to much of the organization's data. For example, a coder reviewing a record might notice that organ donation forms are not being filled out correctly or consistently. This deficiency could have severe consequences; physicians need to be notified and the problem needs to be investigated and corrected. This deficiency is not something a coder needs to review in order to code the medical record, but based on their knowledge, he or she would probably notice the trend and then report it to a supervisor. Knowledge of general good record keeping, as well as knowledge of standards and guidelines, help HIM professionals pinpoint trends and errors that otherwise might go unnoticed.

Problem Resolution and Corrective Action

HIM professionals must play a major role in any corporate compliance program, including the areas of problem resolution and corrective action. By knowing what the accepted practices should be, they can identify areas in which an institution is not in compliance.

When identifying a potential problem or problematic trend, an investigation must take place to determine the seriousness and scope (see "Taking Action" below).

It is vital that an HIM professional sit on the compliance committee. The committee will no doubt discuss many topics that affect the HIM department, and an HIM representative can provide valuable insight. The HIM representative's diverse knowledge can also provide assistance in identifying problem areas and working to resolve problems. HIM professionals can also assist in performing audits to identify problems, look for solutions, and ensure that solutions are working.

All documentation related to potential problems, problem resolution, and corrective action must include a full description of the process, notes from interviews with involved individuals, copies of the guidelines, procedures, etc., and the final results of the investigation. The corporate compliance officer should maintain documentation. HIM professionals should assist in the appropriate storage of these documents, as recovery in the event of an external audit is vital.

Conclusion

Given HIM professionals' training, skills, and commitment to professional ethics, their contribution to the development and implementation of the corporate compliance program is invaluable. HIM professionals should demonstrate their value in corporate compliance by proactively providing information on their capabilities related to each of the seven steps and by providing current information on government initiatives to administration. Develop and implement an HIM compliance program to demonstrate your abilities to top-level management.

When developing and implementing a corporate compliance program, remember that the OIG recognizes the establishment of an effective compliance program. The OIG views it as a sincere effort by the healthcare provider to comply with applicable state and federal standards.

Use existing quality monitoring programs, policies, procedures, education program schedules, etc. to reduce the amount of time and effort needed to develop your HIM or corporate compliance program. The key is not the size of the program manual, but the success it achieves in ensuring compliance through outcomes and ongoing refinement of the processes.

Taking Action

If a routine coding quality audit shows a pattern of coding errors, the HIM professional should take the following action:

- have another HIM professional review the records to verify the existence of the coding problem, and, based on guidelines, verify that the coding practice was truly improper

- notify the compliance committee (or other group, based on organizational structure) of the problem and state that the problem is being investigated

- once approval from the compliance committee and/or the organization's legal counsel is obtained, expand the record sample to include a larger population, in order to determine the true extent of the problem, the number of coders involved, and the number of records

- once the extent of the problem is determined, immediately educate coders (or other staff) to obliterate the problem. Revise procedures to prevent recurrence and take disciplinary action when appropriate

- identify the source of the problem. Document the reason for the error, along with the corrective action taken, in the event of an external audit

- consult legal counsel and report the problem to the payer(s) if advised to do so. In the event of overpayment, work with the business office to ensure immediate refunds

- perform an additional audit within a few months to ensure resolution of the problem. Perform more expansive audits into other potential problem areas to ensure overall coding compliance

Resources

Department of Health and Human Services. 1998a. *Compliance Program Guidance for Home Health Agencies.* Available at http://www.oig.hhs.gov/authorities/docs/cpghome.pdf.

Department of Health and Human Services. 1998b. *Compliance Program Guidance for Hospitals.* Available at http://www.oig.hhs.gov/authorities/docs/cpghosp.pdf.

Department of Health and Human Services. 1998c. *Compliance Program Guidance for Third-Party Medical Billing Companies.* Available at http://oig.hhs.gov/fraud/docs/complianceguidance/thirdparty.pdf

Journal of AHIMA, January 1998 and January 1999 issues

Prophet, Sue. *Health Information Management Compliance—A Model Program for Healthcare Organizations.* Chicago, IL: AHIMA, 1998.

United States Sentencing Commission Guidelines, *Guidelines Manual,* 8A1.2. 2004. Available at http://www.ussc.gov/2004guid/TABCON04.htm.

Prepared by

AHIMA's Compliance Task Force:

Cheryl Hammen, ART (chair, Compliance Task Force)
Gloryanne Bryant, ART, CCS
Rachel Driggs, MBA, RRA
Kathleen Frawley, JD, MS, RRA
Sister M. Nika Lee, RRA
Susan Manning, JD, RRA
Denisha Torres, RRA
LaVonne Wieland, ART
Sue Prophet, RRA, CCS (staff liaison)

AHIMA Practice Briefs

Developing a Coding Compliance Policy Document

Organizations using diagnosis and procedure codes for reporting healthcare services must have formal policies and corresponding procedures in place that provide instruction on the entire process—from the point of service to the billing statement or claim form. Coding compliance policies serve as a guide to performing coding and billing functions and provide documentation of the organization's intent to correctly report services. The policies should include facility-specific documentation requirements, payer regulations and policies, and contractual arrangements for coding consultants and outsourcing services. This information may be covered in payer/provider contracts or found in Medicare and Medicaid manuals and bulletins.

Following are selected tenets that address the process of code selection and reporting. These tenets may be referred to as coding protocols, a coding compliance program, organizational coding guidelines, or a similar name. These tenets are an important part of any organization's compliance plan and the key to preventing coding errors and resulting reimbursement problems. Examples are taken from both outpatient and inpatient coding processes for illustration purposes only. This document cannot serve as a complete coding compliance plan, but will be useful as a guide for creating a more comprehensive resource to meet individual organizational needs.

A coding compliance plan should include the following components:

- A general policy statement about the commitment of the organization to correctly assign and report codes

    Example: Memorial Medical Center is committed to establishing and maintaining clinical coding and insurance claims processing procedures to ensure that reported codes reflect actual services provided, through accurate information system entries.

- The source of the official coding guidelines used to direct code selection

    Example: ICD-9-CM code selection follows the Official Guidelines for Coding and Reporting, developed by the cooperating parties and documented in Coding Clinic for ICD-9-CM, published by the American Hospital Association.

> **Example:** CPT code selection follows the guidelines set forth in the CPT manual and in CPT Assistant, published by the American Medical Association.

- The parties responsible for code assignment. The ultimate responsibility for code assignment lies with the physician (provider). However, policies and procedures may document instances where codes may be selected or modified by authorized individuals

  > **Example:** For inpatient records, medical record analyst I staff are responsible for analysis of records and assignment of the correct ICD-9-CM codes based on documentation by the attending physician.

  > **Example:** Emergency department evaluation and management levels for physician services will be selected by the physician and validated by outpatient record analysts using the HCFA/AMA documentation guidelines. When a variance occurs, the following steps are taken for resolution. (The actual document should follow with procedure details.)

- The procedure to follow when the clinical information is not clear enough to assign the correct code

  > **Example:** When the documentation used to assign codes is ambiguous or incomplete, the physician must be contacted to clarify the information and complete/amend the record, if necessary. (The actual document should follow with details of how the medical staff would like this to occur, e.g., by phone call, by note on the record, etc.) Standard protocols for adding documentation to a record must be followed in accordance with the applicable laws and regulations.

- Specify the policies and procedures that apply to specific locations and care settings. Official coding guidelines for inpatient reporting and outpatient/physician reporting are different. This means that if you are developing a facility-specific coding guideline for emergency department services, designate that the coding rules or guidelines only apply in this setting

  > **Example:** When reporting an injection of a drug provided in the emergency department to a Medicare beneficiary, the appropriate CPT code for the administration of the injection is reported in addition to the evaluation and management service code and drug code. CPT codes are reported whether a physician provides the injection personally or a nurse is carrying out a physician's order. This instruction does not always apply for reporting of professional services in the clinics, because administration of medication is considered bundled with the corresponding evaluation and management service for Medicare patients.

  > **Example:** Diagnoses that are documented as "probable," "suspected," "questionable," "rule-out," or "working diagnosis" are not to have a code assigned as a confirmed diagnosis. Instead, the code for the condition established at the close of the encounter should be assigned, such as a symptom, sign, abnormal test result, or clinical finding. This guideline applies only to outpatient services.

- Applicable reporting requirements required by specific agencies. The document should include where instructions on payer-specific requirements may be accessed

  > **Example:** For patients with XYZ care plan, report code S0800 for patients having a LASIK procedure rather than an unlisted CPT code.

  > **Example:** For Medicare patients receiving a wound closure by tissue adhesive only, report HCPCS Level II code G0168 rather than a CPT code.

Many of these procedures will be put into software databases and would not be written as a specific policy. This is true with most billing software, whether for physician services or through the charge description master used by many hospitals.

- Procedures for correction of inaccurate code assignments in the clinical database and to the agencies where the codes have been reported

  Example: When an error in code assignment is discovered after bill release and the claim has already been submitted, this is the process required to update and correct the information system and facilitate claim amendment or correction. (The actual document should follow with appropriate details.)

- Areas of risk that have been identified through audits or monitoring. Each organization should have a defined audit plan for code accuracy and consistency review and corrective actions should be outlined for problems that are identified

  Example: A hospital might identify that acute respiratory failure is being assigned as the principal diagnosis with congestive heart failure as a secondary diagnosis. The specific reference to Coding Clinic could be listed with instructions about correct coding of these conditions and the process to be used to correct the deficiency.

- Identification of essential coding resources available to and used by the coding professionals

  Example: Updated ICD-9-CM, CPT, and HCPCS Level II code books are used by all coding professionals. Even if the hospital uses automated encoding software, at least one printed copy of the coding manuals should be available for reference.

  Example: Updated encoder software, including the appropriate version of the NCCI edits and DRG and APC grouper software, is available to the appropriate personnel.

  Example: Coding Clinic and CPT Assistant are available to all coding professionals.

- A process for coding new procedures or unusual diagnoses

  Example: When the coding professional encounters an unusual diagnosis, the coding supervisor or the attending physician is consulted. If, after research, a code cannot be identified, the documentation is submitted to the AHA for clarification.

- A procedure to identify any optional codes gathered for statistical purposes by the facility and clarification of the appropriate use of E codes

  Example: All ICD-9-CM procedure codes in the surgical range (ICD-9-CM Volume III codes 01.01-86.99) shall be reported for inpatients. In addition, codes reported from the nonsurgical section include the following. (Completed document should list the actual codes to be reported.)

  Example: All appropriate E codes for adverse effects of drugs must be reported. In addition, this facility reports all E codes, including the place of injury for poisonings, all cases of abuse, and all accidents on the initial visit for both inpatient and outpatient services.

- Appropriate methods for resolving coding or documentation disputes with physicians

  Example: When the physician disagrees with official coding guidelines, the case is referred to the medical records committee following review by the designated physician liaison from that group.

- A procedure for processing claim rejections

  Example: All rejected claims pertaining to diagnosis and procedure codes should be returned to coding staff for review or correction. Any chargemaster issues should be forwarded to appropriate departmental staff for corrections. All clinical codes, including modifiers, must never be changed or added without review by coding staff with access to the appropriate documentation.

  Example: If a claim is rejected due to the codes provided in the medical record abstract, the billing department notifies the supervisor of coding for a review rather than changing the code to a payable code and resubmitting the claim.

- A statement clarifying that codes will not be assigned, modified, or excluded solely for the purpose of maximizing reimbursement. Clinical codes will not be changed or amended merely due to either physicians' or patients' request to have the service in question covered by insurance. If the initial code assignment did not reflect the actual services, codes may be revised based on supporting documentation. Disputes with either physicians or patients are handled only by the coding supervisor and are appropriately logged for review

  Example: A patient calls the business office saying that her insurance carrier did not pay for her mammogram. After investigating, the HIM coding staff discover that the coding was appropriate for a screening mammogram and that this is a noncovered service with the insurance provider. The code is not changed and the matter is referred back to the business office for explanation to the patient that she should contact her insurance provider with any dispute over coverage of service.

  Example: Part of a payment is denied and after review, the supervisor discovers that a modifier should have been appended to the CPT code to denote a separately identifiable service. Modifier –25 is added to the code set and the corrected claim is resubmitted.

  Example: A physician approaches the coding supervisor with a request to change the diagnosis codes for his patient because what she currently has is a pre-existing condition that is not covered by her current health plan. The coding supervisor must explain to the physician that falsification of insurance claims is illegal. If the physician insists, the physician liaison for the medical record committee is contacted and the matter is turned over to that committee for resolution if necessary.

- The use of and reliance on encoders within the organization. Coding staff cannot rely solely on computerized encoders. Current coding manuals must be readily accessible and the staff must be educated appropriately to detect inappropriate logic or errors in encoding software. When errors in logic or code crosswalks are discovered, they are reported to the vendor immediately by the coding supervisor

  Example: During the coding process, an error is identified in the crosswalk between the ICD-9-CM Volume III code and the CPT code. This error is reported to the software vendor, with proper documentation and notification of all staff using the encoder to not rely on the encoder for code selection.

- Medical records are analyzed and codes selected only with complete and appropriate documentation by the physician available. According to coding guidelines, codes are not assigned without physician documentation. If records are coded without the discharge summary or final diagnostic statements available, processes are in place for review after the summary is added to the record

Example: When records are coded without a discharge summary, they are flagged in the computer system. When the summaries are added to the record, the record is returned to the coding professional for review of codes. If there are any inconsistencies, appropriate steps are taken for review of the changes.

Additional Elements

A coding compliance document should include a reference to the AHIMA Standards of Ethical Coding, which can be downloaded from AHIMA's Web site at www.ahima.org. Reference to the data quality assessment procedures must be included in a coding compliance plan to establish the mechanism for determining areas of risk. Reviews will identify the need for further education and increased monitoring for those areas where either coding variances or documentation deficiencies are identified.

Specific and detailed coding guidelines that cover the reporting of typical services provided by a facility or organization create tools for data consistency and reliability by ensuring that all coders interpret clinical documentation and apply coding principles in the same manner. The appropriate medical staff committee should give final approval of any coding guidelines that involve clinical criteria to assure appropriateness and physician consensus on the process.

The format is most useful when organized by patient or service type and easily referenced by using a table of contents. If the facility-specific guidelines are maintained electronically, they should be searchable by key terms. Placing the coding guidelines on a facility intranet or internal computer network is a very efficient way to ensure their use and it also enables timely and efficient updating and distribution. Inclusion of references to or live links should be provided to supporting documents such as Uniform Hospital Discharge Data Sets or other regulatory requirements outlining reporting procedures or code assignments.

AHIMA Coding Practice Team. Practice Brief: Developing a Coding Compliance Policy Document. *Journal of AHIMA* 72, no.7 (2001): 88A–C.

Appendix G

Sample Audit Tools, Forms, and Worksheets

COMPLIANCE AUDIT WORKSHEET

Record #: _____ Staff: _____

Manager: _____ **Mandatory Return Date:** _____

The above record was reviewed for billing and documentation compliance and the following problems were found:

_____ Activity code error _____

_____ Activity not on report of services ☐ (Submit log)

Specify activity as documented in record (date & type of service)

_____

_____ Incorrect CPT code   State code & type of service_____

_____

_____ Missing or incorrect documentation of activity billed

Specify date & type of problem (missing note, incomplete, unsigned, no credentials, incorrect date, and so on)

☐ (addendum note accepted if within legitimate time frame) _____

_____

_____ No valid treatment plan   State date of last plan: _____

Dates of services provided beyond valid dates

_____

_____ Documentation in progress notes do not match interventions on the treatment plan. (Specify problem)

_____

_____ Incorrect diagnosis or diagnosis code   State code and diagnosis _____

_____

_____ Incorrect Social Security #

_____ Other: _____

_____   _____
Reviewer's initials   Date of Review

To Be Completed by Supervisor

Please review these issues with staff and document action taken below.

_____ Corrective action plan (**must check one**) _____ Level one _____ Level two _____ Level three

Specify disciplinary action (verbal, written, and so on) and any remediation plans:

_____

Any additional comments

_____

_____ Date corrective action completed

Signature: Staff _____

Signature: Supervisor _____

To Be Completed by QI Department

Further follow-up required: ___ Y ___ N

If yes, specify:_____

Fiscal Office Response (if necessary) _____

_____
Fiscal Staff Signature/Date

_____   _____
QI Staff Signature/Date   Date Follow-up Completed

REVERSE AUDIT

HI Staff Reviewer _____

Date Reviewed _____

Audit Time Period _____

Client Number	Program RU	Primary Diagnosis	Description of Service Billed	Documentation Required—check the required document(s) for billing								
				ES Assessment	Intake Assessment	Treatment Plan	Clinical Review	Annual Assessment Update	Five Year Assessment	Psych Evaluation	Progress Note	Doc. Consist. w/Billing (Y or N)

Source: South Shore Mental Health Center, Inc.

CLINICAL RECORD REVIEW	Client Name: _____
	Client Number: _____

ASSESSMENT	
• Does the assessment contain all components written or rewritten within the past 5 years?	
• Was each of the eight required components of the assessment written or reviewed within the last year and does it clinically reflect the year's events?	

TREATMENT PLAN	
• Is there a current comprehensive Treatment Plan?	
—Are the goals listed on the Problem Index?	
—Is it based on the most recent assessment?	
—Are the goals specific to the problem?	
—Are the objectives stated in specific and measurable terms?	
• Do the interventions include frequency of services?	
• Are there functional strengths/weaknesses identified?	
• Do the client's symptoms and the recommended interventions bear a clear relationship to the DSM diagnosis?	
• Do the discharge criteria reflect each goal to be met and the specific needs of the program/client?	

CLINICAL REVIEW	
• Does the current Clinical Review reflect the past 6 months events?	
• Has the Treatment Plan been either reviewed or completely rewritten at least every six months and does it clinically reflect the past events?	
• Has the Treatment Plan been reviewed at the following intervals:	
—Upon identification of any major change in the client's *clinical* condition?	
—Upon the achievement of an identified goal(s)?	
• Does the Clinical Review contain an assessment of the individual's current clinical problems/needs? The individual's response to treatment?	

PROGRESS NOTES	
• Do the Progress Notes:	
—Reflect the needs identified in the assessment?	
—Reflect the goals identified in the Treatment Plan?	
—Reflect a professional assessment made by the writer as to why the interventions prescribed *are* or *are not* working?	
—Explain any deviations from the interventions prescribed in the Treatment Plan?	
—Document the response of the client to treatment?	
—Describe the overall outcome of treatment?	
—Avoid being excessively narrative in nature?	
—All white space crossed out?	
—Indicate family/significant other participation?	
—Are they legible?	

CLINICIAN SIGNATURE: _____	DATE: _____
SUPERVISOR/MANAGER SIGNATURE: _____	DATE: _____

Source: South Shore Mental Health Center, Inc.

Month/Year: _____

OUTSTANDING TREATMENT PLAN REPORT

Program	# of Clients With Treatment Plans Due	# of Clients with Outstanding Treatment Plans	# of Clients Who Received Services Outside the Window	Error Rate*	# of Events Outside the Window by Doctor	# of Events Outside the Window by Clinician	Client Contact with Doctor, Clinician, or Both
ES							
OPS							
Addictions							
Elderly							
Psych Only (Children's)							
CIS							
CST A							
CST B							
CAFS							
MTT I							
MTT II							
Residential							
ISMT							
TOTAL							

* Error Rate: Computed by # of Overdue Treatment Plans (Outside the Window) ÷ # of Treatment Plans Due.

Recommend: Annual test of the tracking system on 100% of client treatment plans due in the given month. Any program 5% or less requires no further testing until next annual. Programs resulting in 6% or more will continue to be audited until 5% or less is achieved.

Client Name: _____

Client Number: _____

To: _____

Reviewer Name: _____

Date Reviewed: _____

ADULT DISPOSITION CHART REVIEW

TOPIC	YES	NO	N/A
Health Questionnaire			
History of Clinical High-Risk Behaviors			
Assessment			
Assessment more than 5 years old			
Annual Assessment Update			
Psychopharmacologic Evaluation			
CSP Checklist			
IUR			
ROI signed for past/current treatment providers			
Consent signed			
FOR INTERNAL TRANSFERS ONLY	YES	NO	N/A
MPI			
Master Treatment Plan completed yearly			
Master Treatment Plan Addendum w/in 30 days of Dispo in lieu of full MTP (see Dispo progress note)			
Clinical Review within 6 months of Treatment Plan			
Cleared for disposition			

Other Comments: _____

_____

If corrections have been made, sign below and return this form with the chart to the disposition basket.

_____   _____
Program Manager or Clinician Signature   Date

Client Name: _____

Client Number: _____

To: _____

Reviewer Name: _____

Date Reviewed: _____

CHILDREN'S DISPOSITION CHART REVIEW

TOPIC	YES	NO	N/A
Health Questionnaire			
History of Clinical High-Risk Behaviors			
Assessment			
Assessment more than 5 years old			
Annual Assessment Update			
Psychopharmacologic Evaluation			
IUR			
ROI signed for past/current treatment providers			
Copy of DCYF 004 (foster) or DCYF ROI and DCYF staff ID			
Consent Form signed			
FOR INTERNAL TRANSFERS ONLY	**YES**	**NO**	**N/A**
MPI			
Master Treatment Plan completed yearly			
Clinical Review within 3/6/9 months of Treatment Plan			
Cleared for disposition			

Other Comments: _____

_____

If corrections have been made, sign below and return this form with the chart to the disposition basket.

_____   _____

Program Manager or Clinician Signature   Date

Client Name: _____

Client Number: _____

To: _____

Reviewer Name: _____

Date Reviewed: _____

OUTPATIENT SERVICES CHART REVIEW

TOPIC	YES	NO	N/A
Health Questionnaire			
Initial Intake			
Assessment more than 5 years old			
Annual Assessment Update with all 8 areas			
Psychopharmacologic Evaluation			
CSP Checklist			
CARA			
MPI (dates match treatment plan)			
Treatment Plan completed yearly			
Treatment Plan signed by client If not, progress note documenting refusal			
Treatment Plan signed by Licensed Practitioner of the Healing Arts			
Progress Note documenting client involvement in the treatment plan creation			
Clinical signed by client			
Clinical signed by Licensed Practitioner of the Healing Arts			
Progress notes in DAP/SOAP with problem numbers, date, and duration			
Signed with credentials			
Consent Form			

Other Comments: _____

_____

Please make corrections and return this form to the Reviewed by:

_____   _____
                  Clinician Signature   Date

_____   _____
              Program Manager Signature   Date

EVALUATION AND MANAGEMENT AUDIT TOOL

History
Chief Complaint: Required

History of Present Illness:

Location   Quality   Duration   Timing   Context   Modifiers   S&S

Total: _____

1–3 = Problem/Expanded problem focused.   4 or more elements = Detailed/Comprehensive.

Review of Systems:

Constitutional	CV	GU	Neuro	Hema/lymph
Eyes	Resp	MS	Psych	Allergy/Immuno
ENT	GI	Ekin	Endo	

Total: _____

---

0 elements = Problem focused.   1 = Expanded problem focused.   2–9 = Detailed.   10 = Comprehensive.

Past Family & Social History:

Personal Past History   Family History   Social History   **Total:** _____

---

0 elements = Problem/Expanded problem focused.   1 = Detailed.   3 = Comprehensive.

Examination:

Appearance _____	Insight _____	Memory _____	Speech _____
Fund of Knowledge Associations _____	Judgment _____	Mood/Affect _____	Thought Process _____
	Constitutional _____	Language _____	Orientation _____
Attention Span _____	Abnormal/Psychotic Thoughts _____	Muscoskeletal _____	

1–5 elements = Problem focused.   6 or more elements = Expanded problem focused.   0 = Detailed.
All elements = Comprehensive.

Medical Decision Making:

	1	2	3	4
# of Diagnoses	Minimal	Limited	Multiple	Extensive
Amount/Complexity of Data to be reviewed	None or Minimal	Limited	Moderate	Extensive
Risk of Complication Morbidity or Mortality	Minimal	Low	Moderate	High

---

The documentation supports _____ level of E/M service.

Teaching Physicians:

TP physically present & documents present during one key component of service   Yes   No

---

Psychotherapy:

Time _____	Whom Present _____	Type of Psychotherapy _____
Issue Discussed _____	Patient Response _____	Counseling _____
Recommendations _____	Medication Change _____	Risk and Benefits _____

Comments:

Pocket Guides

(Front)

Butler Hospital E/M Pocket Guide for Psychiatry			
History Elements			
Type of History	HPI	ROS	PFSH
Problem	Brief 1–3	N/A	N/A
Expanded	Brief 1–3	N/A	N/A
Detailed	Extended 4+	Extended 2–9	Problem 1
Comprehensive	Extended 4+	Complete 10	Complete 3
Medical Decision Making			
Decision Making	Straightforward/Low	Moderate	High
# of diagnoses	Minimal (1–2)	Multiple (3)	Extensive (4+)
Amount of data to review	Minimal (1–2)	Multiple (3)	Extensive (4+)
Management Options	Low	Moderate	High

(Back)

Hospitalization CPT Codes

Initial Care		Subsequent Care	
99251	DH, DE, LM	99231	PH, PE, LM
99222	CH, CE, XM	99232	ExH, ExE, LM
99223	CH, CE, HM	99233	DH, DE, HM

Abbreviation Table for CPT Codes

L—Low
X—Moderate
H—High

P—Problem
Ex—Expanded
D—Detailed
C—Comprehensive

H—History
E—Mental Status Exam
M—Medical Decision Making

Single Organ System Exam for Psychiatry

Abnormal/Psychotic thoughts
Appearance
Associations
Attention Span/ Concentration
Constitutional
Fund of Knowledge
Insight
Judgement
Language
Memory
Mood and affect
Muscoskeletal
Orientation
Speech
Thought Processes

Problem focused-1–5 elements
Expanded-6–8 elements
Detailed-9 elements
Comprehensive-All the elements

Psychiatric CPT Codes

(Front)   **(Back)**

PSYCHIATRIC CPT CODES
Types of Psychotherapy
Insight-Oriented Behavior Modifying
and Supportive

*90801	Psychiatric diagnosis interview
90804	Ind. Psychotherapy 20–30 min.
**90805	Ind. Psy. 20–30 min. w/ E&M
90806	Ind. Psychotherapy 45–50 min.
**90807	Ind. Psy. 45–50 minutes w/ E&M
*90808	Ind. Psychotherapy 75–80 min.
**90809	Ind. Psy. 75–80 min. w/ E&M
90847	Family Therapy 45–50 min. w/ Pt.
90846	Family Psychotherapy w/o Pt.
90862	Medication Management
90870	ECT Psychiatric
90899	Unlisted Psy. service/procedure
90853	Group Therapy

* Only once in a treatment episode

** E&M elements required in documentation

CPT Consultation Codes

Written request required from the attending;
One initial consult by consultant per admit.

INPATIENT		OUTPATIENT	
99251	PH, PE, LM	99241	PH, PE, LM
99252	ExH, ExE, LM	99242	ExH, ExE, LM
99253	DH, DE, LM	99243	DH, DE, LM
99254	CH, CE, HM	99244	CH, CE, HM
99255	CH, CE, HM	99245	CH, CE, HM

Guideline and Documentation Tips

Face to Face with the patient
(OP) Unit/Floor (IP)

- Anyone can take history
  (follow-up documentation review)
- Elaborate on all aspects of exam
  (abnormal and normal)
- Refer to other documentation in your notes
  (date & time)
- Condition improving, stable, or worsening
- Treatment regimen, sign, date, and time notes

Appendix G

Appendix G

Audit form from the Rhode Island Medicaid office

MEDICAID RECORD SCORING WORKSHEET

Case #: _____   Client Type: CSP _____ GOP _____

Agency: _____   Date: _____

Reviewer's Name and Degree: _____

Use the following scoring guideline for questions utilizing the 1–4 rating scale unless a separate scale is provided with the question:

1 **Compliance:** In compliance with requirements of item between 85 percent and 100 percent of the time.

2 **Substantial compliance:** In compliance with requirements of item between 70 percent and 84 percent of the time.

3 **Partial compliance:** In compliance with requirements of item between 50 percent and 69 percent of the time.

4 **Noncompliance:** In compliance with requirements of item less than 50 percent of the time.

NA **Not applicable:** Item does not apply to record in question. Rarely used.

Please clarify all items graded 2, 3, or 4 in the "Comments" section of the item.

---

1. Does the record contain a section(s) designated as an assessment of the client's clinical needs? . . . . Y   N
    If "Yes," continue with Item #2. If "No," skip ahead to Item #3.
    Comments: _____
    _____

Use the following scale for Questions #2a and #2b only.

1. Comprehensively lists strengths, weaknesses, and problems.
2. Briefly documents assessment results; would benefit from expansion/clarification.
3. States that assessment was written (2a)/reviewed(2b) but provides inadequate documentation of results.
4. No assessment or documentation that a review was done in this area.

Suggested Content of Individual Components of Assessment:

Psychological:	History, diagnosis, diagnostic formulation, treatment, presenting problem, behavior, affect, mood, mental status if needed, neurological examination if indicated.
Psychosocial:	Functioning, supports, community resources used, environment, leisure activity, cultural, additional functional assessments if required.
Physical:	Physical health review, including listing of current medications and problems, to identify if further medical examination is indicated.
Vocational/Educational:	History, potential for employment/additional education.

2a. Does the assessment contain each of the following components *written or rewritten* within the *past 60 months?*

	Compliance		Noncompliance		Most Recent
Psychological (Behavioral/Emotional)	1	2	3	4	_____
Psychosocial (Environment/Family)	1	2	3	4	_____
Physical (Developmental/Medical)	1	2	3	4	_____
Vocational/Educational (if indicated) . . . . NA	1	2	3	4	_____

2b. Was each of the following components of the assessment either written or reviewed within the last year or, if the client has been discharged, within 12 months prior to the date of discharge?

	Compliance		Noncompliance		Most Recent
Psychological (Behavioral/Emotional)	1	2	3	4	_____
Psychosocial (Environment/Family)	1	2	3	4	_____
Physical (Developmental/Medical)	1	2	3	4	_____
Vocational/Educational (if indicated) . . . . NA	1	2	3	4	_____

Scoring Note: Assessments from other agencies may be used to meet the requirements of these items.

Comments: _____
_____

424

Audit form from the Rhode Island Medicaid office (Continued)

3. Is there a **current** (i.e. written or rewritten *within 12 months* prior to survey date *or,* if the client has been discharged, within 12 months prior to the date of discharge), comprehensive **treatment plan**? . . . . Y   N

    Date of *most recent* treatment plan (MM/DD/YY): _____

    Scoring Note: A preliminary treatment plan will suffice only up to the *4th visit or 30 days after intake,* whichever comes first.

    Comments: _____
    _____

** COMPLETE ITEMS 4–18 ONLY IF THERE IS A *CURRENT* TREATMENT PLAN AS DEFINED ABOVE **
Use The Following Scale For Item 4 Only

1. The treatment plan was reviewed within the last 6 months, and every 6 months within the past year, with the results of the review either entered on the treatment plan itself, as a supplement to the treatment plan, or in a detailed progress note referenced in the treatment plan which is clearly labeled "treatment plan review." The review is comprehensive and updates problem statements, goals, treatment objectives, and evaluates treatment efficiency and effectiveness.

2. The plan was reviewed within the required time frame but not labeled/referenced correctly; or doesn't update problem statements, goals, or treatment objectives; or doesn't evaluate treatment efficiency and effectiveness.

3. The plan was reviewed within the required time frame but documentation is insufficient, e.g., extremely brief or limited to a statement that the plan was reviewed with no further supporting documentation.

4. The plan was not reviewed within the required time frame.

NA It has not been six months since the plan was originally written.

In all cases, please list the review date(s) meeting the requirements. A plan shall be judged to be in compliance with the "6-month review" requirement if it is reviewed within 30 days of the end of the calendar month during which the "sixth month of treatment" occurs. For example, a treatment plan written on either January 1 or January 31 would be due for a review by July 31 but would be found in compliance with the review requirement if it was completed by August 30. That same plan would still be due for a complete re-write on January 31. Once again, however, the 30-day window will allow the agency until March 2 to complete it.

4. Has the treatment plan been either reviewed or completely rewritten at least every six months?. . . . . NA   1   2   3   4
    (Mark NA *only* if this is an *initial* treatment plan written within the last six months.)
    List dates that fulfill the six month review requirement during the past year (MM/DD/YY): _____
    Comments: _____
    _____

---

5. Is the treatment plan/treatment plan review signed *and* dated by a licensed practitioner of the healing arts, as defined in the Community Mental Health Medicaid Procedure Manual, with the practitioner's qualifying degree/title clearly indicated? . . . . Y   N

    Scoring Note: The plan requires that the signature, degree *and* date be present. The plan must also be signed *within two weeks* of its effective date. Grade this item as "N" if any 1 of these 4 requirements is not met. Note that a treatment plan for an MHPRR client requires a *physician's* signature and degree. Use "Comment" section below to detail all records marked "N."

    Detail: ___ Signed/dated outside of two-week window   ___ missing date   ___ missing degree   ___ missing signature
    Comments: _____
    _____

Use The Following Scale For Item 6 Only

1. The diagnosis, goals, and objectives in the treatment plan accurately reflect the current problems and needs as listed in the current assessment.

2. The plan accurately reflects most of the priority problems related to the diagnosis and/or described in the assessment

3. Priority problems that are addressed in the treatment plan are not on the assessment, or priority problems identified elsewhere in the record are not addressed in the plan and/or assessment.

4. The treatment plan is not based on the assessment or there is no assessment.

6. Is the current treatment plan based on the most recent assessment? 1   2   3   4
    Comments: _____
    _____

(Continued on next page)

Audit form from the Rhode Island Medicaid office (Continued)

7. If this is an *initial* treatment plan, was the plan formulated upon completion of the intake process and as soon as possible after the patient's admission? (Score "NA," if this is not an initial plan). . . . . Y   N   NA

   Scoring Note: The treatment plan must have been formulated when clinical information became available and as soon as possible after the client's admission into the program. A preliminary treatment plan will suffice *up to the fourth visit or 30 days after intake,* which ever comes first.

   Comments: _____

   _____

8. Has the treatment plan been reviewed at the following intervals? (circle *one* answer per item)

	Compliance		Noncompliance	
a. Upon transfer between treatment programs.	NA 1		2 3	4
b. Upon any major change in the client's *clinical* condition (i.e. when there has been a significant improvement or decline).	NA 1		2 3	4
c. Upon the achievement of an identified goal (i.e. when goals are meet, discontinued)	NA 1		2 3	4
d. At the end of the estimated length of treatment (i.e. at the target date in the plan)	NA 1		2 3	4

   Scoring Notes: Reviewers should take into account both the *periodicity* and the *quality* of the review. With regard to quality, a good review should document the reason for the review; comment on the client's clinical condition; comment on the results of treatment to date; and both document and justify any changes made to the plan. A simple statement to the effect that "this plan was reviewed on (date) should be graded as a "3."

   Comments: _____

   _____

9. Is there clear evidence in all treatment plan reviews that the reviews are based on:

	Compliance		Noncompliance	
a. An assessment of the individual's current clinical problems/needs?	NA 1		2 3	4
b. The individual's response to treatment? (the outcome of care provided, to what extent were goals reached)	NA 1		2 3	4
c. The overall activity recorded in the progress notes?	NA 1		2 3	4

   Scoring Notes: Reviews must reflect changes in the client's condition, whether the prescribed interventions have been effective or not, and any other pertinent information contained in the progress notes.

   Mark "NA" if there are no reviews contained in the plan.

   Comments: _____

   _____

Use The Following Scale For Items 10a–10c Only

1. Identifies problems/strengths/limitations; behavior oriented; client-focused; individualized to patient; notes severity/impact on life.
2. Items are addressed in the plan but in a brief, generalized manner. Possibly not readily identifiable or clearly documented.
3. Vague or missing major components.
4. No documentation of element at all.

10. Does the treatment plan contain a *clear* indication of the client's:

	Compliance		Noncompliance	
a. Clinical needs/Condition?.	1	2	3	4
b. Functional strengths?	1	2	3	4
c. Limitations?.	1	2	3	4

   Scoring Note: Award a "1" if the items in 10d below are behaviorally focused and clearly describe for each activity, the type of session, treatment methods and procedures.

d. Prescribed services, activities, and programs?	1	2	3	4

   Comments: _____

   _____

Audit form from the Rhode Island Medicaid office (Continued)

11. Does the treatment plan contain a clearly visible DSM-IV diagnosis, *both* written *and* coded?
(Answer "N" if not shown *both* written and coded.). . . . . Y   N
Comments: _____

_____

12. Do the client's symptoms and the recommended interventions bear a clear relationship to the
DSM-IV diagnosis?. 1   2   3   4

Scoring Note Award a "1" only if the client's listed diagnosis is supported by a description of symptoms, other needs and problems which reflect same *and* if the interventions prescribed address the priority behavioral symptoms in relationship to that diagnosis.

Comments: _____

_____

Use The Following Scale For Item 13 Only

1. Contains specific goals/targets that the client must achieve to attain, maintain and/or reestablish emotional and/or physical health, as well as maximum growth and adaptive capabilities. Similar needs identified in the assessment may be grouped and addressed by a single goal that encompasses the entire group.

2. Contains general goals, possibly excessive in number, most of which are reflective of the client's problem and specified treatment regimen.

3. Vague, generalized goals, most of which are not reflective of the client's problem(s) or specified treatment regimen.

4. No goals or goals are not related to the client's problems or treatment regimen.

13. Does the treatment plan clearly indicate specific goals that the patient must achieve during the
course of treatment?. 1   2   3   4
Comments: _____

_____

14. Are the goals in the treatment plan clearly based on the most recent assessment? 1   2   3   4

Scoring Note: Score a "1" only if the plan contains goals that clearly and accurately reflect current problems and needs as listed in the current assessment.

Comments: _____

_____

15. Does the treatment plan contain individualized and realistic objectives for treatment that provide:

Measurable indexes of progress (both individualized and measurable in steps of progress) 1   2   3   4

A projected date of achievement 1   2   3   4

The recommended frequency for each specific treatment procedure. 1   2   3   4

The criteria to be met for terminating specific interventions? (behavioral objective of treatment) 1   2   3   4

Scoring Note: Objectives must be both individualized and current in all cases. They should also be behaviorally focused as well as being specific and measurable. All recommended interventions must have their frequency and duration specified. As an example, the recommendation of "Cognitive & behavioral therapy, aimed at control of inappropriate outbursts, once a week for the next three months, or until the client can attend psychiatric rehabilitation for 3 consecutive days without an outburst, whichever comes first" would meet all criteria.

Comments: _____

_____

16. Does the treatment plan clearly and specifically contain the criteria to be met for terminating the
treatment program? . . . . Y   N

Scoring Note: Answer "Y" only if plan contains specific, individualized criteria for termination of the treatment program which reflects the achievement of the individual's treatment plan goals.

Comments: _____

_____

(Continued on next page)

Audit form from the Rhode Island Medicaid office (Continued)

Use The Following Scale For Item 17 Only	

1. The record documents consistent and adequate efforts to gain the individual's participation in the development of the treatment plans. While this may include a statement signed by the client to the effect that they participated in the development of the plan, a signature alone does not necessarily document the degree of involvement and/or understanding of the planning process.

2. Signed statement by client acknowledging participation in the planning process but no other documentation available.

3. Signed statement by client agreeing to the plan itself but not acknowledging participation.

4. No client participation documented.

---

17. Has the client had the opportunity to participate in the development of the treatment plan as evidenced by specific documentation in the clinical record? 1   2   3   4

    Scoring Note: Score a "1" on this item if you judge that the agency made adequate efforts, well-documented in the medical record, to engage the client in the planning process even if those efforts were not successful.

    Comments: _____

    _____

---

18. Are referrals for services not provided directly by the agency, when required by the client's condition, clearly documented?. . . . . Y   N   NA

    Scoring Note: The treatment plan must include referrals for needed services that are not directly provided by the facility and, if possible, progress notes for those services. Answer "NA" if no referrals were needed.

    Comments: _____

    _____

---

19. Does the client record contain progress notes? . . . . Y   N

    Are the progress notes legible? . . . . Y   N   NA

    If you've answered "Yes" to BOTH of the above, do the progress notes:

    (Leave a–h blank if there are no progress notes or if they are not legible.)

        a. Have signatures, degrees, dates?. 1   2   3   4

        b. Appear in chronological order? 1   2   3   4

        c. Describe significant changes in the client's overall condition or life situation? . . . . NA   1   2   3   4

        d. Describe significant changes in the client's clinical condition?. . . . . NA   1   2   3   4

        e. Provide consistent, periodic documentation of all treatment clearly tied to the objectives contained in the treatment plan? (Score "NA" if no Tx plan.). . . . . NA   1   2   3   4

        f. Document the response of the client to treatment? (Score "NA" if no Tx plan.). . . . . NA   1   2   3   4

        g. Describe the overall outcome of treatment? 1   2   3   4

        h. Avoid being excessively narrative in nature? 1   2   3   4

    Scoring Notes 19c–h: Progress notes should be individualized, specific and avoid excessive repetition.

                   19c: Should document the client's overall situation including significant life events (e.g., death of a parent) even though these changes *do not necessarily* indicate the need for a treatment plan review. Answer "NA" if no significant events occurred.

                   19f: Describes the client's satisfaction, motivation, resistance, etc.

    Comments: _____

    _____

---

20. Do progress notes reflect a professional assessment made by the writer as to why the interventions prescribed *are* or *are not* working? (Score "NA" if no there are no progress notes.). 1   2   3   4   NA

    Scoring Note: Progress notes must reflect the *results* of the treatment rendered, detailing *why* things were done as opposed to simply *what* was done, and record the *effect* that the treatment had on the client's symptomatology. Notes should include documentation of client stressors, limitations, influencing social factors, and an evaluation of the effectiveness/appropriateness of treatment interventions. Finally, there must be a clear path linking the assessment, the treatment plan, the goals, the objectives and the progress notes.

    Comments: _____

    _____

---

21. Do the progress notes explain any significant deviations from the interventions prescribed in the treatment plan? (Answer "NA" if there were no significant deviations or if there are no progress notes.) . . . . NA   1   2   3   4

    Comments: _____

    _____

Audit form from the Rhode Island Medicaid office (Continued)

22. Has the client been discharged? . . . . Y N
If "Yes," date of discharge (MM/DD/YY): _____
If "Yes," is there a discharge summary in the record?. . . . . Y N
If there is a discharge summary, does it:
   a. Appear in the record within 21 days of actual discharge? 1 2 3 4
   b. Contain all significant findings?. 1 2 3 4
   c. Contain the final primary and secondary diagnoses? 1 2 3 4
   d. Contain general observations about the clients' condition at intake, during treatment, and at discharge? . . . 1 2 3 4
   e. Assess the degree of attainment of treatment goals and objectives? 1 2 3 4
   f. Document referral to other programs/agencies as needed? . . . . NA 1 2 3 4
   g. Indicate whether the discharge was planned? . . . . Y N
   Scoring Notes: 22b. Significant findings are pertinent facts relative to either the client's condition
      or illness that have been uncovered during the course of treatment.
      22g. An "unplanned discharge" is one in which the client discontinued treatment.
   Comments: _____

QUESTIONS 23–25 TO BE COMPLETED FOR CLIENTS IN MHPRRS ONLY

23. Does the client's individual record include a current Psychiatric Rehabilitative Residence Individual Care Checklist? Y N
   Comments: _____

24. Has the client's MHPRR service been authorized by a physician as evidenced by having a physician's signature on:
   The client's overall treatment plan? . . . . Y N
   The Psychiatric Rehabilitative Individual Care Checklist? . . . . Y N
   Comments: _____

25. Does the treatment plan contain detailed and specific reasons for which the client is being served in the MHPRR, including the specific aspects of the client's condition that require MHPRR treatment as well as detailed, measurable goals and objectives for that treatment? 1 2 3 4
   Comments: _____

**QUESTIONS 26–27 TO BE COMPLETED FOR CLIENTS WHOSE 6-MONTH TREATMENT **
** PLAN REVIEW DATE IS JANUARY 1, 1999 OR LATER **

26. Was the staff portion of the OEI **fully** completed and received by DBH no later than the end of the calendar month occurring two months after the month during which the treatment plan review was conducted? (Answer "NA" for clients whose treatment plan review date falls in either of the two calendar months preceding that of the site visit. For example, if the site visit takes place during the month of April, use "NA" for all treatment plans due in February or March.) . . . . Y N NA
   Comments: _____

27. Did the client have the opportunity to complete the OEI as evidenced by:
   a) Receipt of a client OEI by DBH that was completed no later than the end of the calendar month occurring two months after the month during which the treatment plan review was conducted? (Answer "NA" for clients whose treatment plan review date falls in either of the two calendar months preceding that of the site visit. For example, if the site visit takes place during the month of April, use "NA" for all treatment plans due in February or March.) . . . . Y N NA
   OR
   b) An entry in the client's individual medical record indicating that the client was given the opportunity to complete the survey during the aforementioned timeframe. (Answer "NA" for clients whose treatment plan review date falls in either of the two calendar months preceding that of the site visit. For example, if the site visit takes place during the month of April, use "NA" for all treatment plans due in February or March.) . . . . Y N NA
   Comments: _____

( ) Check this box if this record is NOT recorded on the OEI Tracking list.

Source: http://www.rules.state.ri.us/rules/released/pdf/MHRH/MHRH_2368.pd

Appendix H

Sample Compliance Plans

AHIMA Sample Compliance and Audit Program

_____ Corporate Compliance and Audit Program (CCAP) is a comprehensive strategy to ensure the submission of consistently accurate claims to the Medicare program, as well as all payers, and will ensure the _____ employees and administrative personnel providing services to _____ comply with the applicable laws relating to its participation in these programs. Fraud and abuse, either inadvertent or purposeful, will not be tolerated by_____. Therefore, the purpose of this compliance program is to meet the government's requirements relating to the delivery and documentation of care and the submission of claims relating to that care.

In order for the final claim to be accurate, the underlying data supporting the claim needs to be accurate as well. Thus, an effective compliance program requires the education of everyone who is directly involved in the patient care process as well as many of those whose jobs are related to that process.

In order to be effective, the **CCAP** is designed in a manner which:

- Addresses the organization's business activities and consequent risks;

- Educates those persons whose jobs could have a material impact on the process;

- Includes auditing and reporting functions designed to measure the effectiveness of the program and to remedy problems as quickly and as efficiently as possible; and

- Contains enforcement and discipline components which ensure that employees and administrators take seriously their compliance responsibilities.

This **CCAP** provides for an extensive and systematic approach on the part of _____ to understand the claim development and submission process, to make employees and administrators aware of how the Medicare laws impact the performance of their job functions and states commitment of the organization to comply with the applicable laws. Employees and administrators must be made aware of the obligation of every employee and administrator to be an active participant in _____ effort to comply with the laws and to participate in the auditing and other activities designed to identify non-compliant behavior or activities.

_____ will ensure that the **CCAP** is consistent and meets the company's goals and strategies with respect to compliance activities. The **CCAP** is important to the company and active participation on the part of employees and administrators is a required part of their job function.

This **CCAP** defines the goals of the compliance program, identifies the necessary participants in the plan, develops the administration process and prescribes the resource needs.

1. Participants—The implementation of the **CCAP** requires participation of individuals involved in or thoroughly familiar with the claim development and submission process, including administrators, and billing and coding personnel. The participants will be involved in the analysis of all steps in the process in order to ensure that the claim which is ultimately submitted is accurate.

2. Resource Needs—_____ will provide information systems resources, and make available the time of its personnel to facilitate the audits, the development and creation of education programs, and the staffing of investigation teams.

3. Elements of _____ **CCAP**

   Compliance Standards and Procedures: Employees and administrators will be held to performance and conduct standards designed to maximize correct billing procedures and eliminate errors. Adherence to the **CCAP** will be an element in evaluating the performance of an individual employee or administrator.

There will be generalized codes of that apply to all employees and administrators and specific rules and procedures which apply to particular employees and administrators and relate to their specific job function.

Here is where each facility must define practices of billing and coding, reporting systems, auditing, employee screening, education and discipline.

The Kent Center's Compliance Program (KCCP)

The Kent Center's Compliance Program (KCCP) defines the Center's commitment to ethical standards and internal compliance monitoring. The guidelines set forth in this plan reflect the Center's dedication to improving the quality of life through its delivery of high quality, cost-effective services to the individuals and communities it serves. The Center's Vision and Guiding Principles further define the Center's commitment to the high professional standards expected of staff, volunteers, students, and business associates.

The Kent Center's Compliance Program (KCCP) has been designed to meet regulatory requirements for professional practices within the healthcare industry, service delivery, documentation of care, and submission of claims related to that care. This program promotes the submission of consistent, accurate claims to payers, as well as compliance with applicable laws and regulations relating to the participation in payer programs. Since data and documentation supporting a claim needs to be accurate, staff directly involved with client care as well as staff whose activities are related to the billing process, must be educated to KCCP. This education includes providing staff with sufficient information to comply with regulations, initial and on-going training in compliance issues, and resources necessary to resolve ethical dilemmas. In no way should staff ever sacrifice ethical and compliant behavior for the purpose of attaining its financial objectives. Fraud and abuse, either inadvertent or purposeful, will not be tolerated by The Kent Center.

The Center's Code of Conduct provides further guidance to its employees, interns, and volunteers in the performance of daily activities and provides guidelines to ensure these activities are within appropriate ethical and legal standards. In addition, professional staff are expected to perform their daily activities within professional practice standards established by their profession and in accordance with regulations promulgated by licensing, accrediting , and funding sources.

Compliance activities will be monitored by the Compliance Officer and reviewed by the Compliance Task Force. The Compliance Officer shall be responsible for oversight of the Center's Compliance Program and reports regularly on the progress of the program to the CEO, Board of Directors, and Compliance Task Force. This oversight shall include the development and implementation of procedures as well as coordination and review of ongoing auditing and monitoring.

The Center's Compliance Program shall include, but not be limited to, the following:

- Standards of Conduct that promote the Center's commitment to ethical conduct and includes rules against conflicts of interests, kickbacks, cross referral relationships, unethical purchasing, marketing, or business practice.

- Development of compliance initiatives at all applicable levels.

- Training, both initial and ongoing, for all staff as well as specific training for clinical and billing staff concerning billing requirements, activity codes, diagnostic coding, and documentation.

- A uniform mechanism for employees to raise questions and receive appropriate guidance concerning professional practices, fee billing, documentation, and other issues as relates to the Center's compliance program.

- Standards and procedures that guide personnel with regard to professional fee billing, documentation, privacy, marketing, purchasing, and other business practices.

- A process for employees to report instances of possible noncompliance and for such reports to be fully and objectively reviewed.

- Regular chart and billing reviews to assess compliance and identify potential issues.

- Regular reviews of overall compliance efforts, centerwide and by program, to ensure billing and documentation practices reflect current requirements, that practice standards are conducted within the established guidelines, and that adjustments are made to improve the program.

- Corrective action plans that address any instance of non-compliance with established standards and procedures and provide for fair disciplinary action consistent with the Center's disciplinary action policies.

- Generation and submission of corrected claims reflecting results of audits or errors identified during the course of business.

- Policies establishing guidelines for reporting and investigating complaints.

It is the policy of The Kent Center that all claims for reimbursement use the proper code for the services provided and that the documentation in the client record supports that code. Procedures concerning billing and documentation are considered an integral part of this plan and can be found in the Billing Procedures and Documentation Guidelines Manuals. The Vice President of Operations shall be responsible for establishing, disseminating, and explaining billing procedures to existing staff and all new personnel. The Vice Presidents for Clinical Programs shall be responsible for ensuring clinical documentation protocols are in place and are followed by clinical staff. A system shall be developed to document that billing and documentation training has occurred.

A random sample of client records and corresponding claims for each program shall be periodically reviewed for compliance with billing and documentation requirements. Each program will be reviewed at least annually, but more frequent reviews may be required. If these reviews result in any instances of non-compliance the Compliance Officer shall report these findings to the CEO in accordance with the procedures for auditing and monitoring.

Employees will be instructed to report any inconsistencies in billing, documentation, business practice, or ethical behavior to the Compliance Officer. Employees who report possible compliance issues will not be subjected to retaliation or harassment as a result of their report. Concerns about possible retaliation or harassment should be reported to either the Director of Human Resources or Human Rights Officer. Whenever inconsistencies are reported, an investigation will be undertaken. The assistance of legal counsel may be sought. Following any investigation a written report will be made to the CEO. Center employees are required to cooperate fully with any investigation undertaken (see procedure on self-reporting of violations).

Whenever non-compliance is identified, corrective action will be taken. The Compliance Officer will meet with the appropriate supervisor to review findings and develop a corrective action plan. If the plan involves overpayments for services, the return of payments will be coordinated with the fiscal department. If it is determined that the remedies decided upon have not corrected the problem(s), further corrective action will be taken depending upon the severity of the offense. Individuals will be given the opportunity to appeal decisions (in writing) of all cases reviewed or investigated.

KCCP is intended to be flexible and readily adaptable to changes in regulatory requirements; therefore this plan will be reviewed regularly and modified as necessary. To ensure appropriate revisions to the plan have been made the Compliance Officer shall submit a report, at least annually, that describes general compliance activities that have occurred and identifies any changes that may be necessary to improve compliance. This report will be distributed to the Compliance Task Force and QI Team for their comments and possible revision to the plan. The plan will then be presented to the CEO and Board of Directors for approval.

The Compliance Program described in this document is intended to establish a framework for effective and legal compliance of The Kent Center. This document is not intended to meet all the procedures designed to achieve compliance. The Center already has numerous policies and procedures, as well as future policies and procedures, which will be a part of its overall legal compliance enforcement program.

Approved by EMT	Initiated 12/99
Approved by Board of Directors	Latest Revision 4/2004

South Shore Mental Health Center Corporate Compliance Plan

Introduction

To realize South Shore Mental Health Center's vision of creating opportunity for wellness and recovery through innovation and the pursuit of excellence, the Center holds its employees to the highest ethical and quality standards. In striving to achieve the mission, South Shore Mental Health Center has set out to implement a Corporate Compliance Program, and appoint a Corporate Compliance Officer to assist in carrying out the program.

Mission of Corporate Compliance

The mission of the Corporate Compliance Program is to strive to protect and promote our integrity and enhance our ability to achieve our business and strategic objectives in a manner consistent with the mission and values of the Center. The four goals of the Compliance Program are:

- To reduce the risk of fraud and abuse,
- To enhance operational functioning,
- To improve the quality of behavioral healthcare services, and
- To reduce the cost of behavioral healthcare.

The mission of the Corporate Compliance Officer is to assist and advise employees to help ensure the Center is compliant with applicable Federal, State and local laws. In this capacity, the Center is committed to providing clear guidelines to train and educate employees regarding applicable laws, regulations, policies and procedures as they pertain to compliance.

The Corporate Compliance Program is intended to promote a culture that encourages employees to conduct activities with integrity and in compliance with laws, regulations, and compliance policies and procedures and to report instances of non-compliance; to educate employees concerning the legal risks of certain business practices; to encourage management to seek appropriate counsel regarding business practices; and to conduct those activities within the requirements of the law and ethical standards of conduct.

Corporate compliance is a partnership with management, to help identify areas of regulatory risk and to help mitigate risk of noncompliance. This partnership enhances management's ability to achieve organizational goals and objectives. Staff will act in a diligent and prudent manner to ensure high standards of creative leadership and fiscal responsibility and will collaborate and network with others who share our values in the provision of behavioral health and health related services.

Organizational Structure

South Shore Mental Health Center has established a Corporate Compliance Committee including the Executive Director as ex-officio member, the Finance Director, the Quality Management Director, who also serves as the Corporate Compliance Officer, the Community Support Program Clinical Director, the Human Resources Director, and the Management of Information Systems Manager. The Committee will have the responsibility of assisting the Corporate Compliance Officer in the implementation of the Compliance Program. The Corporate Compliance Officer/Committee reports to the Executive Director, who in turn reports to the Board of Directors. The Committee shall provide support and feedback for the development of priorities and monitoring of those priorities. In addition, the Committee shall establish priorities for educational programs to be provided and to help identify necessary human and financial resources required for the effective implementation of the Compliance Program.

Elements of the Corporate Compliance Program

- Develop a Code of Conduct, as well as other finance, health information, safety, and human resources policies and procedures that are based on pertinent laws and regulations and are included in the Agency Policy and Procedure Manual and/or the Plan Book.

- Designate a Corporate Compliance Committee and a Corporate Compliance Officer charged with the responsibility of developing, implementing, and monitoring the Compliance Program.

- Design an effective education and training strategy to be implemented upon promulgation of this Plan.

- Design a communication process for reporting any activity by any staff that appears to violate compliance policies, laws, rules, and/or regulations.

- Develop a system to respond to and investigate allegations of improper activities, including appropriate responses to detected offenses, such as the initiation of corrective action, remediation of systemic problems, repayments when appropriate, and preventive measures.

- Develop monitoring and auditing practices designed to monitor compliance, identify problem areas, and assist in the reduction of identified problems.

- Develop policies addressing the nonemployment or retention of excluded individuals or individuals who have had a sanction placed on their license.

Organizational Ethics

An effective Corporate Compliance Program is more than just compliance with laws, regulations, policies, and standards. The Compliance Program is fundamentally about organizational culture. Leadership is charged with instilling an ethical commitment to observe the law and, more generally, to do the right thing. The Center shall implement its Corporate Compliance Program with a balance of regulatory compliance standards and education, and an ethical decision-making structure that promotes the Center's value system as to both business and clinical decisions. The promotion of organizational ethics requires the reflection of such values in the daily leadership example set by management.

_____

Approved by President/CEO

Originated By
Quality Management Director

_____

Source: South Shore Mental Health Center, Inc.

Appendix I

Sample Policies and Procedures

AHIMA Sample Professional Fee Billing Compliance Plan

Foreword

_____ representatives collaborated to develop a Compliance Plan which describes the commitment and procedures for proper billing of physician services.

The Compliance Plan was reviewed by the following:

- _____ Operations Committee
- Hospital Operations Team
- College of Medicine Clinical Administrators
- Legal Counsel

The Compliance Plan was approved by _____ Board of Directors, April 29, 1997, and by _____, Dean of the College of Medicine.

Introduction

_____ have been and continue to be committed to conducting professional fee billing in accordance with applicable regulations. For this purpose, professional fee billing includes the following: proper selection of diagnostic coding, category of service, and level of service; documentation of clinical services; submission of claims; patient billing; collection; payment posting; error correction; and retention of records for physician professional services.

Compliance with laws applicable to professional fee billing is challenging because the regulatory requirements governing reimbursement for professional services are complex and changing. To underscore and enhance the commitment of _____ and to better assist faculty physicians, residents, other healthcare providers and appropriate clinical/billing staff in this area, _____ are implementing an expanded compliance program for professional fee billing. The compliance plan has the following key features:

1. Designation of an official responsible for directing the effort to enhance compliance, including implementation of this plan;

2. Incorporation of standards and policies that guide _____ personnel with regard to professional fee billing;

3. Development of compliance initiatives at all applicable levels;

4. Coordination and enhancement of training of faculty physicians, residents, other healthcare providers, and appropriate clinical/billing staff concerning applicable billing requirements and _____ policies;

5. A uniform mechanism for employees to raise questions and receive appropriate guidance concerning professional fee billing;

6. Regular chart and billing reviews by _____ employees to assess compliance and to identify potential issues; external consultants may be used as needed;

7. A process for employees to report instances of possible noncompliance and for such reports to be fully and objectively reviewed;

8. Regular reviews of the overall compliance effort, including Department/Unit/Section-specific plans, to ensure that billing practices reflect current requirements and that other adjustments are made to improve the program;

9. Formulation of corrective action plans to address any instances of noncompliance with _____ policies or billing requirements.

Chief Compliance Officer

Responsibility for implementing and managing the Compliance Plan will be assigned to the Chief Compliance Officer (CCO). The CCO will function within the _____ organizational structure. A Compliance Plan Implementing Committee, consisting of departmental compliance leaders drawn from clinical departments and other areas across the clinical enterprise will be constituted to implement this Plan, the chair of which will be the CCO. The CCO will, with assistance of counsel when appropriate, perform the following activities:

1. Review, revise, and formulate appropriate policies to guide billing of professional fees;

2. Review, revise, and approve Department/Unit/Section compliance plans, including policies relating to billing and documentation;

3. Assist with the development of training materials and programs, as needed;

4. Review and approve training materials and programs;

5. Oversee chart and billing reviews conducted by both internal and external auditors/consultants;

6. Develop/recommend systems and processes to optimize compliance;

7. Review any inquiries concerning billing or reports of noncompliance by determining whether a compliance issue exists and, if so, developing an appropriate response;

8. Develop appropriate corrective action plans to address any compliance issues;

9. Prepare an annual report that summarizes the compliance effort, both for the _____ and for individual Departments/Sections, and identify changes that will be made to enhance compliance.

The CCO will work closely with the departmental compliance leaders to foster and enhance compliance with all applicable billing requirements. The CCO shall have the authority to direct specific billing practices, including, but not limited to 1) the use of particular codes for designated services, 2) the procedures and practices used to handle billing, and 3) the imposition of restrictions on billing by particular physicians, groups of physicians, or other health professionals. The CCO should consult with other _____ personnel, including, for example, the Chair of the affected department, in an effort to resolve issues through consensus. The authority of the CCO shall extend to all billing for clinical services, whether on a fee for service basis or otherwise provided by _____ employees.

Policy Guidelines

It is the policy of _____ that all claims for professional fee reimbursement use the proper code for the service provided, that the documentation in the medical record supports the code, and that the claim is submitted in the name of the appropriate provider. To guide physicians, residents, other healthcare providers, and appropriate clinical/billing staff in meeting this objective, the CCO shall, with the assistance of legal counsel if necessary, review existing policy statements, revise those statements as necessary, and develop any additional statements that seem advisable. _____ policies concerning billing should be considered an integral part of this plan. These policies may be changed periodically.

Departmental Implementation Plans

Each clinical department shall appoint a physician faculty member to serve as the compliance leader for departmental billing activities. The departmental compliance leader will coordinate departmental compliance activities with the CCO. The CCO shall have regular contact with the compliance leaders. Each clinical department shall prepare a plan to address compliance efforts on a departmental basis. The department plan shall be equal to or more stringent than the _____ plan requirements. Before becoming effective, such plans shall be reviewed and approved by the CCO to ensure consistency with _____ policies. If the CCO has concerns about the content of any departmental plan, he/she should consult with the Department Compliance Leader to explore whether the plan can be modified through mutual agreement. If such consultation fails to resolve the CCO's concerns, the CCO shall have the authority to modify the departmental implementation plan. The departmental implementation plans shall, at a minimum, include the following features:

1. Written policies and procedures for any billing activities;

2. Educational and training programs, as coordinated with the CCO and _____, to address billing issues of particular importance to the department;

3. A program for ensuring and documenting that all physicians, residents, other health-care providers and appropriate clinical/billing staff receive training about proper billing;

4. A program for periodic review of departmental billing;

5. An annual review of the existing compliance plan in order to identify the need for changes and to identify specific compliance objectives during the succeeding year.

Education and Training

The CCO shall be responsible for disseminating and explaining _____ policies concerning billing. To accomplish those objectives, the CCO shall work with representatives of the Deans of the Colleges or their designees, the Departments, and _____ to implement a systematic and ongoing training program to educate existing staff and new personnel about _____ billing policies. All training materials concerning billing issues shall be submitted to the CCO for review and approval before being used.

Training shall be mandatory for all physicians, residents, other health care providers who bill for their services, and billing personnel. A system shall be developed to document that such training has occurred. Moreover, the CCO can require that these individuals attend additional training sessions on particular issues. The training materials shall identify the specific people who should be contacted by physicians, residents, other healthcare providers or appropriate clinical/billing staff about billing questions.

No outside billing consultant may be retained by the _____, or any Department, without the review and concurrence of the CCO. If there is disagreement about the need or appropriateness of seeking such consultation or about the suitability of the proposed consultant, the CCO shall decide whether the consultant should be retained.

Monitoring

Under the supervision of the CCO, a sample of medical records and corresponding bills for each department and section shall be periodically reviewed on a prospective basis for compliance with the _____ billing policies and with legal requirements. Each department shall be reviewed at least annually, but the CCO may require more frequent reviews. Moreover, on an annual basis, the CCO, in consultation with the _____ Executive Committee, may engage an external billing reviewer to review a sample of records drawn from a cross-section of departments. If any of these reviews identify possible instances of noncompliance with _____ billing policies and with legal requirements, the CCO shall report the matter to _____ Executive Committee, the Dean of the college whose billings are at issue, and legal counsel for _____. In consultation with legal counsel, the CCO then shall review the particular matter to determine whether there has been any activity inconsistent with _____ billing policies and legal requirements.

Reporting Compliance Issues

The training materials will direct _____ employees to report to the CCO any activity that employees believe may be inconsistent with _____ policies or legal requirements regarding billing. The training materials will explain how the CCO can be contacted. The training materials will also provide the employees with information about programs and practices of _____ that are designed to achieve compliance with legal requirements. Employees who report possible compliance issues will not be subjected to retaliation or harassment as a result of the report. Concerns about possible retaliation or harassment should be reported to the CCO.

Investigating Compliance Issues

Whenever conduct that may be inconsistent with a billing policy or requirement is reported to or discovered by the CCO, an investigation will be undertaken with the assistance of legal counsel. After review and investigation, the CCO shall prepare a written report of findings for the _____ Executive Committee and the Dean of the appropriate college. _____ employees must cooperate fully with any investigations undertaken by the CCO.

Corrective Action Plans

Whenever noncompliance is identified by the _____ compliance staff, corrective action will be taken. The Chief Compliance Officer will meet with the departmental chair and/or compliance leader to review the findings and develop a corrective action plan within the department. If applicable, overpayments will be returned. If and when the Chief Compliance Officer determines that departmental remedies have not corrected the problem or problems, further corrective action, as described below, will be taken, depending upon the severity of the offense. In all cases, faculty will be given the opportunity to appeal decisions either at the department or _____ level.

Level One Action	
Action	**Responsible Party**
1. Billing is suspended.	1. Chief Compliance Officer initiates billing cessation and notifies Department Chair.
2. Faculty member repeats training session.	2. Department chair and faculty member meet with compliance coordinator to review deficiencies. Note to _____ file. If no further occurrences within 24 months, notation is purged.
3. Billing is resumed.	3. Chief Compliance Officer authorizes resumption of billing.
4. a) Reaudit within the next 60 days; b) If deficiencies are identified, take further action.	4. Chief Compliance Officer

Level Two Action	
1. Faculty member ceases all billing and clinical activity. Intensive remediation (e.g., one-on-one tutoring, intensive review of documentation, more didactic lectures on billing compliance) is undertaken.	1. a) Chief Compliance Officer initiates billing cessation and notifies Department Chair. b) Chair mandates cessation of clinical activity.
2. Department may be fined the greater of $1,000 for aggregated instances of noncompliance identified in the review period or the amount of erroneous billing (over and above repayment). Fine is remitted to _____ to defray compliance monitoring expense.	2. Chief Compliance Officer recommends fine to Dean. Dean levies fine to department.
3. Billing is resumed after steps 1 and 2 in this section are completed.	3. Chief Compliance Officer authorizes resumption of billing and recommends to Chair that clinical activity be resumed.
4. a) Reaudit within next 60 days; b) If deficiencies are identified, take further action.	4. Chief Compliance Officer

Level Three Action	
1. Faculty member ceases all billing and clinical activity.	1. a) Chief Compliance Officer initiates billing cessation and notifies Department Chair. b) Chair mandates cessation of clinical activity.
2. Begin process of termination of medical staff privileges and/or faculty appointment.	2. Chief Compliance Officer recommends actions to Chief of Medical Staff, Dean and Chancellor.
3. Recommend to Chancellor that information regarding noncompliance of faculty member be reported to appropriate government authorities.	3. Chief Compliance Officer and Dean recommend to Chancellor.

Revisions to this Plan

This Compliance Plan is intended to be flexible and readily adaptable to changes in regulatory requirements and in the healthcare system as a whole. The plan shall be regularly reviewed and modified, as necessary. To facilitate appropriate revisions to the plan, the Chief Compliance Officer shall prepare a report, at least annually, that describes the general compliance efforts that have been undertaken during the preceding year and that identifies any changes that might be made to improve compliance. This report shall be circulated to the _____ Executive Committee, _____ CEO, the Deans of the Colleges that utilizes the _____ billing systems, and to others with an interest in compliance for their comments about possible revisions to the plan. This Compliance Plan shall be presented to the _____ Board of Directors and _____ CEO for approval. Revisions to this plan require approval from the _____ Executive Committee and _____ CEO.

Closing Statement

The compliance program described in this document is intended to establish a framework for effective billing and legal compliance by _____. It is not intended to set forth all of the substantive programs and policies of _____ that are designed to achieve compliance. _____ have already established various compliance policies and those policies as well as future policies will be a part of its overall legal compliance enforcement program.

Approved by _____ Executive Committee: 1/20/97

Approved by _____ Board of Directors: 4/29/97

Sample Code of Conduct

Title:	Code of Conduct
Policy Number:	1-015
Date Established:	8/28/90
Date of Latest Review:	11/02/04
Date of Latest Revision:	11/01/04
Date:	10/27/04

Purpose: The purpose of this policy is to establish standards of conduct, which shall govern all staff, volunteers, and other individuals representing The Kent Center. These standards provide a uniform set of guidelines consistent with the mission and guiding principles of the Center and reflect specific policies and procedures adopted by The Kent Center and its Board of Directors.

Policy: All Kent Center staff, trainees, and representatives (referred to as individuals hereafter) are expected to conform to and comply with these standards as a condition of employment with the Center. Violation of the code of conduct is considered just cause for the Center to invoke disciplinary action in accordance with the policy on Disciplinary Procedures (see policy #3-007—Disciplinary Procedures) or initiate termination based on any existing service agreement. Staff who have questions about the code of conduct or the appropriateness of any activity should consult with their supervisor, VP, Compliance Officer, or CEO. Supervision should be utilized when necessary to clarify any of the points listed in this Code of Conduct. Any individual who becomes aware of a violation of the law or standards set forth in this Code of Conduct is responsible for reporting this to the Compliance Officer or CEO. The Center will take no adverse action against any person making such reports in good faith.

Code of Conduct/Personal Conduct:

1. The dignity and worth of every individual shall be recognized. Individuals covered by this policy shall not discriminate against clients, collaterals, other staff, or other members of the community on the basis of race, color, religion, handicap, sex, sexual orientation, ancestry, marital status, national origin, veteran's status, or age.

2. Individuals shall demonstrate an ongoing awareness of the client's right to an objective, professional relationship. Individuals will demonstrate their awareness of this by:

    a. Focusing on the client's goals, needs, concerns and problems and delivering services in accordance with best practice standards of their profession.

    b. Assuring that all individuals receive access to high-quality professional assessments, necessary and appropriate services, and termination from services in accordance with standards of care and approved Center criteria. Decisions for such services will be made without bias or discrimination, but solely on the basis of The Kent Center's approved practices and criteria.

    c. Responding to all requests for information and access to care in accordance with privacy protocols and in a timely and customer-friendly manner, including contacting or providing referrals to other individuals or organizations when the Center cannot provide the requested services or information.

d. Ensuring personal and professional biases do not affect the therapeutic relationship and that professional boundaries are maintained.

e. Not entering into personal relationships with clients whom they have met in the workplace. Individuals who find themselves in contact with clients through their nonwork activities and circle of friends must maintain confidentiality of the client's status and a friendly professional distance must be maintained in that relationship. Dual relationships (e.g. therapist/Tupperware party consultant, case manager/real estate agent) should be avoided if possible. If you find yourself in a situation that is a dual relationship, you should consult your VP or CEO immediately.

f. Never dating and or having sexual involvement with a client.

g. Never borrowing or lending money to a client.

h. Never giving, or accepting gifts without exploring their significance with the staff person's supervisor and the client.

i. Insuring the client's right to privacy is maintained at all times and that confidentiality applies even after the individual or representative is no longer employed/associated with The Kent Center.

3. All parties shall demonstrate an ongoing awareness of the client's rights to privacy as stipulated in both State and Federal law. All communication whether verbal, written, or electronic is strictly confidential and must be shared on a "need to know basis" (see Minimum Necessary Policy # 4-113). Individuals shall not:

a. Reveal the names of clients utilizing the Center's services to unauthorized persons, including fellow staff members who do not have the need to know (see Policy #4-113), or agencies, or acknowledge whether a person is or is not a Center client. No information, including confirmation or denial of client status, may be released except as outlined in The Kent Center policies and procedures.

b. Talk about clients at home, or with friends, or convey information that could specifically identify a client.

c. Mention client's names in public places, such as the staff lounge, corridors, or other public areas at the Center, or nonsecure, nonprivate areas in the community or over any cordless or nondigital cellular telephone or via electronic mail on the Internet.

d. Provide verbal, written, or electronic information to anyone without a signed authorization from the client, except as provided by law (see Center Policies Section 4.1).

4. Displays of negative, destructive, or socially inappropriate behavior, which might have a negative impact on morale, efficiencies, or the ability of other staff to perform their assigned duties are not acceptable.

a. Individuals shall use language that communicates respect.

b. Physical or verbal abuse is not permitted between any individuals. Clinical staff on occasion may be required to place verbal or physical limits on client behavior. Such limitations must be consistent with service plans and physical/nonphysical restraints (see Restraint Policy # 4-203).

c. Sexual harassment of any individual is strictly prohibited at The Kent Center (see Sexual Harassment Policy 3-013).

d. Individuals will not use alcohol or any legal or illegal substances that could impair ones ability to perform his/her duties during working hours (see Drug and Alcohol Free Work Place Policy 1-008).

e. Individuals are expected to respect the work environment provided by The Kent Center and are to avoid any activity that interferes with others ability to work. This sensitivity includes the use of personal electronic devices (i.e., radio, TV, phone, etc.), wearing of fragrances, soliciting for non-Center sponsored activities or anything that adversely impacts the work environment for others.

f. Individuals shall dress appropriately for their role/setting and conduct themselves in a dignified and respectful manner at all times.

g. Individuals shall not participate in the spreading of rumors.

h. Individuals shall not discuss personal, private, or financial information about other individuals without their specific permission.

i. Individuals shall not read correspondence intended for others unless identified as an appropriate authorized person.

j. Individuals shall only share sensitive, personal, financial or proprietary information on a "need to know" basis.

5. Individuals of the Center have a responsibility to ensure services are provided in a healthy and safe environment. Individuals are expected to follow Center health and safety practices, to assist in keeping working environments clean, and to report promptly conditions that present a risk to one's health and safety.

6. Each individual is expected to adhere to the Center's guiding principles and to all Center policies and procedures at all times. Each individual is expected to:

a. Thoroughly acquaint himself/herself with all policies, procedures and standards of the Center and the programs he/she is assigned to;

b. Voice disagreement with other staff only for the positive purpose of resolving misunderstandings or conflicts, raising the possibility of revision of outdated policies, improving internal systems/protocols, or concerns related to "best practice" issues;

c. Never undermining the confidence of clients in The Kent Center by voicing disagreement with Center policies in the presence of clients collaterals, or non–Kent Center staff, and;

d. Resign his/her position at the Center if there is an unresolvable conflict between the Center's policies and his/her own personal or professional standards.

7. In all decisions about use of resources, Kent Center staff will use funds in an efficient, effective and ethical manner within the scope for which the funds were authorized.

a. Individuals will not use Center resources for personal purposes unless authorized by the CEO or designee.

b. Claims for payment must accurately represent the services provided.

c. Purchasing and referral decisions will be made without conflict of interest or kickbacks of any kind.

8. Conflicts of interest and any appearance of conflict are to be avoided.

9. Individuals with authority over agency's funds and resources will abide by the conflict of interest policy.

10. Individuals with business interests outside The Kent Center must refrain from any clinical or administrative referrals to those businesses.

11. Individuals with a conflict of interest will disclose the conflict and excuse themselves from the discussion of a decision involving the conflict.

12. Individuals may not accept material gifts from other individuals or organizations that might in any way benefit from a clinical or administrative decision made by Kent Center staff.

13. Marketing and fund-raising activities are conducted in accordance with Center policies and comply with federal and state laws (e.g., antikickback statutes, referral relationships, etc).

14. Staff shall never knowingly falsify any entry in

    • a client's record,

    • an activity log,

    • time sheet,

    • mileage sheet,

    • or any other Center document used for billing, fee generation, to procure services, or reimburse an employee for authorized expenses incurred in the performance of their job.

15. Individuals are to perform only those duties within the scope of their professional training, job duties, and responsibilities (i.e., case managers/therapists should refrain from offering advice on medication not sanctioned by a licensed prescriber). Staff whose job description requires credentialing will restrict their activity to the practice for which they are credentialed.

16. Employees have a responsibility to know and understand the laws and other regulations governing the provision of clinical and administrative services and must, at all times, perform their job duties in accordance with all applicable State and Federal statutes and regulations. Employees are obligated to immediately report any known or suspected violations of State or Federal regulations or any known or suspected occurrences of erroneous claims for service to management.

17. Individuals who know or suspect violations of this Code of Conduct shall report the violation either directly to the Center's Compliance Officer at 738-4229, Ext. 216 or call the anonymous confidential hotline at 738-1338, Ext #444. Any false accusations with the intent of harassing or retaliating against another person are a violation of the Code of Conduct.

18. The Compliance Officer will notify the CEO immediately of any allegation and will investigate, evaluate, and make recommendations to the CEO and other appropriate managers.

19. Disciplinary action for violations of the Code of Conduct and other laws, regulations, or policies shall be carried out in accordance with the Center's existing disciplinary policies and procedures and will be based on the nature, severity, and frequency of the violation.

Note: Prior to any suspension or discharge of an individual or termination of contract an explanation will be given of the evidence supporting the allegations and an opportunity to respond to the allegations and evidence.

_____   _____
President/CEO   Date

* For the purpose of this policy Code of Conduct and Code of Ethics is one in the same.

_____

South Shore Mental Health Center
Policy and Procedure Manual

SECTION: RISK MANAGEMENT

Policy No.: 5.9/CODE OF CONDUCT

The true foundation of South Shore Mental Health Center has always been its commitment to provide quality care to our clients. As part of this, the Center strives to ensure an ethical and compassionate approach to healthcare delivery and management. This Code of Conduct provides guidance to ensure that our work is done in an ethical and legal manner. These obligations apply to our clients, the communities we serve, third-party payors, regulators, accreditors, suppliers, and our staff.

While all staff is obligated to follow our Code, leadership is expected to set the example, to be in every respect a model. Leaders must ensure that those on their teams have sufficient information to comply with law, regulation, and policy. They must help to create a culture within South Shore Mental Health Center that promotes the highest standards of ethics and compliance. This culture must encourage everyone in the organization to raise concerns when they arise.

We affirm the following commitments to South Shore Mental Health Center stakeholders:

To Our Clients: We are committed to providing quality care that is sensitive, compassionate, promptly delivered, and cost effective. We treat all clients with respect and dignity and provide care that is both necessary and appropriate. We make no distinction in the admission, transfer, or discharge of clients or in the care we provide based on race, color, religion, or national origin.

Upon intake, each client is provided a written statement of client rights. We assure clients' involvement in all aspects of their care and obtain informed consent for treatment. Each client is provided with a clear explanation of care including, but not limited to, diagnosis, treatment plan, right to refuse or accept care, associated fees of treatment, and an explanation of the risks and benefits associated with medications, if prescribed.

Clients will be accorded appropriate confidentiality, privacy, and opportunity for resolution of complaints. We do not release or discuss client-specific information with others unless it is by client written consent, or as otherwise authorized or required by law.

To the Communities We Serve: We are committed to understanding the particular needs of the communities we serve and to provide these communities with quality, cost-effective healthcare. South Shore Mental Health Center is an integral part of its community and serves as a primary resource for mental health treatment and education to children, adolescents, families, and adults. The Center continuously assesses the priorities, needs, and expectations of the community and works cooperatively with other healthcare providers and resources to meet community needs.

To Our Third Party Payors: We will take great care to assure that all billings to government and to private insurance payors reflect truth and accuracy and conform to all pertinent federal and state laws and regulations. We will prohibit any Center staff person from knowingly presenting or causing to be presented claims for payment or approval that are false, fictitious, or fraudulent.

We will operate oversight systems designed to verify that claims are submitted only for services actually provided and that services are billed as provided. These systems will emphasize the critical nature of complete and accurate documentation of services provided.

Our business involves reimbursement under government programs, which require the submission of certain reports of our costs of operation. We will comply with federal and state laws relating to all cost reports. These laws and regulations define what costs are allowable and outline appropriate methodologies to claim reimbursement for the cost of services. Given their complexity, all issues related to the completion and settlement of cost reports must be communicated through or coordinated with the Finance Director.

To Our Regulators and Accreditors: South Shore Mental Health Center services may be provided only pursuant to appropriate federal, state, and local laws and regulations. Such laws and regulations may include subjects such as licenses, permits, access to treatment, consent to treatment, medical record-keeping, confidentiality, client rights, clinical privileges, and Medicare and Medicaid regulations. The Center is subject to numerous other laws in addition to these healthcare regulations.

We will comply with all applicable laws and regulations. All staff must be knowledgeable about and comply with all laws and regulations. The Center will provide its employees the information and education they need to comply fully with all applicable rules.

South Shore Mental Health Center will be forthright in dealing with any billing inquiries. We will cooperate with and be courteous to all government inspectors and provide them with the information to which they are entitled during an inspection. During a government inspection, staff will not conceal, destroy, or alter any documents, lie or make misleading statements to a government representative.

We will deal with all accrediting bodies in a direct, open, and honest manner. No action should ever be taken in relationships with accrediting bodies that would mislead the accreditor or survey team, either directly or indirectly. Where South Shore Mental Health Center determines to seek any form of accreditation, all standards of the accrediting group are important and must be followed.

To Our Suppliers: We are committed to fair competition among prospective suppliers.

To Our Staff: South Shore Mental Health Center ensures to our staff that our information systems, business operations, employment practices, development activities, and environments of care are consistent with all applicable federal, state, and local laws and regulations. Each Center staff person is responsible for the integrity and accuracy of our organization's documents and records, not only to comply with regulations but also to ensure that records are available to defend our business practices and actions. It is critical that staff actively engaged in service provision document care according to agency policy. Staff are held accountable to documentation standards. Any intentional misrepresentation of documentation is considered a major offense in the Progressive Discipline Policy and Procedure.

The Center has established policies and procedures for the management of health information, financial and business operations, safety, workplace conduct, and human resources that provide guidance beyond the scope of this Code but can be referred to for additional information.

PROCEDURES:

License and Certification Renewals: Staff employed in positions that require professional licenses, certifications, or other credentials are responsible for maintaining the current status of their credentials and shall comply at all times with federal and state requirements applicable to their respective disciplines. To assure compliance, South Shore Mental Health Center requires evidence of the individual having a current license or credential status.

Conflict of Interest: A conflict of interest may occur if your outside activities or personal interests influence or appear to influence your ability to make objective decisions in the course of your job responsibilities. A conflict of interest may also exist if the demands of any outside activities hinder or distract you from the performance of your job or cause you to use South Shore Mental Health Center resources for other than Center purposes. It is your obligation to ensure that you remain free of conflicts of interest in the performance of your responsibilities at the Center. If you have any question about whether an outside activity might constitute a conflict of interest, you must obtain the approval of your supervisor before pursuing the activity.

Political Activities and Contributions: The organization's political participation is limited by law. South Shore Mental Health Center funds or resources are not to be used to contribute to political campaigns or for gifts or payments to any political party or any of their affiliated organizations. It is important to separate personal and corporate political activities in order to comply with the appropriate rules and regulations relating to lobbying or attempting to influence government officials. You may, of course, participate in the political process on your own time and at your own expense. While you are doing so, it is important not to give the impression that you are speaking on behalf of or representing the Center in these activities.

At times, the Center may ask colleagues to make personal contact with government officials or to write letters to present our position on specific issues. In addition, it is a part of the role of some South Shore Mental Health Center management to interface on occasion with government officials. If you are making these communications on behalf of the organization, be certain that you are familiar with any regulatory constraints and observe them.

Marketing and Advertising: We may use marketing and advertising activities to educate the public, provide information to the community, increase awareness of our services, and to recruit colleagues. We will present only truthful, fully informative, and nondeceptive information in these materials and announcements. Marketing materials will reflect services available and the level of licensure and certification, when appropriate.

The South Shore Mental Health Center Ethics and Corporate Compliance Program Structure: The intent of this program is to demonstrate in the clearest possible terms the absolute commitment of the organization to the highest standards of ethics and compliance. This commitment permeates all leaders of the organization. There is an oversight committee including the President/CEO as ex-officio member, the Finance Director, and the Quality Management Director, who also serves as the Corporate Compliance Officer, the Community Support Program Clinical Director, the Human Resources Director, and the Management of Information Systems Manager. These individuals are prepared to support you in meeting the standards of this Code.

Personal Obligation to Report: Each staff person has an individual responsibility for reporting any activity by any colleague, physician, subcontractor, or vendor that appears to violate applicable laws, rules, regulations, or this Code. To obtain guidance on an ethics or compliance issue or to report a suspected violation, staff may choose from several options.

We encourage the resolution of issues at a local level whenever possible. It is expected and good practice, when you are comfortable with it and appropriate under the circumstances, to raise concerns first with your supervisor. If this is uncomfortable or inappropriate, another option is to discuss the situation with your respective Director. You are always free to contact a member of the corporate compliance committee noted above. Staff are not obligated to identify themselves when making a report of possible misconduct. The attached form may be completed and forwarded to any member of the corporate compliance team anonymously.

The Corporate Compliance Officer will be responsible to maintain documentation of all contacts. The nature and extent of any investigation will rest on the judgement of the corporate compliance committee. The corporate compliance committee will meet monthly and, on an emergency basis, more frequently as necessary, to review contacts and otherwise maintain the integrity of the corporate compliance program.

South Shore Mental Health Center will make every effort to maintain, within the limits of the law, the confidentiality of the identity of any individual who reports possible misconduct. There will be no retribution or discipline for anyone who reports a possible violation in good faith. Any staff person who deliberately makes a false accusation with the purpose of harming or retaliating against another staff person will be subject to discipline.

Investigation, Corrective Action, and Discipline: South Shore Mental Health Center is committed to investigate all reported concerns promptly. The corporate compliance committee will coordinate any findings from the investigation and recommend corrective action or changes that need to be made. Violators of this Code will be subject to disciplinary action. The precise discipline utilized will depend on the nature, severity, and frequency of the violation and may result in any of the following disciplinary actions: verbal warning, written warning, suspension, termination, and/or restitution.

Acknowledgment Process: South Shore Mental Health Center requires all staff to sign an acknowledgment that they have received the Code and understand it represents mandatory policies of the Center. New staff will be required to sign this acknowledgement as a condition of employment at the time of orientation with the Human Resources Director.

STATUTES, REGULATIONS, AND STANDARDS:

South Shore Mental Health Center complies with all federal, state, and local laws and regulations, and maintains compliance with the Joint Commission Accreditation of Healthcare Organization's standards.

STAFF DEVELOPMENT AND TRAINING REQUIREMENTS:

Upon initial implementation of the policy, and annually thereafter, all Directors, Managers, and Supervisors will receive a structured orientation and training.

These leaders will be expected to relay pertinent information to their respective teams. All new South Shore Mental Health Center staff will be responsible for reviewing this policy and procedure on hire with the Human Resources Director, and for attending the next scheduled Center Orientation and annual corporate compliance training.

MONITORING REQUIREMENTS:

The corporate compliance leadership team will monitor this policy. This policy will be reviewed on an annual basis by the corporate compliance leadership team who will forward to Center Management for review, and conclude with final approval verified by the signature of the President/CEO.

FORMS AND ATTACHMENTS:

Attachment A — Acknowledgement Form

Attachment B — Corporate Compliance Contact Form

Attachment C — Questions and Answers

ORIGINATED BY:

Quality Management Director

_____
President/CEO

Source: South Shore Mental Health Center, Inc.

Appendix J

Glossary

Access: The ability of a subject to view, change, or communicate with an object in a computer system

Accreditation: A voluntary process of institutional or organizational review in which a quasi-independent body created for this purpose periodically evaluates the quality of the entity's work against preestablished written criteria; also, a determination by an accrediting body that an eligible organization, network, program, group, or individual complies with applicable standards

Accreditation standards: Preestablished statements of the criteria against which the performance of participating healthcare organizations will be assessed during a voluntary accreditation process

Accrediting body: A professional organization that establishes the standards against which healthcare organizations are measured and conducts periodic assessments of the performance of individual healthcare organizations

Admitting diagnosis: A provisional description of the reason why a patient requires care in an inpatient hospital setting

Advance directive: A legal, written document that describes the patient's preferences regarding future healthcare or stipulates the person who is authorized to make medical decisions in the event the patient is incapable of communicating his or her preferences

Aggregate data: Data extracted from individual health records and combined to form de-identified information about groups of patients that can be compared and analyzed

Ambulatory surgery: An elective surgical procedure performed on a patient who is classified as an outpatient and who is usually released from the surgical facility on the day of surgery

American College of Surgeons (ACS): The scientific and educational association of surgeons formed to improve the quality of surgical care by setting high standards for surgical education and practice

American Health Information Management Association (AHIMA): The professional membership organization for managers of health record services and healthcare information systems as well as coding services; provides accreditation, certification, and educational services

American Hospital Association (AHA): The national trade organization that provides education, conducts research, and represents the hospital industry's interests in national legislative matters; membership includes individual healthcare organizations as well as individual healthcare professionals working in specialized areas of hospitals, such as risk management

American Medical Association (AMA): The national professional membership organization for physicians that distributes scientific information to its members and the public, informs members of legislation related to health and medicine, and represents the medical profession's interests in national legislative matters

American Osteopathic Association (AOA): The professional association of osteopathic physicians, surgeons, and graduates of approved colleges of osteopathic medicine that inspects and accredits osteopathic colleges and hospitals

American Psychiatric Association (APA): The international professional association of psychiatrists and related medical specialists that works to ensure humane care and effective treatment for all persons with mental disorders, including mental retardation and substance-related disorders.

American Psychological Association (APA): The professional organization that aims to advance psychology as a science and profession and as a means of promoting health, education, and human welfare.

Appeal: A request for reconsideration of a negative claim decision

Application service provider (ASP): A third-party service company that manages, delivers, and remotely hosts standardized software-based services to customers across a wide-area network from a central data center through an outsourcing contract based on a fixed, monthly usage or transaction-based pricing

Architecture: The configuration, structure, and relationships of hardware (the machinery of the computer including input/output devices, storage devices, and so on) in an information system

Assessment: The systematic collection and review of patient-specific data

Assisted living: A type of freestanding long-term care facility where residents receive necessary medical services but retain a degree of independence

Attending physician: The physician primarily responsible for the care and treatment of a patient

Audit: A review process conducted by healthcare organizations (internally and/or externally) to identify variations from established baselines

Audit trail: A chronological set of computerized records that provides evidence of information system activity (log-ins and log-outs, file accesses) that is used to determine security violations

Authentication: The process of identifying the source of health record entries by attaching a handwritten signature, the author's initials, or an electronic signature; also, proof of authorship that ensures, as much as possible, that log-ins and messages from a user originate from an authorized source

Author: The originator of a health record entry

Authorization: The granting of permission to disclose confidential information; as defined in terms of the HIPAA privacy rule, written permission by an individual to use or disclose his or her personally identifiable health information for purposes other than treatment, payment, or healthcare operations

Average length of stay (ALOS): The mean length of stay for hospital inpatients discharged during a given period of time

Behavioral health: A broad array of psychiatric services provided in acute, long-term, and ambulatory care settings; includes treatment of mental disorders, chemical dependency, mental retardation, and developmental disabilities as well as cognitive rehabilitation services

Behavioral healthcare organization: An organization that can provide a wide array of services, including diagnosis and treatment for mental disorders, chemical dependency, mental retardation, developmental disabilities, and cognitive rehabilitative services in either an acute, long-term, or ambulatory care setting.

Benchmarking: Comparing data against a predetermined reference point, either internal or external

Best practice: Term used to refer to services that have been deemed effective and efficient with certain groups of clients

Board of directors: The elected or appointed group of officials who bear ultimate responsibility for the successful operation of a healthcare organization

Business associate: According to the HIPAA privacy rule, an individual (or group) who is not a member of the covered entity's workforce, but who helps the covered entity in the performance of various functions involving access, use, or disclosure of protected health information

Case management: The ongoing, concurrent review performed by clinical professionals to ensure the necessity and effectiveness of the clinical services being provided to a patient; also, a term used to describe a process that integrates and coordinates patient care and needs across a continuum of care settings or the process of developing a specific care plan for a patient that serves as a communication tool to improve quality of care and reduce cost

Case manager: A medical professional (usually a nurse or a social worker) who reviews cases to determine the necessity of care and to advise providers on payer's utilization restrictions

Case study: A type of nonparticipant observation in which researchers investigate one person, one group, or one institution in depth

Centers for Medicare and Medicaid Services (CMS): The division of the Department of Health and Human Services that is responsible for developing healthcare policy in the United States and for administering the Medicare program and the federal portion of the Medicaid program; called the Health Care Financing Administration (HCFA) prior to 2001

Certification: The process by which a duly authorized body evaluates and recognizes an individual, institution, or educational program as meeting predetermined requirements; also, an evaluation performed to establish the extent to which a particular computer system, network design, or application implementation meets a prespecified set of requirements

Certification standards: Detailed compulsory requirements for participation in Medicare and Medicaid programs

Chargemaster: A financial management form that contains information about the organization's charges for the healthcare services it provides to patients

Chart: The health record of a patient (noun); to document information about a patient in a health record (verb)

Check sheet: A tool that permits the systematic recording of observations of a particular phenomenon so that trends or patterns can be identified

Child Welfare League of America (CWLA): An association of public and private nonprofit agencies and organizations across the U.S. and Canada devoted to improving life for abused, neglected, and otherwise vulnerable children and young people and their families

Claim: A billing statement submitted to a third-party payer by a healthcare provider to describe the services that were provided to a patient

Classification system: A system for grouping similar diseases and procedures and organizing related information for easy retrieval; also, a system for assigning numeric or alphanumeric code numbers to represent specific diseases and/or procedures

Client: A patient who receives behavioral or mental health services

Clinic: An outpatient facility providing a limited range of healthcare services and assuming overall healthcare responsibility for patients

Clinical Context Object Workgroup (CCOW): A standard protocol developed by HL7 to allow clinical applications to share information at the point of care

Clinical decision support system (CDSS): A special subcategory of clinical information systems that is designed to help healthcare providers make knowledge-based clinical decisions

Clinical information system (CIS): A category of a health information system that includes systems that directly support patient care

Clinical messaging: The function of electronically delivering data and automating the work flow around the management of clinical data

Clinical practice guideline: A detailed, step-by-step guide used by healthcare practitioners to make knowledge-based decisions related to patient care; also called clinical protocol

Clinical pertinence review: A review of medical records performed to assess the quality of information using criteria determined by the healthcare organization

Clinician: A healthcare provider, including physicians and others, who treats patients

Closed-record review: A review of records after a patient has been discharged from the organization or treatment has been terminated

Code: In information systems, software instructions that direct computers to perform a specified action; in healthcare, an alphanumeric representation of the terms in a clinical classification or vocabulary

Code of Federal Regulations (CFR): The official collection of legislative and regulatory guidelines that are mandated by final rules published in the *Federal Register*

Coding: The process of assigning numeric representations to clinical documentation

Commission on Accreditation of Rehabilitation Facilities (CARF): A private, not-for-profit organization that develops customer-focused standards for behavioral healthcare and medical rehabilitation programs and accredits such programs on the basis of its standards

Compliance: The process of establishing an organizational culture that promotes the prevention, detection, and resolution of instances of conduct that do not conform to federal, state, or private payer healthcare program requirements or the healthcare organization's ethical and business policies

Computer-based patient record (CPR): An electronic patient record housed in a system designed to provide users with access to complete and accurate data, practitioner alerts and reminders, clinical decision support systems, and links to medical knowledge; also called electronic health record or computerized patient record

Computer-based Patient Record Institute (CPRI): A private organization founded in 1992 to develop a strategy to support the development and adoption of computer-based patient records

Concept: A unit of knowledge created by a unique combination of characteristics

Conditions of Participation: The administrative and operational guidelines and regulations under which facilities are allowed to take part in the Medicare and Medicaid programs; published by the Centers for Medicare and Medicaid Services, a federal agency under the Department of Health and Human Services

Confidentiality: A legal and ethical concept that establishes the healthcare provider's responsibility for protecting health records and other personal and private information from unauthorized use or disclosure

Consent to treatment: Legal permission given by a patient or a patient's legal representative to a healthcare provider that allows the provider to administer care and/or treatment or to perform surgery and/or other medical procedures

Context: The text that illustrates a concept or the use of a designation

Continuous quality improvement (CQI): A management philosophy that emphasizes the importance of knowing and meeting customer expectations, reducing variation within processes, and relying on data to build knowledge for process improvement; also, a continuous cycle of planning, measuring, and monitoring performance and making knowledge-based improvements

Continuum of care: The range of healthcare services provided to clients, from routine ambulatory care to intensive acute care

Control chart: A run chart with lines on it called control limits that provides information to help predict the future outcome of a process with a high degree of accuracy

Corporate compliance program: A facilitywide program that comprises a system of policies, procedures, and guidelines that are used to ensure ethical business practices

Corrective action plan (CAP): A written plan of actions to be taken in response to identified issues or citations from an accrediting or licensing body

Council on Accreditation for Children and Family Services (COA): A private not-for-profit organization that accredits child and family service programs using preestablished standards and criteria

Covered entity: According to the HIPAA privacy rule, any health plan, healthcare clearinghouse, or healthcare provider that transmits specific healthcare transactions in electronic form

Credentialing: The process of reviewing and validating the qualifications (degrees, licenses, and other credentials) of healthcare practitioners, granting medical staff membership, and awarding specific clinical privileges to licensed, independent practitioners

Crosswalks: Lists of translating codes from one system to another

Data: The dates, numbers, images, symbols, letters, and words that represent basic facts and observations about people, processes, measurements, and conditions

Data accuracy: The extent to which data are free of identifiable errors

Data analysis: The process of translating data into information that can be used by an application

Data collection: The process by which data are gathered

Data comparability: The standardization of vocabulary such that the meaning of a single term is the same each time the term is used. Data comparability produces consistency in information derived from the data

Data confidentiality: The extent to which personal health information is kept private

Data element: An individual fact or measurement that is the smallest unique subset of a database

Data integrity: The extent to which healthcare data are complete, accurate, consistent, and timely; also, a security principle that keeps information from being modified or otherwise corrupted either maliciously or accidentally

Data mining: The process of extracting information from a database and then quantifying and filtering discrete, structured data

Data quality management: A managerial process that ensures the integrity (accuracy and completeness) of an organization's data during data collection, application, warehousing, and analysis

Data repository: An open-structure database that is not dedicated to the software of any particular vendor or data supplier, in which data from diverse sources are stored so that an integrated, multidisciplinary view of the data can be achieved; also called a central data repository or, when related specifically to healthcare data, a clinical data repository

Data security: The process of keeping data safe from unauthorized alteration or destruction

Data warehouse: A database that makes it possible to access data from multiple databases and combine the results into a single query and reporting interface

Database: An organized collection of data, text, references, or pictures in a standardized format, typically stored in a computer system for multiple applications

Decision support system (DSS):   A computer-based system that gathers data from a variety of sources and assists in providing structure to the data by using various analytical models and visual tools in order to facilitate and improve the ultimate outcome in decision-making tasks associated with nonroutine and nonrepetitive problems

Deemed status: An official designation that a healthcare organization is in compliance with the Medicare *Conditions of Participation*

Deficiency analysis: An audit process designed to ensure that all services billed have been documented in the health record

Deidentify: The act of removing from a health record or data set any information that could be used to identify the individual to whom the data apply in order to protect his or her confidentiality

Demographic information: Information used to identify an individual, such as name, address, gender, age, and other information linked to a specific person

Department of Health and Human Services (HHS):   The cabinet-level federal agency that oversees all of the health- and human-services–related activities of the federal government and administers federal regulations

Diagnosis: A word or phrase used by a physician to identify a disease from which an individual patient suffers or a condition for which the patient needs, seeks, or receives medical care

Diagnostic and Statistical Manual of Mental Disorders, Fourth Revision (DSM-IV):   A nomenclature developed by the American Psychiatric Association to standardize the diagnostic process for patients with psychiatric disorders; includes codes that correspond to ICD-9-CM codes

Diagnostic codes: Numeric or alphanumeric characters used to classify and report diseases, conditions, and injuries

Discharge summary: The final conclusions at the termination of a facility stay or treatment

Discrete data: Data that may be represented as separate and distinct values

Documentation: The recording of pertinent healthcare findings, interventions, and responses to treatment as a business record and form of communication among caregivers

Electronic data interchange (EDI):   A standard transmission format using strings of data for business information communicated among the computer systems of independent organizations

Electronic health record (EHR): A computerized record of health information and associated processes; also called computer-based patient record

Electronic medical record (EMR): A form of computer-based health record in which information is stored in whole files instead of by individual data element

Encoder: Specialty software used to facilitate the assignment of diagnostic and procedural codes according to the rules of the coding system

Encounter: The direct personal contact between a patient and a physician or other person who is authorized by state licensure law and, if applicable, by medical staff bylaws to order or furnish healthcare services for the diagnosis or treatment of the patient

Episode of care: A period of relatively continuous medical care performed by healthcare professionals in relation to a particular clinical problem or situation

Evaluation and management (E/M Codes): Current Procedural Terminology (CPT) codes that describe client encounters with healthcare professionals for assessment counseling and other routine healthcare services

Evidence-based practices: Services that use decision support systems and best practices in medicine rather than relying on subjective information

Executive information system (EIS): An information system designed to combine financial and clinical information for use in the management of business affairs of a healthcare organization; also called executive decision support system

Federal Register: The daily publication of the U.S. Government Printing Office that reports all changes in regulations and federally mandated standards, including HCPCS and ICD-9-CM codes

Fee for service: A method of reimbursement through which providers receive reimbursement on either billed charges for services provided or on annually updated fee schedules

Focused review: The process whereby a health record is analyzed to gather specific information about diagnoses, treatments, or providers

Formulary: A list of drugs that a pharmacy stocks; under pharmacy benefits management programs, the drugs that are covered under a health plan

42 CFR Part 2: Federal confidentiality regulations governing and protecting records of clients receiving treatment for alcohol and drug abuse–related conditions

Health information: According to the HIPAA privacy rule, any information (verbal or written) created or received by a healthcare provider, health plan, public health authority, employer, life insurer, school or university, or healthcare clearinghouse that relates to the physical or mental health of an individual, provision of healthcare to an individual, or payment for provision of healthcare

Health information management (HIM): An allied health profession that is responsible for ensuring the availability, accuracy, and protection of the clinical information that is needed to deliver healthcare services and to make appropriate healthcare-related decisions

Health information management (HIM) professional: An individual who has received professional training at the associate or baccalaureate degree level in the management of health data and information flow throughout healthcare delivery systems; formerly known as medical record technician or administrator

Health Insurance Portability and Accountability Act of 1996 (HIPAA): The federal legislation enacted to provide continuity of health coverage, control fraud and abuse in healthcare, reduce healthcare costs, and guarantee the security and privacy of health information

Health record: A paper- or computer-based tool for collecting and storing information about the healthcare services provided to a patient in a single healthcare facility; also called a patient record, medical record, resident record, or client record, depending on the healthcare setting

Health record number: A unique numeric or alphanumeric identifier assigned to each patient's record upon admission to a healthcare organization

Healthcare Facilities Accreditation Program (HFAP): The AOA survey program to monitor the quality of care in hospitals providing postdoctoral training for osteopathic physicians, ambulatory care/surgery, substance abuse, mental health, physical rehabilitation organizations, and critical access hospitals

Healthcare Information and Management Systems Society (HIMSS):   A national membership association that provides leadership in healthcare for the management of technology, information, and change

Healthcare provider: A provider of diagnostic, medical, and surgical care as well as the services or supplies related to the health of an individual and any other person or organization that issues reimbursement claims or is paid for healthcare in the normal course of business

Histogram: A graphic technique used to display the frequency distribution of continuous data (interval or ratio data) as either numbers or percentages in a series of bars

Hospital: A healthcare organization that has an organized medical staff and permanent facilities that include inpatient beds and continuous medical/nursing services and that provides diagnostic and therapeutic services for patients as well as overnight accommodations and nutritional services

Human–computer interface: The device used by humans to access and enter data into a computer system, such as a keyboard on a PC, personal digital assistant, voice recognition system, and so on

Incident report: A quality/performance management tool used to collect data and information about potentially compensable events (events that may result in death or serious injury)

Indicator: An activity, event, occurrence, or outcome that is to be monitored and evaluated under a JCAHO standard in order to determine whether those aspects conform to standards; commonly relates to the structure, process, and/or outcome of an important aspect of care

Individually identifiable data: Personal information that can be linked to a specific patient, such as age, gender, date of birth, and address

Individually identifiable health information: The term used in the HIPAA privacy rule to indicate any patient-identifiable health information, including demographic and/or payment information, that relates to the past, present, or future condition or treatment of an individual and that can be used to identify the individual

Information: Factual data that have been collected, combined, analyzed, interpreted, and/or converted into a form that can be used for a specific purpose

Information management: The acquisition, organization, analysis, storage, retrieval, and dissemination of information to support decision-making activities

Information system (IS):   An automated system that uses computer hardware and software to record, manipulate, store, recover, and disseminate data (that is, a system that receives and processes input and provides output); often used interchangeably with information technology

Information technology (IT):   Computer technology (hardware and software) combined with telecommunications technology (data, image, and voice networks); often used interchangeably with information system

Institute of Medicine (IOM):   A branch of the National Academy of Sciences whose goal is to advance and distribute scientific knowledge with the mission of improving human health

Integration: The complex task of ensuring that all elements and platforms in an information system communicate and act as a uniform entity; or the combination of two or more benefit plans to prevent duplication of benefit payment

Integrity: The state of being whole or unimpaired

Interface: The zone between different computer systems across which users want to pass information (for example, a computer program written to exchange information between systems or the graphic display of an application program designed to make the program easier to use)

***International Classification of Diseases, Ninth Revision, Clinical Modification* (ICD-9-CM):** A classification system used in the United States to report morbidity and mortality information

Interoperability: The ability, generally by adoption of standards, of systems to work together

Intranet: A private information network that is similar to the Internet and whose servers are located inside a firewall or security barrier so that the general public cannot gain access to information housed within the network

Joint Commission on Accreditation of Healthcare Organizations (JCAHO):   A private, not-for-profit organization that evaluates and accredits hospitals and other healthcare organizations that provide acute care, home care, mental healthcare, ambulatory care, and long-term care services

Knowledge: The information, understanding, and experience that give individuals the power to make informed decisions

Knowledge management: The process by which data are acquired and transformed into information through the application of context, which in turn provides understanding; also, a management philosophy that promotes an integrated and collaborative approach to the process of information asset creation, capture, organization, access, and use

Knowledge sources: Various types of reference material and expert information that are compiled in a manner accessible for integration with patient care information to improve the quality and cost-effectiveness of healthcare provision

Knowledge-based assets: Assets that are the sources of knowledge for an organization (for example, printed documents; unwritten rules; work flows; customer knowledge; data in databases and spreadsheets; and the human expertise, know-how, and tacit knowledge within the minds of the organization's workforce)

Length of stay (LOS):   The total number of patient days for an inpatient episode, calculated by subtracting the date of admission from the date of discharge

Licensure: The legal authority or formal permission from authorities to carry on certain activities that, by law or regulation, require such permission (applicable to institutions as well as individuals)

Licensure requirements: Criteria healthcare providers must meet in order to gain and retain state licensure to provide specific services

Longitudinal: A type of time frame for research studies during which data are collected from the same participants at multiple points in time

Long-term care: Healthcare services provided in a nonacute care setting to chronically ill, aged, disabled, or mentally handicapped individuals

Managed behavioral healthcare organization (MBHO):   A type of healthcare organization that delivers and manages all aspects of behavioral healthcare or the payment for care by limiting providers of care, discounting payment to providers of care, and/or limiting access to care

Managed care: A generic term for reimbursement and delivery systems that integrate the financing and provision of healthcare services by means of entering into contractual agreements with selected providers to furnish comprehensive healthcare services and developing explicit criteria for the selection of healthcare providers, formal programs of ongoing quality improvement and utilization review, and significant financial incentives for members to use providers associated with the plan

Managed care organization (MCO):   A type of healthcare organization that delivers medical care and manages all aspects of care or the payment for care by limiting providers of care, discounting payment to providers of care, and/or limiting access to care

Medicaid: An entitlement program that oversees medical assistance for individuals and families with low incomes and limited resources; jointly funded between state and federal governments

Medical record: *See* Health record

Medical staff: A formal organization of physicians (or other professionals such as dentists) with the delegated authority and responsibility to maintain proper standards of medical care and to plan for continued betterment of that care

Medicare: A federally funded health program established in 1965 to assist with the medical care costs of Americans sixty-five years of age and older as well as other individuals entitled to Social Security benefits owing to their disabilities

Medicare *Conditions of Participation* (COP):   A publication that describes the requirements that institutional providers (such as hospitals, skilled nursing facilities, and home health agencies) must meet to receive reimbursement for services provided to Medicare beneficiaries

Migration path: A series of steps required to move from one situation to another

National Committee for Quality Assurance (NCQA):   A private not-for-profit accreditation organization whose mission is to evaluate and report on the quality of managed care organizations in the United States

Natural language processing: In healthcare applications, the communications technology used to extract unstructured or structured medical word data from free text and then to translate the information into diagnostic or procedural codes for clinical and administrative applications

Needs assessment: A procedure performed to determine what is required, lacking, or desired by an employee, a group, or an organization

Network: A type of information technology that connects different computers and computer systems so that they can share information

Nomenclature: A recognized system of terms used in a science or art that follows preestablished naming conventions

On-line analytical processing (OLAP):   A data access architecture that exploits multidimensional data structure to allow the user to drill down into the data by selecting and summarizing them along any combination of their dimensions and permitting the retrieval and summary of large volumes of data; also called on-line/real-time analytical processing

ORYX initiative: A JCAHO initiative that supports the integration of outcomes data and other performance measurement data into the accreditation process

Outcome: The end result of healthcare treatment; also, the performance (or nonperformance) of one or more processes, services, or activities by healthcare providers

Outcomes management: The process of systematically tracking a patient's clinical treatment and responses to that treatment, including measures of morbidity and functional status, for the purpose of improving care; also called outcomes measurement

Outsourcing: The hiring of an individual or company external to an organization to perform a function either on-site or off-site

Pareto chart: A bar graph that includes bars arranged in order of descending size to show decisions on the prioritization of issues, problems, or solutions

Patient: A living or deceased individual who is receiving or has received healthcare services

Patient care charting: A system in which caregivers enter data into health records

Patient Self-Determination Act (PSDA):   The federal legislation that requires healthcare facilities to provide written information on the patient's right to issue advance directives and to accept or refuse medical treatment

Peer review: An evaluation of professional performance by other people of equal standing within the same profession; also, the process by which experts in the field evaluate the quality of a manuscript for publication in a scientific or professional journal

Peer review organization (PRO):   Until 2002, a medical organization that performs a professional review of medical necessity, quality, and appropriateness of healthcare services provided to Medicare beneficiaries; now called quality improvement organization (QIO)

Performance improvement: The continuous study and adaptation of a healthcare organization's functions and processes to increase the likelihood of achieving desired outcomes

Performance measure: A quantitative tool used to assess the clinical, financial, and utilization aspects of a healthcare provider's outcomes or processes

Personal health record (PHR):   An electronic health record maintained and updated by an individual for himself or herself

Physician's order: A physician's written or verbal instructions to the other caregivers involved in a patient's care

Plan–Do–C–Act (PDCA) cycle: A performance improvement model developed by Walter Shewhart, but popularized in Japan by W. Edwards Deming

Plan–Do–Study–Act (PDSA) cycle: A performance improvement model designed specifically for healthcare organizations

Planning: An examination of the future and preparation of action plans to attain goals; also, one of the four traditional management functions

Platform: The combination of hardware and operating system on which an application program can run

Policy: A statement that describes how a department or an organization is supposed to handle a specific situation

Population: The universe of data under investigation from which a sample is taken

461

Practice guidelines: Protocols of care that guide the clinical care process; also known as Care Maps™, critical paths, and clinical practice guidelines

Preferred provider organization (PPO): A managed care arrangement based on a contractual agreement between healthcare providers (professional and/or institutional) and employers, insurance carriers, or third-party administrators to provide healthcare services to a defined population of enrollees at established fees that may or may not be a discount from usual and customary or reasonable charges

Priority focus areas (PFAs): Processes, systems, or structures of an organization that impact on quality and safety of care for which JCAHO has standards; also a part of the PFP

Priority focus process (PFP): A process used by the JCAHO to collect, analyze, and create information about a specific organization being accredited to tailor the survey to meet the organization's needs

Privacy: The quality or state of being hidden from, or undisturbed by, the observation or activities of other persons or freedom from unauthorized intrusion; in healthcare-related contexts, the right of a patient to control disclosure of personal information

Privacy Act of 1974: The legislation that gave individuals some control over information collected about them by the federal government

Privacy officer: The individual responsible for the development and implementation of an organization's privacy policies and procedures

Privacy rule: The federal regulations created to implement the privacy requirements of the simplification subtitle of the Health Insurance Portability and Accountability Act of 1996

Procedure: A document that describes the steps involved in performing a specific function

Process: A systematic series of actions taken to create a product or service; a formal writing (writ) issued by authority of law; any means used by the court to acquire or to exercise jurisdiction over a person or a specified property; a term from Donabedian's model of quality assessment that focuses on how care is provided

Progress note: The documentation of a patient's care, treatment, and therapeutic response that is entered into the health record by all of the clinical professionals involved in a patient's care, including nurses, physicians, therapists, and social workers

Prospective payment: A method of determining reimbursement based on predetermined factors, not individual services

Protected health information (PHI): All patient-identifiable health information, whether oral or recorded in any form or medium, electronic or not, that is created or received by a healthcare provider or another entity subject to the requirements of the Health Insurance Portability and Accountability Act

Protocol: In healthcare, a detailed plan of care for a specific medical condition based on investigative studies; in medical research, a rule or procedure to be followed in a clinical trial; in a computer network, a protocol is used to address and ensure delivery of data

Providers: A generic term that refers to individual clinical practitioners and organizations that deliver healthcare services

Psychiatric hospital: A hospital that provides diagnostic and treatment services to patients with mental or behavioral disorders

Psychiatry: The study, treatment, and prevention of mental disorders

Psychotherapy notes: Notes recorded in any medium by a mental health professional to document or analyze the contents of conversations between therapists and clients during private or group counseling sessions

Quality assurance: A set of activities designed to measure the quality of a service, product, or process with remedial action, as needed, to maintain a desired standard

Quality improvement organization (QIO): An organization under contract with the Centers for Medicare and Medicaid Services to ensure that Medicare beneficiaries receive high-quality healthcare that is medically necessary and appropriate and meets professionally recognized standards of care; until 2002, called peer review organization

Quality indicator: A standard against which actual care may be measured to identify a level of performance for that standard

Quantitative audit: An audit that compares a report of services billed for a specific client and within a specific time frame against the health record documentation; sometimes called a billing audit

Qui tam litigation: "Provisions within the law that allow for persons or entities with evidence of fraud against federal programs or contracts to sue the wrongdoer on behalf of the government" (Source: The False Claims Act Legal Center)

Regulation: A rule or order having the force of law issued by executive authority of the government

Reimbursement: A payment for services provided

Release of information (ROI): The process of disclosing patient-identifiable information from the health record to another party

Request for proposal (RFP): A type of business correspondence asking for very specific product or contract information that is often sent to a narrow list of vendors that have been preselected after a review of requests for information

Residential care: Services, including board and lodging, provided in a protective environment, but with minimal supervision, to residents who are not in an acute phase of illness and would be capable of self-preservation during an emergency

Responsibility: The accountability required as part of a job, such as supervising work performed by others or managing assets or funds

Retrospective review: The part of the utilization review process that concentrates on a review of clinical information following patient discharge

Rules engine: A computer program that applies sophisticated mathematical models to data that generate alerts and reminders to support healthcare decision making

Run chart: A type of graph that shows data points collected over time and identifies emerging trends or patterns

Sanctions: Penalties or other mechanisms of enforcement used to provide incentives for obedience with the law or with rules and regulations

Security: The means to control access and protect information from accidental or intentional disclosure to unauthorized persons and from unauthorized alteration, destruction, or loss; also, the physical protection of facilities and equipment from theft, damage, or unauthorized access; collectively, the policies, procedures, and safeguards designed to protect the confidentiality of information, maintain the integrity and availability of information systems, and control access to the content of these systems

Security officer: The person assigned responsibility for managing the organization's information security program

Security rule: The federal regulations created to implement the security requirements of the Health Insurance Portability and Accountability Act of 1996

Service: An act performed by a person on behalf of another person

SOAP: An acronym for a component of the problem-oriented medical record that refers to how each progress note contains documentation relative to **s**ubjective observations, **o**bjective observations, **a**ssessments, and **p**lans

Software: A program that directs the hardware components of a computer system to perform the tasks required

Source systems: *See* Feeder systems.

Stakeholder: An individual within the organization who has an interest in, or is affected by, the results of a project

Standard: A scientifically based statement of expected behavior against which structures, processes, and outcomes can be measured; also, a model or example established by authority, custom, or general consent or a rule established by an authority as a measure of quantity, weight, extent, value, or quality

Standing orders: Orders the medical staff or an individual physician has established as routine care for a specific diagnosis or procedure

Statute: A law enacted by a legislative body of a unit of government (for example, the U.S. Congress, state legislatures, and city councils)

Strategic information systems (IS) planning: A process for setting IS priorities within an organization; the process of identifying and prioritizing IS needs based on the organization's strategic goals with the intent of ensuring that all IS technology initiatives are integrated and aligned with the organization's overall strategic plan

Strategic management: The art and science of formulating, implementing, and evaluating cross-functional decisions that enable an organization to achieve its objectives

Strategic plan: A broad organizationwide plan by which the organization accomplishes its strategic goals

Strategic planning: A disciplined effort to produce fundamental decisions that shape and guide what an organization is and does and why

Structured data: Binary, computer-readable data

System: A set of related and highly interdependent components that are operating for a particular purpose

Systematized Nomenclature of Human and Veterinary Medicine (SNOMED): A comprehensive clinical vocabulary developed by the College of American Pathologists that is the most promising set of clinical terms available for a controlled vocabulary for healthcare

Taxonomy: A term referring to the principles of a classification system, such as data classification

Terminal: A term used to describe the hardware in a mainframe computer system by which data may be entered or retrieved

Third-party payer: An insurance company (for example, Blue Cross/Blue Shield) or healthcare program (for example, Medicare) that reimburses healthcare providers and/or patients for the delivery of medical services

Tracer methodology: An evaluation process used by the JCAHO to evaluate care and services provided by using the individual's record and retracing specific care areas and processes that patients/clients encounter

Train-the-trainer: A method of training certain individuals who, in turn, will be responsible for training others on a task or skill

Unstructured data: Nonbinary, human-readable data

Utilization management (UM): The planned, systematic review of the patients in a healthcare facility against care criteria for admission, continued stay, and discharge; also, a collection of systems and processes to ensure that facilities and resources, both human and nonhuman, are used maximally and are consistent with patient care needs

Utilization review (UR): The process of determining whether the medical care provided to a specific patient is necessary according to preestablished objective screening criteria at time frames specified in the organization's utilization management plan

Variable: A factor

Variance: A measure of variability that gives the average of the squared deviations from the mean; in financial management, the difference between the budgeted amount and the actual amount of a line item

Visit: A single encounter with a healthcare professional that includes all of the services supplied during the encounter

Vocabulary: A list or collection of clinical words or phrases and their meanings

Work flow: Any work process that must be handled by more than one person

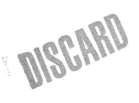

Index

(Continued on next page)

(Continued on next page)

(Continued on next page)

(Continued on next page)